DIAGNOSIS AND MANAGEMENT OF PITUITARY DISORDERS

CONTEMPORARY ENDOCRINOLOGY

P. Michael Conn, SERIES EDITOR

DIAGNOSIS AND MANAGEMENT OF PITUITARY DISORDERS

Edited by

BROOKE SWEARINGEN, MD
Department of Neurosurgery, Massachusetts General Hospital, Harvard Medical School, Boston, MA

and

BEVERLY M. K. BILLER, MD
Neuroendocrine Unit, Department of Medicine, Massachusetts General Hospital, Harvard Medical School, Boston, MA

⁂ Humana Press

Editors
Brooke Swearingen
Department of Neurosurgery
Massachusetts General Hospital
Harvard Medical School
Boston, MA
USA

Beverly M. K. Biller
Neuroendocrine Unit
Department of Medicine
Massachusetts General Hospital
Harvard Medical School
Boston, MA
USA

Series Editor
P. Michael Conn, PhD
Associate Director and Senior Scientist
Oregon National Primate Research Center
Professor
Oregon Health and Science University
505 NW 185th Ave.
Beaverton, OR 97006

ISBN: 978-1-58829-922-2   e-ISBN: 978-1-59745-264-9

Library of Congress Control Number: 2007942035

Cover illustration: Chapter 4, Fig. 3 by John T. Lysack et al.

Printed on acid-free paper

9 8 7 6 5 4 3 2 1

springer.com

Preface

This book presents a comprehensive update on the current diagnostic and treatment options for the management of disease of the sella, with an emphasis on pituitary adenomas. Over the past several decades, the techniques of molecular biology have been employed to investigate the pathogenesis of these tumors, as discussed by Drs. Lania, Mantovani, and Spada in Chapter 1. Their pathological analysis is discussed by Drs. Gejman and Hedley-Whyte in Chapter 2. The evaluation of patients presenting with sellar disease is based both on modern endocrine techniques, as discussed by Dr. Snyder in Chapter 3, as well as new imaging modalities, as discussed by Drs. Lysack and Schaefer in Chapter 4. Since Harvey Cushing first plotted visual fields, the intimate anatomic relationship between the sella and the optic structures has required careful neuro-ophthalmologic evaluation in these cases; this is discussed by Drs. Cestari and Rizzo in Chapter 5. The management of secretory adenomas remains challenging. Prolactinomas, since the introduction of medical treatment in the 1980s, have been primarily managed with dopamine agonists as discussed by Drs. Shibli-Rahhal and Schlechte in Chapter 6. The diagnosis of acromegaly, discussed by Dr. Clemmons in Chapter 7, is made by hormonal testing and depends on reliable GH and IGF-1 assays. The treatment of acromegaly, once primarily a surgical disease, is now increasingly amenable to new medical agents, including somatostatin analogs and growth hormone receptor antagonists. The relative advantages of these approaches are discussed by Dr. Freda, and Drs. Buchfelder and Nomikos, in Chapters 8 and 9, respectively. The patient with Cushing's disease requires an extensive and sophisticated endocrine evaluation before undergoing transsphenoidal surgery, as outlined by Drs. Findling and Raff in Chapter 10. The surgical approach is described by Dr. Kelly in Chapter 11, with options for medical treatment discussed by Drs. Lindsay and Nieman in Chapter 12. The diagnosis and treatment of the uncommon TSH adenomas is described by Drs. Zemskova and Skarulis in Chapter 13. Nonfunctioning tumors currently remain the province of the neurosurgeon, as discussed by Drs. Muh and Oyesiku in Chapter 14. Drs. Chandler and Barkan describe the surgical techniques used to remove sellar tumors in Chapter 15, while Drs. Barkan, Blank, and Chandler address the perioperative management of patients with these lesions in Chapter 16. Although advances in medical treatment and surgical techniques have made its use less frequent, radiation therapy continues to have an important role in the management of these patients, as described by Drs. Shih and Loeffler in Chapter 17. Finally, a number of specialized and clinically important topics arise in caring for patients with pituitary disorders. The diagnosis and management of inflammatory disease of the pituitary is discussed by Drs. Ulmer and Byrne in Chapter 18, the management of apoplexy by Drs. Russell and Miller in Chapter 19, and the management of pituitary disease during pregnancy by Dr. Molitch in Chapter 20. Modern imaging techniques will sometimes demonstrate an incidental sellar abnormality when none was suspected; the evaluation of these patients is described by Dr. Frohman in Chapter 21. Although pituitary adenomas are relatively less common in children, other sellar pathologies, especially craniopharyngiomas, are more important and their endocrine management is critical in the developing child; these topics are discussed by Drs. Stanley, Prabhakaran, and Misra in Chapter 22. Finally, the management of cystic disease of the sella can be an especially thorny problem, and therapeutic options are described by Drs. Snyder, Naidich, and Post in Chapter 23.

It has been a pleasure to work with some of the leading authorities in the field of pituitary disease in the preparation of this volume and we would like to thank them both for their contributions to this volume and their commitment to the field of pituitary education. In addition, we would like to thank Dr. Michael Conn and Richard Lansing of Springer publishing for conceiving this project and asking us to participate in it, and the editorial staff at Springer for their expert assistance in preparing the volume.

Brooke Swearingen, MD
Beverly M. K. Biller, MD

Contents

Contributors

ARIEL L. BARKAN, MD • *Professor, Departments of Internal Medicine and Neurosurgery, University of Michigan Medical Center, Ann Arbor, MI*

HOWARD BLANK, MD • *Fellow, Division of Metabolism, Endocrinology, and Diabetes, University of Michigan Medical Center, Ann Arbor, MI*

MICHAEL BUCHFELDER, MD, PhD • *Professor and Chairman, Department of Neurosurgery, University of Erlangen-Nuremberg, Erlangen, Germany*

THOMAS N. BYRNE, MD • *Clinical Professor of Neurology and Health Sciences and Technology, Harvard Medical School, Massachusetts General Hospital, Boston, MA*

DEAN M. CESTARI, MD • *Assistant Professor of Ophthalmology, Massachusetts Eye & Ear Infirmary, Harvard Medical School, Boston, MA*

WILLIAM F. CHANDLER, MD • *Professor, Departments of Neurosurgery and Internal Medicine, University of Michigan Medical Center, Ann Arbor, MI*

DAVID R. CLEMMONS, MD • *Kenan Professor of Medicine, UNC School of Medicine, Chapel Hill, NC*

JAMES W. FINDLING, MD • *Director, Endocrine-Diabetes Center, Aurora St. Luke's Medical Center, Clinical Professor of Medicine, Medical College of Wisconsin, Milwaukee, WI*

PAMELA U. FREDA, MD • *Associate Professor of Medicine, Columbia University, College of Physicians and Surgeons, New York, NY*

LAWRENCE A. FROHMAN, MD • *Professor Emeritus of Medicine, Section of Endocrinology, Metabolism, and Diabetes, University of Illinois at Chicago, Chicago, IL*

ROGER GEJMAN, MD • *Research Fellow in Neuropathology, Massachusetts General Hospital, Research Fellow in Pathology, Harvard Medical School, Boston, MA*

E. TESSA HEDLEY-WHYTE, MD • *Professor of Pathology, Harvard Medical School, Neuropathologist, Massachusetts General Hospital, Boston, MA*

DANIEL F. KELLY, MD • *Director, Neuroendocrine Tumor Center, John Wayne Cancer Institute at Saint John's Health Center, Santa Monica, CA*

ANDREA LANIA, MD, PhD • *Endocrine Unit, Department of Medical Sciences, Fondazione Policlinico, IRCCS, University of Milan, Milan, Italy*

JOHN R. LINDSAY, MD • *Altnagelvin Hospital, Western Health and Social Care Trust, Londonderry, UK*

JAY S. LOEFFLER, MD • *Herman and Joan Suit Professor of Radiation Oncology, Harvard Medical School, Chair, Department of Radiation Oncology, Massachusetts General Hospital, Boston, MA*

JOHN T. LYSACK, MD, FRCPC • *Clinical Assistant in Neuroradiology, Massachusetts General Hospital, Harvard Medical School, Boston, MA*

GIOVANNA MANTOVANI, MD, PHD • *Endocrine Unit, Department of Medical Sciences, Fondazione Policlinico, IRCCS, University of Milan, Milan, Italy*

KAREN KLAHR MILLER, MD • *Neuroendocrine Unit, Massachusetts General Hospital, Harvard Medical School, Boston, MA*

MADHUSMITA MISRA, MD, MPH • *Assistant in Pediatrics, Pediatric Endocrinology Unit, MassGeneral Hospital for Children, Assistant in Biology, Neuroendocrine Unit, Massachusetts General Hospital, Assistant Professor of Pediatrics, Harvard Medical School, Boston, MA*

MARK E. MOLITCH, MD • *Professor of Medicine, Division of Endocrinology, Metabolism, and Molecular Medicine, Northwestern University Feinberg School of Medicine, Chicago, IL*

CARRIE R. MUH, MD, MS • *Department of Neurological Surgery, Emory University School of Medicine, Atlanta, GA*

THOMAS P. NAIDICH, MD • *Director of Neuroradiology, Professor of Radiology and Neurosurgery, Irving and Dorothy Regenstreif Research Professor of Neuroscience (Neuroimaging), Mount Sinai Medical Center, New York, NY*

LYNNETTE K. NIEMAN, MD • *Senior Investigator, RBMB, NICHD, Associate Director, IETP, NICHD-NIDDK, Reproductive Biology and Medicine Branch, NICHD, National Institutes of Health, Bethesda, MD*

PANAGIOTIS NOMIKOS, MD • *Senior Neurosurgeon, Department of Neurosurgery, Hygeia Hospital, Marousi, Greece*

NELSON M. OYESIKU, MD, PHD, FACS • *Professor and Vice-Chairman, Department of Neurological Surgery, Emory University School of Medicine, Atlanta, GA*

KALMON D. POST, MD • *Professor of Neurosurgery, Mount Sinai Medical Center, New York, NY*

RAJANI PRABHAKARAN, MD • *Fellow, Pediatric Endocrinology, MassGeneral Hospital for Children, Harvard Medical School, Boston, MA*

HERSHEL RAFF, PHD • *Director, Endocrine Research Laboratory, Aurora St. Luke's Medical Center, Professor of Medicine, Medical College of Wisconsin, Milwaukee, WI*

JOSEPH F. RIZZO III, MD • *Associate Professor of Ophthalmology, Massachusetts Eye & Ear Infirmary, Harvard Medical School, Boston, MA*

STEVEN J. RUSSELL, MD, PhD • *Instructor in Medicine, Harvard Medical School, Assistant in Medicine, Massachusetts General Hospital, Boston, MA*

PAMELA W. SCHAEFER, MD • *Associate Director of Neuroradiology, Clinical Director of MRI, Massachusetts General Hospital, Associate Professor of Radiology, Harvard Medical School, Boston, MA*

JANET A. SCHLECTE, MD • *Professor of Medicine, University of Iowa Hospitals and Clinics, Iowa City, IA*

AMAL SHIBLI-RAHHAL, MD • *Assistant Professor of Medicine, University of Iowa Hospitals and Clinics, Iowa City, IA*

HELEN A. SHIH, MD, MS, MPH • *Instructor in Radiation Oncology, Massachusetts General Hospital, Harvard Medical School, Boston, MA*

MONICA C. SKARULIS, MD • *Clinical Endocrinology Branch, National Institute of Diabetes, Digestive and Kidney Diseases, National Institutes of Health, Bethesda, MD*

BRIAN J. SNYDER, MD • *Department of Neurosurgey, Mount Sinai Medical Center, New York, NY*

PETER J. SNYDER, MD • *Professor of Medicine, University of Pennsylvania, Philadelphia, PA*

ANNA SPADA, MD • *Professor of Endocrinology, Endocrine Unit, Department of Medical Sciences, Fondazione Policlinico, IRCCS, University of Milan, Milan, Italy*

TAKARA STANLEY, MD • *Fellow, Pediatric Endocrinology, MassGeneral Hospital for Children, Harvard Medical School, Boston, MA*

STEPHAN ULMER, MD • *Institute of Neuroradiology, University Hospital of Schleswig-Holstein, Kiel, Germany*

MARINA S. ZEMSKOVA, MD • *Associate Investigator, Clinical Endocrinology Branch, National Institute of Diabetes, Digestive and Kidney Diseases, National Institutes of Health, Bethesda, MD*

Color Plate

The following color illustrations are printed in the insert.

Chapter 2

Fig. 1: Prolactinoma composed of cells with chromophobic cytoplasm arranged in a diffuse architectural pattern (A). Prolactinoma with small, hyperchromatic cells after dopamine agonist therapy (B). Positive immunohistochemical reaction for PRL with diffuse (C) and paranuclear patterns (D) in two prolactinomas.

Fig. 2: Densely granulated somatotroph pituitary adenoma with acidophilic and densely granulated cytoplasm (A), strong positive immunoreaction for GH (B) and diffuse immunohistochemical staining pattern for CAM 5.2 (C). Sparsely granulated somatotroph pituitary adenoma with a chromophobic and less granular cytoplasm (D). The same tumor as in (D) with slightly positive reaction for GH (E) and the dot-like positive reaction with CAM 5.2 corresponding to fibrous bodies (F).

Fig. 3: ACTH-producing pituitary tumor composed of densely granular basophilic cells (A) with strong positive immunohistochemical reaction for ACTH (B).

Fig. 4: Gonadotropic pituitary adenoma with a papillary pattern (A); perivascular pseudorosettes (B); and focal and weak expression of beta-FSH (C). Ultrastructural appearance of a tumor cell with oncocytic changes, i.e., many mitochondria (D).

Fig. 5: Craniopharyngioma composed of cords and islands of squamoid epithelium limited by columnar cells (A). Some cavities contain keratin material (*) (B). A cystic area has a thin epithelial wall(C) and adjacent inflammatory reaction with many foamy macrophages (D) (hematoxylin and eosin stain).

Fig. 6: Germinoma with a dense lymphocytic population and scattered groups of bigger round tumor cells with clear cytoplasm (arrows) (hematoxylin and eosin stain).

Fig. 7:   Granular cell tumor composed of closely apposed acidophilic cells with bland nuclei and granular cytoplasm (hematoxylin and eosin stain).

Fig. 9:   Lymphocytic hypophysitis with a dense inflammatory infiltrate including lymphocytes and plasma cells. Scattered pituitary cells are seen between the inflammatory cells (arrows) (hematoxylin and eosin stain).

Chapter 5

Fig. 6:   Horizontal section of the visual pathways. The visual fields demonstrate the correlation of lesion site and field defect. (Reproduced with permission, Yanoff M, Duker JS, editors. Ophthalmology, 2nd ed. St Louis, Mo: Mosby; 2004.)

Fig. 7:   Localization and probable identification of masses by pattern of field loss. Junctional scotomas occur with compression of the anterior angle of the chiasm (sphenoid meningiomas). Bitemporal hemianopia results from compression of the body of the chiasm from below (e.g., pituitary adenoma, sellar meningiomas). Compression of the posterior chiasm and its decussating nasal fibers may cause central bitemporal scotomas (e.g., hydrocephalus, pinealoma, craniopharyngioma). (Reproduced with permission, Yanoff M, Duker JS, editors. Ophthalmology, 2nd ed. St Louis, Mo: Mosby; 2004.)

Fig. 9:   Parasympathetic and sympathetic innervation of the iris muscles. (Reproduced with permission, Yanoff M, Duker JS, editors. Ophthalmology, 2nd ed. St Louis, Mo: Mosby; 2004.)

Fig. 10: (A) Early papilledema. The optic disk of an 18-year-old man 2 weeks after he had complained of diplopia arising from sixth cranial nerve palsies caused by increased intracranial pressure. Note the minimal evidence of edema. (Reproduced with permission, Yanoff M, Duker JS, editors. Ophthalmology, 2nd ed. St Louis, Mo: Mosby; 2004.) (B) Developed papilledema. The optic disk of a 36-year-old woman who suffered headache and blurred vision for 2 months. Fully developed disk edema present—note the engorged veins and peripapillary hemorrhages. (Reproduced with permission, Yanoff M, Duker JS, editors. Ophthalmology, 2nd ed. St Louis, Mo: Mosby; 2004.) (C) Chronic papilledema. Severe and chronic disk edema in a 27-year-old very obese woman who has pseudotumor cerebri. Note that the disk cup is obliterated and hard exudates are present. (Reproduced with permission, Yanoff M, Duker JS,

1

Molecular Pathogenesis of Pituitary Adenomas

Andrea Lania, MD, PhD,
Giovanna Mantovani, MD, PhD,
and Anna Spada, MD

CONTENTS

Summary

The genesis of pituitary tumors is still under debate. Although these neoplasia are monoclonal in origin, mutations of GNAS1, the gene encoding the α subunit of Gs is the only mutational change unequivocally associated with GH-secreting adenomas. In addition, multiple events, including the overexpression of cell cycle regulators, growth factors, and stimulatory hormones together with epigenetic disruption of genes with antioncogenic properties, frequently occur in pituitary tumors; their relative importance is still uncertain.

Key Words: Pituitary adenomas, Tumorigenesis, Oncogene, Oncosuppressor genes, *gsp.*

1. INTRODUCTION

The pathogenesis of pituitary tumors remains controversial. The respective role and importance of intrinsic alterations of the pituicytes themselves, dysregulation of hypothalamic hormones, and autocrine/paracrine action of locally produced growth factors are still under debate *(1–4).* The demonstration by X-chromosome inactivation analysis that the majority of pituitary adenomas

From: *Contemporary Endocrinology: Diagnosis and Management of Pituitary Disorders*
Edited by: B. Swearingen and B. M. K. Biller © Humana Press, Totowa, NJ

are monoclonal in origin represents a milestone in this debate *(5,6)*. Indeed, these data unequivocally indicate that pituitary neoplasia arise from the replication of a single mutated cell, suggesting that growth advantage results from either activation of protooncogenes or inactivation of tumor-suppressor genes. Both in vivo and in vitro evidence suggest that, in addition to mutational changes, tumor formation requires a secondary event for clonal expansion and progression. The need for a "second hit" is indicated by the clinical observation that high-resolution neuroradiological imaging "incidentally" detects pituitary microadenomas in about 20% of subjects without signs or symptoms of pituitary disorders, a value that is about 1,000-fold higher than the clinical prevalence of the disease and approaches the incidence of pituitary adenomas found in unselected autopsies *(7,8)*. In this chapter we will summarize the molecular abnormalities that have been proposed to be responsible for pituitary tumor formation and progression.

2. ACTIVATION OF PROTOONCOGENES IN PITUITARY TUMORS

Pituitary tumors may originate from genetic abnormalities able to confer gain of function of either common or pituitary-specific protooncogenes. Moreover, in the absence of genetic abnormalities, dysregulation or overexpression of signal molecules that are components of proliferative pathways may promote cell growth (Table 1).

Table 1
Gain-of-function Events in Pituitary Tumors

Human pituitary tumor	Gene	Defect
ACTH-omas	Cyclin E	Increased expression
GH-omas	GNAS1	Somatic mutations
NFPA, GH-omas	Gi2α	Somatic mutations
PRL-omas	HMGA2	Increased expression
All types	PTTG	Increased expression
All types	FGFR4	Alternative transcription initiation
Pituitary carcinoma metastases; Aggressive PRL-omas	Ras	Somatic mutations
Aggressive adenomas	Cyclin D1	Increased expression
Invasive NFPA	PKC	Somatic mutations

FGFR4, fibroblast growth factor receptor 4; PKC, protein kinase C; PTTG, pituitary tumor transforming gene; NFPA, nonfunctioning pituitary adenoma.

2.1. Genetic Abnormalities of Protooncogenes

Common and pituitary specific protooncogenes have been extensively screened for genetic abnormalities in pituitary tumors during the past two decades. This extensive search has failed to identify the initial pathogenetic event in most tumors, and at present few genetic defects in protooncogenes are unequivocally associated with pituitary tumorigenesis.

2.1.1. Gain-of-Function Mutations of Monomeric and Heterotrimeric GTP-Binding Proteins

The family of RAS protooncogene encodes a 21-kD monomeric GDP/GTP-binding protein mainly involved in the activation of the mitogen activated protein kinase (MAPK) cascade and growth factor signaling. This protooncogene may acquire mitogenic properties by point mutations in codons 12 and 13 that increase the affinity for GTP, or mutations in codon 61 that prevent GTPase activity. RAS mutations are present with relatively high frequency in human malignancies, while they are uncommon in pituitary tumors. Indeed, a Gly12 to Val substitution has been observed in one single, unusually aggressive, and ultimately fatal prolactinoma resistant to dopaminergic inhibition *(9)*. Consistent with the view that this mutational change probably represents a late event associated with unusual malignant features, RAS mutations have been detected in metastases of pituitary carcinomas, but not in the primitive tumors *(10,11)*.

In contrast to the rare occurrence of RAS mutations, mutations in the gene encoding the α subunit of Gs (GNAS1) are frequent events, occurring in about 30–40% of GH-secreting adenomas *(12,13)*. Gs is a ubiquitously expressed protein that belongs to the family of heterotrimeric G proteins and is constituted by the specific α subunit and the common βγ subunits. Gs protein mediates the activation of adenylyl cyclase and generation of cAMP in pituitary target cells in response to several hormones. In particular, by interacting with specific G protein-coupled receptors, hypothalamic releasing hormones such as GH-releasing hormone (GHRH), corticotroph-releasing hormone (CRH), pituitary adenylate cyclase activating peptide (PACAP) and vasoactive intestinal peptide (VIP) activate the cAMP-dependent pathway. Although in vitro mutagenesis studies have documented a number of possible activating substitutions in the GNAS1 gene, the only amino acid changes so far reported replace either Arg 201 with Cys or His or Ser, or, less frequently, Gln 227 with Arg or Leu. These changes result in the constitutive activation of the subunit due to the reduction of GTPase activity *(12,13)*. Since somatotrophs belong to a set of cells that recognize cAMP as a mitogenic signal, Gsα may be considered the product of a protooncogene that is converted into an oncogene, designated *gsp* (for Gs protein) in selected cell types. Although this oncogene has been demonstrated to confer growth advantage in vitro, patients carrying *gsp*-positive or *gsp*-negative tumors have the same clinical and biochemical phenotype, recurrence rate, and outcome *(14–17)*. The discrepancy between the mitogenic action of the mutant Gsα observed in vivo and in vitro strongly suggests the presence of events able to counteract in vivo the putative growth advantage conferred by the *gsp* oncogene. In this respect, some counteracting mechanisms, such as the instability of the mutant protein and the expression of cAMP-regulated genes with opposing actions, i.e., cAMP-specific phosphodiesterase isoforms and the inducible cAMP early repressor, have been identified in *gsp*-positive tumors *(18–22)*.

The phenotype of pituitary tumors is also related to the imprinting of GNAS1. The GNAS1 locus that maps on human chromosome 20q13 is under a complex imprinting control, with multiple maternally, paternally and bi-allelically alternatively spliced transcripts *(23,24)*. Recent reports demonstrated a predominant, though not exclusive, maternal origin of Gsα in adult human thyroid, gonad, and pituitary tissue *(25–27)*. Almost all *gsp*-positive tumors show mutations on the maternal allele *(25,27)*. Moreover, a partial loss of GNAS1 imprinting, resulting in Gsα overexpression, has been found in *gsp*-negative GH-secreting adenomas, although subsequent studies did not confirm this observation *(25,27)*.

Following the first identification in GH-secreting adenomas, *gsp* mutations have been infrequently detected also in other pituitary tumors, i.e., in about 10% of nonfunctioning pituitary adenomas and < 5% of ACTH-secreting adenomas *(28,29)*.

At present, Gsα is the only G protein that has been identified as target for activating mutations unequivocally associated with pituitary tumors. In fact, data concerning mutations of Gi2α protein, a protein involved in the inhibition of adenylyl cyclase and calcium influx, are discordant. Previous screening studies reported amino acids substitutions of Gln 205 (corresponding to Gln 227 of the Gsα sequence) with Arg in a subset of pituitary tumors; these studies were not confirmed by subsequent reports *(30,31)*. Despite the absence of mutations in Gq and G11 genes that are involved in Ca^{2+}/calmodulin and phospholipid-dependent protein kinase C activation, some reports suggested an overactivity of this pathway due to mutations of protein kinase Cα gene in pituitary adenomas. In particular, point mutations replacing Gly 294, a domain containing the calcium-binding site, with Asp have been identified in four invasive pituitary tumors *(28)*, an observation not confirmed by subsequent studies *(32,33)*.

2.1.2. GENETIC ABNORMALITIES OF GROWTH FACTORS

The normal pituitary and pituitary tumors produce a wide number of growth factors and express their specific receptors *(3,4)*. In contrast to other human neoplasms, genetic abnormalities of these factors and receptors are a rare event in pituitary tumorigenesis, the only alteration occurring in fibroblast growth factor (FGF) signaling. Indeed, about 40% of pituitary adenomas show the aberrant expression of an *N*-terminally truncated variant of FGF receptor-4. This variant is constitutively phosphorylated in the absence of the ligand and causes transformation in vitro and in vivo *(34)*. Interestingly, in contrast to previous models of pituitary tumorigenesis, the expression of the truncated receptor in the pituitary of transgenic mice results in tumor formation in the absence of massive hyperplasia, a phenomenon similar to that observed in human pituitary adenomas *(34)*. Moreover, disruption of FGF receptor 4 signaling seems to be associated with tumor invasion, since this receptor is required, together with other molecules, such as *N*-cadherin, phospholipase C-γ, and tumor-suppressor neural cell-adhesion molecule, for normal cell contact *(34,35)*.

2.2. Overexpression of Protooncogenes and Proliferative Signals

In contrast to the few molecular changes detected in pituitary tumors, in these neoplasms amplification of proliferative signals frequently occurs by overexpression. While the resulting phenotypes and their clinical correlations have been extensively investigated, the molecular mechanisms responsible for this dysregulation remain largely undefined.

2.2.1. OVEREXPRESSION OF CELL CYCLE REGULATORS

The expression of genes involved in cell progression to replication has been extensively investigated in pituitary tumors. Pituitary adenomas overexpress cyclins, particularly cyclin D1 and cyclin E. In particular, in a screening study reporting the expression of cyclins in about 100 pituitary tumors, cyclin D1 was overexpressed in aggressive functioning and nonfunctioning tumors, while cyclin E was preferentially present in corticotroph adenomas *(36)*. Moreover, using a frequent polymorphism in cyclin D1 gene (CCND1), allelic imbalance indicative of gene amplification has been found in about 25% of pituitary tumors, despite the absence of a clear increase of cyclin D1 protein *(37)*.

Almost all pituitary adenomas overexpress the pituitary tumor transforming gene (PTTG), an estrogen-inducible gene with high transforming properties originally isolated from the rat pituitary cell line and subsequently found to be expressed at high levels particularly in invasive hormone-secreting tumors *(38,39)*. Structural characterization has identified PTTG as a member of the securin family. PTTG is an anaphase inhibitor that prevents premature chromosome separation through inhibition of separase activity *(39)*. Therefore, its degradation is required to start anaphase and separation of sister chromatids during mitosis. Due to the critical role of PTTG in maintaining genomic stability, it has been proposed that PTTG overexpression may be, at least in part, responsible for the aneuploidy frequently observed in pituitary tumors. Moreover, PTTG participates in cellular responses to DNA damage in humans, since it has been demonstrated that securin is a downstream target of the oncosuppressor p53 *(40)*. Finally, PTTG mediates the estrogen-induced upregulation of growth factors with potent mitogenic and angiogenic activity, such as FGF-2.

The high mobility group A nonhistone chromosomal protein 2 (HMGA2) is a nuclear architectural factor that plays a critical role in a wide range of biological processes including regulation of gene expression, embryogenesis, and neoplastic transformation. Overexpression of this protein is characteristic of rapidly dividing cells in embryonic tissues and in tumors and is probably related to interaction with the retinoblastoma gene (RB). Consistent with the observations that HMGA2 overexpression causes GH-secreting and PRL-secreting adenomas in transgenic animals and that high levels of HMGA2 protein are present in human prolactinomas, it has been suggested that this protein may be implicated in lactotroph proliferation *(41,42)*.

2.2.2. OVEREXPRESSION OF GROWTH FACTORS

Several growth factors are overexpressed in pituitary tumors. In particular, transforming growth factor-α, epidermal growth factor, and their common tyrosine kinase receptor are overexpressed in pituitary adenomas, particularly in those with high aggressiveness *(3,4)*. Although in the pituitary, unlike other tissues, vascularization is lower in adenomas compared to the normal gland, high levels of growth factors with angiogenic properties such as FGF and vascular endothelial growth factor (VEGF) are detected in pituitary tumors and particularly in aggressive prolactinomas *(3,4)*. In pituitary tumors derived from the gonadotroph lineage, activin/inhibin subunits appear highly expressed together with the specific type I and type II receptors, while follistatin, which prevents activin action by binding this subunit, is reduced *(43,44)*. Accordingly, it has been proposed that the imbalanced expression of these proteins, resulting in an enhanced activin signaling, may represent a pathogenetic mechanism in the development of this adenoma subtype.

2.2.3. OVEREXPRESSION OF RECEPTORS FOR HYPOTHALAMIC RELEASING HORMONES

Pituitary function is under the strict control of hypothalamic neurohormones that are required for pituitary cell commitment and growth as well as hormone synthesis and release. It is a common clinical observation that ectopic overproduction of releasing hormones, such as GHRH or CRH, results in proliferation of the target cells. However, the vast majority of sporadic pituitary tumors do not show hyperplasia in the surrounding tissue. Although these data suggest that hormonal stimulation is not a primary etiologic mechanism in pituitary tumorigenesis, it is worth noting that aggressive GH-secreting adenomas frequently express high intrapituitary amounts of GHRH *(45)*.

Receptors of hypothalamic neurohormones have been extensively investigated for either activating mutations or overexpression, both of which could mimic states of hormone excess. Studies carried out on a large series of functioning and nonfunctioning adenomas failed to identify mutational changes in the genes encoding TRH, GnRH, CRH and V3 receptors, while variants of the GHRH receptor devoid of any pathogenetic relevance have been found in about 20% of GH-secreting adenomas *(46)*. In contrast to the absence of mutational changes, these receptors are frequently overexpressed. Indeed, high levels of V3 and CRH receptor have been detected in ACTH-secreting adenomas, whereas most functioning and nonfunctioning adenomas possess TRH, GnRH, VIP, and PACAP receptors, normally coupled to intracellular effectors *(47,48)*.

3. LOSS OF ANTIPROLIFERATIVE SIGNALS

Proliferation may result from either inactivating mutations of common tumor suppressors or specific pituitary inhibitors, or epigenetic disruption of gene expression at mRNA or protein levels (Table 2).

3.1. Inactivating Mutations of Antiproliferative Signals

Few genetic defects have been so far identified in tumor-suppressor genes to confer constitutive activation of protooncogenes, while downregulation of inhibitory molecules at mRNA or protein levels is not a rare event.

3.1.1. INACTIVATING MUTATIONS OF TUMOR-SUPPRESSOR GENES

According to the "two-hit" hypothesis, loss of tumor-suppressor genes requires a first "hit," represented by a germline or a somatic mutation, followed by a second "hit," that is usually a somatic deletion of the second allele in the involved tissue. This results in loss of heterozygosity (LOH), although evidence suggests other pathogenetic mechanisms beyond this hypothesis *(49)*. In pituitary tumors, LOH occurs with relatively high frequency (15–30%) and in several loci, such as 10q26, 11q13, 11p, 13q, and 22q13 *(2)*. However, the search for mutations of known antioncogenes in the retained allele has failed to reveal inactivating mutations in most cases. Indeed, in contrast to the pituitary tumor development observed in the knockout mice for RB and for p27Kip1, a cyclin-dependent kinase inhibitor that induces G1 arrest by RB hypophosphorylation, and the frequent LOH on chromosomes where these

Table 2
Loss-of-function Events In sporadic Pituitary Tumors

Human pituitary tumor	Gene	Defect
Aggressive adenomas	RB	Promoter methylation
All types	p16INK4a	Promoter methylation
ACTH-omas	p27Kip1	Reduced expression
TSH-omas	TRβ	Inactivating mutations
GH-omas	AIP	Inactivating mutations
NFPA	ZAC	LOH
ACTH-omas	GR	LOH
GH-omas	PRKAR1A	Reduced expression (in sporadic tumors) Inactivating mutation (in Carney Complex)
Resistant PRL-omas	D2R	Reduced expression
Resistant GH-omas	Sst2	Reduced expression

RB, retinoblastoma; LOH, loss of heterozygosity; D2R, dopamine receptor type 2; sst2, somatostatin receptor type 2; TRβ, thyroid hormone receptor β; GR, glucocorticoid receptor; AIP, aryl hydrocarbon receptor interacting protein; PRKAR1A, type 1 alpha regulatory subunit of protein kinase A.

genes are located *(50,51)*, no inactivating mutation of these genes has been reported so far *(50–52)*. Similarly, no mutation in the tumor-suppressor *p53* gene, the most frequently altered oncosuppressor gene in human neoplasia, has been ever found in human pituitary tumors *(53)*.

Since pituitary tumors are part of multiple endocrine neoplasia syndromes, such as MEN1 and Carney complex, the two genes responsible for the diseases, i.e., MEN1 and type 1α regulatory subunit of protein kinase A (PRKAR1A), have been screened for mutations in sporadic pituitary adenomas, yielding negative results *(54,55)*. However, consistent with the finding that LOH in the region 11q13, where MEN1 locus is located, is present in 10–20% of sporadic pituitary adenomas, genetic abnormalities in this region have been reported recently *(56)*. By combining chip-based technologies with genealogy data, germline loss-of-function mutations in the aryl hydrocarbon receptor (AHR) interacting protein (AIP) gene in individuals with pituitary adenoma predisposition have been reported recently. In particular, in a population-based series from Northern Finland, two AIP mutations accounted for 16% of all patients diagnosed with GH-secreting adenomas and for 40% of the affected patients younger than 35 years of age. AIP forms a complex with the AHR, a ligand-activated transcription factor that regulates a variety of xenobiotic metabolizing enzymes and mediates most of the toxic responses of dioxin-like chemicals.

However, the mechanisms by which AIP exerts its tumor-suppressive action in the pituitary remain to be determined. Recently, the occurrence of inactivating mutations of this tumor-suppressor gene was not confirmed in a series of US patients *(57)*.

3.1.2. Inactivating Mutations of Components of the Negative Feedback

It is well established that negative feedback is a potent inhibitory mechanism of both hormone secretion and cell growth. However, few genetic mutations have been identified to support the hypothesis that poor sensitivity to peripheral hormones is responsible for pituitary cell proliferation. Only one mutation of the glucocorticoid receptor (GR) has been far reported in one macroadenoma from a patient with Nelson's syndrome *(58)*. However, LOH at the GR gene locus is present in about a third of ACTH-secreting adenomas, suggesting a possible role of GR allelic deletion in glucocorticoid resistance and corticotroph tumorigenesis *(59)*. Similarly, the reduced inhibition of TSH secretion by T3 in TSH-secreting adenomas has been associated with mutations in the thyroid hormone receptor β isoform (TRβ), causing lack of T3 binding in two tumors *(60)*.

3.2. Downregulation of Antiproliferative Signals

The infrequent occurrence of mutations in genes encoding components of antiproliferative pathways strongly suggests that posttrascriptional events may cause antioncogene silencing by reducing mRNA/protein expression or stability. Indeed, epigenetic disruption and downregulation of common tumor-suppressor genes, probably due to gene promoter methylation as well as pituitary specific inhibitory signals, frequently occurs in pituitary tumors, although its relevancy in pituitary tumorigenesis remains uncertain.

3.2.1. Downregulation of Tumor-Suppressor Genes

Investigation of possible defects in RB occurring at the RNA or protein level in pituitary tumor tissues yielded contradictory results, with some immuno-histochemical studies reporting low RB protein levels and other studies not confirming these data *(52,61)*. The low expression of p27Kip1 protein found in recurrent pituitary tumors and pituitary carcinomas by immunohistochemistry and not by mRNA analysis was consistent with protein degradation rather than reduced transcription *(62)*. A similar reduced expression, probably depending on methylation within the exon 1 CpG island, affects p16INK4a, another cyclin-dependent kinase inhibitor that prevents RB phosphorylation *(63)*. A widely expressed zinc finger protein named ZAC that shows transactivation and DNA-binding activities and that, like p53, inhibits tumor cell proliferation has been found highly expressed in the normal anterior pituitary gland but downregulated in most pituitary adenomas *(64)*.

3.2.2. DOWNREGULATION OF INHIBITORY SIGNALS

In addition to the component of the negative feedback, other hormones and receptors that physiologically inhibit pituitary hormone secretion may be considered as possible targets for inactivating mutations with pathogenetic impact. The best candidates among these are the dopaminergic D2 receptor (D2R) and the somatostatin receptor (sst) type 1–3 and 5.

Although the development of prolactinomas in D2R-deficient mice strongly suggests that inactivating mutations of this receptor might results in lactotroph proliferation *(65)*, studies carried out on prolactinomas, including those resistant to dopaminergic drugs, failed to find mutations in the D2R gene *(66)*. Conversely, resistant prolactinomas frequently show a reduction of D2R transcript, and particularly of the shortest isoform that is more efficiently coupled to phospholipase C *(67)*. In addition to the defect in D2R mRNA splicing and expression, the absence of D2R protein due to increased instability and degradation has been observed in metastases of a malignant prolactinoma resistant to different dopamine agonists *(68)*.

In analogy with the poor, if any, evidence of mutations in D2R, mutational changes of the sst genes seem to occur rarely. In fact, only one mutation in the sst5 gene has been identified so far in one octreotide-resistant acromegalic patient *(69)*. In the absence of mutations, several expression studies suggest that the different degree of responsiveness to somatostatin analog observed in acromegalic patients is probably related to the level of expression of somatostatin receptors. In particular, poor responsiveness to treatment seems to correlate with a low expression of sst2, while the role of sst5, the most highly expressed somatostatin receptor in normal and adenomatous somatotrophs, is still controversial *(70)*.

In addition to receptors, molecules that participate in the transduction of extracellular signals may have inhibitory functions. In particular, molecules that are involved in the negative control of the cAMP cascade may be considered as putative antioncogenes in tissues where cAMP is mitogenic, such as the pituitary. Accordingly, inactivating mutations of PRAKAR1A, the gene encoding the type 1A regulatory subunit of protein kinase A, that render the catalytic subunit more susceptible to activation by cAMP have been identified in patients with Carney complex, a multiple neoplasia syndrome that includes pituitary tumors. Although subsequent studies failed to identify mutations of PRKAR1A in sporadic pituitary adenomas *(54,55)*, the low expression of the wild-type subunit due to proteasome-mediated degradation induces cAMP-dependent cell proliferation in GH-secreting adenomas *(71)*.

4. CONCLUSIONS

In the last years several candidate factors have been implicated in the genesis and progression of pituitary adenomas. To date, GNAS1 is the only gene that has been identified as a target for activating mutations that unequivocally cause cell proliferation in about 30–40% of GH-secreting adenomas. Abnormalities in the expression of cell cycle regulators, receptors, and growth factors and their signaling have been proposed to play a relevant role in cell transformation and/or clonal expansion. It is tempting to speculate that no single factor might effectively explain tumorigenesis in the pituitary.

REFERENCES

1. Farrel WE, Clayton RN. Molecular pathogenesis of pituitary tumors. Front Neuroendocrinol 2000;21:174–98.
2. Lania A, Mantovani G, Spada A. G protein mutations in endocrine diseases. Eur J Endocrinol 2001145, 543–59.
3. Asa SL, Ezzat S. The pathogenesis of pituitary tumours. Nat Rev Cancer 2002;2:836–49.
4. Ezzat S, Asa SL. Mechanisms of disease: The pathogenesis of pituitary tumors. Nat Clin Pract 2006;2:220–30.
5. Alexander JM, Biller BMK, Bikkal H, Zervas NT, Arnold A, Klibanski A. Clinically non functioning pituitary adenomas are monoclonal in origin. J Clin Invest 1990; 86:336–40.
6. Herman V, Fagin J, Gonsky R, Kovacs K, Melmed S. Clonal origin of pituitary adenomas. J Clin Endocrinol Metab 1990;71:1427–33.
7. Burrow GN, Wortzman G, Rewcastle NB, Hodgate RC, Kovacs K. Microadenomas of the pituitary and abnormal sella tomograms in an unselected autopsy series. N Engl J Med 1981;304:156–8.
8. Elster AD. Modern imaging of the pituitary. Radiology 1993;187:1–14.
9. Karga HJ, Alexander JM, Hedley-Whyte ET, Klibanski A, Jameson JL. Ras mutations in human pituitary tumors. J Clin Endocrinol Metab 1992;74:914–9.
10. Cai WY, Alexander JM, Hedley-Whyte ET, et al. Ras mutations in human prolactinomas and pituitary carcinomas. J Clin Endocrinol Metab 1994;78:89–93.
11. Pei L, Melmed S, Scheithauer B, Kovacs K, Prager D. H-ras mutations in human pituitary carcinoma metastasis. J Clin Endocrinol Metab 1994;78:842–6.
12. Vallar L, Spada A, Giannattasio G. Altered Gs and adenylate cyclase activity in human GH-secreting pituitary adenomas. Nature 1987;330:566–7.
13. Landis C, Masters SB, Spada A, Pace AM, Bourne HR, Vallar L. GTPase inhibiting mutations activate the alpha chain of Gs and stimulate adenylyl cyclase in human pituitary tumours. Nature 1989;340:692–6.
14. Spada A, Arosio M, Bochicchio D, et al. Clinical, biochemical, and morphological correlates in patients bearing growth hormone-secreting pituitary tumors with or without constitutively active adenylyl cyclase. J Clin Endocrinol Metab 1990;71:1421–6.

15. Adams EF, Brockmeier S, Friedmann E, Roth M, Buchfelder M, Fahlbusch R. Clinical and biochemical characteristics of acromegalic patients harboring gsp-positive and gsp-negative pituitary tumors. Neurosurgery 1993;33:198–201.

16. Yang I, Park S, Ryu M, et al. Characteristics of gsp-positive growth hormone-secreting pituitary tumors in Korean acromegalic patients Eur J Endocrinol 1996;134:720–6.

17. Barlier A, Gunz G, Zamora AJ, et al. Prognostic and therapeutic consequences of Gs alpha mutations in somatotroph adenomas. J Clin Endocrinol Metab 1998;83:1604–10.

18. Lania A, Persani L, Ballaré E, Mantovani S, Losa M, Spada A. Constitutively active $G_{s\alpha}$ is associated with an increased phosphodiesterase activity in human growth hormone secreting adenomas. J Clin Endocrinol Metab 1998;83:1624–8.

19. Persani L, Borgato S, Lania A, et al. Relevant cAMP-specific phosphodiesterase isoforms in human pituitary: effect of Gs(alpha) mutations. J Clin Endocrinol Metab 2001;86: 3795–800.

20. Bertherat J, Chanson P, Montiminy M. The cyclic adenosine 3'-5'-monophosphate-responsive factor CREB is constitutively activated in human somatotrophs. Mol Endocrinol 1995;9:777–83.

21. Peri A, Conforti B, Baglioni-Peri S, et al. Expression of cyclic adenosine 3',5'-monophosphate (cAMP)-responsive element binding protein and inducible-cAMP early repressor genes in growth hormone-secreting pituitary adenomas with or without mutations of the Gs alpha gene. J Clin Endocrinol Metab 2001;86:2111–7.

22. Ballare E, Mantovani S, Lania A, Di Blasio AM, Vallar L, Spada A. Activating mutations of the Gs alpha gene are associated with low levels of Gs alpha protein in growth hormone-secreting tumors. J Clin Endocrinol Metab 1998;83:4386–90.

23. Hayward BE, Kamiya M, Strain L, et al. The human GNAS1 gene is imprinted and encodes distinct paternally and biallelically expressed G proteins. Proc Natl Acad Sci USA 1998;95:10038–43.

24. Hayward B, Bonthron DT. An imprinted antisense transcript at the human GNAS1 locus. Hum Mol Genet 2000;9:835–41.

25. Hayward BE, Barlier A, Korbonits M, et al. Imprinting of the G(s)alpha gene GNAS1 in the pathogenesis of acromegaly. J Clin Invest 2001;107:R31–6.

26. Mantovani G, Ballare E, Giammona E, Beck-Peccoz P, Spada A. The $G_{s\alpha}$ gene: predominant maternal origin of transcription in human thyroid gland and gonads. J Clin Endocrinol Metab 2002;87:4736–40.

27. Mantovani G, Bondioni S, Lania AG, et al. Parental origin of Gsalpha mutations in the McCune-Albright syndrome and in isolated endocrine tumors. J Clin Endocrinol Metab 2004;89:3007–9.

28. Tordjman K, Stern N, Ouaknine G, et al. Activating mutations of the Gs alpha gene in non functioning pituitary adenomas. J Clin Endocrinol Metab 1993;77:765–9.

29. Williamson EA, Ince PG, Harrison D, Kendall-Taylor P, Harris PE. G-protein mutations in human adrenocorticotrophic (ACTH) hormone-secreting adenomas. Eur J Clin Invest 1995;25:128–31.

30. Williamson EA, Daniels M, Foster S, Kelly WF, Kendall-Taylor P, Harris PE. Gs alpha and Gi alpha mutations in clinically non-functioning pituitary tumours. Clin Endocrinol 1994;41:815–20.

31. Petersenn S, Heyens M, Ludecke DK, Beil FU, Schulte HM. Absence of somatostatin receptor type 2 A mutations and gip oncogene in pituitary somatotroph adenomas Clin Endocrinol (Oxf) 2000;52, 35–42.

32. Alvaro V, Levy L, Dubray C, et al. Invasive human pituitary tumors express a point-mutated alpha-protein kinase C. J Clin Endocrinol Metab 1993;77:1125–9.

33. Dong Q, Brucker-Davis F, Weintraub BD, et al. Screening of candidate oncogenes in human thyrotroph tumors: absence of activating mutations of the G alpha q, G alpha 11, G alpha s, or thyrotropin-releasing hormone receptor genes. J Clin Endocrinol Metab 1996;81:1134–40.

34. Ezzat S, Zheng L, Zhu XF, Wu GE, Asa SL. Targeted expression of a human pituitary tumor-derived isoform of FGF receptor-4 recapitulates pituitary tumorigenesis. J Clin Invest 2002;109:69–78.

35. Cavallaro U, Niedermeyer J, Fuxa M, Christofori G. N-CAM modulates tumour-cell adhesion to matrix by inducing FGF-receptor signalling. Nat Cell Biol 2001;3:650–7.

36. Jordan S, Lidhar K, Karbonits M, Lowe DG, Grossman AB. Cyclin D and cyclin E expression in normal and adenomatous pituitary. Eur J Endocrinol 2000;143:R1–6.

37. Hibberts NA, Simpson DJ, Bicknell JE, et al. Analysis of cyclin DI (CCND1) allelic imbalance and overexpression in sporadic pituitary tumors. Clin Cancer Res 1999;5: 2133–9.

38. Pei L, Melmed S. Isolation and characterization of a pituitary tumor-transforming gene (PTTG). Mol Endocrinol 1997;11:433–41.

39. Chen LL, Puri R, Lefkowitz EJ, Kakar SS. Identification of the human pituitary tumor transforming gene (HPTTG) family: molecular structure, expression, and chromosomal localization. Gene 2000;246:41–50.

40. Zhou Y, Mehta KR, Choi AP, Scolavino S, Zhang X. DNA damage-induced inhibition of securin expression is mediated by p53. J Biol Chem 2003;278:462–70.

41. Fedele M, Battista S, Kenyon L, et al. Overexpression of the HMGA2 gene in transgenic mice leads to the onset of pituitary adenomas. Oncogene 2002;21:3190–8.

42. Finelli P, Pierantoni GM, Giardino D, et al. The High Mobility Group A2 gene is amplified and overexpressed in human prolactinomas. Cancer Res 2002;62, 2398–405.

43. Danila DC, Inder WJ, Zhang X, et al. Activin effects on neoplastic proliferation of human pituitary tumors. J Clin Endocrinol Metab 2000;85:1009–15.

44. Wessels HT, Hofland LJ, van der Wal R, et al. In vitro secretion of FSH by cultured clinically nonfunctioning and gonadotroph pituitary adenomas is directly correlated with locally produced levels of activin A. Clin Endocrinol (Oxf) 2001;54:485–92.

45. Thapar K, Kovacs K, Stefaneau L, et al. Overexpression of the growth-hormone-releasing hormone gene in acromegaly associated pituitary tumors. An event associated with neoplastic progression and aggressive behavior. Am J Pathol 1997;151:769–84.

46. Lee EJ, Kotlar TJ, Ciric I, et al. Absence of constitutively activating mutations in the GHRH receptor in GH-producing pituitary tumors. J Clin Endocrinol Metab 2001;86:3989–95.

47. de Keyzer Y, Rene P, Beldjord C, Lenne F, Bertagna X. Overexpression of vasopressin (V3) and corticotrophin-releasing hormone receptor genes in corticotroph tumours. Clin Endocrinol (Oxf) 1998;49:475–82.

48. Spada A, Reza Elahi F, Lania A, Gil del Alamo P, Bassetti M, Faglia G. Hypothalamic peptides modulate cytosolic free Ca^{2+} levels and adenylyl cyclase activity in human nonfunctioning pituitary adenomas. J Clin Endocrinol Metab 1991;71:913–8.

49. Tucker T, Friedman JM. Pathogenesis of hereditary tumors: beyond the "two-hit" hypothesis. Clin Genet 2002;62:345–57.

50. Jacks T, Fazeli A, Schmitt EM, Bronson RT, Goodell MA, Weinberg RA Effects of an Rb mutation in the mouse. Nature 1992;359:295–300.

51. Nakayama K, Ishida N, Shirane M, et al. Mice lacking p27(Kip1) display increased body size, multiple organ hyperplasia, retinal dysplasia, and pituitary tumors. Cell 1996;85: 707–72.

52. Simpson DJ, Magnay J, Bicknell JE, et al. Chromosome 13q deletion mapping in pituitary tumors: infrequent loss of the retinoblastoma susceptibility gene (RB1) despite loss of RB1 product in somatotropinomas. Cancer Res 1999;59:1562–6.
53. Levy A, Hall L, Yeudall WA, Lightman SL. p53 gene mutations in pituitary adenomas: rare events. Clin. Endocrinol 1994;41:809–14.
54. Tanaka C, Kimura T, Yang P, et al. Analysis of loss of heterozygosity on chromosome 11 and infrequent inactivation of the MEN-1 gene in sporadic pituitary adenomas. J Clin Endocrinol Metab 1998;83:2631–4.
55. Kaltsas GA, Kola B, Borboli N, et al. Sequence analysis of the PRKAR1A gene in sporadic somatotroph and other pituitary tumours. Clin Endocrinol (Oxf) 2002;57:443–8.
56. Vierimaa O, Georgitsi M, Lehtonen R, et al. Pituitary adenoma predisposition caused by germline mutations in the AIP gene. Science 2006;312:1228–30.
57. Yu R, Bonert V, Saporta I, Raffel LJ, Melmed S. Aryl hydrocarbon receptor protein variants in sporadic pituitary sporadic adenomas. J Clin Endocrinol Metab 2006;91:5126–9.
58. Karl M, Lamberts SW, Koper JW, et al. Cushing's disease preceded by generalized glucocorticoid resistance: clinical consequences of a novel, dominant-negative glucocorticoid receptor mutation. Proc Assoc Am Physicians 1996;108:296–307.
59. Huizenga NA, de Lange P, Koper JW, et al. Human adrenocorticotropin-secreting pituitary adenomas show frequent loss of heterozygosity at the glucocorticoid receptor gene locus. J Clin Endocrinol Metab 1998;83:917–21.
60. Ando S, Sarlis NJ, Oldfield EH, Yen PM. Somatic mutation of TRbeta can cause a defect in negative regulation of TSH in a TSH-secreting pituitary tumor. J Clin Endocrinol Metab 2001;86:5572–6.
61. Simpson DJ, Hibberts NA, McNicol AM, Clayton RN, Farrell WE. Loss of pRb expression in pituitary adenomas is associated with methylation of the RB1 CpG island. Cancer Res 2000;60:1211–6.
62. Bamberger CM, Fehn M, Bamberger AM, et al. Reduced expression levels of the cell-cycle inhibitor p27Kip1 in human pituitary adenomas. Eur J Endocrinol 1999;140:250–5.
63. Simpson DJ, Bicknell JE, McNicol AM, Clayton RN, Farrell WE. Hypermethylation of the p16/CDKN2A/MTSI gene and loss of protein expression is associated with nonfunctional pituitary adenomas but not somatotrophinomas. Genes Chromosomes Cancer 1999;24:328–36.
64. Pagotto U, Arzberger T, Theodoropoulou M, et al. The expression of the antiproliferative gene ZAC is lost or highly reduced in nonfunctioning pituitary adenomas. Cancer Res 2000;60:6794–9.
65. Asa SL, Kelly MA, Grandy DK, Low MJ. Pituitary lactotroph adenomas develop after prolonged lactotroph hyperplasia in dopamine D2 receptor-deficient mice. Endocrinology 1999;140:5348–55.
66. Friedman E, Adams EF, Hoog A, et al. Normal structural dopamine type 2 receptor gene in prolactin-secreting and other pituitary tumors. J Clin Endocrinol Metab 1994;78:568–74.
67. Caccavelli L, Feron F, Morange I, et al. Decreased expression of the two D2 dopamine receptor isoforms in bromocriptine-resistant prolactinomas. Neuroendocrinology 1994;60:314–22.
68. Winkelmann J, Pagotto U, Theodoropoulou M, et al. Retention of dopamine 2 receptor mRNA and absence of the protein in craniospinal and extracranial metastasis of a malignant prolactinoma: a case report. Eur J Endocrinol 2002;146:81–8.
69. Ballare E, Persani L, Lania AG, et al. Mutation of somatostatin receptor type 5 in an acromegalic patient resistant to somatostatin analog treatment. J Clin Endocrinol Metab. 2001;86:3809–14.

70. Jaquet P, Saveanu A, Gunz G, et al. Human somatostatin receptor subtypes in acromegaly: distinct patterns of messenger ribonucleic acid expression and hormone suppression identify different tumoral phenotypes. J Clin Endocrinol Metab 2000;85:781–92.
71. Lania AG, Mantovani G, Ferrero S, et al. Proliferation of transformed somatotroph cells related to low or absent expression of protein kinase a regulatory subunit 1A protein. Cancer Res 2004;64:9193–8.

2 Pathology of Pituitary Adenomas

Roger Gejman, MD,
and E. Tessa Hedley-Whyte, MD

CONTENTS

1. INTRODUCTION
2. TYPES OF PITUITARY ADENOMAS
3. PATHOLOGY OF OTHER SELLAR LESIONS

Summary

Pituitary adenomas are the most common tumors of the sella and are manifest by either symptoms of mass effect or symptoms of hormone overproduction or underproduction. The histological and functional classification of pituitary adenomas is reviewed in relation to their clinical presentation and potential therapies. The pathological classification of pituitary tumors is complex. The role of immunohistochemical markers is discussed, but their value remains controversial. The pathological characteristics of other sellar lesions that enter into the differential diagnosis of pituitary tumors are described.

Key Words: Pituitary adenomas, Pathology, Chromophobe, Basophil.

1. INTRODUCTION

Pituitary adenomas are the most common tumors of the sella. It is difficult to determine their true incidence as they are often asymptomatic. The prevalence is about 14% in postmortem studies and about 22% in imaging studies *(1)*. The majority of pituitary adenomas are slow-growing tumors, but some have a higher growth rate and can be invasive. Pituitary carcinomas are very rare and are defined by the presence of metastasis or cerebrospinal fluid dissemination *(2)*. Pituitary adenomas are clinically significant because they may

From: *Contemporary Endocrinology: Diagnosis and Management of Pituitary Disorders*
Edited by: B. Swearingen and B. M. K. Biller © Humana Press, Totowa, NJ

present with symptoms of mass effect, especially visual compromise, and symptoms of endocrine dysfunction.

Pituitary adenomas have been classified in various ways. The original classification was based on the staining affinity of the tumor cells, i.e., acidophilic, basophilic, and chromophobic adenomas. There is some correlation between the cytoplasmic staining characteristics and the type of hormone produced, but this rule is not useful in all cases, since adenomas with different hormonal production can have similar morphological and staining patterns. For example, the acidophilic tumors are typical of acromegaly, but there are cases of chromophobic growth hormone (GH)-producing tumors. Assignment to classification categories changed with the introduction of immunohistochemical techniques and electron microscopy. Using those techniques and clinical data have enabled a morphofunctional classification (Table 1) that regroups the pituitary adenomas by functional or clinical status, correlated with immunohistochemical and electron microscopic characteristics (3). Although this classification is familiar to most endocrinologists and pathologists, for practical reasons it is not very useful in daily practice. The main difficulty is the requirement of electron microscopy for subclassification of some adenoma categories. This technique is expensive, and requires a relatively long time

Table 1
Functional Classification of Pituitary Adenomas

Sparsely granulated PRL cell adenoma
Densely granulated PRL cell adenoma
Sparsely granulated GH cell adenoma
Densely granulated GH cell adenoma
Mixed GH cell–PRL cell adenoma
Mamosomatotroph adenoma
Acidophil stem cell adenoma
Corticotroph adenoma
Thyrotroph adenoma
Gonadotroph adenoma
Silent corticotroph adenoma subtype 1
Silent corticotroph adenoma subtype 2
Silent corticotroph adenoma subtype 3
Null cell adenoma
Oncocytoma
Unclassified

Source: Kovacs and Horvath (1986) (3).

Table 2
Tumors of Pituitary

Pituitary adenomas
    PRL-producing tumors
    Growth hormone-producing tumors
    Adrenocorticotropin-producing tumor
    Gonadotropin-producing tumor
    Thyrotropin producing adenomas
    Null cell adenomas
    Plurihormonal adenomas
Pituitary carcinoma
Gangliocytoma
Mesenchymal tumors
    Chordoma
    Meningioma
Granular cell tumors
Secondary tumors

Source: Tumors of Endocrine Organs, WHO Classification (2004) *(2)*.

to process tissue. In addition, since the biopsies tend to be small, there is a potential sampling problem particularly when a mix of normal gland and tumor tissue is present. The latest Endocrine Tumors Classification of the WHO *(2)* includes a pituitary adenoma classification based on the previous morphofunctional classification, but it gives more importance to the classical types of adenomas with clear definitions, providing an easier approach to these tumors (Table 2). The remaining pathologic categories are included, but at a secondary level as microscopic variants.

2. TYPES OF PITUITARY ADENOMAS

2.1. Prolactin-Producing Adenomas

Definition: The WHO definition includes benign pituitary tumors producing prolactin (PRL) originating from the PRL adenohypophyseal cells. These tumors are also known as lactotroph adenomas or prolactinomas. They are the most common pituitary adenoma comprising 45% of the clinical cases with an incidence of 6 to 10 per million per year and a prevalence of 60 to 100 cases per million in clinical series *(4)*. The number of these tumors in surgical series is very low, less than 10% in our series, due to the success of dopamine agonist therapy. The tumors can often be grossly distinguished from the normal anterior gland because the tumors are softer and have a reddish or tan color. Some of the macroadenomas may have fibrosis and a cystic component. Microscopically, the majority of prolactinomas are chromophobic (*see* Fig. 1A and Color Plate 1). They show a wide variation in architecture including trabecular, papillary, or solid patterns. Sometimes these tumors have a prominent fibrous stroma with psammomatous calcifications. The cells become smaller and hyperchromatic following treatment with dopamine agonists (Fig. 1B). Rare densely granulated adenomas have acidophilic characteristics. Some authors include as prolactinomas the stem cell adenomas that will be described with the GH-producing adenomas.

Immunohistochemistry shows positive immunostaining for PRL (Fig. 1C), sometimes with paranuclear pattern corresponding to the Golgi area (Fig. 1D). Ultrastructural study reveals a prominent rough endoplasmic reticulum (RER) forming concentric whorls and Golgi apparatus with immature and mature granules with diameters between 150 and 300 nm. A common finding is the presence of granule exocytosis at the lateral cell borders. The highly granulated variant has less RER and mature large granules.

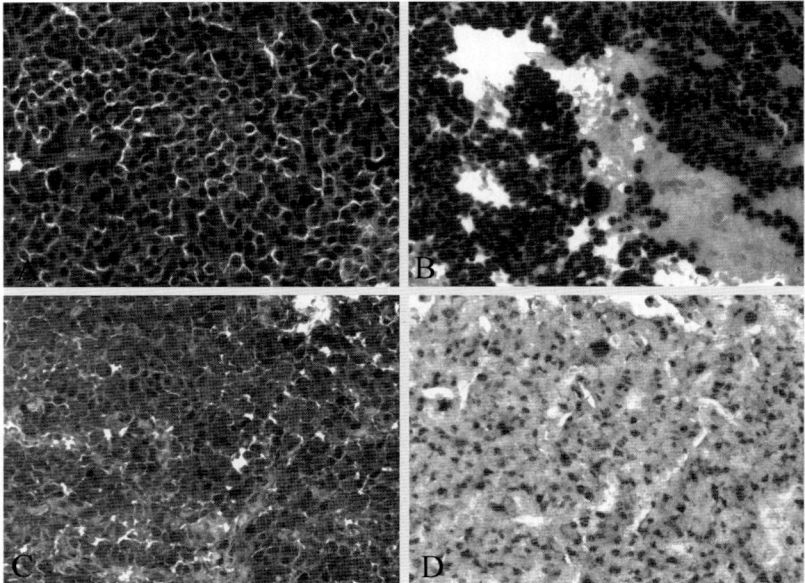

Fig. 1. Prolactinoma composed of cells with chromophobic cytoplasm arranged in a diffuse architectural pattern (A). Prolactinoma with small, hyperchromatic cells after dopamine agonist therapy (B). Positive immunohistochemical reaction for PRL with diffuse (C) and paranuclear patterns (D) in two prolactinomas. (*See* Color Plate 1.)

2.2. GH-Producing Adenomas

Definition: Pituitary adenomas producing GH in excess and clinically associated with gigantism in young patients and acromegaly in adults. Adenomas expressing GH immunohistochemically without clinical evidence of overproduction are very rare. The incidence of acromegaly is about 2 to 4 per million with a mean age at presentation of 40–50 years *(5)*. These tumors represent about 9–10% of resected pituitary tumors in our series. The WHO definition includes pure GH-producing tumors, mammosomatotroph adenomas, and acidophil stem cell adenomas. Morphologically, the majority of these tumors are macroadenomas and frequently have suprasellar growth and expansion to the lateral sellar wall. Subtype variants include densely granulated somatotroph adenomas and sparsely granulated somatotroph adenomas. Fortunately, they can be distinguished without electron microscopy, since there is a strong correlation between the cytokeratin pattern and the tumor type. The densely granulated variant is a classical acidophilic adenoma and may have a solid, trabecular, or sinusoidal architecture (*see* Fig. 2A and Color Plate 2). In general, this variant shows strong positive immunostaining for GH (Fig. 2B) and variable positivity for alpha-subunit. Immunostaining for cytokeratins, CAM 5.2, reveals a diffuse cytoplasmic pattern in the tumor cells (Fig. 2C). They have strong nuclear positivity for the transcription factor

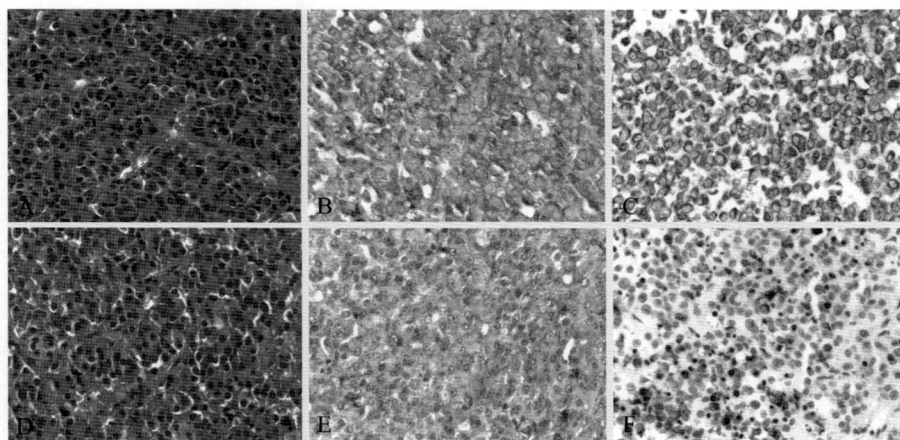

Fig. 2. Densely granulated somatotroph pituitary adenoma with acidophilic and densely granulated cytoplasm (A), strong positive immunoreaction for GH (B) and diffuse immunohistochemical staining pattern for CAM 5.2 (C). Sparsely granulated somatotroph pituitary adenoma with a chromophobic and less granular cytoplasm (D). The same tumor as in (D) with slightly positive reaction for GH (E) and the dot-like positive reaction with CAM 5.2 corresponding to fibrous bodies (F). (*See* Color Plate 2.)

Pit-1 *(6)*, a common transcription factor for GH, as well as PRL and thyroid stimulating hormone (TSH)-producing adenomas. Ultrastructural study reveals a well-developed Golgi apparatus and RER and many granules 300 to 400 nm in diameter similar to normal somatotrophs. The sparsely granulated variant is less acidophilic or even chromophobic and sometimes has a marked pleomorphism, making it difficult to differentiate from metastatic carcinoma (Fig. 2D). The immunohistochemical expression of GH in this variant is weak and focal (Fig. 2E), with variable expression of alpha-subunit and Pit-1. This type has a strong dot-like pattern of positivity with low molecular weight cytokeratins (CAM 5.2), reflecting intracytoplasmic fibrous bodies (Fig. 2F). Ultrastructural studies show a few small secretory granules (100–250 nm) and whorls of intermediate filaments corresponding to the fibrous bodies in the cytoplasm. The incidence of mammosomatotroph adenomas has increased in the last 10 years probably due to improvements in immunocytochemistry. Some normal pituitary cells also produce both hormones. These tumors can also express alpha-subunit and Pit-1 and more rarely express TSH. The cells that produce GH, PRL, and TSH have a similar origin, which may explain why there is coexpression of these hormones. According to the WHO classification, these tumors should not be included, therefore, in the plurihormonal pituitary adenomas. Another variant of GH-producing tumors is the acidophil stem cell adenoma. This type of adenoma is associated with hyperprolactinemia and minor symptoms of acromegaly. The tumor cells have slightly acidophilic cytoplasm sometimes with clear vacuoles that correspond to giant mitochondria. The architecture is diffuse or in solid sheets. Immunohistochemistry is positive for PRL and faintly positive for GH. The definition is based on ultrastructural characteristics that show a mix between sparsely granulated GH-producing cells and PRL-producing cells. Some interesting characteristics include the presence of numerous mitochondria, including giant ones that are the hallmark of this tumor. CAM 5.2 is useful for demonstrating fibrous bodies.

2.3. TSH-Producing Adenomas

These tumors are rare and account for about 1% of pituitary adenomas *(7)*. They can present with hyperthyroidism, but the majority are clinically nonfunctioning *(8)*. A few cases are associated with primary hypothyroidism, which might be the stimulating factor in adenoma development *(7)*. Some TSH-producing tumors may also demonstrate immunohistochemical positivity for GH or PRL.

These tumors in general are macroadenomas and are found to be invasive at the time of surgery. Their color and consistency are generally similar to other pituitary adenomas, but occasionally they can be very firm. Microscopically, the tumors can have either a sinusoidal or a solid pattern. The cells are chromophobic and can have small cytoplasmic granules with PAS stain. Characteristically, the cells have a polygonal or elongated shape. The cell shape is more evident with TSH immunostaining, because the cell boundaries are often indistinct with hematoxylin and eosin staining. Some cases have small psammomatous calcifications and fibrosis. Immunohistochemistry shows positivity for TSH and variable staining for alpha-subunit; some also express GH and PRL. Ultrastructural study reveals characteristics of thyrotrophs including long cellular prolongations, abundant RER with electron-lucent material. The cells also have a prominent Golgi apparatus, lysosomes, and small granules in the range of 150 to 250 nm adjacent to the plasmalemma.

2.4. ACTH-Producing Adenomas

The ACTH-producing adenomas comprise tumors that are derived from corticotrophs, the cells that produce propriomelanocortin, from which ACTH and beta-endorphin are cleaved, together with several other peptides. These tumors comprise about 15% of the clinical cases of pituitary tumors. Corticotroph hyperplasia may be another cause of Cushing's disease, but the biopsy diagnosis is difficult to make due to the small size of the surgical specimen. Some clinically nonfunctioning macroadenomas express ACTH, and may have varying degrees of invasion. The clinically nonfunctioning cases correspond to the silent adenomas type 1 and type 2 (Table 1) (3). The majority of ACTH adenomas are very small microadenomas, softer and paler than the normal gland. Microscopically, the typical tumor has a densely granulated basophilic cytoplasm apparent with the classical hematoxylin and eosin stain (see Fig. 3A and Color Plate 3). The cytoplasm also is strongly PAS (periodic acid Schiff stain)-positive. The less common macroadenomas are more chromophobic and less PAS-positive. The most important pathologic consideration

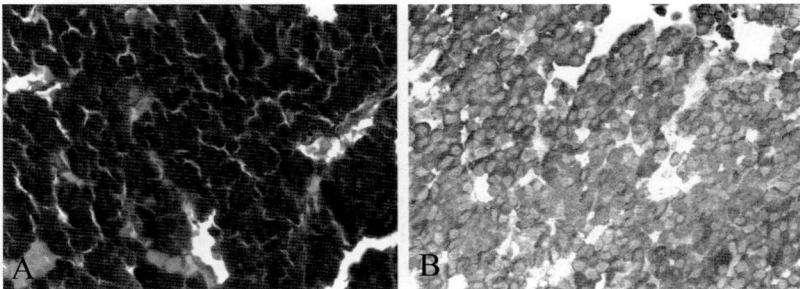

Fig. 3. ACTH-producing pituitary tumor composed of densely granular basophilic cells (A) with strong positive immunohistochemical reaction for ACTH (B). (*See* Color Plate 3.)

in distinguishing the tumor from the normal gland is the overall architecture. These adenomas may not have well-defined margins and tumor cells can be intermixed with the normal gland. The tumor cells are round and arranged in a sinusoidal pattern. The nucleus is centrally placed with a conspicuous nucleolus. Immunohistochemistry shows variable degrees of positive staining for ACTH and also beta-endorphin (Fig. 3B). Ultrastructural study reveals granules between 150 and 450 nm in diameter that sometimes have an irregular shape. The cells contain a well-developed RER and Golgi apparatus as well as bundles of intermediate filaments.

The normal corticotroph cells respond to high levels of cortisol by developing Crooke's hyalinization corresponding to intracytoplasmic accumulation of low molecular weight cytokeratins. Occasionally, the adenoma cells may have the same change and are then designated Crooke's cell adenomas *(3)*.

2.5. Gonadotropin-Producing Adenomas

These comprise the majority of clinically nonfunctioning adenomas, about 80% of pituitary adenomas in our surgical series. Clinical manifestations of gonadotropin excess are not evident and some patients have evidence of gonadal dysfunction, presumably from mass effect. Usually these tumors are macroadenomas with a rich vascular network, frequent necrosis, and hemorrhagic areas. Microscopically, they can have different patterns, but the sinusoidal and papillary pattern is the most common often with perivascular pseudorosettes (*see* Fig. 4A and B and Color Plate 4). The cells are chromophobic with focal oncocytic transformation in some cases. The cells are tall and sometimes elongated, giving an ependymoma-like appearance. The immunohistochemistry is unpredictable with variable degrees of positive reaction for FSH (Fig. 4C), LH, or alpha-subunit. The ultrastructural characteristics include few secretory granules, a poorly developed Golgi apparatus, and RER. Secretory granules are small, about 250 nm. Cell processes are also faint. Some cells are oncocytic and about 50% of their cytoplasm is occupied by mitochondria (Fig. 4D).

2.6. Null Cell Adenomas

Under this denomination are the adenomas without any clinical or immunohistochemical evidence of hormonal production. It is difficult to determine the real incidence because the sensitivity of immunohistochemistry continues to improve. They tend to occur in elderly patients, in the sixth decade of life or older. Usually they are macroadenomas and frequently have suprasellar or lateral extension and invasion.

Microscopically, the tumors are chromophobic. Immunohistochemistry can show scattered beta-FSH-positive or alpha-subunit-positive cells. Electron microscopy reveals poorly differentiated cells with scattered small electron

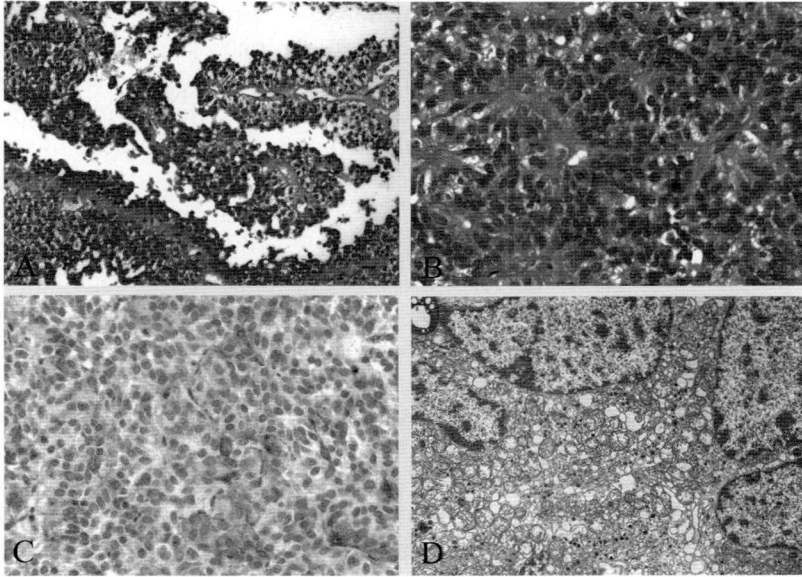

Fig. 4. Gonadotropic pituitary adenoma with a papillary pattern (A); perivascular pseudorosettes (B); and focal and weak expression of beta-FSH (C). Ultrastructural appearance of a tumor cell with oncocytic changes, i.e., many mitochondria (D). (*See* Color Plate 4.)

dense granules, mostly close to the plasmalemma. The latest WHO classification includes the oncocytoma as a null cell adenoma variant. Oncocytomas have hypereosinophilic cytoplasm and a high number of mitochondria using electron microscopy.

2.7. Plurihormonal Adenomas

The 2004 WHO classification includes in this category only tumors with coexpression of pituitary hormones that cannot be explained by a common cellular origin, which excludes tumors with any combination of GH, PRL and TSH, or FSH and LH. By this definition these tumors are rare.

2.8. Pituitary Carcinomas

Primary carcinomas are very rare. There are about 100 published cases, which represents approximately 0.2% of operated pituitary neoplasms (9). The definition of pituitary carcinoma is based on the presence of metastases in other organs including brain or evidence of cerebrospinal fluid dissemination. The majority are clinically functioning tumors, with those producing PRL and ACTH most common. These tumors are often invasive and sometimes discontinuous growth in adjacent meninges or brain invasion is present. Microscopically, the tumors have different degrees of high cell density, pleomorphism, necrosis, and invasion, but all of these characteristics can also be found in benign pituitary adenomas. Proliferation markers and mitotic index are high in these cases, but are not always useful diagnostic criteria because of overlap in the results with those of invasive adenomas.

2.9. Morphologic Prognostic Factors in Pituitary Adenomas

No single histological characteristic appears to be associated with more aggressive clinical behavior. Some immunohistochemical markers may be independent risk factors for progression or invasion. It has been shown that a Ki-67 labeling index greater than 3% and extensive p53 positivity correlate with progression as well as with invasion *(2)*. Other studies have produced somewhat different results, suggesting that the Ki-67 labeling index threshold should be lower, probably around 2% *(10,11)*. Another marker that has shown similar results to Ki-67 is PCNA *(12)*. Some histological types, such as the sparsely granulated somatotroph adenoma, have been associated with a worse outcome. These tumors tend to be larger and more aggressive, with a lower surgical cure rate *(13)*.

2.10. Morphological and Diagnostically Useful Characteristics of Pituitary Adenomas

The complete pathological classification and subclassification, using electron microscopy, is often difficult due to small sample sizes. Table 3 shows some of the more relevant morphological characteristics in each category using light microscopy alone.

3. PATHOLOGY OF OTHER SELLAR LESIONS

The sellar and parasellar region can be the site of other neoplastic and nonneoplastic mass lesions that should be considered in the differential diagnosis of pituitary adenomas (Table 4).

3.1. Tumors

3.1.1. CRANIOPHARYNGIOMA

These tumors are solid or partially cystic masses derived from Rathke's pouch. Craniopharyngiomas account for 1.2–4.6% of all intracranial tumors *(14)*. These tumors have a bimodal age distribution with peaks in children between 5 and 14 years and adults over 50 years old *(15)*. The clinical features include visual disturbances and endocrine deficiencies, the latter more frequently in children. Cognitive deterioration and personality changes have

Table 3
Morphological Characteristics Using Light Microscopy

Type	Cytoplasm	Architecture	Additional Characteristics	Immunohistochemistry
Growth hormone-producing adenoma— densely granulated	Acidophilic and granular	Diffuse		GH alpha-subunit; diffuse pattern with CAM 5.2
Growth hormone-producing adenoma—sparsely granulated	Chromophobic and hypogranular	Diffuse	Variable pleomorphism	GH, fibrous bodies with CAM 5.2
Mammosomatotroph adenoma	Chromophobic or acidophilic	Variable		GH and PRL in the same cells
Acidophil stem cell adenomas	Slightly acidophilic cytoplasm	Diffuse	Sometimes clear vacuoles (giant mitochondria)	PRL and faint reaction for GH
PRL-producing adenoma—sparsely granulated	Chromophobic cytoplasm	Wide variation	Psammomatous calcifications	PRL (paranuclear pattern), alpha-subunit rarely found
PRL-producing adenoma— highly granulated	Acidophil and granular	Wide variation		PRL (diffuse)

(Continued)

Table 3
(Continued)

Type	Cytoplasm	Architecture	Additional Characteristics	Immunohistochemistry
TSH-producing adenoma	Chromophobic	Variable		TSH and alpha-subunit
Gonadotroph adenoma	Chromophobic focal oncocytic changes	Sinusoidal with perivascular pseudorosettes papillary pattern		Variable positivity for FSH, LH, and alpha-subunit
ACTH producing tumors	Basophilic or amphophilic macroadenomas. may be chromophobic.	Sinusoidal	Crooke's hyalinization in adjacent pituitary tissue	ACTH
Null Cell Adenoma	Chromophobic	solid sheets. sometimes perivascular pseudorosettes		negative

Table 4
Other Lesions in the Sellar Location

Tumors
   Craniopharyngioma
   Meningiomas
   Neurohypophyseal gangliocytoma
   Neurohypophyseal glioma
   Granular cell tumors
   Germ cell tumors
   Chordomas and other soft tissue and bone tumors
   Metastatic tumors
Cysts and malformations
   Rathke's cleft cyst
   Arachnoid cyst
   Epidermoid cyst
   Dermoid cyst
Empty sella syndrome
Vascular lesions
   Saccular aneurysm
   Cavernous malformation
Inflammatory conditions
   Lymphocytic hypophysitis
   Granulomatous hypophysitis

been found in half of the patients. Some patients present with symptoms of intracranial hypertension and diabetes insipidus. Craniopharyngiomas can be either retro or prechiasmatic and occasionally wholly intrasellar. Macroscopically, the tumor has well-defined borders but is often adherent to adjacent structures. The cut surface is heterogeneous with fibrotic and calcified areas. The cystic areas are filled with a liquid with a "machine oil" appearance, which produces a severe irritative meningitis when spilled into the subarachnoidal space. Microscopically, there are two types of craniopharyngioma. The adamantinomatous type, the most common variant in children, is composed of nests and cords of squamoid epithelium with a peripheral palisade of columnar cells (*see* Fig. 5A and Color Plate 5). This pattern is similar to odontogenic tumors such as ameloblastoma or adamantinoma. The epithelium produces keratin often referred to as wet keratin (Fig. 5B), which can calcify. Frequently, necrotic debris, cholesterol clefts, and ossification of wet keratin are also present. When this cyst material contacts connective or pituitary tissue, it generates an inflammatory reaction rich in foamy macrophages, foreign body giant cells, and cholesterol crystals (Fig. 5D). The second type is the papillary

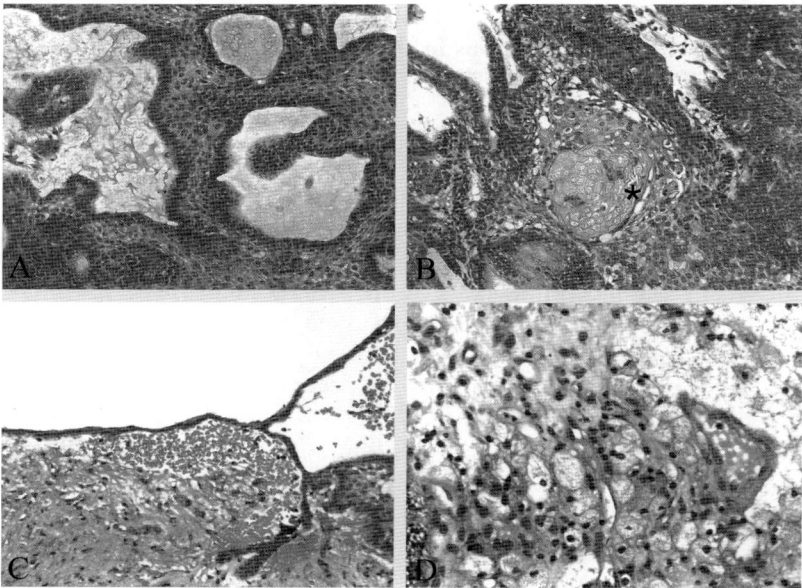

Fig. 5. Craniopharyngioma composed of cords and islands of squamoid epithelium limited by columnar cells (A). Some cavities contain keratin material (*) (B). A cystic area has a thin epithelial wall(C) and adjacent inflammatory reaction with many foamy macrophages (D) (hematoxylin and eosin stain). (*See* Color Plate 5.)

craniopharyngioma, a variant almost exclusively seen in adult patients. When a craniopharyngioma grows into brain the surrounding compressed tissue is gliotic with abundant Rosenthal fibers and eosinophilic granular bodies. These tumors have no obvious histological characteristics that predict progression.

3.1.2. GERM CELL TUMORS

These tumors arise in the midline and are more common before the third decade of life and in male more frequently than female patients. They comprise about 1% of intracranial tumors in adults and 6% in children. The sella is the second most common location after the pineal gland. Morphologically, these tumors are similar to their gonadal counterparts (*see* Fig. 6 and Color Plate 6). Germinomas are equivalent to seminomas and are the most common germ cell tumors, followed by teratomas. The other categories include embryonal carcinomas, yolk sac tumors, and choriocarcinomas. The last three types are generally mixed with germinomatous or teratomatous elements and may not be initially recognized in a small biopsy. The tumor cells express placental alkaline phosphatase and CD30 by immunohistochemistry *(16)*. Other useful markers in the differential diagnosis are alpha-fetoprotein,

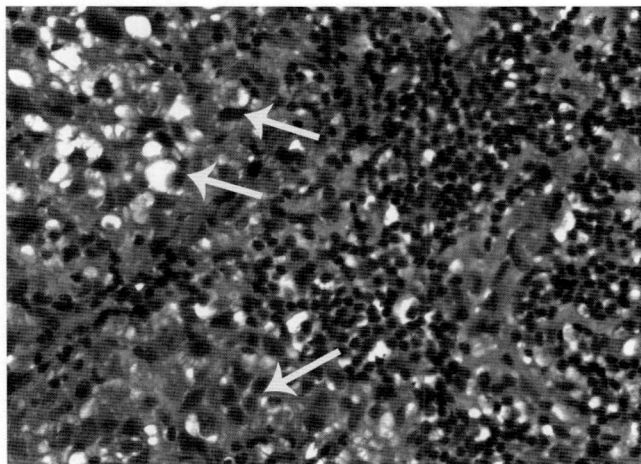

Fig. 6. Germinoma with a dense lymphocytic population and scattered groups of bigger round tumor cells with clear cytoplasm (arrows) (hematoxylin and eosin stain). (*See* Color Plate 6.)

carcinoembryonic antigen, and cytokeratins, which are positive in the majority of nongerminomatous tumors. Immunohistochemistry for chorionic gonadotropin is positive in choriocarcinomas, but can also be positive in isolated syncytiotrophoblast cells in germinomas or other germ cell tumors. The histological type determines the prognosis and therapy. Germinomas are radiosensitive with a long-term remission in approximately 70% of cases.

3.1.3. PRIMARY TUMORS OF THE HYPOTHALAMUS AND NEUROHYPOPHYSIS

These tumors are rare but can mimic a pituitary adenoma with the clinical presentation of hypopituitarism or chiasm compression. Diabetes insipidus, when present, should suggest that the lesion is not a pituitary adenoma. In this category the main types of tumors are granular cell tumors, neurohypophyseal astrocytoma, and ganglion cell lesions.

Granular Cell Tumors. These present at a mean age of about 50 years, typically with symptoms of pituitary hypofunction, visual disturbances, and headache *(2,17)*. Macroscopically, they are well-defined gray or tan suprasellar and intrasellar masses. Microscopically, the cells are polygonal having round nuclei with prominent nucleoli, abundant eosinophilic granular cytoplasm, and variable degrees of pleomorphism (*see* Fig. 7 and Color Plate 7). Mitoses are not usually found. Perivascular lymphocytes are common. This tumor has an uncertain histogenesis but is believed to originate from the normal glial cells of the posterior gland (pituicytes) as it has a different immunoprofile

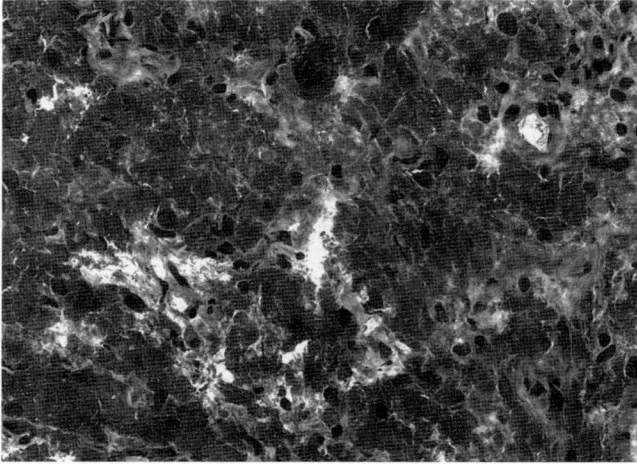

Fig. 7. Granular cell tumor composed of closely apposed acidophilic cells with bland nuclei and granular cytoplasm (hematoxylin and eosin stain). (*See* Color Plate 7.)

in comparison to granular tumors in other locations. Granular cell tumors in other locations are S-100-positive and are thought to arise from Schwann cells. Sellar granular cell tumors are glial fibrillary acid protein (GFAP)-positive in some cases, supporting their origin from pituicytes. In other reports the tumors have been GFAP-negative; thus the controversy about the cell of origin remains. Tumor cells are also positive for CD68, alpha-1-antitrypsin, and alpha-1-antichemotrypsin. One case of atypical granular cell tumor with marked pleomorphism and increased mitotic activity has been reported *(18)*.

Sellar Gliomas. Gliomas in the sellar location are very rare but the complete spectrum, from typical pilocytic astrocytomas, probably arising from the third ventricle or optic chiasm, to ependymomas or glioblastomas, has been reported. Aggressive sellar gliomas have been associated with prior radiation for a pituitary adenoma *(19)*.

Gangliocytoma/Hypothalamic Hamartoma. There is controversy about the real nature of this category variously classified as ganglioglioma, gangliocytoma, hypothalamic hamartoma, choristoma. The WHO classification includes this lesion as a benign tumor, the gangliocytoma. Characteristics favoring a hamartomatous condition include their occurrence in children and pathological findings not present in other classical glioneuronal tumors. These include the similarity of the ganglionic component to the normal hypothalamic cells, including the presence of hypothalamic hormones. Some cases have been associated with other malformations. A high proportion of sellar gangliocytomas is associated with pituitary adenoma. Morphologically, gangliocytoma/hypothalamic hamartomas are well-delineated lesions consisting of ganglion cells with dysplastic features such as multinucleation and large size. Sometimes the ganglionic cells are in a neuropil but in other cases they are intermixed with pituitary cell or pituitary adenoma cells (20,21). There is some evidence that neuronal differentiation in pituitary adenomas is a possible explanation for the combined tumors (22). Tumor cells express neuronal markers such as synaptophysin, chromogranin, and neurofilament. Tumor cells can also be positive for hypothalamic hormones including GnRH, GHRH, TRH, and CRH. The coexistence of a pituitary adenoma, most frequently GH producing, may be due to the secretion of hypothalamic factors by the tumor. Prolactinomas and corticotrophin-producing tumors have also been reported (23,24).

Spindle Cell Oncocytoma. This apparently benign tumor of the anterior pituitary has been described recently. The reported patients have been aged 26 and 76 years, with tumor sizes between 1.5 and 6.5 cm. The clinical symptoms included hypopituitarism and chiasm compression. The tumor is composed of spindle-shaped cells with a fascicular arrangement having abundant granular, eosinophilic cytoplasm with immunocytochemical expression of S-100, epithelial membrane antigen, and vimentin. In the majority of cases, immunohistochemistry for the pituitary hormones, chromogranin, CD68, and CD34 has been negative (25–28).

3.1.4. MESENCHYMAL TUMORS

Meningiomas. Meningiomas originate in the parasellar leptomeninges and make up 15% of intracranial meningiomas. There are no differences between meningiomas in this location and other intracranial locations. Morphologically, they are usually well circumscribed and have a granular to fibrous cut surface. The three main histological variants are meningothelial, fibroblastic, and transitional. The WHO classification includes three grades: grade I or benign meningioma, grade II or atypical meningioma, and grade III or malignant meningioma. Atypical meningiomas are associated with a high rate of recurrence. The grade III or malignant meningioma is defined by a high mitotic index (over 20 mitotic figures in 10 high-power fields) and behaves like a sarcoma with a high recurrence rate and short survival, commonly less than 2 years.

Chordomas. Chordomas are locally aggressive, slowly growing malignant tumors. They originate from notochordal elements found in the sella. They are more common in adults after the fourth decade, but can occur in children. Pure intrasellar tumors are very rare. More commonly, they are parasellar or suprasellar.

Other Rare Mesenchymal Tumors. Sarcomas in patients without a previous history of radiation are very rare (29). Various types of sellar sarcomas have been reported *(29–31)*. Chondrosarcomas are important in the differential diagnosis of chordomas.

3.1.5. METASTATIC TUMORS

Metastatic tumors to the sella are rare, but in autopsy series range from 0.14% to 28.1% of all brain metastases *(32)*. Compromise of the posterior lobe is the most common presentation. In women they arise from carcinomas of the lung, breast, and gastrointestinal tract, while in men the most common origins are lung and prostate.

3.2. Cystic Lesions with Sellar Location

3.2.1. RATHKE'S CLEFT CYSTS

Normally small Rathke's cleft remnant cysts exist in the pars intermedia, some of which may be visible to the naked eye at autopsy. The cysts can become large enough to produce symptoms of chiasm compression and hypopituitarism. Cases associated with pituitary adenomas have been reported *(33)*. Macroscopically, the unilocular cysts are between the anterior and posterior pituitary lobes and have a watery to proteinaceous content that is sometimes brown due to secondary hemorrhage. Microscopically, the cyst wall is composed of cuboidal and ciliated cells, with occasional goblet cells and metaplastic squamous epithelium. The cyst wall may be surrounded by variable degrees of fibrosis and inflammation (Fig. 8).

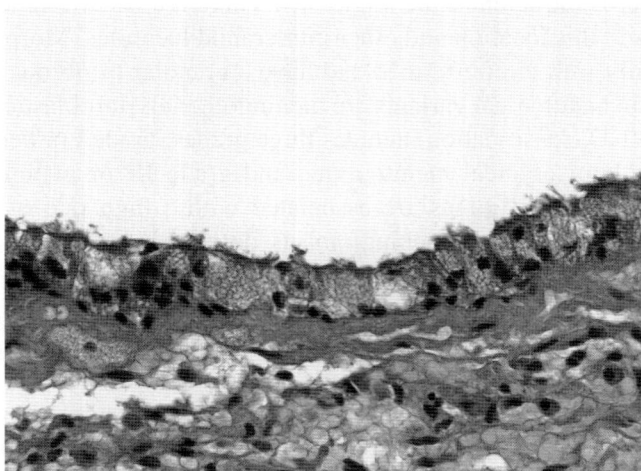

Fig. 8. Colloid and mucinous content with a piece of columnar epithelium with some goblet cells (hematoxylin and eosin stain).

3.2.2. Epidermoid and Dermoid Cysts

Epidermoid and dermoid cysts are developmental lesions and not true tumors; they originate from misplaced squamous or dermoid tissue. Rare cases are thought to be due to secondary trauma. Purely intrasellar epidermoid cysts are uncommon. Intracranially, this lesion tends to surround rather than displace adjacent structures. Symptoms can occur if the cyst enlarges to compress adjacent structures.

3.2.3. Arachnoidal Cysts

Arachnoidal cysts are congenital or acquired lesions that can be above or inside the sella. If they reach a large size they can be symptomatic. The content is similar to CSF. Microscopically, the wall is composed of a flattened connective tissue with a monolayer of arachnoidal cells.

3.2.4. The Empty Sella Syndrome

The Empty Sella Syndrome may potentially arise in two situations. The first is a developmental disorder consistent with incomplete development of the diaphragma sellae with secondary invagination of arachnoid and compression of the pituitary. The second condition is secondary to pituitary surgery, irradiation or infarction of pituitary.

3.3. Vascular Lesions

Pituitary infarction is ischemic necrosis of pituitary gland secondary to shock, head trauma, and hemorrhage. The clinical manifestation is hypopituitarism. Pituitary apoplexy is a medical emergency presenting with headache and sometimes visual loss and is secondary to hemorrhage or infarction of a pituitary macroadenoma. It is described in detail in Chapter 19. Sheehan's syndrome with hypopituitarism is due to necrosis of the pituitary associated with postpartum hemorrhage.

3.4. Inflammatory Conditions

3.4.1. Lymphocytic Hypophysitis

This condition is a rare inflammatory disease that can be confused with a tumor because it is characterized by an increase in the gland size, sometimes extending outside the sella, and may be associated with hyperprolactinemia. Most cases occur in women, either during pregnancy or postpartum. Many patients also have a concomitant autoimmune disorder such as thyroiditis, adrenalitis, or atrophic gastritis (34). The hyperprolactinemia may be secondary to pregnancy, stalk compression, or stimulation by autoantibodies such as in Grave's disease. Morphologically, the gland can be edematous and enlarged but

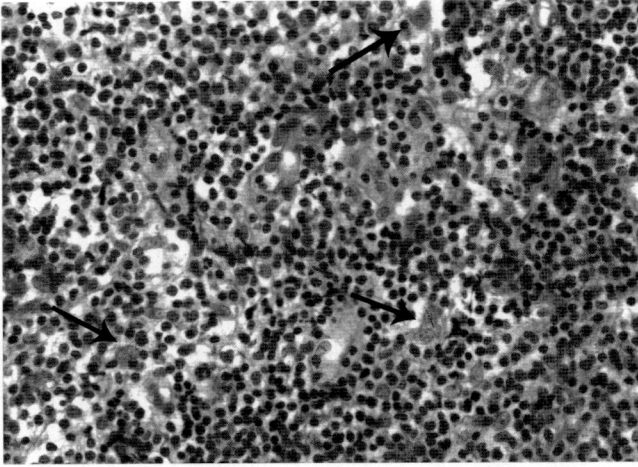

Fig. 9. Lymphocytic hypophysitis with a dense inflammatory infiltrate including lympho-cytes and plasma cells. Scattered pituitary cells are seen between the inflammatory cells (arrows) (hematoxylin and eosin stain). (*See* Color Plate 8.)

in more advanced stages it becomes atrophic and fibrotic. A diffuse lympho-cytic and plasmacytic infiltrate is associated with islands of atrophic pituitary tissue (*see* Fig. 9 and Color Plate 8). Focal oncocytic change is sometimes present. In later stages it may be necessary to use immunohistochemistry with cytokeratins to find the pituitary cells.

3.4.2. GRANULOMATOUS HYPOPHYSITIS

Granulomatous hypophysitis can be idiopathic, similar to lymphocytic hypophysitis, but without differences in gender distribution. The clinical presentation includes variable degrees of hypopituitarism, diabetes insipidus, headache, or hyperprolactinemia. Granulomatous inflammation in the pituitary gland can be due to infections such as tuberculosis, fungal infections, and syphilis, or to sarcoidosis. Sarcoidosis is a systemic disease that includes compromise of the central nervous system structures in a small proportion of cases, with special predilection for the basal cerebral structures affecting meninges, cranial nerves, and pituitary.

REFERENCES

1. Ezzat S, Asa SL, Couldwell WT, et al. The prevalence of pituitary adenomas: a systematic review. Cancer 2004;101:613–9.
2. DeLellis. Pathology and Genetics of Tumours of Endocrine Organs, WHO Classification of Tumours. Lyon: IARC Press; 2004.

3. Kovacs K, Horvath E. Tumors of Pituitary Gland. Washington DC: Armed Force Institute of Pathology; 1986.
4. Ciccarelli A, Daly AF, Beckers A. The epidemiology of prolactinomas. Pituitary 2005;8: 3–6.
5. Holdaway IM, Rajasoorya C. Epidemiology of acromegaly. Pituitary 1999;2:29–41.
6. Pellegrini I, Barlier A, Gunz G, et al. Pit-1 gene expression in the human pituitary and pituitary adenomas. J Clin Endocrinol Metab 1994;79:189–96.
7. Bertholon-Gregoire M, Trouillas J, Guigard MP, Loras B, Tourniaire J. Mono- and pluri-hormonal thyrotropic pituitary adenomas: pathological, hormonal and clinical studies in 12 patients. Eur J Endocrinol 1999;140:519–27.
8. Smallridge RC. Thyrotropin-secreting pituitary tumors. Endocrinol Metab Clin North Am 1987;16:765–92.
9. Pernicone PJ, Scheithauer BW, Sebo TJ, et al. Pituitary carcinoma: a clinicopathologic study of 15 cases. Cancer 1997;79:804–12.
10. Schreiber S, Saeger W, Ludecke DK. Proliferation markers in different types of clinically non-secreting pituitary adenomas. Pituitary 1999;1:213–20.
11. Gejman R, Swearingen B, Hedley-Whyte ET. Role of Ki67 proliferation index and p53 expression in predicting progression of pituitary adenomas Brain Pathol 2006;16(s1):S110.
12. Hsu DW, Hakim F, Biller BM, et al. Significance of proliferating cell nuclear antigen index in predicting pituitary adenoma recurrence. J Neurosurg 1993;78:753–61.
13. Yamada S, Aiba T, Sano T, et al. Growth hormone-producing pituitary adenomas: corre-lations between clinical characteristics and morphology. Neurosurgery 1993;33:20–7.
14. Prabhu VC, Brown HG. The pathogenesis of craniopharyngiomas. Childs Nerv Syst 2005;21:622–7.
15. Bunin GR, Surawicz TS, Witman PA, Preston-Martin S, Davis F, Bruner JM. The descriptive epidemiology of craniopharyngioma. J Neurosurg 1998;89:547–51.
16. Cossu-Rocca P, Jones TD, Roth LM, et al. Cytokeratin and CD30 expression in dysger-minoma. Hum Pathol 2006;37:1015–21.
17. Schaller B, Kirsch E, Tolnay M, Mindermann T. Symptomatic granular cell tumor of the pituitary gland: case report and review of the literature. Neurosurgery 1998;42:166–70.
18. Kasashima S, Oda Y, Nozaki J, Shirasaki M, Nakanishi I. A case of atypical granular cell tumor of the neurohypophysis. Pathol Int 2000;50:568–73.
19. Simmons NE, Laws ER, Jr. Glioma occurrence after sellar irradiation: case report and review. Neurosurgery 1998;42:172–8.
20. Perry DI, McGinn GJ, Del Bigio MR. Mixed gangliocytoma – adenoma of the sella: case report. Can Assoc Radiol J 2002;53:303–6.
21. Castillo M, Mukherji SK. Intrasellar mixed gangliocytoma-adenoma. Am J Roentgenol 1997;169:1199–200.
22. Kontogeorgos G, Mourouti G, Kyrodimou E, Liapi-Avgeri G, Parasi E. Ganglion cell containing pituitary adenomas: signs of neuronal differentiation in adenoma cells. Acta Neuropathol (Berl) 2006;112:21–8.
23. Asa SL, Scheithauer BW, Bilbao JM, et al. A case for hypothalamic acromegaly: a clinicopathological study of six patients with hypothalamic gangliocytomas producing growth hormone-releasing factor. J Clin Endocrinol Metab 1984;58:796–803.
24. Puchner MJ, Ludecke DK, Valdueza JM, et al. Cushing's disease in a child caused by a corticotropin-releasing hormone-secreting intrasellar gangliocytoma associated with an adrenocorticotropic hormone-secreting pituitary adenoma. Neurosurgery 1993;33:920–4.
25. Vajtai I, Sahli R, Kappeler A. Spindle cell oncocytoma of the adenohypophysis: Report of a case with a 16-year follow-up. Pathol Res Pract 2006;202:745–50.

26. Dahiya S, Sarkar C, Hedley-Whyte ET, et al. Spindle cell oncocytoma of the adenohypophysis: report of two cases. Acta Neuropathol (Berl) 2005;110:97–9.
27. Kloub O, Perry A, Tu PH, Lipper M, Lopes MB. Spindle cell oncocytoma of the adenohypophysis: report of two recurrent cases. Am J Surg Pathol 2005;29:247–53.
28. Roncaroli F, Scheithauer BW, Cenacchi G, et al. "Spindle cell oncocytoma" of the adenohypophysis: a tumor of folliculostellate cells? Am J Surg Pathol 2002;26:1048–55.
29. Lopes MB, Lanzino G, Cloft HJ, Winston DC, Vance ML, Laws ER, Jr. Primary fibrosarcoma of the sella unrelated to previous radiation therapy. Mod Pathol 1998;11: 579–84.
30. Arita K, Sugiyama K, Tominaga A, Yamasaki F. Intrasellar rhabdomyosarcoma: case report. Neurosurgery 2001;48:677–80.
31. Inenaga C, Morii K, Tamura T, Tanaka R, Takahashi H. Mesenchymal chondrosarcoma of the sellar region. Acta Neurochir (Wien) 2003;145:593–7.
32. Komninos J, Vlassopoulou V, Protopapa D, et al. Tumors metastatic to the pituitary gland: case report and literature review. J Clin Endocrinol Metab 2004;89:574–80.
33. Sumida M, Migita K, Tominaga A, Iida K, Kurisu K. Concomitant pituitary adenoma and Rathke's cleft cyst. Neuroradiology 2001;43:755–9.
34. Thodou E, Asa SL, Kontogeorgos G, Kovacs K, Horvath E, Ezzat S. Clinical case seminar: lymphocytic hypophysitis: clinicopathological findings. J Clin Endocrinol Metab 1995;80:2302–11.

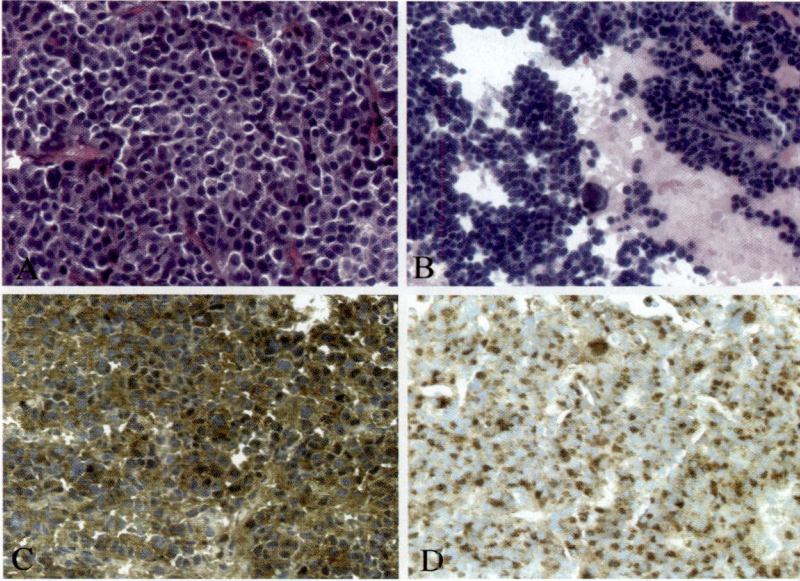

Color Plate 1. Prolactinoma. (Chapter 2, Fig. 1; *see* complete caption and discussion on p. 20).

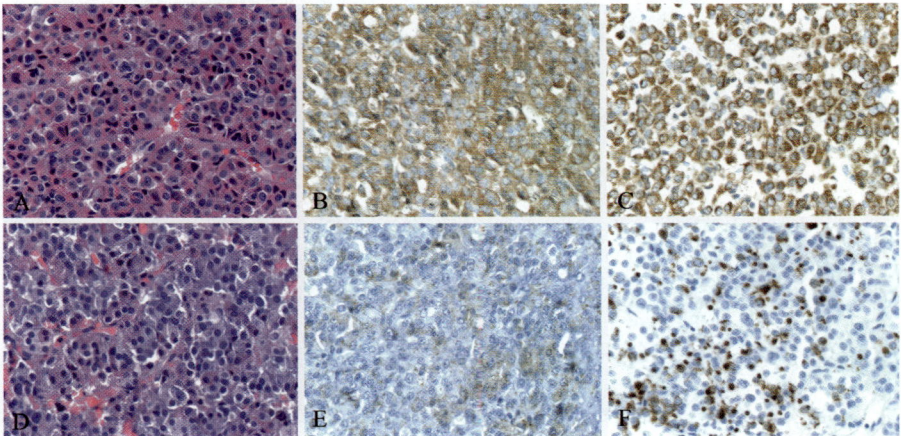

Color Plate 2. Somatotroph pituitary adenoma. (Chapter 2, Fig. 2; *see* complete caption and discussion on p. 21).

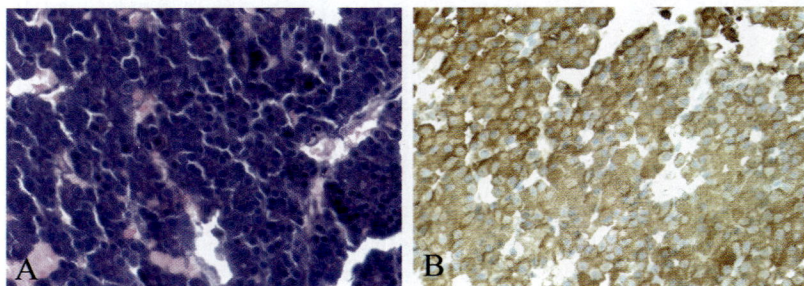

Color Plate 3. ACTH-producing pituitary tumor. (Chapter 2, Fig. 3; *see* complete caption and discussion on p. 23).

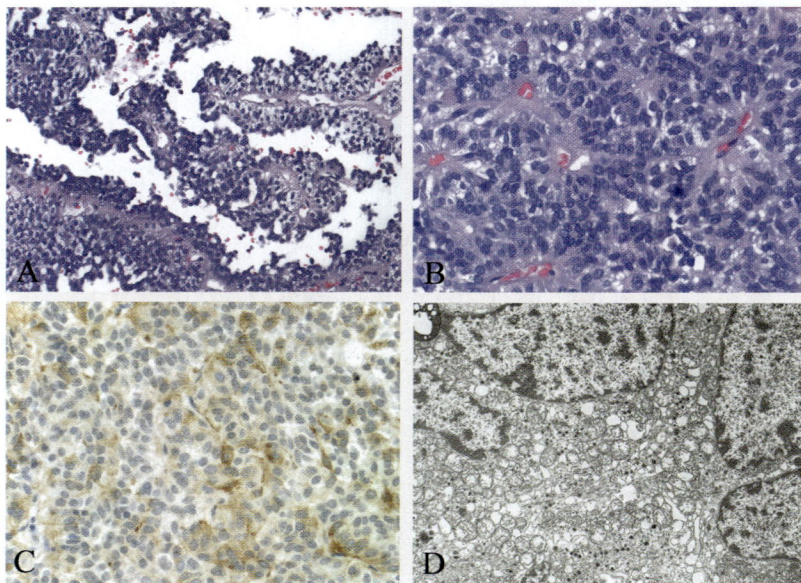

Color Plate 4. Gonadotropic pituitary adenoma. (Chapter 2, Fig. 4; *see* complete caption on p. 25 and discussion on p. 24).

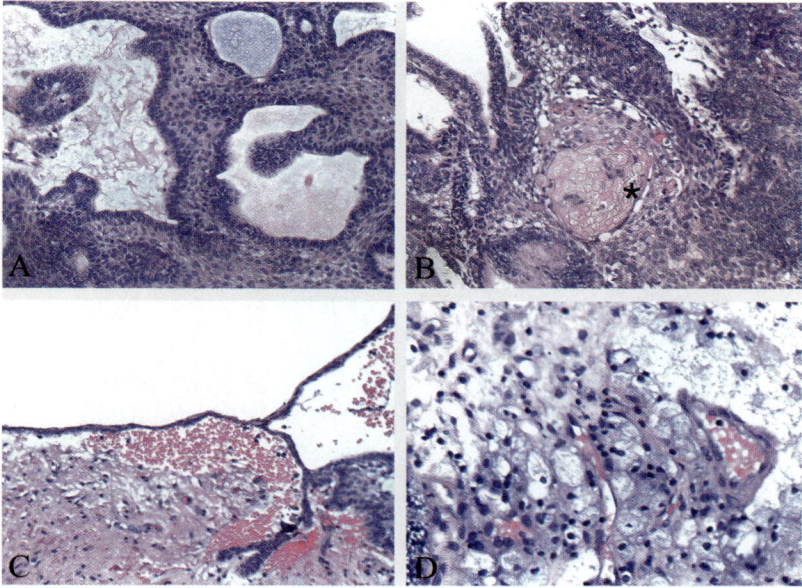

Color Plate 5. Craniopharyngioma. (Chapter 2, Fig. 5; *see* complete caption on p. 30 and discussion on p. 29).

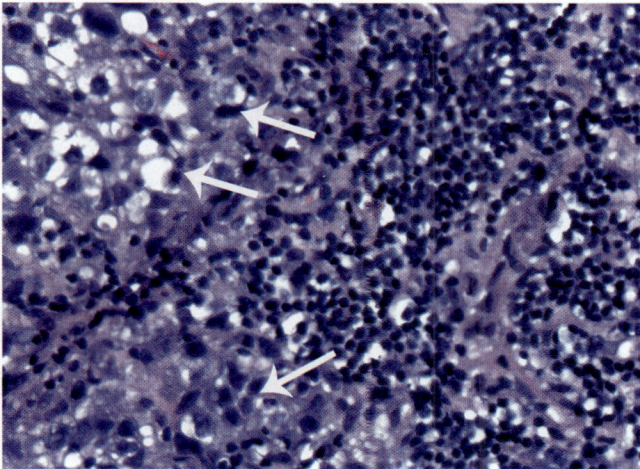

Color Plate 6. Germinoma. (Chapter 2, Fig. 6; *see* complete caption on p. 31 and discussion on p. 30).

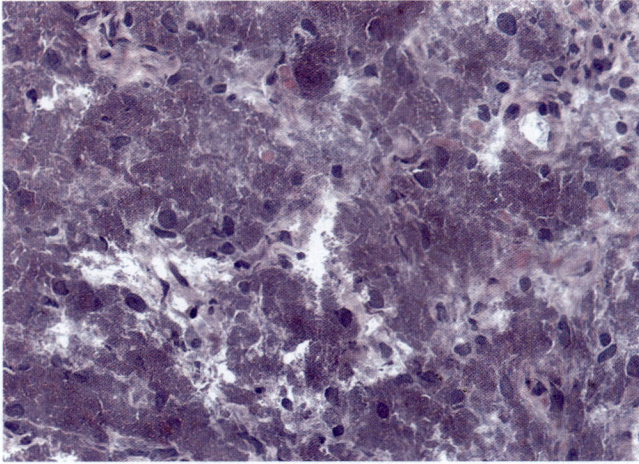

Color Plate 7. Granular cell tumor. (Chapter 2, Fig. 7; *see* complete caption on p. 31 and discussion on p. 32).

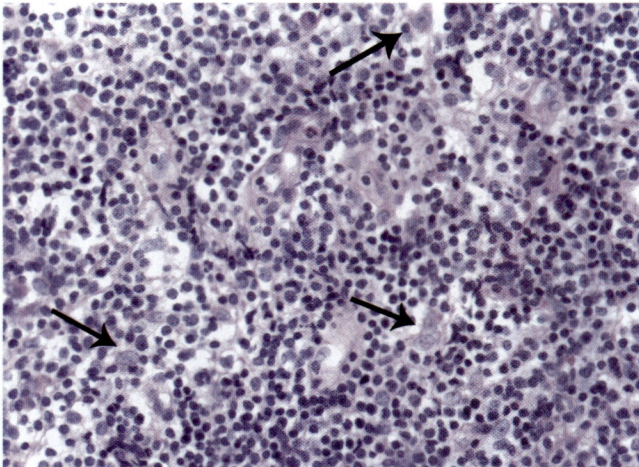

Color Plate 8. Lymphocytic hypophysitis. (Chapter 2, Fig. 9; *see* complete caption and discussion on p. 36).

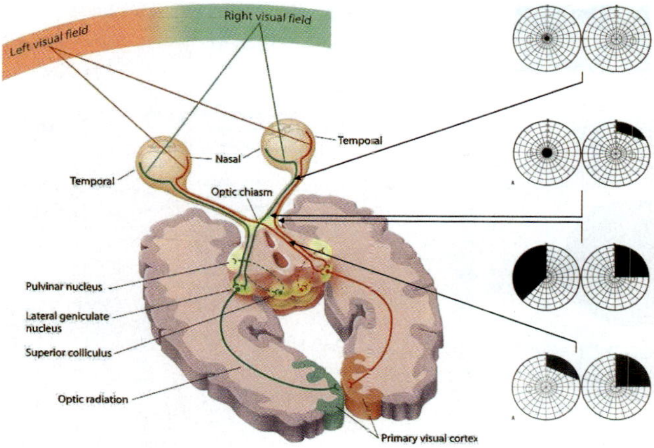

Color Plate 9. Visual pathways. (Chapter 5, Fig. 6; *see* complete caption on p. 99 and discussion on p. 98).

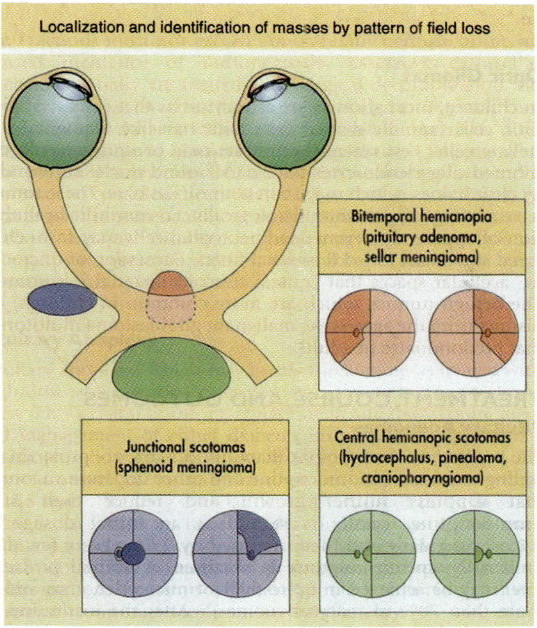

Color Plate 10. Localization and probable identification of masses by pattern of field loss. (Chapter 5, Fig. 7; *see* complete caption on p. 100 and discussion on p. 98).

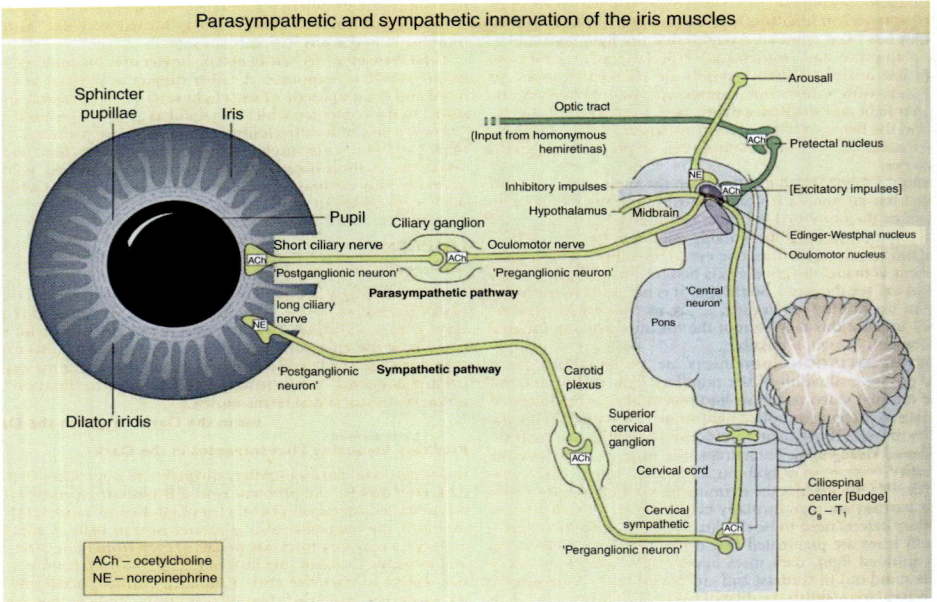

Parasympathetic and sympathetic innervation of the iris muscles

Arousall

Sphincter pupillae

Iris

Optic tract

(Input from homonymous hemiretinas)

Pretectal nucleus

Inhibitory impulses

[Excitatory impulses]

Pupil

Hypothalamus

Midbrain

Edinger-Westphal nucleus

Short ciliary nerve

Ciliary ganglion

Oculomotor nerve

Oculomotor nucleus

'Postganglionic neuron'

'Preganglionic neuron'

Parasympathetic pathway

'Central neuron'

long ciliary nerve

Pons

'Postganglionic neuron'

Sympathetic pathway

Carotid plexus

Dilator iridis

Superior cervical ganglion

Cervical cord

Ciliospinal center [Budge] $C_8 - T_1$

Cervical sympathetic

'Perganglionic neuron'

ACh – ocetylcholine
NE – norepinephrine

Color Plate 11. Parasympathetic and sympathetic innervation of the iris muscles. (Chapter 5, Fig. 9; *see* discussion on p. 104).

(A)

(C)

(B)

(D)

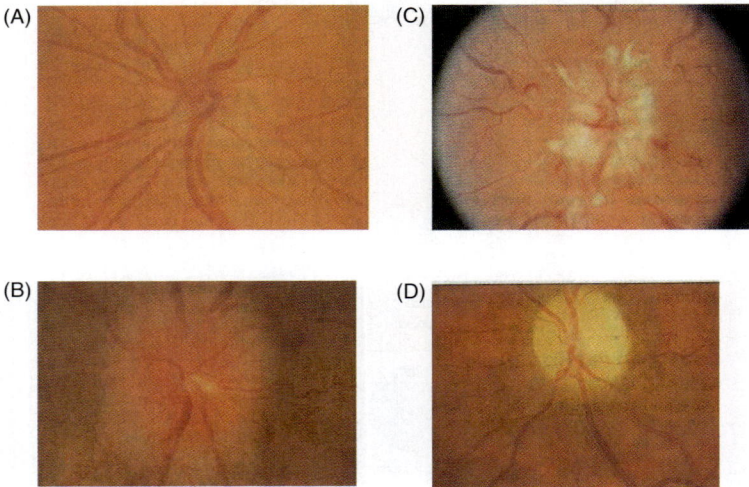

Color Plate 12. Papilledema. (Chapter 5, Fig. 10; *see* complete caption on p. 107 and discussion on p. 106).

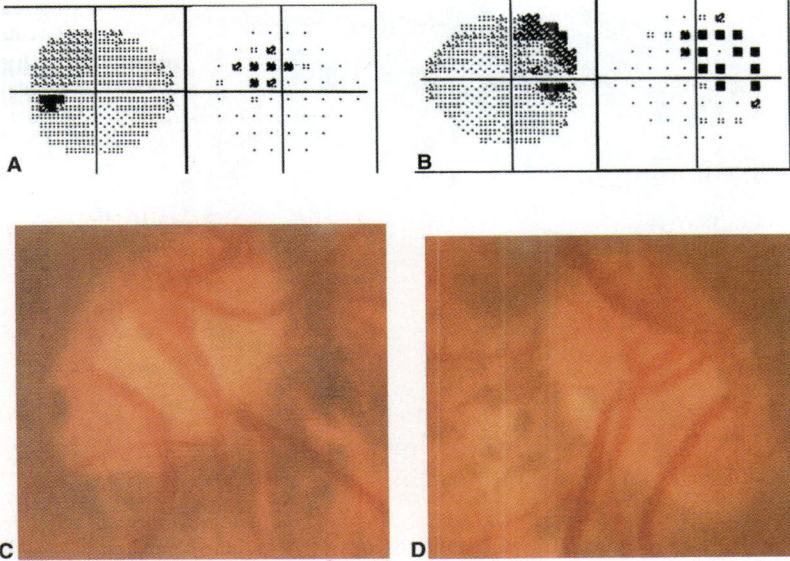

Color Plate 13. Optic disk tilting and the resulting visual field defects. (Chapter 5, Fig. 11; *see* complete caption and discussion on p. 108).

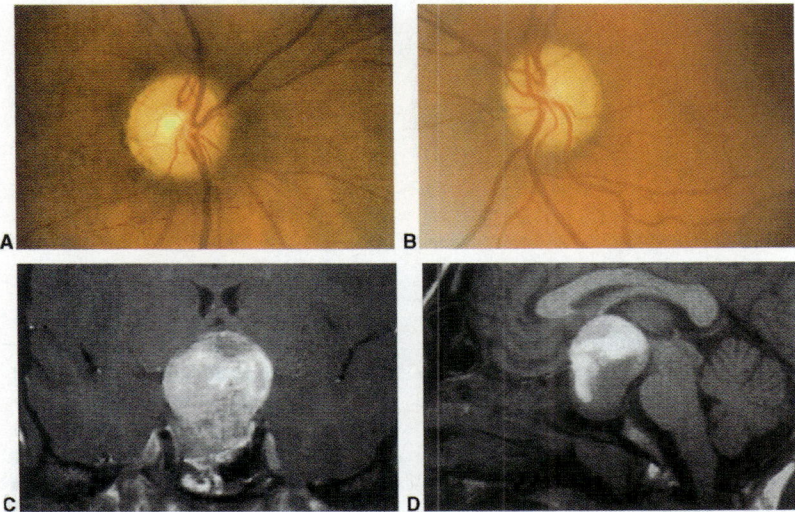

Color Plate 14. Acute compressive optic neuropathy in pituitary apoplexy. (Chapter 5, Fig. 18; *see* complete caption on p. 122 and discussion on p. 121).

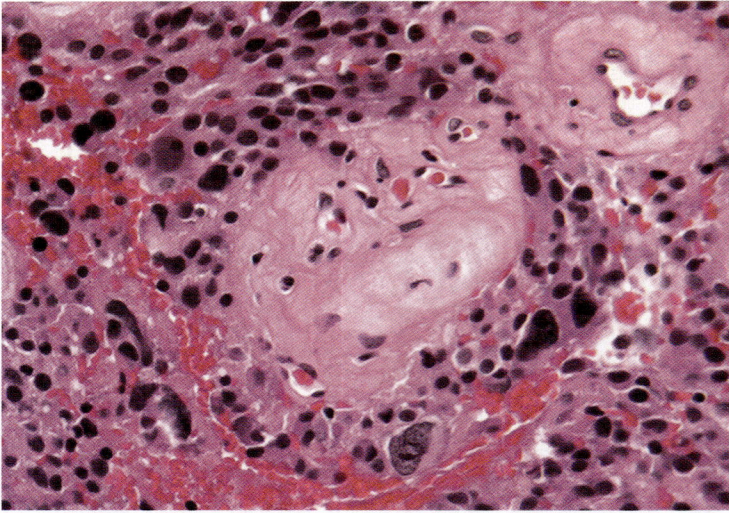

Color Plate 15. TSH-oma cells by light microscopy (40× magnification). H&E stain shows significant cytological and nuclear pleomorphism of tumor cells (Chapter 13, Fig. 1; *see* discussion on page p. 239).

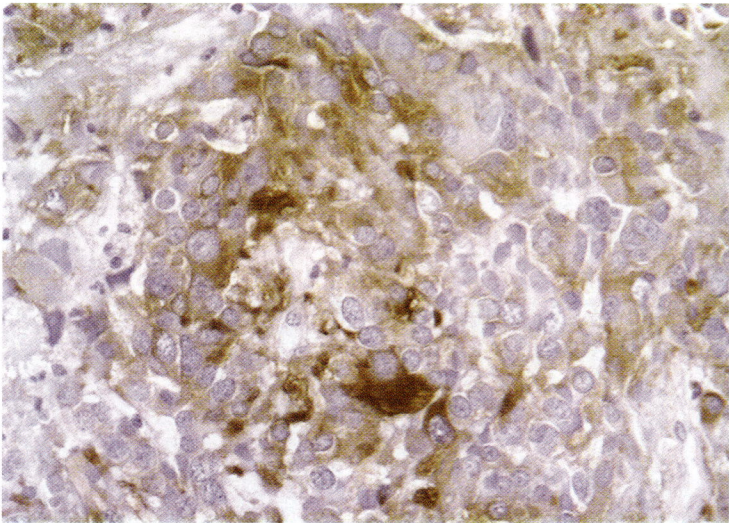

Color Plate 16. Immunohistochemical staining of TSH-oma (40× magnification). Tumor cells show positive reaction for TSH. The intensity of staining is variable from cell to cell (Chapter 13, Fig. 2; *see* discussion on page p. 239).

3 Endocrinologic Approach to the Evaluation of Sellar Masses

Peter J. Snyder, MD

CONTENTS

1. INTRODUCTION
2. IDENTIFICATION OF A SELLAR MASS AS
   A PITUITARY ADENOMA BY ITS HORMONAL
   HYPERSECRETION
3. LABORATORY EVALUATION OF HORMONAL
   HYPERSECRETION BY PITUITARY ADENOMAS
4. CLINICAL VALUE OF IDENTIFYING
   PITUITARY ADENOMAS
5. EVALUATION OF HORMONAL DEFICIENCIES
   ASSOCIATED WITH A SELLAR MASS
6. SUMMARY

Summary

The patient with a sellar mass requires endocrine evaluation for syndromes of hypoproduction and hyperproduction of pituitary hormones. This chapter describes the appropriate endocrine evaluation to delineate these syndromes.

Key Words: Lactotroph adenomas, somatotroph adenomas, corticotroph adenomas, gonadotroph adenomas, and thyrotroph adenomas.

1. INTRODUCTION

When a sellar mass is identified by magnetic resonance imaging (MRI)—no matter if the MRI was performed because of related neurologic symptoms, such as visual field loss, or because of an unrelated symptom—endocrinologic evaluation should be performed for two reasons: to attempt to identify the

From: *Contemporary Endocrinology: Diagnosis and Management of Pituitary Disorders*
Edited by: B. Swearingen and B. M. K. Biller © Humana Press, Totowa, NJ

nature of the mass by its hormonal hypersecretion and to determine if the mass
is causing hyposecretion from the normal pituitary gland. Among sellar masses,
only pituitary adenomas generally cause hypersecretion, but any sellar mass
can interfere with secretion from the nonadenomatous pituitary, by damage to
the hypothalamus, or by pressure on the hypothalamic–pituitary stalk or on the
pituitary itself, and thereby cause hyposecretion.

2. IDENTIFICATION OF A SELLAR MASS AS A PITUITARY ADENOMA BY ITS HORMONAL HYPERSECRETION

A pituitary adenoma can arise from any cell in the anterior pituitary gland,
so the adenoma can, potentially, secrete an excessive amount of whatever
hormone is normally made by the cell from which the adenoma arose.

2.1. Types of Pituitary Adenomas

Adenomas that arise from cells that produce peptide hormones typically
secrete relatively efficiently and cause clinical syndromes, whereas adenomas
that arise from cells that produce glycopeptide hormones are typically ineffi-
cient and do not usually cause clinical syndromes. For example, somatotroph
adenomas typically secrete growth hormone excessively and cause acromegaly
even when the adenoma is too small to cause neurologic symptoms, and corticotroph adenomas cause Cushing's syndrome even when they are so small
they cannot readily be identified by MRI. There are exceptions to this generalization, and occasional somatotroph (1) and corticotroph adenomas (2) are so
inefficient as to be called "silent." Lactotroph adenomas are usually efficient,
so that in premenopausal women they cause hypogonadism even when they are
very small. At the other end of the spectrum are gonadotroph and thyrotroph
adenomas, which typically are quite inefficient and whose secretory products
usually do not cause clinical syndromes (3). These adenomas are usually not
detected until they become so large that they cause neurologic symptoms,
such as visual field impairment. There are exceptions to this generalization as
well; gonadotroph adenomas that produce FSH excessively may cause ovarian
hyperstimulation in premenopausal women (4,5), and thyrotroph adenomas
that produce intact TSH may cause hyperthyroidism (6,7).

2.2. Clinical Evaluation of Hormonal Hypersecretion by Pituitary Adenomas

Patients who present with sellar masses by MRI should be evaluated by
history and physical examination for evidence of hormonal hypersecretion.
Even though most somatotroph adenomas cause acromegaly, sometimes the
clinical features are not recognized prior to finding the adenoma as a sellar

mass on MRI *(1)*. Therefore, all patients who are found to have a sellar mass should be asked about change in ring and shoe size and symptoms of sleep apnea and carpal tunnel syndrome. They should also be examined for typical physical features of acromegaly, including frontal bossing, prognathism, and large hands and feet.

Similarly, even though most corticotroph adenomas secrete efficiently and cause Cushing's syndrome when they are < 1 cm in diameter, some are less efficient and first come to medical attention as a sellar mass > 1 cm *(2)*. Consequently, all patients who present with a sellar mass should be asked about the new development of diabetes, hypertension, and osteoporosis and should be examined for manifestations of centripetal obesity, such as round and red face, supraclavicular fat pads, and truncal adiposity; thin limbs; ecchymoses; and wide, purple striae. Usually, however, the patient who has a corticotroph macroadenoma that presents as a sellar mass will have a relatively subtle degree of Cushing's syndrome.

Lactotroph adenomas are a third example of adenomas that usually secrete efficiently and cause symptoms when small, but less commonly are ineffi-cient and present as a sellar mass. The typical clinical presentation of lactotroph adenomas depends on gender and, for women, menopausal status. A premenopausal woman should be asked about oligomenorrhea or amenorrhea and galactorrhea. A postmenopausal woman should be asked about her age of menopause and if it was earlier than that of other women in her family. Men should be asked about erectile dysfunction, decreased libido, and infertility.

Most gonadotroph adenomas secrete inefficiently, and the secreted products, intact gonadotropins and their subunits, usually cause no symptoms or signs, at least not in men and postmenopausal women *(3)*. In premenopausal women, however, secretion of intact FSH continuously by a gonadotroph adenoma causes ovarian hyperstimulation, which is manifest clinically by oligomen-orrhea or amenorrhea and infertility *(4,5)*.

Most thyrotroph adenomas also secrete inefficiently, but those that secrete intact TSH cause hyperthyroidism, so patients with sellar masses should be asked about typical symptoms of hyperthyroidism *(6,7)*.

3. LABORATORY EVALUATION OF HORMONAL HYPERSECRETION BY PITUITARY ADENOMAS

Every sellar mass should be evaluated by laboratory tests for the possi-bility that it is a pituitary adenoma, even if the history and physical exami-nation give no clues of hormonal hypersecretion, because many pituitary adenomas, especially those that present as a sellar mass, are clinically silent. The possibility of a lactotroph adenoma should be evaluated by measuring the serum prolactin concentration. If the result is > 200 ng/ml, the mass is likely a lactotroph adenoma. If the result is lower, the test should be repeated at 1:10 and 1:100 dilutions to determine if the actual concentration is higher but masked by the "hook effect" *(8,9)*. If the result is still < 200 ng/ml, the mass could still be an inefficiently secreting lactotroph adenoma or another kind of sellar mass causing hyperprolactinemia by stalk compression.

The possibility that the mass is a somatotroph adenoma should be evaluated by measuring the serum concentration of IGF-1. An elevated value very likely indicates that the mass is a somatotroph adenoma, even if the patient does not appear acromegalic.

The possibility that the mass is a corticotroph adenoma should be evaluated by measuring 24-h excretion of cortisol. If the value is elevated, at least two more determinations should be made, and plasma ACTH should be measured.

The possibility that the mass is a gonadotroph adenoma should be evaluated by measuring the serum concentrations of FSH, LH, and alpha-subunit *(8)*. In countries where synthetic TRH is available, testing the serum LHβ subunit response to a bolus dose of TRH should be considered, because it is the most sensitive in vivo marker *(10,11)*. Premenopausal women who have oligomenorrhea or amenorrhea should also be evaluated by measurement of estradiol and, if elevated, ultrasound of the ovaries *(4,5)*.

The possibility that the mass is a thyrotroph adenoma should be evaluated by measurement of the serum concentrations of thyroxine and TSH. A serum concentration of thyroxine that is elevated but TSH that is not suppressed suggests that the mass is a thyrotroph adenoma *(6,7)*. An elevated molar ratio of alpha-subunit to TSH would support this diagnosis.

4. CLINICAL VALUE OF IDENTIFYING PITUITARY ADENOMAS

There are two major reasons why identifying a sellar mass as a pituitary adenoma is clinically useful. The first is that knowing that a mass is a certain kind of adenoma allows consideration of specific medical treatment of the adenoma, such as dopamine agonist treatment of a lactotroph or somatotroph adenoma and somatostatin analog treatment of a somatotroph or thyrotroph adenoma. In the future there may be other possibilities as well. Even when the kind of adenoma is not one currently amenable to medical treatment, knowing that the lesion is a pituitary adenoma can influence surgical treatment. For example, if a sellar mass is identified as a gonadotroph adenoma biochemically when it had been thought to be a craniopharyngioma by MRI, the treatment will still be surgery, but the approach will more likely be transsphenoidal knowing that it is a pituitary adenoma rather than transcranial for a craniopharyngioma.

The second major reason that identifying a lesion as a pituitary adenoma is clinically useful is finding a tumor marker by which to monitor the response to whatever treatment is chosen. If, for example, the serum concentration of prolactin, or IGF-1, or alpha-subunit is elevated prior to treatment, that hormone or subunit can be used to monitor treatment, whether it be surgery, medication or radiation.

5. EVALUATION OF HORMONAL DEFICIENCIES ASSOCIATED WITH A SELLAR MASS

Any kind of sellar mass can cause a deficiency of one or more anterior pituitary hormones by damage to the hypothalamus, compression of the stalk, or compression of or damage to the pituitary gland itself. Consequently, part of the evaluation of any sellar mass, and especially those > 1 cm in diameter, should include determination of the deficiencies of any hormones secreted or controlled by the pituitary. Measurements should include the serum concentrations of thyroxine, cortisol at 8 a.m. on more than one occasion, testosterone in men, and estradiol in women of premenopausal age. Following treatment, these functions should be reevaluated and, if persistent, treated.

Evaluation for the possible deficiency of vasopressin, i.e., diabetes insipidus, is important not only because it needs to be treated if present but because its presence helps identify the type of sellar mass. Only sellar masses that arise in the hypothalamus or high in the stalk generally cause diabetes insipidus; pituitary lesions, such as pituitary adenomas, do not. Patients should be asked about polydipsia and polyuria, especially about nocturia, and, if present, should be asked to measure their 24-h urine volume. If it is > 3 l, a water deprivation test should be considered.

6. SUMMARY

Sellar masses should be evaluated hormonally to determine if they are pituitary adenomas that are hypersecreting and/or if they are causing hyposecretion of pituitary hormones by the nonadenomatous pituitary. Identifying a sellar mass as a specific kind of pituitary adenoma may influence treatment of the adenoma, e.g., permitting specific pharmacologic treatment, and may provide a tumor marker by which to follow response to treatment. Hormonal hyposecretion should be reevaluated after treatment and, if persistent, treated.

REFERENCES

1. Klibanski A, Zervas NT, Kovacs K, Ridgway, EC. Clinically silent hypersecretion of growth hormone in patients with pituitary tumors J Neurosurg 1987;66:806–11.
2. Horvath E, Kovacs K, Killinger, DW, Smyth HS, Platts ME, Singer, W. Silent corticotropic adenomas of the human pituitary gland. A histologic study, immunocytologic, and ultrastructural study Am J Pathol 1980;98: 617–38.

3. Snyder, PJ. Gonadotroph cell adenomas of the pituitary Endocr Rev 1985;6:552–63.

4. Djerassi A, Coutifaris C, West V A, et al. Gonadotroph adenoma in a premenopausal woman secreting follicle- stimulating hormone and causing ovarian hyperstimulation. J Clin Endocrinol Metab 1995;80:591–4.

5. Mor E, Rodi IA, Bayrak A, Paulson R J, Sokol R Z. Diagnosis of pituitary gonadotroph adenomas in reproductive-aged women Fertil Steril 2005;84:757.

6. Brucker-Davis F, Oldfield EH, Skarulis MC, Doppman JL, Weintraub BD. Thyrotropin-secreting pituitary tumors: diagnostic criteria, thyroid hormone sensitivity, and treatment outcome in 25 patients followed at the National Institutes of Health J Clin Endocrinol Metab 1999;84:476–86.

7. Beck-Peccoz P, Brucker-Davis F, Persani L, Smallridge RC, Weintraub BD. Thyrotropin-secreting pituitary tumors Endocr Rev 1996;17:610–38.

8. Petakov MS, Damjanovic SS, Nikolic-Durovic MM, et al. Pituitary adenomas secreting large amounts of prolactin may give false low values in immunoradiometric assays: the hook effect. J Endocrinol Invest 1998;21:184–8.

9. St-Jean E, Blain F, Comtois R. High prolactin levels may be missed by immunoradiometric assay in patients with macroprolactinomas. Clin Endocrinol (Oxf) 1996;44:305–9.

10. Daneshdoost L, Gennarelli TA, Bashey HM, et al. Recognition of gonadotroph adenomas in women. N Engl J Med 1991;324:589–94.

11. Daneshdoost L, Gennarelli TA, Bashey HM, et al. Identification of gonadotroph adenomas in men with clinically nonfunctioning adenomas by the LHβ subunit response to TRH J Clin Endocrinol Metab 1993;77:1352–5.

4

Imaging of the Pituitary Gland, Sella, and Parasellar Region

John T. Lysack, MD, FRCPC,
and Pamela W. Schaefer, MD

CONTENTS

1. INTRODUCTION
2. ANATOMY
3. IMAGING MODALITIES AND TECHNIQUES
4. NORMAL VARIATION IN IMAGING APPEARANCE OF
   THE PITUITARY GLAND
5. NEOPLASTIC LESIONS
6. CONGENITAL AND BENIGN CYSTIC LESIONS
7. INFLAMMATORY AND INFECTIOUS LESIONS
8. HEMORRHAGIC AND VASCULAR LESIONS

Summary

This chapter discusses the anatomy of the sellar region, as well as the optimal imaging techniques and radiographic findings typical of sellar disease. Based on the imaging characteristics, a practical differential diagnosis can be constructed to guide appropriate therapy.

Key Words: magnetic resonance imaging, pituitary adenoma.

1. INTRODUCTION

Familiarity with the anatomy of the pituitary gland, sella, and parasellar region is of primary importance when approaching imaging interpretation of pathology affecting these areas. An understanding of the normal variation in appearance of the pituitary gland, sella, and parasellar region is crucial to avoid the false-positive identification of pathology.

From: *Contemporary Endocrinology: Diagnosis and Management of Pituitary Disorders*
Edited by: B. Swearingen and B. M. K. Biller © Humana Press, Totowa, NJ

Computed tomography (CT) is useful for preoperative planning, identification of calcium, and evaluation of osseous structures. However, magnetic resonance imaging (MRI) remains the single most useful diagnostic imaging modality because it allows precise delineation of the pituitary gland and adjacent parenchyma, cerebrospinal fluid (CSF), soft tissue structures, and bone marrow.

Imaging is often performed to evaluate pituitary adenomas, the most common tumor affecting the sellar/parasellar region. Knowledge of the imaging features typical or suggestive of less common sellar/parasellar neoplastic lesions, congenital and benign cystic lesions, inflammatory and infectious lesions, and hemorrhagic and vascular lesions allows for the generation of a practical differential diagnosis.

2. ANATOMY

2.1. Sella Turcica

The sella turcica, a bilaterally symmetric depression in the posteromedian aspect of the sphenoid bone, takes its name from the Latin for "Turkish saddle." Its anterior margin is defined by the tuberculum sellae in the midline and by the anterior clinoid processes bilaterally. Its posterior margin is defined by the dorsum sellae in the midline and by the posterior clinoid processes bilaterally. Inferiorly, the floor of the sella turcica is a thin layer of bone that also forms the roof of the sphenoid sinus. The diaphragma sellae is a dural membrane contiguous with the tentorium cerebelli that lies between the superior margin of the pituitary gland and the inferior aspect of the suprasellar cistern. The lateral margins of the sella are defined by the cavernous sinuses, each of which extends from the superior orbital fissure back to the petrous apex.

2.2. Pituitary Gland and Infundibulum

The pituitary gland (hypophysis cerebri) lies within the sella turcica (Fig. 1), which is therefore also known as the pituitary (hypophyseal) fossa. The pituitary gland consists of an anterior lobe (the adenohypophysis), a posterior lobe (the neurohypophysis), and an intermediate lobe (the pars intermedia). Embryologically, the adenohypophysis and pars intermedia are derived from the stomodeal ectoderm lining the anterior and posterior walls of Rathke's pouch, respectively, while the neurohypophysis is derived from the diencephalic neuroectoderm.

The bulk of the adenohypophysis lies within the anterior aspect of the pituitary fossa and is called the pars distalis. A thin superior extension of the pars distalis is known as the pars tuberalis, which lies at the anterior margin of the

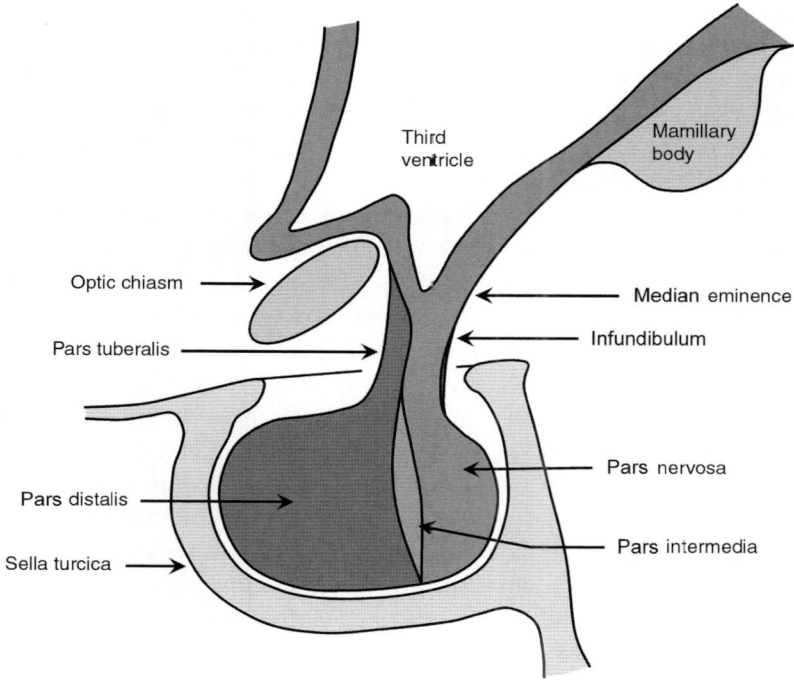

(A)

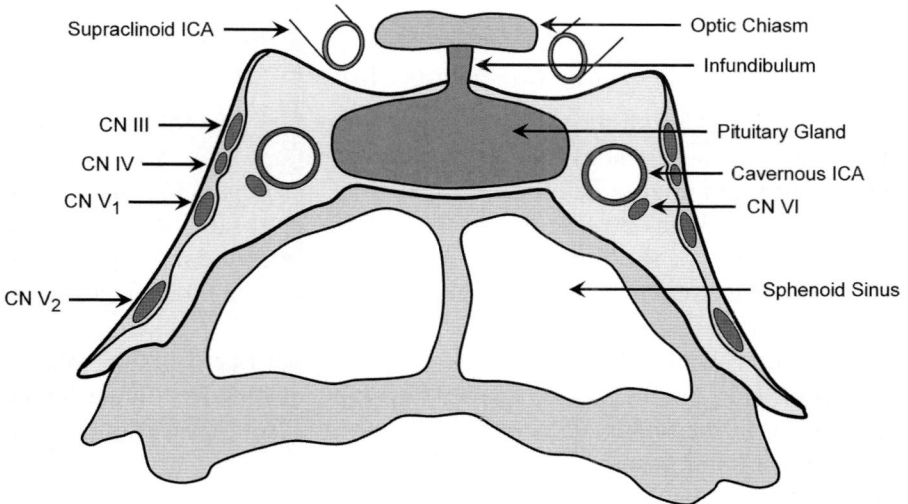

(B)

Fig. 1. Anatomy. (A) Schematic midline sagittal view of the sella turcica, pituitary gland, and infundibulum. (B) Schematic coronal view of the cavernous sinuses. ICA, internal carotid artery; CN, cranial nerve.

infundibulum and median eminence (a small swelling on the tuber cinereum, itself a gray matter structure of the hypothalamus located posterior to the optic chiasm and anterior to the mamillary bodies that contributes to the floor of the third ventricle). The adenohypophysis is responsible for the production of prolactin, adrenocorticotropin (ACTH), growth hormone (GH), thyroid-stimulating hormone (TSH), follicle-stimulating hormone (FSH), luteinizing hormone (LH) and, from the pars intermedia, melanocyte-stimulating hormone (MSH).

The portion of the neurohypophysis that lies within the posterior aspect of the pituitary fossa is called the pars nervosa. The pars nervosa is contiguous with the infundibulum, which extends superiorly through a defect in the diaphragma sellae to become contiguous with the median eminence of the hypothalamus. Therefore, the neurohypophysis is effectively a projection of the hypothalamus; it does not produce hormones (in contradistinction to the adenohypophysis) but stores and releases antidiuretic hormone (ADH) and oxytocin.

The blood supply to the neurohypophysis is via the inferior hypophyseal artery, a branch of the cavernous segment of the internal carotid artery. The superior hypophyseal artery, a branch of the supraclinoid segment of the internal carotid artery, supplies the median eminence and infundibulum. The superior hypophyseal artery also feeds the capillary network of the hypophyseal-portal system, which in turn supplies the adenohypophysis. These capillaries are fenestrated and lack a blood–brain barrier, allowing for the intravascular diffusion of pituitary hormones.

2.3. Cavernous Sinuses

The lateral margins of the sella turcica are formed by the cavernous sinuses. These are extradural venous sinuses that receive blood from the ophthalmic veins, middle and inferior cerebral veins, and the sphenoparietal sinuses. Each cavernous sinus drains posteriorly via the superior petrosal sinus to the transverse sinus and via the inferior petrosal sinus to the internal jugular vein. A network of intercommunicating sinuses beneath the diaphragma sellae also connects the cavernous sinuses to each other.

The medial wall of the cavernous sinus is formed by the sphenoid periosteum. The lateral wall of the cavernous sinus is formed by dura extending anteriorly from the tentorium cerebelli and extends from the petrous apex to the superior orbital fissure.

Cranial nerves III (oculomotor nerve), IV (trochlear nerve), V_1 (ophthalmic branch of the trigeminal nerve), and V_2 (maxillary branch of the trigeminal nerve) occupy the lateral aspect of the cavernous sinus where they can be found to lie in that order from top to bottom. The cavernous segment of the internal carotid artery occupies the inferomedial aspect of the cavernous sinus. Cranial nerve VI (abducens nerve) lies at the inferolateral aspect of the cavernous carotid artery.

At the posterior aspect of the cavernous sinus, near the petrous apex, lies Dorello's canal, through which cranial nerve VI passes before entering the cavernous sinus. Just superior to this is Meckel's cave, which contains the Gasserian cistern and the trigeminal ganglion. At the anterior aspect of the cavernous sinus, cranial nerves III, IV, V_1, and VI enter the orbit via the superior orbital fissure. The maxillary nerve (V_2) passes anteriorly through the foramen rotundum where it crosses the pterygopalatine fossa before entering the infraorbital canal.

3. IMAGING MODALITIES AND TECHNIQUES

3.1. Magnetic Resonance Imaging

MRI is the single most useful modality for imaging the pituitary gland, sella, and parasellar region. The primary sequences are high-resolution (e.g., 16-cm field of view; 192 × 256 matrix size; 2 excitations), thin-section (2–3 mm slice thickness) T1-weighted imaging in the coronal and sagittal planes before and after the administration of intravenous gadolinium (0.05 mmol/kg body weight).

Precontrast and postcontrast T1-weighted imaging in the axial plane, fast spin-echo (FSE) T2-weighted imaging, fluid-attenuated inversion recovery (FLAIR), diffusion-weighted imaging (DWI), and GRE susceptibility-weighted sequences may provide additional information in selected cases. Dynamic contrast-enhanced imaging employing a thin-section coronal gradient echo (GRE) technique may improve detection of some microadenomas. Evaluation of the intracranial vasculature can be achieved using MR angiography (MRA) and MR venography (MRV).

3.2. Computed Tomography

The main role of CT in this region is to assist in preoperative planning. Thin-section imaging using a low-dose technique and a bone/detail algorithm/kernel allows for high-quality multiplanar reformatting. When transsphenoidal surgery is planned, evaluation of the nasal cavity, ethmoid sinuses, and sphenoid sinuses is necessary. Osseous coverage of the carotid arteries and optic nerves should be specifically evaluated.

From a diagnostic standpoint, noncontrast CT may be used to assess for the presence of calcification within a sellar or suprasellar mass. CT is also the modality of choice for evaluating hyperostosis, invasion, destruction, and/or remodeling of adjacent osseous structures. These findings can be very helpful for narrowing the differential diagnosis in some cases.

In patients who cannot undergo MRI (e.g., cardiac pacemaker), thin-section CT before and after the administration of contrast can be performed. Imaging during the arterial phase of enhancement may increase detection of microadenomas. High-resolution coronal and sagittal reformations should be obtained. CT angiography (CTA) and CT venography (CTV) can be used to assess the intracranial arterial and venous structures, respectively.

4. NORMAL VARIATION IN IMAGING APPEARANCE OF THE PITUITARY GLAND

In general, the normal adult pituitary gland has a flat superior margin and is no thicker (superoinferior dimension) than 8 mm in males and 10 mm in females (1,2). The adenohypophysis is homogeneous in density (CT) and signal (MRI) and enhances homogeneously following the intravenous administration of contrast. The infundibulum should be in the midline and should smoothly taper from a maximum 3.8 mm in diameter at the level of the optic chiasm to a maximum 2.3 mm in diameter at its insertion on the pituitary gland (3).

During periods of increased hormonal activity (neonatal period and early infancy, adolescence, pregnancy, postpartum period), the pituitary gland may be relatively hyperintense on T1-weighted imaging and may have a superior convex margin (1). The infundibulum can measure up to 4 mm in diameter during pregnancy and the pituitary gland can measure up to 12 mm in height during the immediate postpartum period (4).

The posterior pituitary bright spot refers to the T1-weighted hyperintensity of the normal neurohypophysis (5). It is thought that the presence of ADH and/or phospholipid vesicles within the neurohypophysis is responsible for this appearance (6–8). The posterior pituitary bright spot is absent in 10–20 % of normal adult patients (9) and in 33 % of normal infants (10), although at least part of this can be explained by technical factors such as choice of frequency encoding gradient direction (11).

The dynamic enhancement pattern of the normal pituitary gland reflects its arterial blood supply via the inferior and superior hypophyseal branches of the internal carotid artery and the hypophyseal-portal system; the neurohypophysis enhances first, the infundibulum enhances approximately 4 s later, and the adenohypophysis enhances following an additional 10–15 s (12,13).

5. NEOPLASTIC LESIONS

5.1. Pituitary Adenoma

Pituitary adenomas are slowly growing benign epithelial tumors. They are the most common sellar/parasellar lesions in the adult population, with an estimated prevalence of 15–20 % (14).

Pituitary adenomas are classified by size and functional activity. Lesions that are smaller than 10 mm are called microadenomas, while lesions that are 10 mm or larger are called macroadenomas. Hormone-secreting lesions are called functioning adenomas, while those that do not secrete hormones are called nonfunctioning adenomas.

5.1.1. MICROADENOMAS

Microadenomas are more likely to be functioning than nonfunctioning, probably because the presence of hormone-mediated signs and symptoms leads to a relatively early diagnosis. Microadenomas are usually rounded or ovoid, but are occasionally flattened or triangular, intrasellar lesions (15). Prolactinomas are the most common functioning microadenomas and tend to occur in the inferolateral aspect of the adenohypophysis (16). ACTH-secreting microadenomas tend to occur centrally (17), are typically very small, and are the most difficult microadenomas to accurately identify on imaging (18). GH-secreting and TSH-secreting adenomas tend to occur in the lateral and central aspects of the adenohypophysis, respectively (17). Microadenomas are usually hypointense on T1-weighted images relative to normal anterior pituitary tissue, but are isointense on T1-weighted imaging in approximately 25 % of cases (15). Intrinsic T1-weighted hyperintensity, probably secondary to internal hemorrhage, is occasionally seen, particularly in prolactinomas (15). The T2-weighted signal characteristics of microadenomas are highly variable. However, it has been observed that greater than 80 % of prolactinomas are hyperintense on T2-weighted imaging and approximately 67 % of GH-secreting microadenomas are isointense or hypointense on T2-weighted imaging (15). Regardless of their location or imaging characteristics, however, *functioning* adenoma subtypes are differentiated biochemically.

Since normal pituitary tissue enhances earlier and more intensely than most microadenomas (19), early-phase dynamic gadolinium-enhanced images are particularly useful for the identification of microadenomas, which appear hypointense relative to the normal gland (Fig. 2) (20). For ACTH-secreting pituitary tumors, which are typically very small, gadolinium-enhanced spoiled gradient recalled acquisition in the steady state (SPGR) imaging has been advocated because of its increased sensitivity (21), but this increased sensitivity may lead to decreased specificity and increased identification of "incidentalomas" in normal individuals.

On CT, which is generally much less sensitive than MRI, microadenomas are usually hypodense and enhance relatively later and less intensely than the surrounding normal pituitary tissue. Secondary signs of a pituitary microadenoma include focal upward convexity of the superior margin of the pituitary gland and deviation of the infundibulum away from the lesion (16).

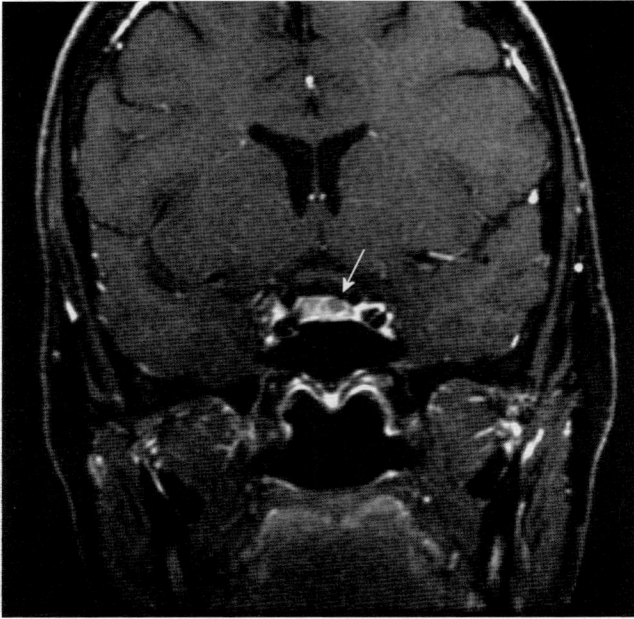

Fig. 2. Microadenoma in a 61-year-old female with the finding of a pituitary lesion during imaging evaluation for dizziness. Early-phase dynamic gadolinium-enhanced coronal T1-weighted image. A small well-defined ovoid lesion (arrow), which enhances less than the surrounding pituitary gland, is seen within the left aspect of the pituitary gland.

5.1.2. MACROADENOMAS

Macroadenomas are more likely to be nonfunctioning than functioning probably because a lack of hormone-mediated signs and symptoms leads to a relatively late diagnosis. Because they remain clinically silent from a hormonal perspective, the first signs and symptoms produced by nonfunctioning macroadenomas are related to mass effect (e.g., headache and/or visual field defects).

By definition, macroadenomas usually extend beyond the sella, and remodeling with enlargement of the sella is almost invariably present *(22)*. The most common pattern is suprasellar extension, in which case the adenoma usually has a polycyclic shape *(15)*. A waist may be seen where the lesion extends through the diaphragma sellae (Fig. 3). There may be mass effect on the overlying optic apparatus and extension into one or both cavernous sinuses.

It can be remarkably difficult to accurately differentiate between compression and invasion of the cavernous sinus *(15)*. Interposition of normal pituitary tissue between the lesion and the cavernous sinus excludes cavernous sinus invasion, while complete carotid artery encasement is diagnostic for

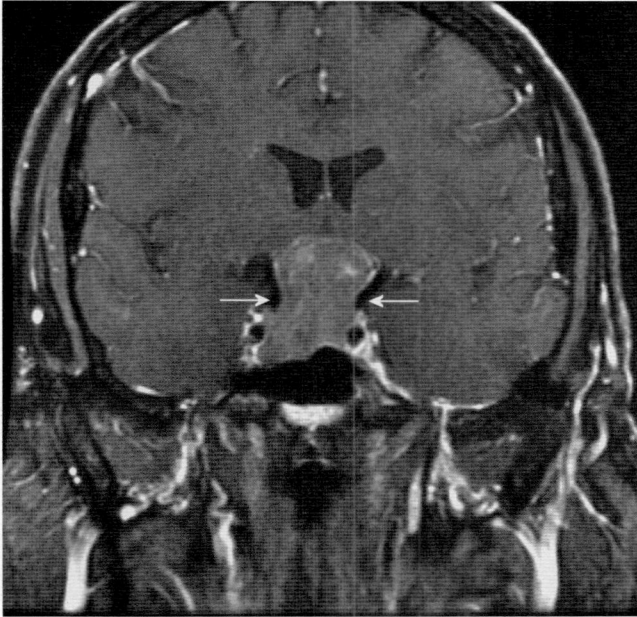

Fig. 3. Macroadenoma in a 57-year-old male with progressive vision loss. Coronal gadolinium-enhanced T1-weighted image. There is a large, heterogeneously enhancing sellar lesion with suprasellar extension. A waist is seen (arrows) where the lesion extends through the diaphragma sellae.

cavernous sinus invasion (Fig. 4) *(23,24)*. When there is less than 25 % encasement of the carotid artery, cavernous sinus invasion is usually not present. Conversely, when there is greater than 67 % encasement of the carotid artery, cavernous sinus invasion is usually present *(24,25)*. Even when there is cavernous sinus invasion, however, macroadenomas tend not to constrict the carotid artery *(22)* or cause cranial nerve dysfunction.

The MRI signal characteristics of macroadenomas are quite variable. They may be homogeneous or heterogeneous and can have cystic components, but generally are hypointense relative to normal pituitary tissue on both nonenhanced and enhanced T1-weighted images and are relatively hyperintense on T2-weighted images. DWI with apparent diffusion coefficient (ADC) maps can provide information about the consistency of macroadenomas. Relatively lower ADC values have been correlated with softer tumor consistency at surgery and higher cellularity at pathology *(26)*.

Macroadenomas also have a variable appearance on CT. Like microadenomas, they are usually hypodense and enhance relatively later and less intensely than the surrounding normal pituitary tissue.

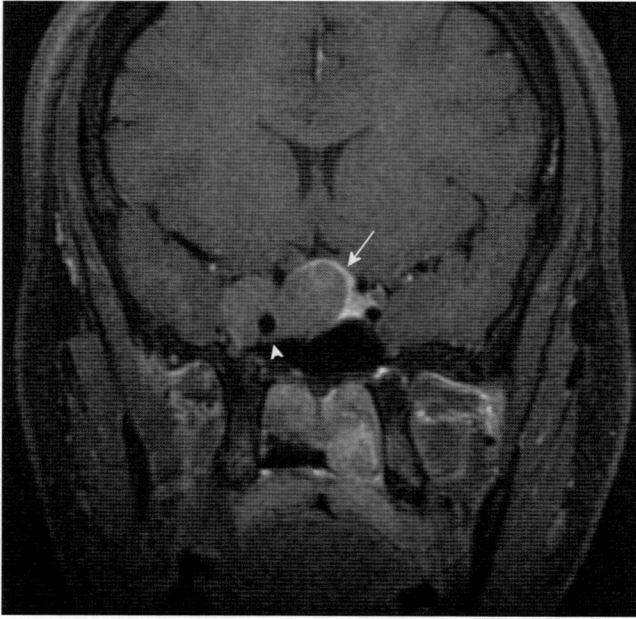

Fig. 4. Macroadenoma in a 26-year-old female with headache. Coronal gadolinium-enhanced T1-weighted image. There is a heterogeneously enhancing sellar/parasellar lesion with encasement of the right carotid artery (arrowhead) indicating cavernous sinus invasion. Note the normally enhancing pituitary tissue within the left sella and along the superior margin of the lesion (arrow).

Hemorrhage into a pituitary macroadenoma is relatively common. In one study, pituitary apoplexy developed in 9.5% of patients with a pituitary macroadenoma during a 5-year period *(27)*.

5.2. *Craniopharyngioma*

Craniopharyngiomas are the most common sellar/parasellar masses in children *(17)*. They are slowly growing squamous epithelial tumors that arise from cell rests embryologically related to Rathke's pouch. While usually histologically benign, they may be locally aggressive and tend to recur after surgery *(16)*. They are usually suprasellar (90–95%) in location. Extension down into the sella is common (50–70%), but isolated intrasellar craniopharyngiomas are relatively rare (5–10%) *(16,28)*.

Craniopharyngiomas have a bimodal incidence. The major peak is at 5–10 years of age; the secondary peak is at 40–60 years of age *(16,28)*. Clinical symptoms, particularly in childhood, are usually related to increased intracranial pressure. Visual changes related to compression of the optic apparatus or endocrine dysfunction may also occur.

Craniopharyngiomas can be solid, cystic, or mixed solid and cystic *(29)*. Cysts and calcifications occur in the majority of lesions (80–90 %), particularly in children *(16,17)* who usually have adamantinomatous craniopharyngiomas (Fig. 5). Purely solid lesions are more commonly seen in adults who usually have papillary craniopharyngiomas (Fig. 6) *(28)*.

The cystic lesions have variable MR signal intensity depending on protein content. Cysts with low protein concentration are relatively hypointense on T1-weighted images while cysts with high protein concentration are T1-weighted hyperintense *(29)*. On CT, the cystic areas are usually slightly higher in density than CSF, reflecting increased protein content. The solid components have variable density on CT, but are usually hypodense relative to normal gray matter. They are usually hypointense or isointense relative to gray matter on T1-weighted imaging and hyperintense on T2-weighted imaging. Enhancement

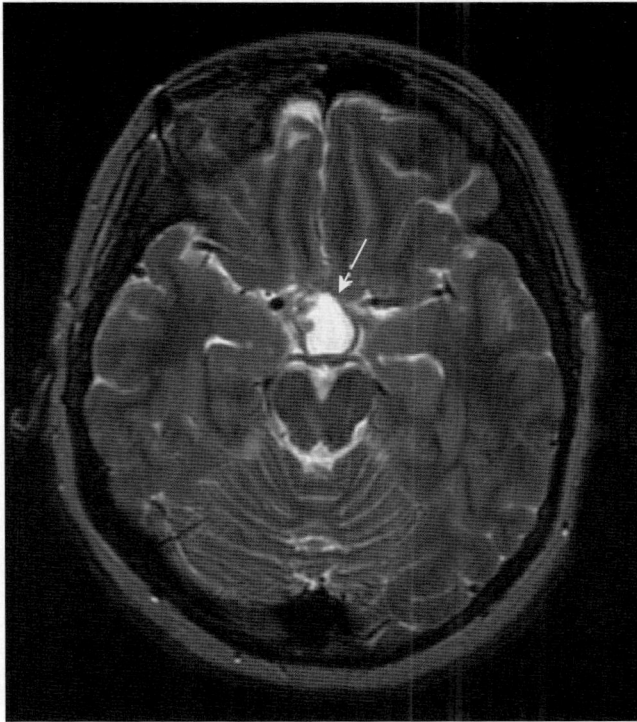

(A)

Fig. 5. (Continued)

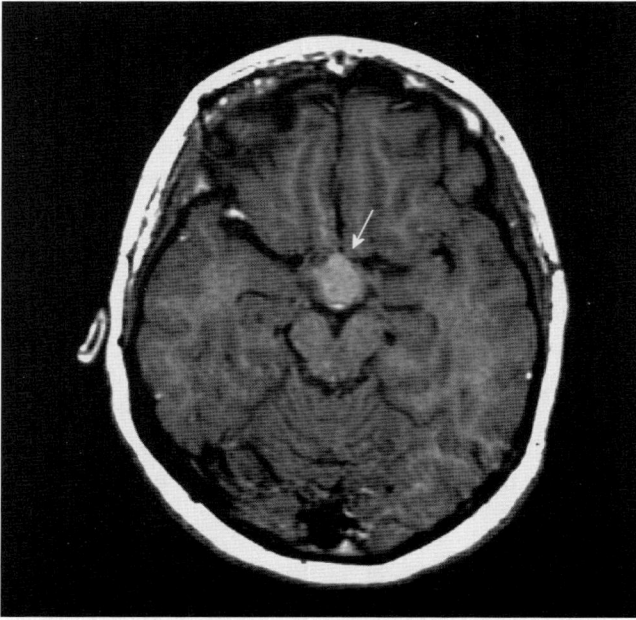

(B)

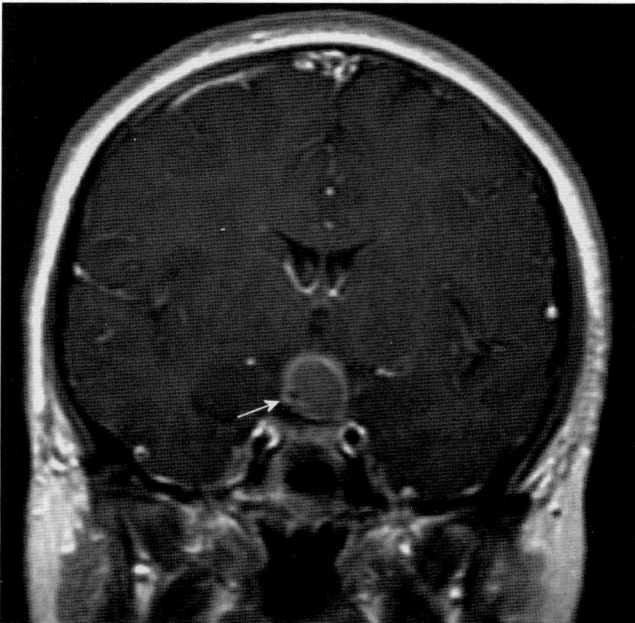

(C)

Fig. 5. (Continued)

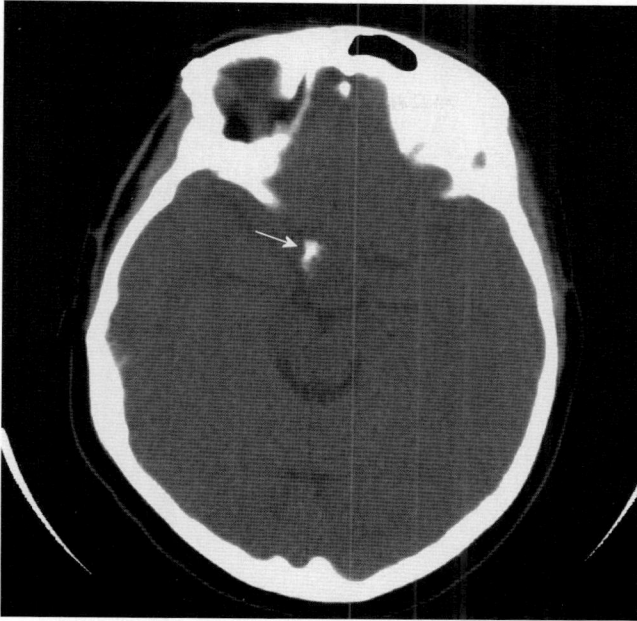

(D)

Fig. 5. Craniopharyngioma (adamantinomatous) in a 15-year-old female with growth delay and primary amenorrhea. (A) Axial T2-weighted image. A primarily cystic lesion (arrow) is seen within the suprasellar cistern. (B) Axial T1-weighted image. The cystic lesion contains hyperintense material (arrow), compatible with proteinaceous fluid. (C) Coronal gadolinium-enhanced T1-weighted image. There is enhancement of the cyst wall and a small focus of signal dropout (arrow) that is suggestive of calcification. (D) Nonenhanced axial CT. This confirms the presence of calcification (arrow).

of the cyst walls and solid components can be seen on both contrast-enhanced CT and gadolinium-enhanced MRI *(30)*.

The most characteristic imaging finding is the presence of calcification, which can involve areas of solid tumor and/or cyst wall. Calcification is seen in up to 90% of childhood craniopharyngiomas and in 50% of adult tumors *(28)*. CT is the preferred modality for the evaluation of calcification, although T1-weighted hyperintensity or areas of signal dropout on both T1-weighted and T2-weighted MRI can be identified in some cases.

5.3. Germ Cell Tumors

Intracranial germ cell tumors are usually midline pineal or suprasellar lesions, and typically present in children and young adults. The most common suprasellar germ cell tumor is the germinoma. Teratomas are the second most

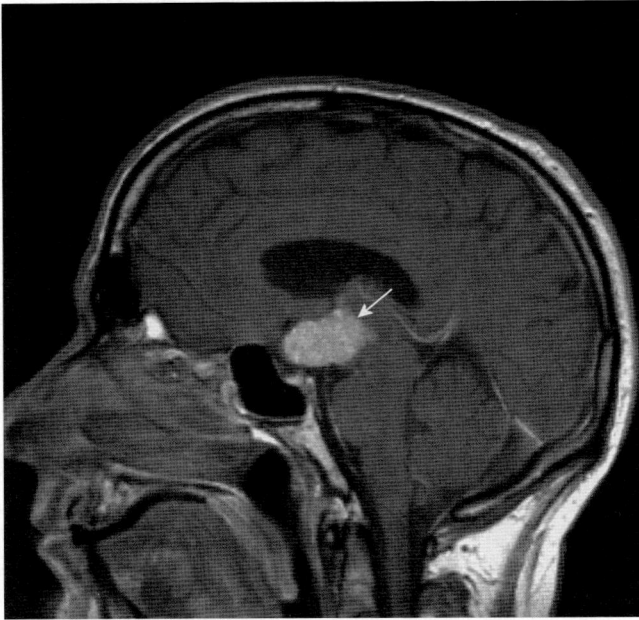

(A)

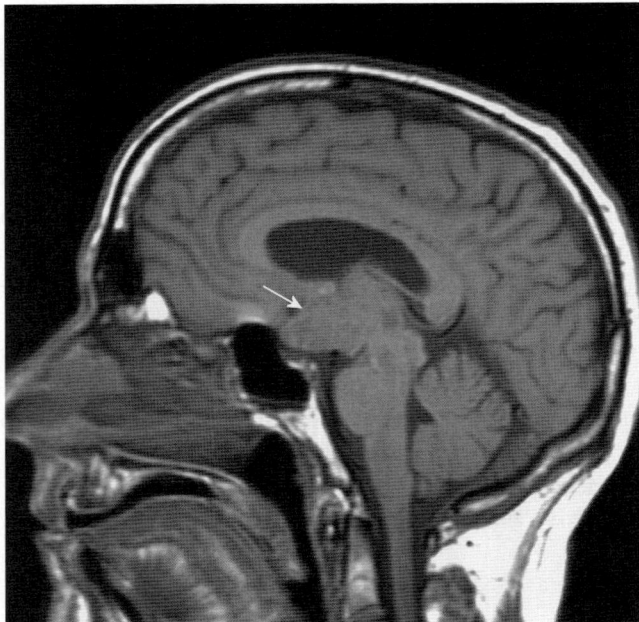

(B)

Fig. 6. (Continued)

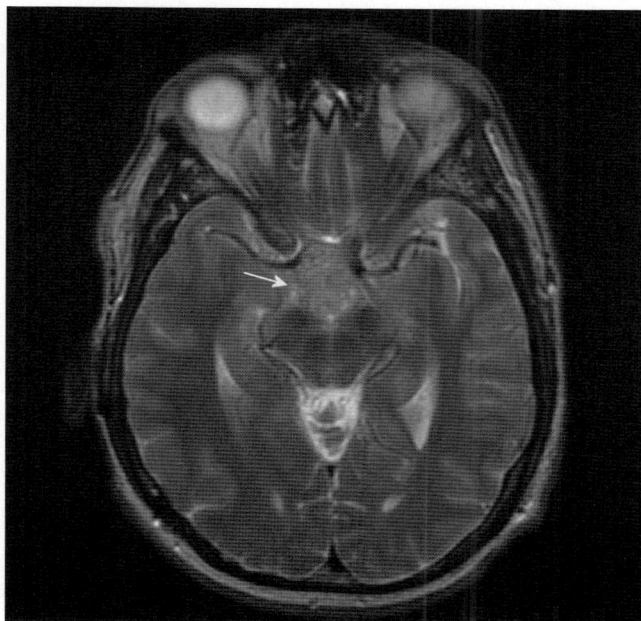

(C)

Fig. 6. Craniopharyngioma (papillary) in a 42-year-old male with an incidental finding of a suprasellar mass during imaging follow-up for a middle ear cholesteatoma (not shown). (A) Sagittal gadolinium-enhanced T1-weighted image. An enhancing suprasellar mass is seen extending back to the third ventricle (arrow). (B) Sagittal T1-weighted image without gadolinium. The lesion is isointense relative to gray matter (arrow). (C) Axial T2-weighted image. The solid mass is slightly hyperintense relative to gray matter (arrow).

common suprasellar germ cell tumor. Other suprasellar germ cell tumors, including embryonal cell carcinoma, yolk sac tumor, and choriocarcinoma, are extremely rare. Suprasellar germ cell tumors usually involve the infundibulum (Fig. 7) and/or median eminence of the hypothalamus (i.e., the ADH pathway), and are often associated with central diabetes insipidus *(28)*.

Germinomas are relatively fast-growing lesions and can therefore be large at presentation. On noncontrast CT, they are typically hyperdense lesions. On MRI, they are isointense or slightly hypointense on T1-weighted images, and isointense or hyperintense on T2-weighted images *(31)*. Germinomas characteristically are homogeneous and enhance intensely and homogeneously *(32)*, although cystic degeneration and heterogeneous enhancement can occur *(33)*. Calcification and hemorrhage are atypical, and should suggest an alternative diagnosis *(28)*.

Teratomas have heterogeneous attenuation, signal intensity, and enhancement at CT and MR imaging. The presence of macroscopic fat (hypodense on CT and hyperintense on T1-weighted images) and calcification is characteristic *(34)*.

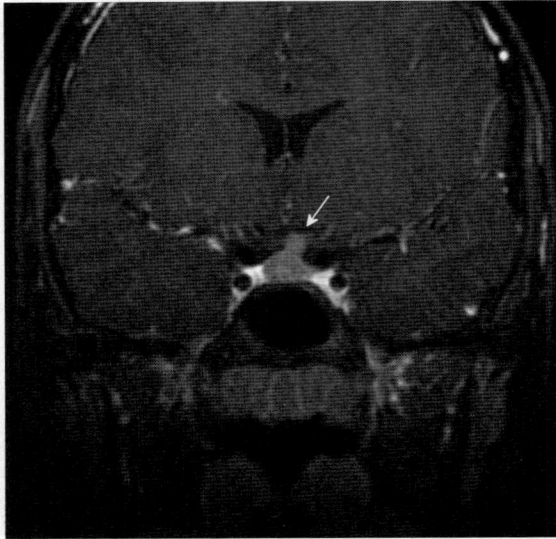

(A)

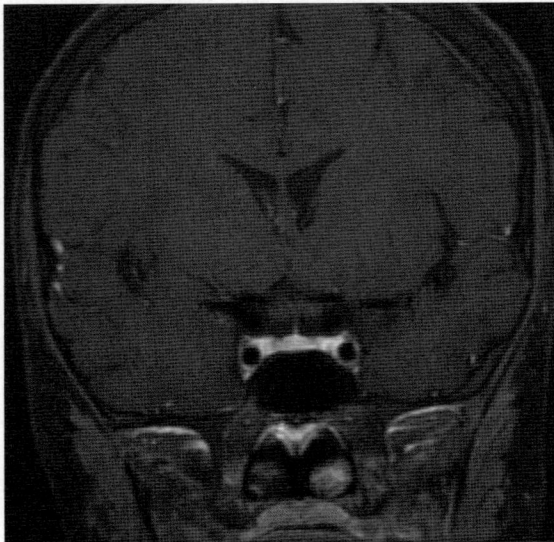

(B)

Fig. 7. Germinoma in a 10-year-old female with diabetes insipidus and elevated CSF human chorionic gonadotropin (HCG). (A) Coronal gadolinium-enhanced T1-weighted image. There is a homogeneously enhancing mass infiltrating the infundibulum (arrow) and pituitary gland. (B) Coronal gadolinium-enhanced T1-weighted image. Following 8 weeks of chemotherapy, symptoms resolved and imaging returned to normal.

5.4. Optic Pathway Glioma

Optic pathway gliomas are of three general types – generally benign childhood tumors associated with neurofibromatosis type 1 (NF1), generally benign childhood tumors not associated with NF1, and generally malignant adult tumors. The appearance of these lesions on CT and MRI is variable. In general, they are isodense to hypodense on CT, isointense to hypointense on T1-weighted imaging, and hyperintense on T2-weighted imaging (Fig. 8). There is variable enhancement. Compared to those seen with NF1, optic pathway gliomas that are not associated with NF1 are larger, faster-growing, more heterogeneous, and often have prominent cystic components *(35)*.

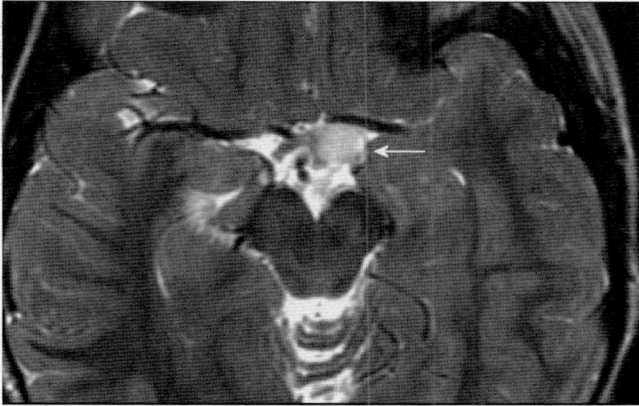

(A)

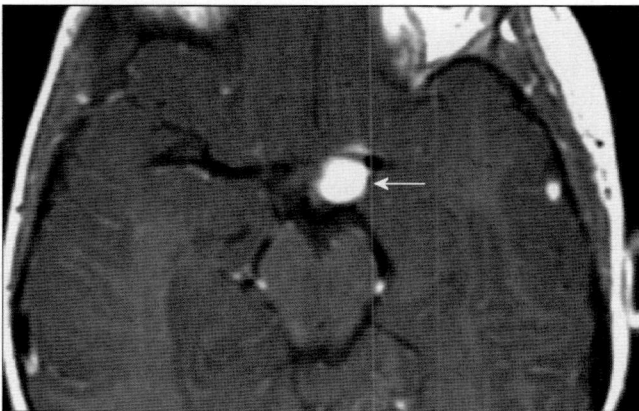

(B)

Fig. 8. (Continued)

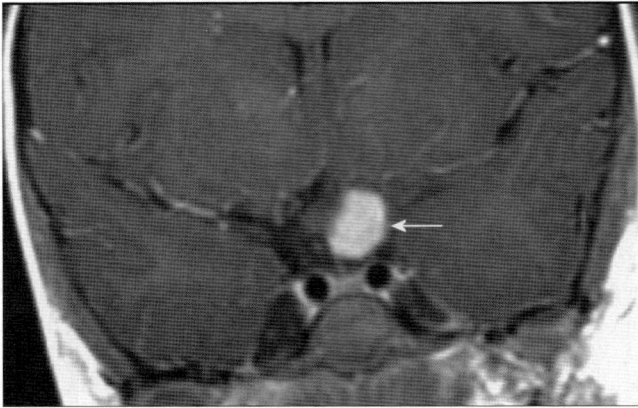

(C)

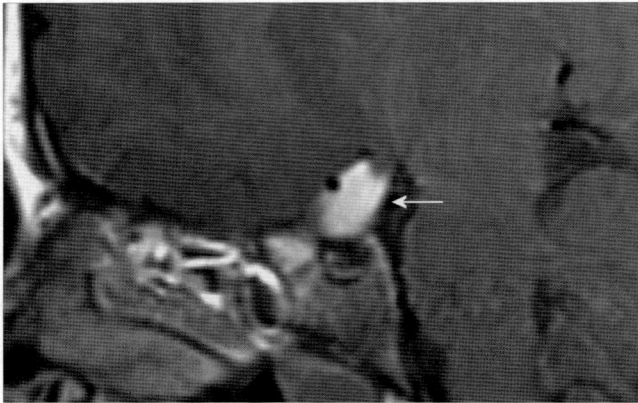

(D)

Fig. 8. Optic pathway glioma In a 5-year-old male with vision loss. (A) Axial T2-weighted image. A hyperintense lesion (arrow) is seen within the left aspect of the suprasellar cistern. (B) Axial gadolinium-enhanced T1-weighted image. The suprasellar lesion (arrow) intensely enhances. (C) Coronal gadolinium-enhanced T1-weighted image. The enhancing suprasellar lesion (arrow) is centered in the left aspect of the optic chiasm. (D) Sagittal gadolinium-enhanced T1-weighted image. The optic pathway glioma (arrow) extends from the optic chiasm back along the anterior aspect of the left optic tract.

The generally malignant adult gliomas are typically larger, faster–growing, and more heterogeneous than the usually benign childhood lesions.

5.5. Meningioma

Meningiomas are slow-growing benign neoplasms that arise from dura. They are the second most common sellar/parasellar neoplasm in adults (behind adenomas), with a peak incidence between 40 and 70 years of age and a female to male ratio of 2:1 *(16,17)*. Approximately 10% of all meningiomas arise in the parasellar region, and may involve the tuberculum sellae (Fig. 9), diaphragma sellae, planum sphenoidale (Fig. 10), sphenoid wing, anterior clinoid process, clivus, cavernous sinus, or optic nerve sheath. Clinically, these tumors frequently present with progressive visual impairment secondary to compression of the optic apparatus, or with endocrine dysfunction secondary to compression of the pituitary gland, infundibulum, or hypothalamus.

On CT, meningiomas are typically isodense to slightly hyperdense relative to gray matter. They may calcify and cause hyperostosis of adjacent bone. On MRI, they are typically isointense to slightly hypointense on both T1-weighted and T2-weighted sequences. They homogeneously and intensely enhance. A dural tail (contiguous tapering dural enhancement representing hypervascularity and/or tumor) is often seen but is not specific *(15,17)*.

Meningiomas can be locally aggressive, with encasement of the optic apparatus and invasion of the cavernous sinus. Rarely, meningiomas invade the skull base, sphenoid sinus, or orbit. Unlike macroadenomas, meningiomas

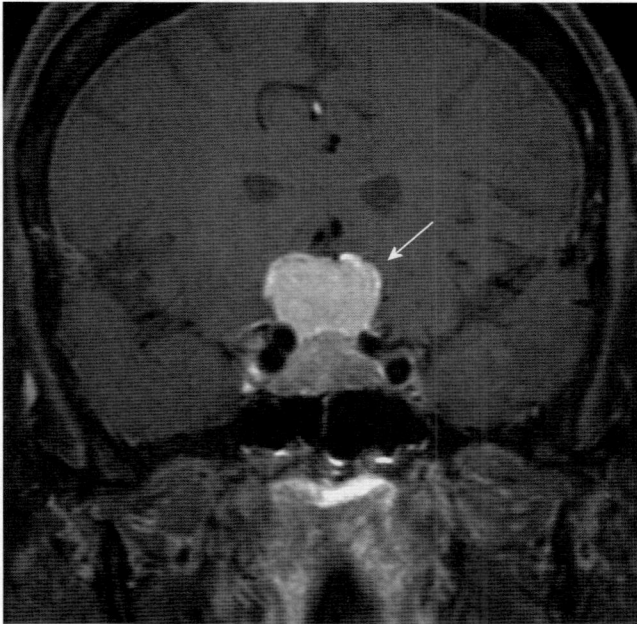

(A)

Fig. 9. (Continued)

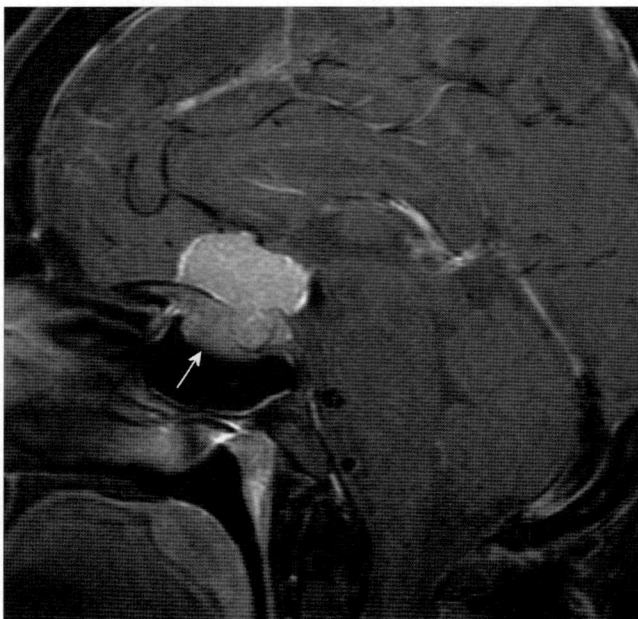

(B)

Fig. 9. Meningioma of the tuberculum sellae in a 69-year-old female with progressive visual loss. (A) Coronal gadolinium-enhanced T1-weighted image. An intensely enhancing extra-axial tumor (arrow) centered at the tuberculum sellae is demonstrated. (B) Sagittal gadolinium-enhanced T1-weighted image. The meningioma extends anteriorly to the planum sphenoidale and posteriorly over the dorsum sellae. It involves the sella and suprasellar region and is inseparable from the pituitary gland. There is associated hyperostosis and enhancement of the adjacent sphenoid bone (arrow).

extending into the cavernous sinus tend to constrict the carotid artery *(22)*. MRA or CTA may be helpful in delineating the degree of carotid narrowing.

5.6. Metastatic Disease

The most common primary tumors that metastasize hematogenously to the pituitary gland and infundibulum are breast and lung carcinoma *(36,37)* followed by leukemia *(38,39)* and lymphoma (Fig. 11) *(40)*. The neurohypophysis, infundibulum, and tuber cinereum are thought to be more susceptible to hematogenous metastatic disease due to their rich blood supply and the lack of a blood–brain barrier *(16,36)*. An intrasellar metastasis can mimic a pituitary macroadenoma. Expansion of the infundibulum, bone destruction, and rapid growth are all features that favor metastatic disease (macroadenomas tend to displace the infundibulum, remodel the sella, and grow slowly).

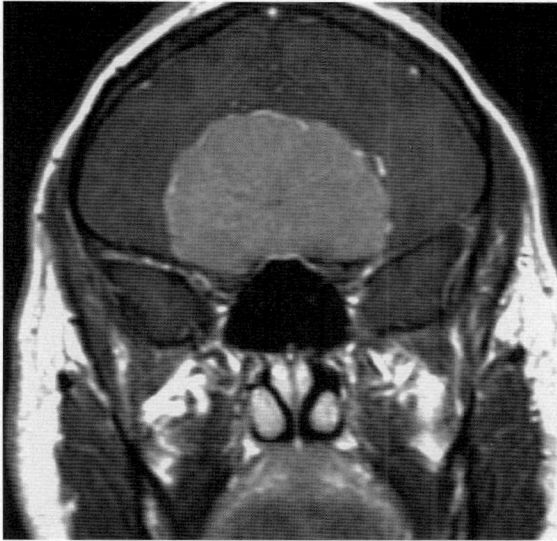

(A)

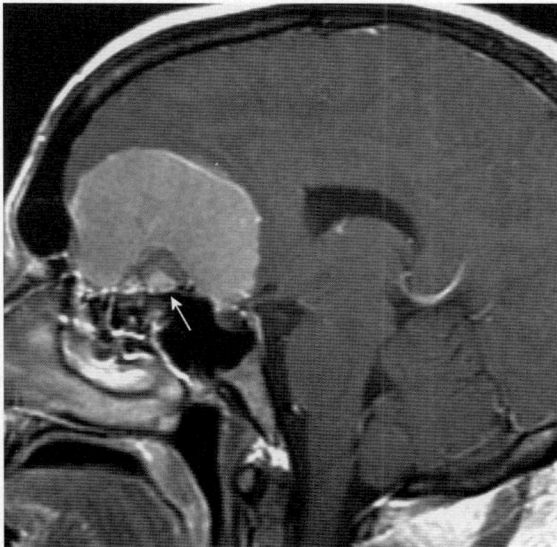

(B)

Fig. 10. Meningioma of the planum sphenoidale in a 36-year-old male with anosmia and headache. (A) Coronal gadolinium-enhanced T1-weighted image. This shows an intensely enhancing extra-axial tumor centered over the planum sphenoidale. (B) Sagittal gadolinium-enhanced T1-weighted image. Associated hyperostosis and enhancement of the cribriform plate (arrow) is demonstrated.

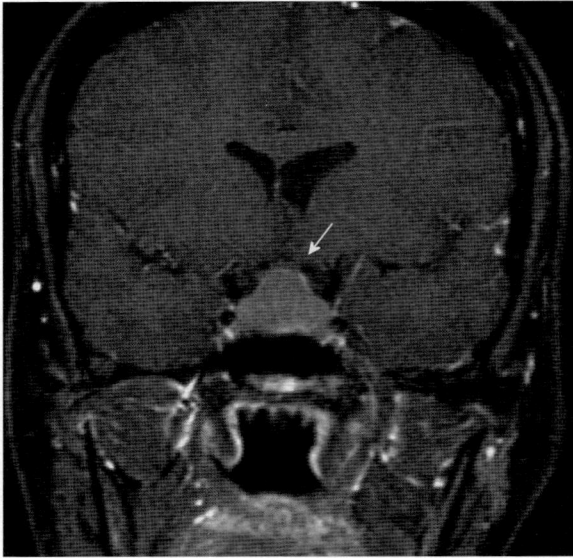

(A)

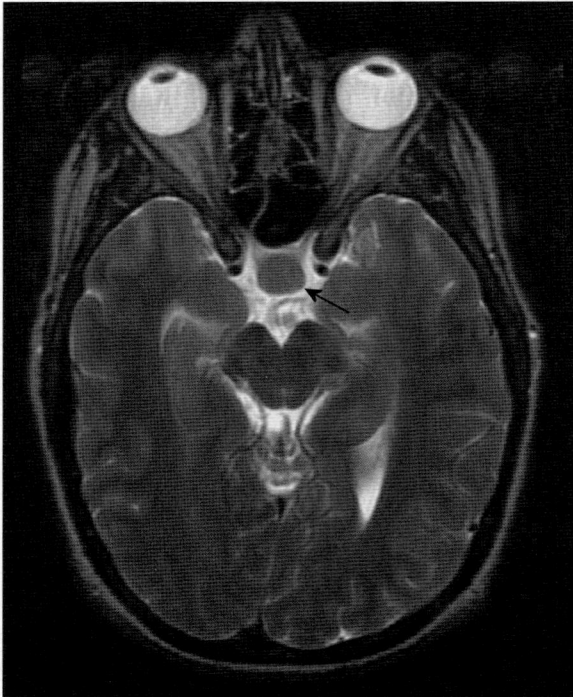

(B)

Fig. 11. (Continued)

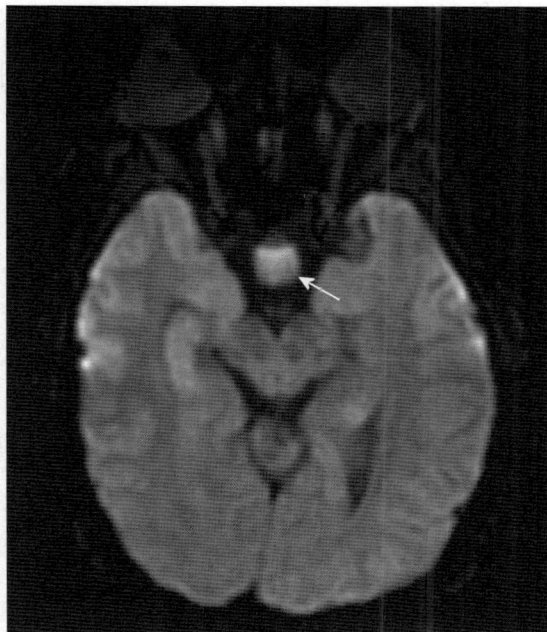

(C)

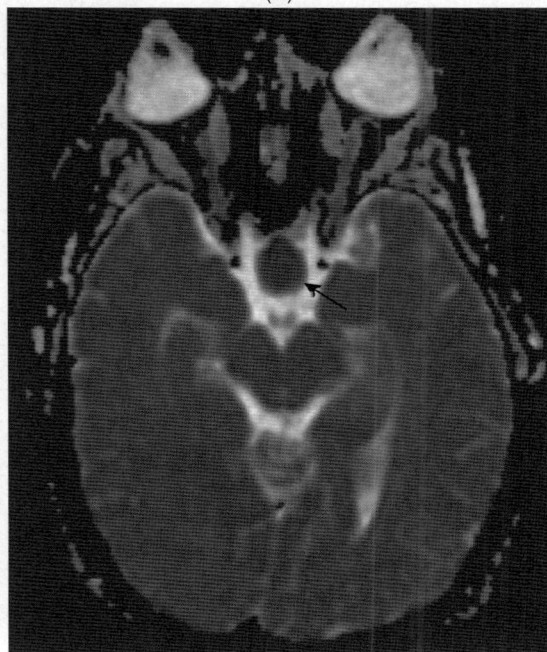

(D)

Fig. 11. (Continued)

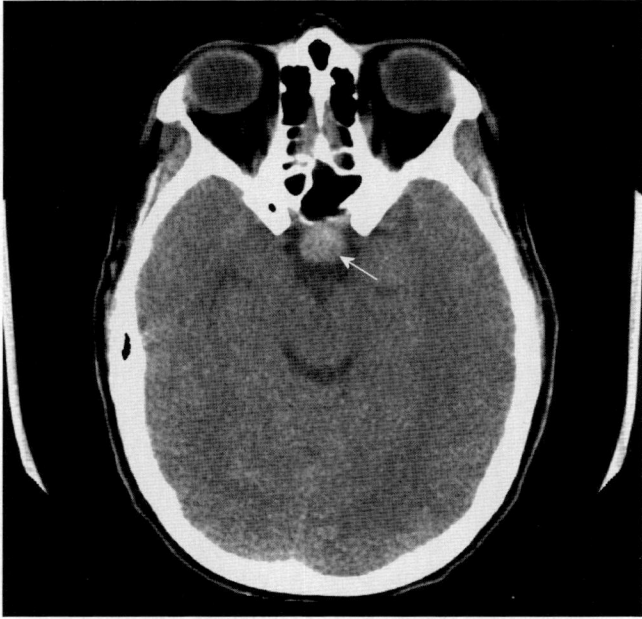

(E)

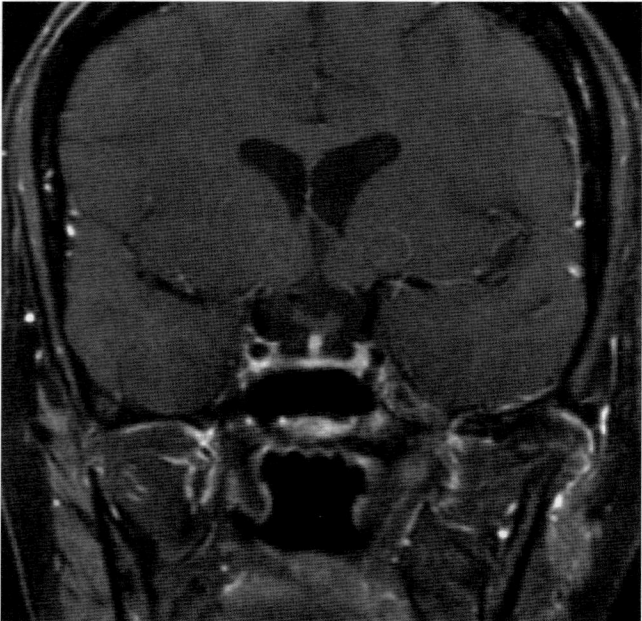

(F)

Fig. 11. (Continued)

Parasellar osseous and/or dural metastatic disease with intrasellar extension is more common than hematogenous spread of tumor to the pituitary gland. The most common associated primary tumors are breast, prostate, and lung carcinoma (Fig. 12) *(41)*; less common primary tumors include follicular carcinoma of the thyroid gland *(42)*, hepatocellular carcinoma *(43)*, and renal cell carcinoma *(44)*. Parasellar metastatic disease can mimic a parasellar meningioma. Bone destruction and rapid growth favor the diagnosis of metastatic disease.

5.7. Schwannoma

Schwannomas are benign slowly growing nerve sheath tumors. In the parasellar region, they usually arise from the trigeminal nerve within the cavernous sinus *(45)*. On MRI, schwannomas are typically isointense to hypointense on T1-weighted images, hyperintense on T2-weighted images, and enhance intensely. Cavernous sinus schwannomas tend to cause mesial displacement of the cavernous internal carotid artery and may result in erosion and/or remodeling of adjacent osseous structures. Expansion of the superior orbital fissure, foramen rotundum, or foramen ovale can also be seen *(28)*.

5.8. Osseous Tumors

Primary osseous neoplasms affecting the sellar/parasellar region include chordoma, chondrosarcoma, plasmacytoma, and lymphoma *(16)*. Clivus chordomas are relatively rare, slowly growing, but locally aggressive tumors arising from remnants of primitive notochord in the region of the sphenooccipital synchondrosis. On CT, a midline soft tissue mass with associated bone destruction is seen (Fig. 13). On MRI, chordomas are hypointense on T1-weighted sequences, heterogeneously hyperintense on T2-weighted images, and enhance *(46)*.

Chondrosarcomas are usually more laterally located because they are thought to arise from cartilaginous rests in the region of the petroclival

---

Fig. 11. Metastatic disease (lymphoma) in a 43-year-old female with gamma–delta T-cell lymphoma and a previous history of meningeal lymphomatosis. (A) Coronal gadolinium-enhanced T1-weighted image. This demonstrates an enhancing sellar lesion with suprasellar extension (arrow). (B) Axial T2-weighted image. The lesion (arrow) is hypointense relative to gray matter. (C) Axial diffusion-weighted image (DWI). The lesion (arrow) is hyperintense relative to gray matter. (D) Axial apparent diffusion coefficient (ADC) map. The lesion (arrow) has a low apparent diffusion coefficient relative to gray matter. (E) Axial nonenhanced CT. The lesion (arrow) is hyperdense relative to gray matter. These are all features of a small cell tumor with dense cell packing such as lymphoma. (F) Coronal gadolinium-enhanced T1-weighted image. Following 8 weeks of intrathecal chemotherapy, imaging returned to normal.

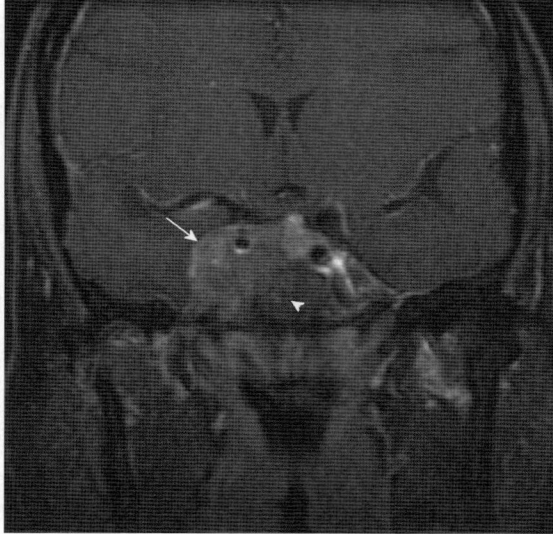

(A)

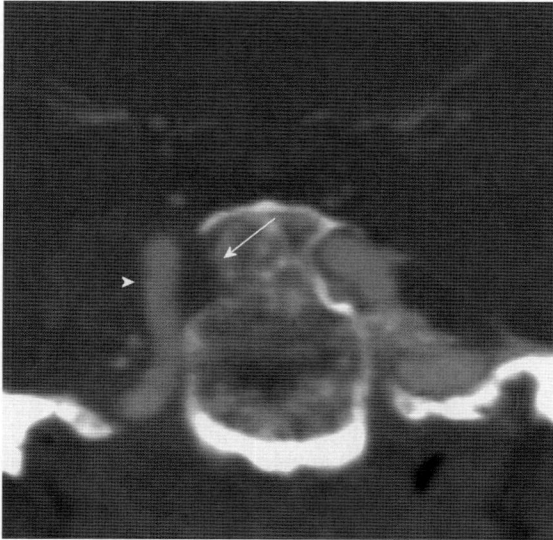

(B)

Fig. 12. Metastatic disease (lung cancer) in a 37-year-old female with metastatic non-small cell lung cancer (NSCLC). (A) Coronal gadolinium-enhanced T1-weighted image. There is an enhancing parasellar lesion (arrow) with right cavernous sinus invasion and abnormal enhancement of the underlying sphenoid bone (arrowhead). (B) Coronal maximum intensity projection (MIP) CTA reconstruction. This confirms cortical destruction (arrow) adjacent to the encased and narrowed right carotid artery (arrowhead).

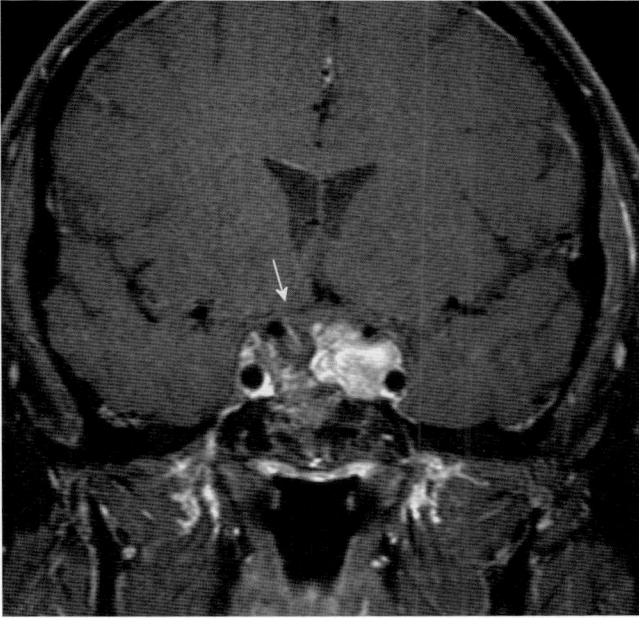

(A)

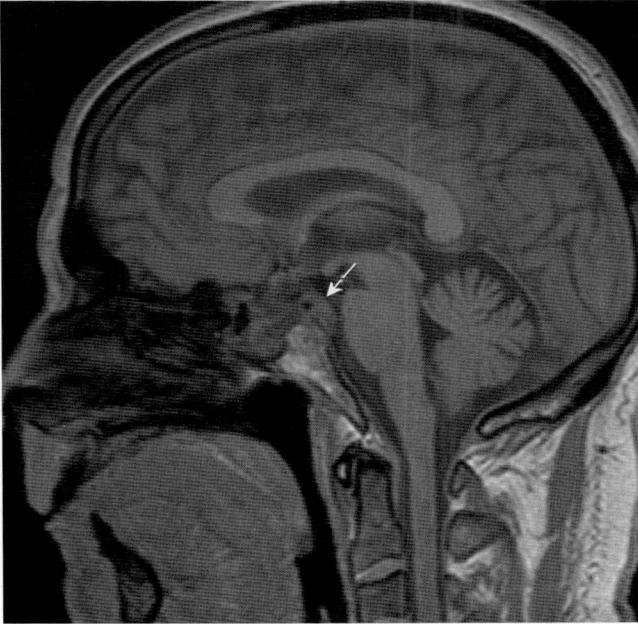

(B)

Fig. 13. (continued)

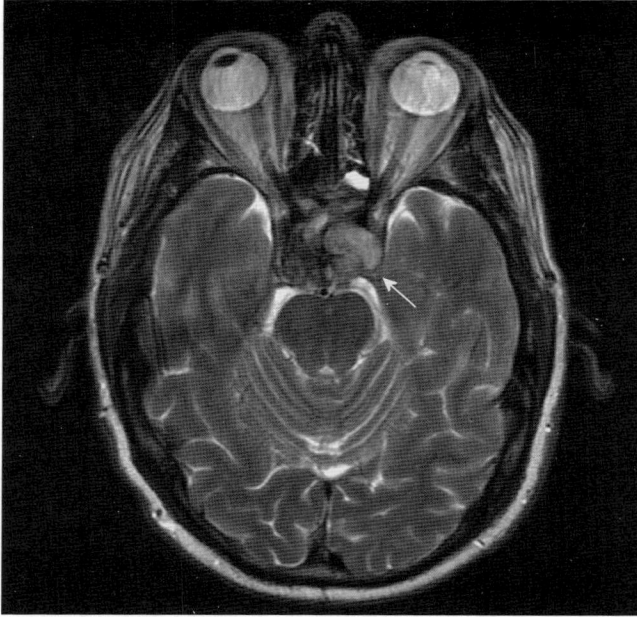

(C)

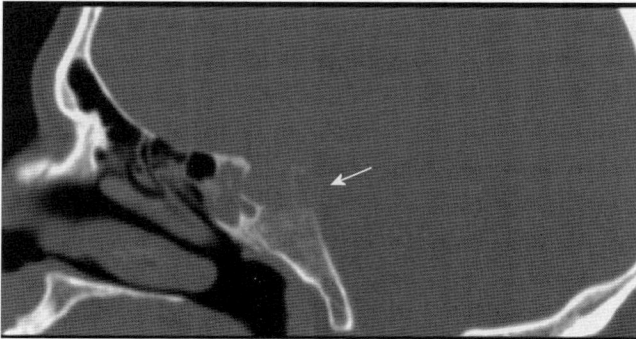

(D)

Fig. 13. Chordoma in a 56-year-old male with visual loss. (A) Coronal gadolinium-enhanced T1-weighted image. A heterogeneously enhancing sellar/parasellar lesion (arrow) is demonstrated. (B) Sagittal T1-weighted image without gadolinium. A heterogeneous predominantly hypointense lesion (arrow) is associated with destruction of the superior clivus. (C) Axial T2-weighted image. The sellar/parasellar mass (arrow) is heterogeneous but predominantly hyperintense. (D) Sagittal nonenhanced CT reconstruction. Osseous destruction of the superior clivus (arrow) is confirmed.

suture. Compared to chordomas, chondrosarcomas more commonly calcify, but the two tumors cannot be accurately differentiated based on their imaging features *(47)*.

Lymphomas and plasmacytomas tend to be relatively hypointense on both T1-weighted and T2-weighted imaging and enhance, but otherwise have nonspecific imaging features.

6. CONGENITAL AND BENIGN CYSTIC LESIONS

6.1. Tuber Cinereum Hamartoma

The tuber cinereum is a gray matter structure of the inferior hypothalamus located posterior to the optic chiasm and anterior to the mamillary bodies. It is continuous with the infundibulum inferiorly (via the median eminence), with the anterior perforated substances bilaterally, and with the lamina terminalis anteriorly.

Tuber cinereum hamartomas are rare congenital gray matter lesions that may present with the classic triad of gelastic epilepsy, central precocious puberty, and developmental delay *(48)*.

MRI typically shows a pedunculated mass interposed between the superior aspect of the infundibulum (anteriorly) and the mamillary bodies (posteriorly) (Fig. 14). The mass is isointense to gray matter on T1-weighted images, isointense or slightly hyperintense to gray matter on T2-weighted images, and does not enhance *(49,50)*.

6.2. Rathke's Cleft Cyst

Rathke's cleft cysts are benign lesions that arise from primitive vesicles that lie between the pars intermedia and the pars distalis (Fig. 15) *(51)*. They can be entirely intrasellar or intrasellar with suprasellar extension. They are relatively common, with a 4% prevalence at autopsy *(52)*. They are usually small and asymptomatic, and are often incidental findings. When large enough to be symptomatic, they can cause headache, endocrine dysfunction, or visual disturbances.

As opposed to craniopharyngiomas, Rathke's cleft cysts rarely calcify. They can have a thin rim of peripheral enhancement due to enhancement of the cyst wall or of normal surrounding pituitary tissue *(53,54)*. Thick or nodular enhancement is atypical, and should suggest an alternative diagnosis *(17)*. The internal density and signal characteristics vary with protein content. Low protein content results in relatively low density on CT and low signal on T1-weighted images while high protein content results in relatively high density on CT and relatively high signal on T1-weighted images *(53,55)*. An intracystic nodule having high signal intensity on T1-weighted images and low

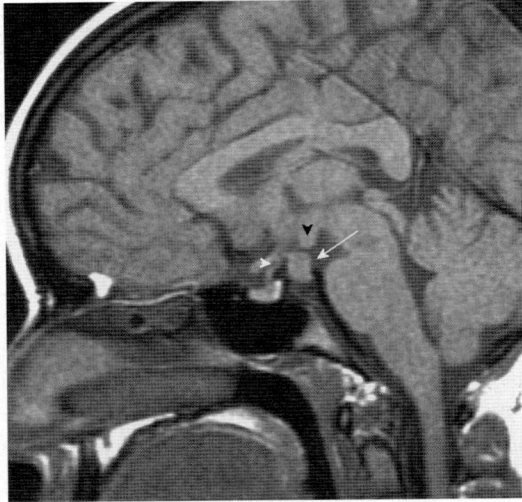

(A)

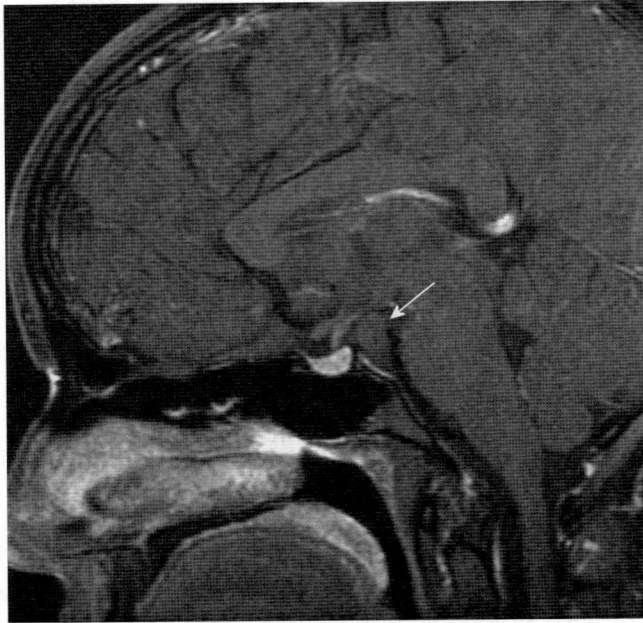

(B)

Fig. 14. Tuber cinereum hamartoma in a 15-year-old female with a past medical history of precocious puberty diagnosed at 13 months of age. (A) Sagittal T1-weighted image. A pedunculated mass (arrow) that is isointense to gray matter is interposed between the superior aspect of the infundibulum (white arrowhead) and the mamillary bodies (black arrowhead). (B) Sagittal gadolinium-enhanced T1-weighted image. The lesion (arrow) does not enhance.

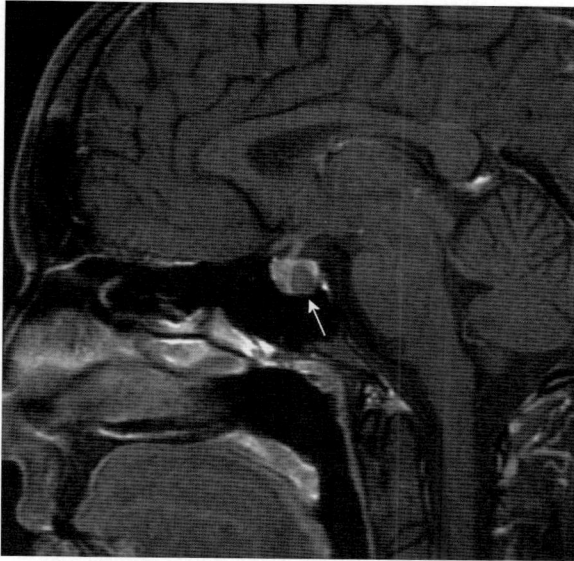

(A)

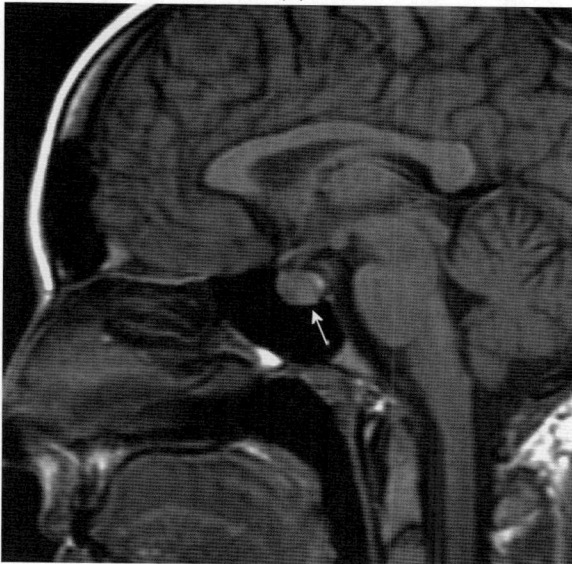

(B)

Fig. 15. Rathke's cleft cyst in a 22-year-old female with an incidental finding of a pituitary lesion on an MRI of the cervical spine (not shown) obtained for neck pain. (A) Sagittal gadolinium-enhanced T1-weighted image. A small well-defined nonenhancing lesion (arrow) is seen in the expected location of the pars intermedia. (B) Sagittal T1-weighted image without gadolinium. The lesion contains relatively high-signal material (arrow), consistent with proteinaceous fluid.

signal intensity on T2-weighted images may be characteristic *(56,57)*. Unlike intrasellar/suprasellar arachnoid cysts, Rathke's cleft cysts typically displace the adenohypophysis and infundibulum anteriorly *(58)*.

6.3. Arachnoid Cyst

Suprasellar arachnoid cysts usually occur in children and may present with hydrocephalus, spasticity, gait disturbance, and visual impairment *(16)*. There are thought to be two types of suprasellar arachnoid cysts: a noncommunicating intraarachnoid cyst of the diencephalic membrane of Liliequist and a communicating cystic dilation of the interpeduncular cistern *(59)*.

Intrasellar arachnoid cysts are rarer and are usually seen in adults *(32,60)*. They are thought to arise from herniation of an arachnoid diverticulum through an incomplete diaphragma sellae *(61)*.

On MRI, arachnoid cysts are well-circumscribed lesions that are isointense (or near isointense) to CSF on all sequences. On CT, they are isodense (or near isodense) to CSF and there may be remodeling of the surrounding bone. They do not enhance or calcify. The presence of peripheral calcification or enhancement suggests an alternative diagnosis, such as a cystic pituitary adenoma, Rathke's cleft cyst, or craniopharyngioma *(60)*. Unlike Rathke's cleft cysts, intrasellar/suprasellar arachnoid cysts typically displace the adenohypophysis and infundibulum posteriorly *(58)*.

6.4. Dermoid Inclusion Cyst

Dermoid inclusion cysts are slowly growing benign lesions that contain keratinizing squamous epithelium, cholesterol, sebaceous and sweat glands, fat, and hair. They are classically midline lesions, but can be seen in a parasellar location. They can present with headache, endocrine dysfunction, or visual disturbances due to mass effect on adjacent structures. Rarely, they rupture and present as a chemical meningitis *(34)*.

On MRI, dermoids are usually hyperintense on T1-weighted imaging secondary to the presence of cholesterol and fat *(5,34)*. Rarely, a fat-fluid level is seen. CT typically shows very low attenuation due to fat and can show peripheral calcification *(34)*.

6.5. Epidermoid Inclusion Cyst

Epidermoid inclusion cysts are slowly growing benign lesions that contain keratinizing squamous epithelium and cholesterol. Unlike dermoids, epidermoids are classically paramedian lesions *(34)*.

On CT, epidermoids have densities similar to CSF, but may be slightly hyperdense or hypodense depending on the relative amounts of keratin and cholesterol *(34)*. They are usually isointense to slightly hyperintense relative to

CSF on T1-weighted and T2-weighted MRI. When epidermoids appear similar to CSF on CT as well as T1-weighted and T2-weighted MRI, they are difficult to differentiate from arachnoid cysts. In these instances, hyperintensity on FLAIR and DWI strongly suggests the diagnosis of epidermoid *(62,63)*.

6.6. Empty Sella

An empty sella (or partially empty sella) is defined as a sella that is completely (or partially) filled with CSF. It may be primary (idiopathic) or secondary (e.g., due to surgical resection or radiation necrosis). Primary causes have not been well established. Theories include a normal variant, CSF pulsations causing herniation of the arachnoid membrane through an incompetent diaphragma sellae, and spontaneous necrosis of a preexisting pituitary adenoma *(17)*. The end result is flattening of the pituitary gland (which is pressed down into the floor of the sella) and, at times, expansion of the sella (Fig. 16). The infundibulum remains in the midline. Patients with an empty sella are often asymptomatic *(64)* but may present with symptoms related to elevated intracranial pressure *(65)*. Rarely, patients may present with visual impairment related to prolapse of the optic chiasm down through the incompetent diaphragma sellae *(66)*.

7. INFLAMMATORY AND INFECTIOUS LESIONS

7.1. Lymphocytic Hypophysitis

Lymphocytic hypophysitis is a rare inflammatory autoimmune disorder that typically affects women in the peripartum period, although it can occur in both sexes. Clinically, there may be endocrine dysfunction, visual impairment, or headache. On MRI, the infundibulum is characteristically thickened and densely enhances (Fig. 17). The pituitary gland can also be enlarged but otherwise has a normal appearance and enhances normally. The clinical symptoms and imaging findings typically wax and wane; there is controversy about the role of steroids in management *(67)*.

7.2. Granulomatous Hypophysitis

7.2.1. SARCOIDOSIS

Involvement of the central nervous system (CNS) by sarcoidosis is relatively rare, but when it does occur, it usually manifests as basilar leptomeningitis with parenchymal spread via the perivascular (Virchow–Robin) spaces. Marked T2-weighted hypointensity, thickening, and enhancement of the infundibulum and hypothalamus can be seen with or without basilar leptomeningitis *(68)*.

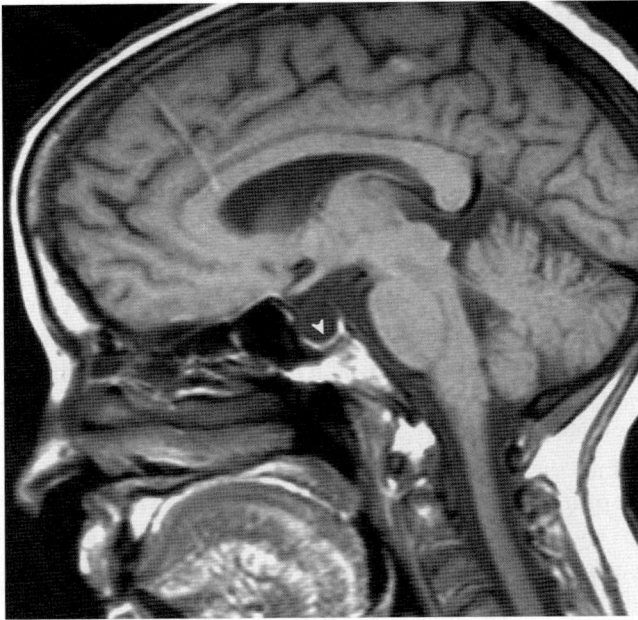

(A)

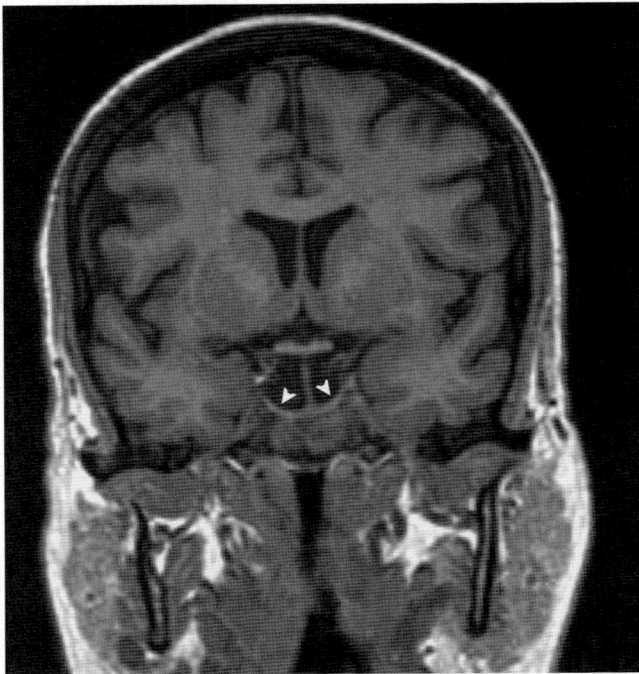

(B)

Fig. 16. (Continued)

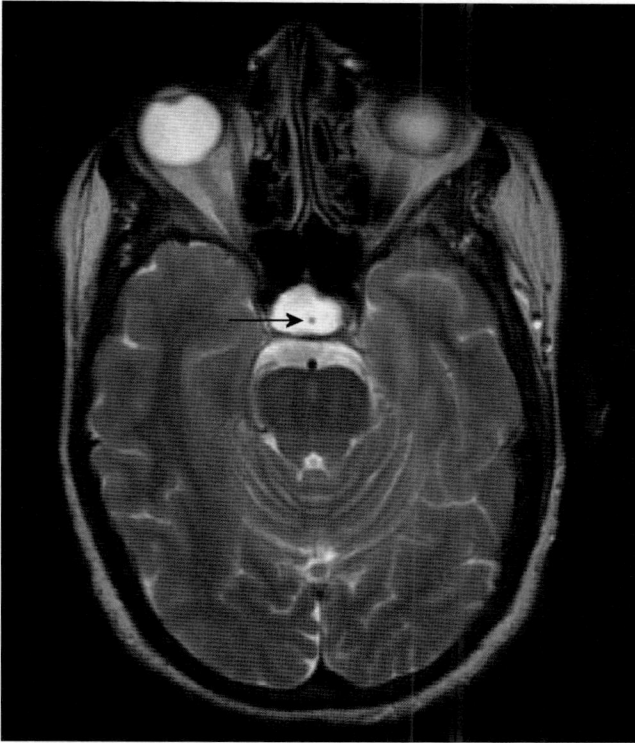

(C)

Fig. 16. Empty sella in a 55-year-old female with pseudodementia associated with depression. (A) Sagittal T1-weighted image. The pituitary gland (arrowhead) is flattened. (B) Coronal T1-weighted image. The pituitary gland (arrowheads) is pressed down into the floor of an expanded sella. Note that the infundibulum remains near the midline. (C) Axial T2-weighted image. CSF surrounds the infundibulum (arrow) and fills the sella.

7.2.2. Tuberculosis

CNS involvement by tuberculosis is similar to that by sarcoidosis, in that it typically manifests as basilar meningitis *(69)*. Tuberculomas of the pituitary gland and/or infundibulum may occur with or without tubercular meningitis *(70)*. Usually, this manifests as thickening and intense enhancement of the infundibulum.

7.2.3. Langerhans Cell Histiocytosis

Langerhans cell histiocytosis (LCH) is an inflammatory disorder of unknown etiology that primarily affects children and young adults. Multifocal LCH

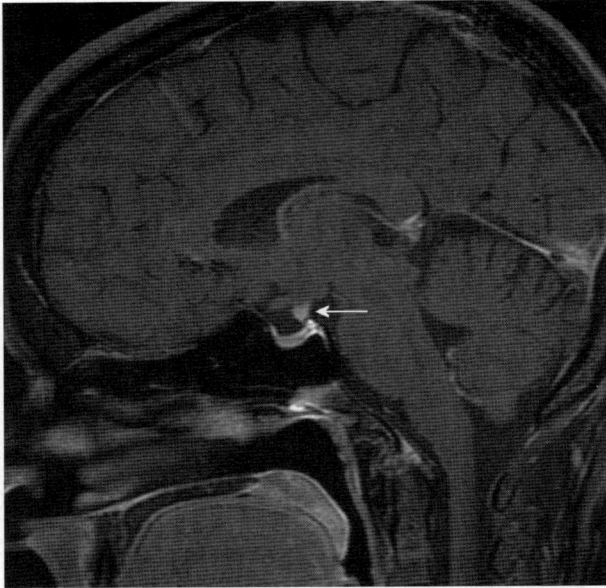

(A)

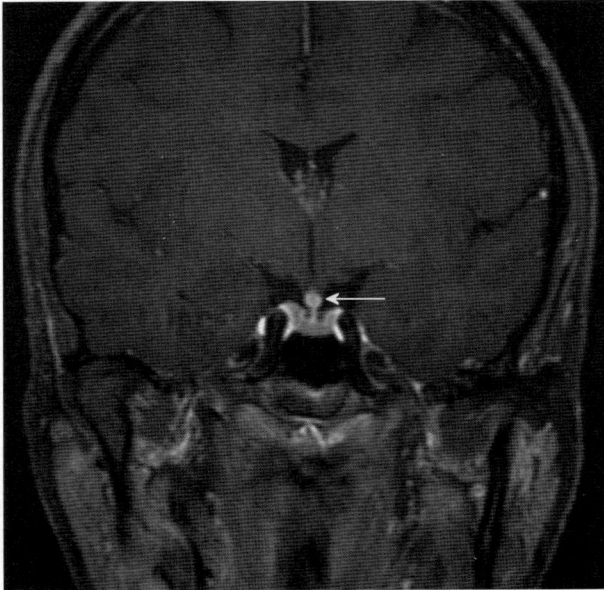

(B)

Fig. 17. Lymphocytic hypophysitis in a 38-year-old postpartum female with headache, diabetes insipidus, and elevated antinuclear antibodies (ANA). (A) Sagittal gadolinium-enhanced T1-weighted image. This demonstrates nodular thickening and dense enhancement of the infundibulum (arrow). (B) Coronal gadolinium-enhanced T1-weighted image. Nodular thickening and dense enhancement of the infundibulum (arrow) are seen.

(previously called Hand–Schüller–Christian disease) may present with a classic triad of diabetes insipidus, exophthalmos, and lytic bone lesions. In multifocal LCH, CNS involvement is usually secondary to direct extension from skull lesions. However, unifocal LCH (previously called eosinophilic granuloma) or multifocal LCH can primarily affect the infundibulum, pituitary gland, and/or hypothalamus. In these cases, MRI typically demonstrates infundibular thickening and enhancement (Fig. 18) *(71,72)*.

7.3. Tolosa–Hunt Syndrome

Tolosa–Hunt syndrome is painful ophthalmoplegia secondary to an idiopathic inflammatory disorder that affects the cavernous sinus and promptly responds to steroids *(73)*. On MRI, the lesion is usually hypointense relative to fat and isointense relative to muscle on T1-weighted images, isointense relative to fat on T2-weighted images, and intensely enhances. Extension into the orbital apex is a common feature *(74)*. It has been suggested that Tolosa–Hunt syndrome and idiopathic inflammatory pseudotumor of the orbit are two forms of the same pathological process *(73)*.

7.4. Pituitary Abscess

A pituitary abscess is usually secondary to contiguous extension of infection from the sphenoid sinuses *(32)*. Like brain abscesses elsewhere, they typically are rounded T2-weighted hyperintense and ring-enhancing lesions and may have internal restricted diffusion *(75)*. Associated findings can include meningitis, epidural abscess, and cavernous sinus thrombosis.

8. HEMORRHAGIC AND VASCULAR LESIONS

8.1. Pituitary Apoplexy and Infarction

Pituitary apoplexy is a clinical syndrome that includes headache, visual deficits, ophthalmoplegia, altered mental status, and/or hormonal dysfunction secondary to acute hemorrhage into the pituitary gland *(76)*. This usually occurs in the presence of a preexisting pituitary adenoma but may also occur during pregnancy when the gland is enlarged and hypervascular. The characteristics of hemorrhage on MRI vary depending on its stage. Patients are typically imaged during the acute stage when deoxyhemoglobin predominates (isointense to pituitary gland on T1-weighted images and hypointense on T2-weighted images), or during the early subacute stage when intracellular methemoglobin predominates (hyperintense on T1-weighted images and

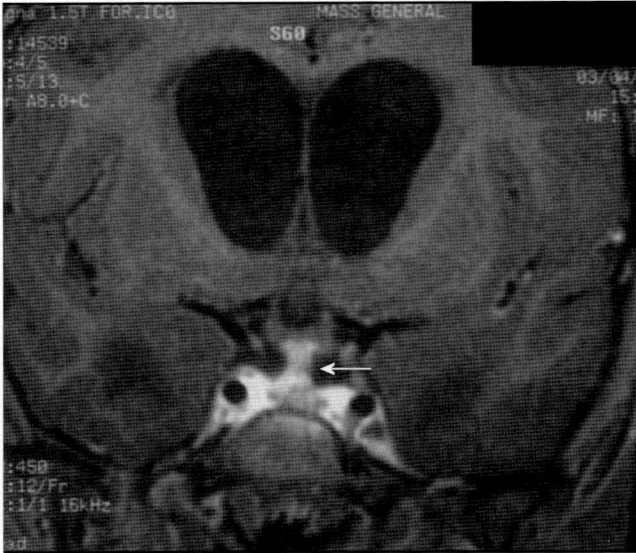

(A)

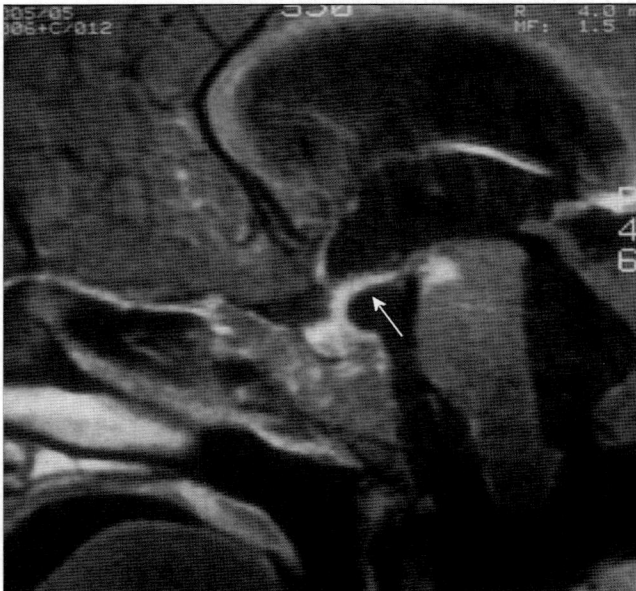

(B)

Fig. 18. Langerhans cell histiocytosis in a 14-year-old male with diabetes insipidus and hydrocephalus. (A) Coronal gadolinium-enhanced T1-weighted image. There is thickening and enhancement of the infundibulum (arrow). (B) Sagittal gadolinium-enhanced T1-weighted image. Enhancement extends back along the hypothalamus (arrow). Note also the distended ventricles.

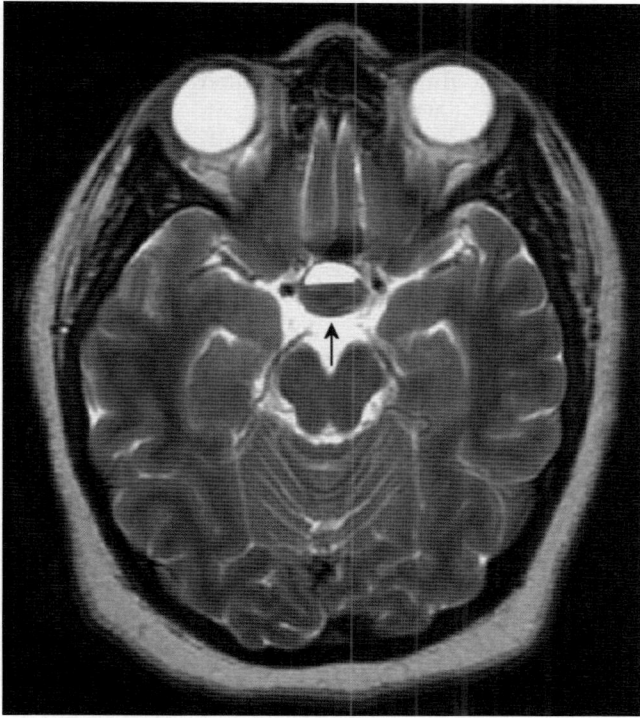

(A)

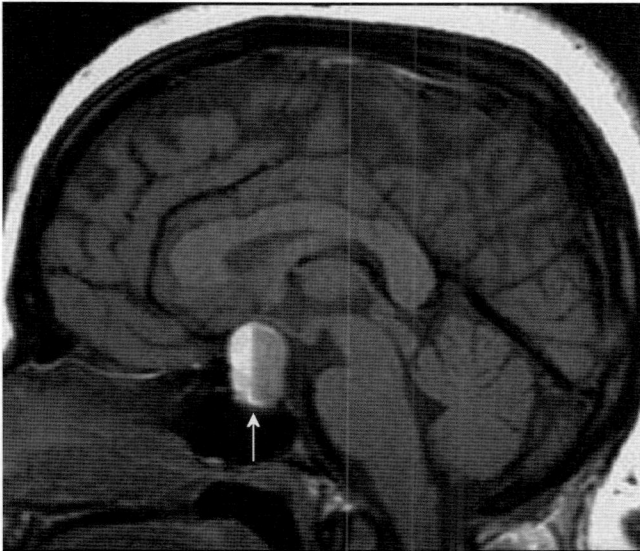

(B)

Fig. 19. (Continued)

hypointense on T2-weighted images). In the late subacute stage, extracellular methemoglobin predominates (hyperintense on both T1-weighted and T2-weighted images). A fluid–fluid (hematocrit) level can also be seen (Fig. 19).

Acute pituitary infarction usually occurs in the peripartum period (Sheehan's syndrome) *(77)*. The pituitary gland is typically enlarged and isointense relative to gray matter on T1-weighted and T2-weighted images *(76,77)* and demonstrates restricted diffusion *(76)*. Thin peripheral enhancement may be seen *(76,77)*.

8.2. Aneurysms

Aneurysms are important mimics of parasellar tumors. They can involve the cavernous carotid (Fig. 20), ophthalmic, posterior communicating, or anterior communicating arteries. Routine MRI may demonstrate a focally enlarged flow void, peripheral lamellated thrombus, or an associated phase encoding flow artifact. CT may demonstrate wall calcification or erosion of adjacent osseous structures (e.g., the posterior clinoid process with posterior communicating artery aneurysms). MRA, CTA, and/or conventional angiography may be employed for diagnostic, screening, and treatment planning purposes.

8.3. Cavernous Sinus Thrombosis

Cavernous sinus thrombosis is often associated with clinical and imaging evidence of paranasal sinusitis and orbital cellulitis *(78)*. Routine MRI may demonstrate absence of the normal flow voids. Thin-section coronal gadolinium-enhanced MRI will demonstrate a lack of normal contrast enhancement. CTV and/or conventional venography can be used to confirm the diagnosis, assess the degree of extension into the other intracranial/cervical venous structures, and monitor the effect of treatment.

◄──

Fig. 19. Pituitary apoplexy in a 21-year-old female with the sudden onset of headache during the second trimester of pregnancy. (A) Axial T2-weighted image. There is a suprasellar lesion (arrow) containing a fluid–fluid (hematocrit) level. (B) Sagittal T1-weighted image without gadolinium. A hematocrit level (arrow) is present. The dependent fluid is hypointense on the T2-weighted image and is isointense on the T1-weighted image, consistent with deoxyhemoglobin (acute stage blood). The nondependent fluid is hyperintense on both the T2-weighted and T1-weighted images, consistent with extracellular methemoglobin (late subacute stage blood). Images courtesy of Arastoo Vossough, PhD, MD.

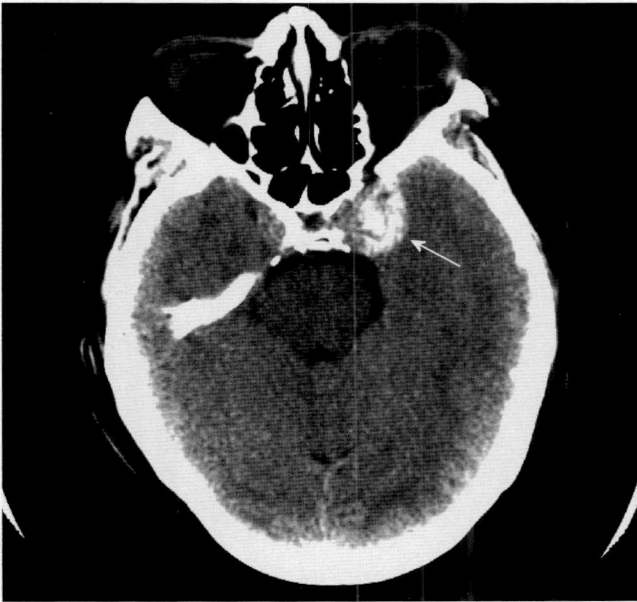

(A)

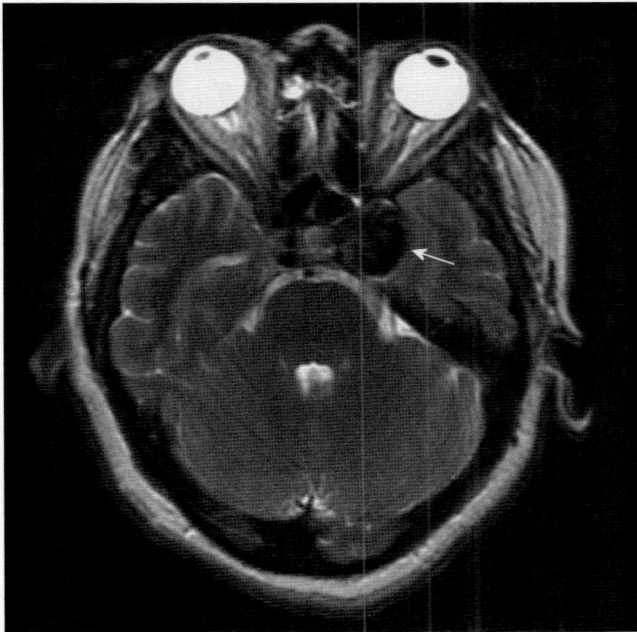

(B)

Fig. 20. (Continued)

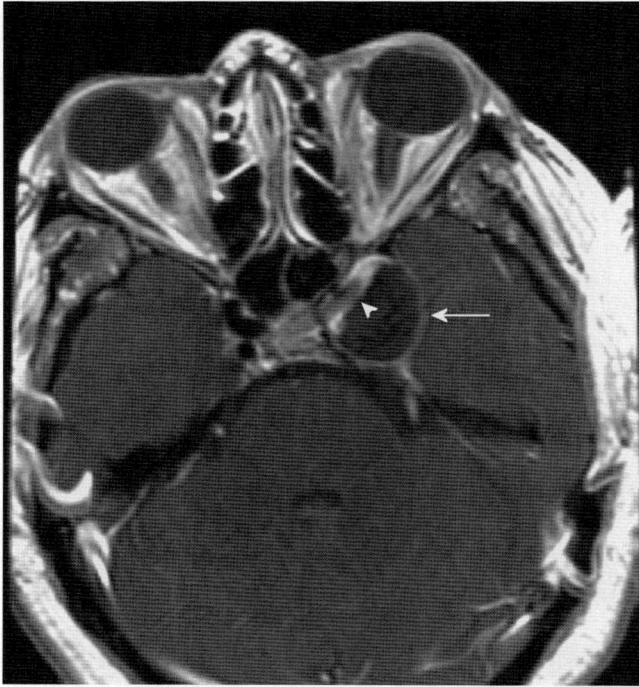

(C)

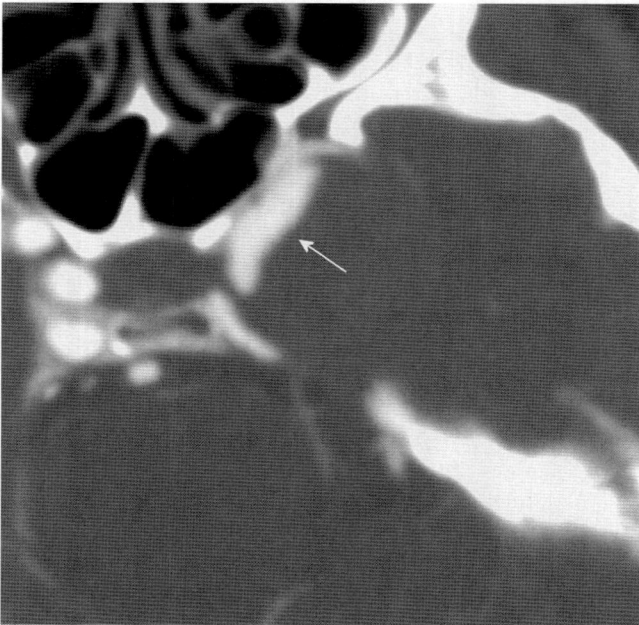

(D)

Fig. 20. (Continued)

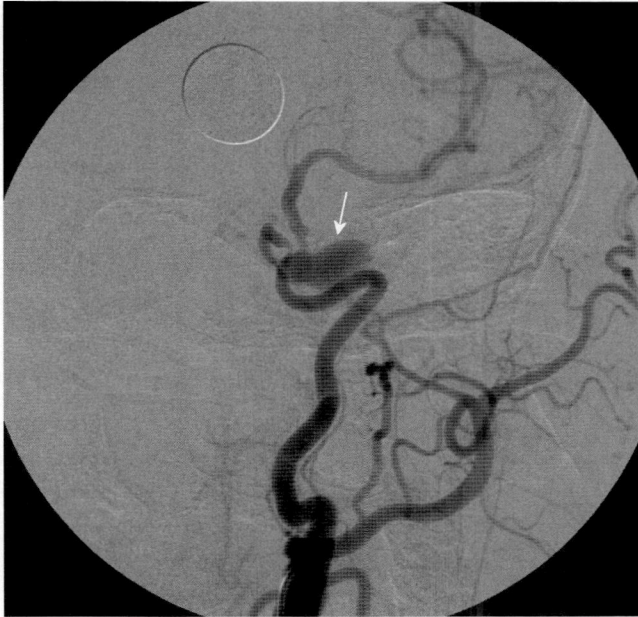

(E)

Fig. 20. Aneurysm of the cavernous carotid artery in a 51-year-old female with left ptosis, diplopia, and headache. (A) Axial nonenhanced CT. A hyperdense lesion (arrow) is centered along the lateral aspect of the left cavernous sinus. (B) Axial T2-weighted image. The lesion (arrow) involves the left cavernous sinus. A normal left cavernous carotid artery flow void is not seen. (C) Axial gadolinium-enhanced T1-weighted image. There is thin linear peripheral enhancement (arrow) with more prominent tubular enhancement at the anteromedial aspect of the lesion (arrowhead). (D) Axial maximum intensity projection (MIP) CTA reconstruction. Contrast fills the anteromedial aspect (arrow) of a partially thrombosed left cavernous carotid artery aneurysm. (E) Catheter angiogram. A lobulated cavity (arrow) communicates with an irregular left cavernous carotid artery.

REFERENCES

1. Elster AD, Chen MY, Williams DW 3rd, Key LL. Pituitary gland: MR imaging of physiologic hypertrophy in adolescence. Radiology 1990;174:681–5.
2. Suzuki M, Takashima T, Kadoya M, et al. Height of normal pituitary gland on MR imaging: age and sex differentiation. J Comput Assist Tomogr 1990;14:36–9.
3. Simmons GE, Suchnicki JE, Rak KM, Damiano TR. MR imaging of the pituitary stalk: size, shape, and enhancement pattern. AJR Am J Roentgenol 1992;159:375–7.
4. Elster AD, Sanders TG, Vines FS, Chen MY. Size and shape of the pituitary gland during pregnancy and post partum: measurement with MR imaging. Radiology 1991;181:531–5.
5. Bonneville F, Cattin F, Marsot-Dupuch K, Dormont D, Bonneville JF, Chiras J. T1 signal hyperintensity in the sellar region: spectrum of findings. Radiographics 2006;26:93–113.

6. Kucharczyk J, Kucharczyk W, Berry I, de Groot J, Kelly W, Norman D. and Newton TH. Histochemical characterization and functional significance of the hyperintense signal on MR images of the posterior pituitary. AJR Am J Roentgenol 1989;152:153–7.

7. Kucharczyk W, Lenkinski RE, Kucharczyk J. and Henkelman RM. The effect of phospholipid vesicles on the NMR relaxation of water: an explanation for the MR appearance of the neurohypophysis? AJNR Am J Neuroradiol 1990;11:693–700.

8. Kurokawa H, Fujisawa I, Nakano Y, et al. Posterior lobe of the pituitary gland: correlation between signal intensity on T1-weighted MR images and vasopressin concentration. Radiology 1998;207:79–83.

9. Elster AD. Imaging of the sella: anatomy and pathology. Semin Ultrasound CT MR 1993;14:182–94.

10. Cox TD, Elster AD. Normal pituitary gland: changes in shape, size, and signal intensity during the 1st year of life at MR imaging. Radiology 1991;179:721–4.

11. Sato N, Ishizaka H, Matsumoto M, Matsubara K, Tsushima Y. and Tomioka K. MR detectability of posterior pituitary high signal and direction of frequency encoding gradient. J Comput Assist Tomogr 1991;15:355–8.

12. Tien RD. Sequence of enhancement of various portions of the pituitary gland on gadolinium-enhanced MR images: correlation with regional blood supply. AJR Am J Roentgenol 1992;158:651–4.

13. Yuh WT, Fisher DJ, Nguyen HD, Tali ET, Gao F, Simonson TM, Schlechte JA. Sequential MR enhancement pattern in normal pituitary gland and in pituitary adenoma. AJNR Am J Neuroradiol 1994;15:101–8.

14. Ezzat S, Asa SL, Couldwell WT, Barr CE, Dodge WE, Vance ML, McCutcheon IE. The prevalence of pituitary adenomas: a systematic review. Cancer 2004;101:613–19.

15. Bonneville JF, Bonneville F. and Cattin F. Magnetic resonance imaging of pituitary adenomas. Eur Radiol 2005;15:543–8.

16. Zee CS, Go JL, Kim PE, Mitchell D, Ahmadi J. Imaging of the pituitary and parasellar region. Neurosurg Clin N Am 2003;14:55–80.

17. Naidich MJ, Russell EJ. Current approaches to imaging of the sellar region and pituitary. Endocrinol Metab Clin North Am 1999;28:45–79.

18. Buchfelder M, Nistor R, Fahlbusch R. and Huk WJ. The accuracy of CT and MR evaluation of the sella turcica for detection of adrenocorticotropic hormone-secreting adenomas in Cushing disease. AJNR Am J Neuroradiol 1993;14:1183–90.

19. Sakamoto Y, Takahashi M, Korogi Y, Bussaka H. and Ushio Y. Normal and abnormal pituitary glands: gadopentetate dimeglumine-enhanced MR imaging. Radiology 1991;178:441–5.

20. Bartynski WS, Lin L. Dynamic and conventional spin-echo MR of pituitary microlesions. AJNR Am J Neuroradiol 1997;18:965–72.

21. Patronas N, Bulakbasi N, Stratakis CA, et al. Spoiled gradient recalled acquisition in the steady state technique is superior to conventional postcontrast spin echo technique for magnetic resonance imaging detection of adrenocorticotropin-secreting pituitary tumors. J Clin Endocrinol Metab 2003;88:1565–9.

22. Donovan JL, Nesbit GM. Distinction of masses involving the sella and suprasellar space: specificity of imaging features. AJR Am J Roentgenol 1996;167:597–603.

23. Scotti G, Yu CY, Dillon WP, et al. MR imaging of cavernous sinus involvement by pituitary adenomas. AJR Am J Roentgenol 1988;151:799–806.

24. Vieira JO Jr, Cukiert A. and Liberman B. Evaluation of magnetic resonance imaging criteria for cavernous sinus invasion in patients with pituitary adenomas: logistic regression analysis and correlation with surgical findings. Surg Neurol 2006;65:130–5.

25. Cottier JP, Destrieux C, Brunereau L, et al. Cavernous sinus invasion by pituitary adenoma: MR imaging. Radiology 2000. 215, 463–9.
26. Pierallini A, Caramia F, Falcone C, et al. Pituitary macroadenomas: preoperative evaluation of consistency with diffusion-weighted MR imaging—initial experience. Radiology 2006;239:223–31.
27. Arita K, Tominaga A, Sugiyama K, et al. Natural course of incidentally found nonfunctioning pituitary adenoma, with special reference to pituitary apoplexy during follow-up examination. J Neurosurg 2006;104:884–91.
28. FitzPatrick M, Tartaglino LM, Hollander MD, Zimmerman RA, Flanders AE. Imaging of sellar and parasellar pathology. Radiol Clin North Am 1999;37:101–21.
29. Molla E, Marti-Bonmati L, Revert A, et al. Craniopharyngiomas: identification of different semiological patterns with MRI. Eur Radiol 2002;12:1829–36.
30. Curran JG, O'Connor E. Imaging of craniopharyngioma. Childs Nerv Syst 2005;21:635–9.
31. Fujimaki T, Matsutani M, Funada N, et al. CT and MRI features of intracranial germ cell tumors. J Neurooncol 1994;19:217–26.
32. Connor SE, Penney CC. MRI in the differential diagnosis of a sellar mass. Clin Radiol 2003;58:20–31.
33. Tomura N, Takahashi S, Kato K, et al. and Mizoi K. Germ cell tumors of the central nervous system originating from non-pineal regions: CT and MR features. Comput Med Imaging Graph 2000;24:269–76.
34. Smirniotopoulos JG, Chiechi MV. Teratomas, dermoids, and epidermoids of the head and neck. Radiographics 1995;15:1437–55.
35. Kornreich L, Blaser S, Schwarz M, et al. Optic pathway glioma: correlation of imaging findings with the presence of neurofibromatosis. AJNR Am J Neuroradiol 2001;22:1963–9.
36. Kurkjian C, Armor JF, Kamble R, Ozer H. and Kharfan-Dabaja MA. Symptomatic metastases to the pituitary infundibulum resulting from primary breast cancer. Int J Clin Oncol 2005;10:191–4.
37. Teears RJ, Silverman EM. Clinicopathologic review of 88 cases of carcinoma metastatic to the pituitary gland. Cancer 1975;36:216–20.
38. Frangoul HA, Shaw DW, Hawkins D, Park J. Diabetes insipidus as a presenting symptom of acute myelogenous leukemia. J Pediatr Hematol Oncol 2000;22:457–9.
39. Rye AD, Stitson RN, Dyer MJ. Pituitary infiltration in B-cell chronic lymphocytic leukaemia. Br J Haematol 2001;115:718.
40. Megan Ogilvie C, Payne S, Evanson J, Lister TA, Grossman AB. Lymphoma metastasizing to the pituitary: an unusual presentation of a treatable disease. Pituitary 2005;8:139–46.
41. Laigle-Donadey F, Taillibert S, Martin-Duverneuil N, Hildebrand J. and Delattre JY. Skull-base metastases. J Neurooncol 2005;75:63–9.
42. Yilmazlar S, Kocaeli H. and Cordan T. Sella turcica metastasis from follicular carcinoma of thyroid. Neurol Res 2004;26:74–8.
43. Aung TH, Po YC, Wong WK. Hepatocellular carcinoma with metastasis to the skull base, pituitary gland, sphenoid sinus, and cavernous sinus. Hong Kong Med J 2002;8:48–51.
44. Endo K, Okano R, Kuroda Y, Yamada S. and Tabei K. Renal cell carcinoma with skull base metastasis preceded by paraneoplastic signs in a chronic hemodialysis patient. Intern Med 2001;40:924–30.
45. Eisenberg MB, Al-Mefty O, DeMonte F, and Burson GT. Benign nonmeningeal tumors of the cavernous sinus. Neurosurgery 1999;44:949–54.
46. Meyers SP, Hirsch WL Jr, Curtin HD, Barnes L, Sekhar LN, Sen C. Chordomas of the skull base: MR features. AJNR Am J Neuroradiol 1992;13:1627–36.

47. Pamir MN, Ozduman K. Analysis of radiological features relative to histopathology in 42 skull-base chordomas and chondrosarcomas. Eur J Radiol 2006;58:461–70.

48. Maixner W. Hypothalamic hamartomas—clinical, neuropathological and surgical aspects. Childs Nerv Syst 2006;22:867–73.

49. Boyko OB, Curnes JT, Oakes WJ, Burger PC. Hamartomas of the tuber cinereum: CT, MR, and pathologic findings. AJNR Am J Neuroradiol 1991;12:309–14.

50. Burton EM, Ball WS, Jr., Crone K. and Dolan LM. Hamartoma of the tuber cinereum: a comparison of MR and CT findings in four cases. AJNR Am J Neuroradiol 1989;10: 497–501.

51. Rottenberg GT, Chong WK, Powell M. and Kendall BE. Cyst formation of the craniopharyngeal duct. Clin Radiol 1994;49:126–9.

52. Teramoto A, Hirakawa K, Sanno N. and Osamura Y. Incidental pituitary lesions in 1,000 unselected autopsy specimens. Radiology 1994;193:161–4.

53. Kucharczyk W, Peck WW, Kelly WM, Norman D. and Newton TH. Rathke cleft cysts: CT, MR imaging, and pathologic features. Radiology 1987;165:491–5.

54. Naylor MF, Scheithauer BW, Forbes GS, Tomlinson FH, Young WF. Rathke cleft cyst: CT, MR, and pathology of 23 cases. J Comput Assist Tomogr 1995;19:853–9.

55. Sumida M, Uozumi T, Mukada K, Arita K, Kurisu K, Eguchi K. Rathke cleft cysts: correlation of enhanced MR and surgical findings. AJNR Am J Neuroradiol 1994;15: 525–32.

56. Byun WM, Kim OL, Kim D. MR imaging findings of Rathke's cleft cysts: significance of intracystic nodules. AJNR Am J Neuroradiol 2000;21:485–8.

57. Binning MJ, Gottfried ON, Osborn AG, Couldwell WT. Rathke cleft cyst intracystic nodule: a characteristic magnetic resonance imaging finding. J Neurosurg 2005;103:837–40.

58. Nomura M, Tachibana O, Hasegawa M, et al. Contrast-enhanced MRI of intrasellar arachnoid cysts: relationship between the pituitary gland and cyst. Neuroradiology 1996;38:566–8.

59. Miyajima M, Arai H, Okuda O, Hishii M, Nakanishi H. and Sato K. Possible origin of suprasellar arachnoid cysts: neuroimaging and neurosurgical observations in nine cases. J Neurosurg 2000;93:62–7.

60. Shin JL, Asa SL, Woodhouse LJ, Smyth HS, Ezzat S. Cystic lesions of the pituitary: clinicopathological features distinguishing craniopharyngioma Rathke's cleft cyst, and arachnoid cyst. J Clin Endocrinol Metab 1999;84:3972–82.

61. Harter LP, Silverberg GD, Brant-Zawadzki M. Intrasellar arachnoid cyst: case report. Neurosurgery 1980;7:387–90.

62. Bergui M, Zhong J, Bradac GB, Sales S. Diffusion-weighted images of intracranial cyst-like lesions. Neuroradiology 2001;43:824–9.

63. Ikushima I, Korogi Y, Hirai T, et al. MR of epidermoids with a variety of pulse sequences. AJNR Am J Neuroradiol 1997;18:1359–63.

64. Agid R, Farb RI, Willinsky RA, Mikulis DJ, Tomlinson G. Idiopathic intracranial hypertension: the validity of cross-sectional neuroimaging signs. Neuroradiology 2006;48:521–7.

65. Maira G, Anile C. and Mangiola A. Primary empty sella syndrome in a series of 142 patients. J Neurosurg 2005;103:831–6.

66. Bursztyn EM, Lavyne MH, Aisen M. Empty sella syndrome with intrasellar herniation of the optic chiasm. AJNR Am J Neuroradiol 1983;4:167–8.

67. Rivera JA. Lymphocytic hypophysitis: Disease spectrum and approach to diagnosis and therapy. Pituitary 2006;9:35–45.

68. Smith JK, Matheus MG, Castillo M. Imaging manifestations of neurosarcoidosis. AJR Am J Roentgenol 2004;182:289–95.

69. Bernaerts A, Vanhoenacker FM, Parizel PM, et al. Tuberculosis of the central nervous system: overview of neuroradiological findings. Eur Radiol 2003;13:1876–90.
70. Desai KI, Nadkarni TD, Goel A. Tuberculomas of the hypophysis cerebri: report of five cases. J Clin Neurosci 2003;10:562–6.
71. Prayer D, Grois N, Prosch H, Gadner H. and Barkovich AJ. MR imaging presentation of intracranial disease associated with Langerhans cell histiocytosis. AJNR Am J Neuroradiol 2004;25:880–91.
72. Makras P, Samara C, Antoniou M, et al. Evolving radiological features of hypothalamo-pituitary lesions in adult patients with Langerhans cell histiocytosis (LCH). Neuroradiology 2006;48:37–44.
73. Wasmeier C, Pfadenhauer K. and Rosler A. Idiopathic inflammatory pseudotumor of the orbit and Tolosa–Hunt syndrome—are they the same disease? J Neurol 2002;249:1237–41.
74. Yousem DM, Atlas SW, Grossman RI, Sergott RC, Savino PJ, Bosley TM. MR imaging of Tolosa–Hunt syndrome. AJNR Am J Neuroradiol 1989;10:1181–4.
75. Takayasu T, Yamasaki F, Tominaga A, Hidaka T, Arita K, Kurisu KA. Pituitary abscess showing high signal intensity on diffusion-weighted imaging. Neurosurg Rev 2006;29:246–8.
76. Rogg JM, Tung GA, Anderson G. and Cortez S. Pituitary apoplexy: early detection with diffusion-weighted MR imaging. AJNR Am J Neuroradiol 2002;23:1240–5.
77. Lavallee G, Morcos R, Palardy J, Aube M. and Gilbert D. MR of nonhemorrhagic postpartum pituitary apoplexy. AJNR Am J Neuroradiol 1995;16:1939–41.
78. Eustis HS, Mafee MF, Walton C, Mondonca J. MR imaging and CT of orbital infections and complications in acute rhinosinusitis. Radiol Clin North Am 1998;36:1165–83.

5   Neuro-ophthalmology of Sellar Disease

Dean M. Cestari, MD, and Joseph F. Rizzo III, MD

CONTENTS

Summary

The degree to which a patient with sellar pathology has been neurologically affected by the lesion can be best determined with a neuro-ophthalmic examination, which traditionally includes a detailed historical assessment and physical examination. With lesions in the sellar region, the clinical neuro-ophthalmologic examination often reveals neural dysfunction because several important afferent and efferent visual pathways course near this area. The combination of neuroradiological, neuroendocrinological, and neuro-ophthalmological assessment is needed to properly manage the typical patient with a parasellar lesion. This chapter will provide an overview of the relevant anatomy and clinical neuro-ophthalmic features of lesions that affect the sellar region.

From: *Contemporary Endocrinology: Diagnosis and Management of Pituitary Disorders*
Edited by: B. Swearingen and B. M. K. Biller © Humana Press, Totowa, NJ

Key Words: vision, Visual field, chiasm.

1. INTRODUCTION

The pituitary gland sits in the skull base in a bony indentation called the sella turcica. Many different types of lesions can present within the sella turcica or the surrounding parasellar areas (Fig. 1). Pituitary adenomas are by far the most common lesion to arise in this area, accounting for over 90 % of masses

Intrasellar

Common
  Physiologic hypertrophy
  Microadenoma
  Cyst (Rathke's cleft, pars intermedia)
Rare
  Craniopharyngioma
  Metastasis
Rare but important
  Aneurysm
  Paramedian internal carotid artery

Infundibular stalk

Uncommon
  Germinoma
  Lymphoma/leukemia
  Sarcoid
  Histiocytosis
  Metastasis
  Meningitis
  Astrocytoma
Rare
  Hypophysitis
  Pituicytoma
  Choristoma

Suprasellar

Common
  Macroadenoma (upward extension)
  Meningioma
  Aneurysm
  Craniopharyngioma
  Glioma (usually pilocytic astrocytoma)
Uncommon
  Lipoma
  Dermoid/epidermoid
  Cyst (arachnoid, Rathke cleft, inflammatory)
  Focal meningitis
  Metastasis
  Ectopic neurohypophysis
Rare
  Hamartoma (tuber cinereum)
  Hypophysitis

Anterior third ventricle/optic chiasm

Common
  Glioma
Uncommon
  Germinoma
  Metastasis
  Colloid cyst (foramen of Monró)
  Glioependymal cyst

Sphenoid/cavernous sinus

Common
  Metastasis (direct, hematogenous)
  Sinusitis/osteomyelitis
  Meningioma
Uncommon
  Schwannoma
  Thrombosis
  Lymphoma
Rare
  Chordoma
  Osteocartilaginous tumors

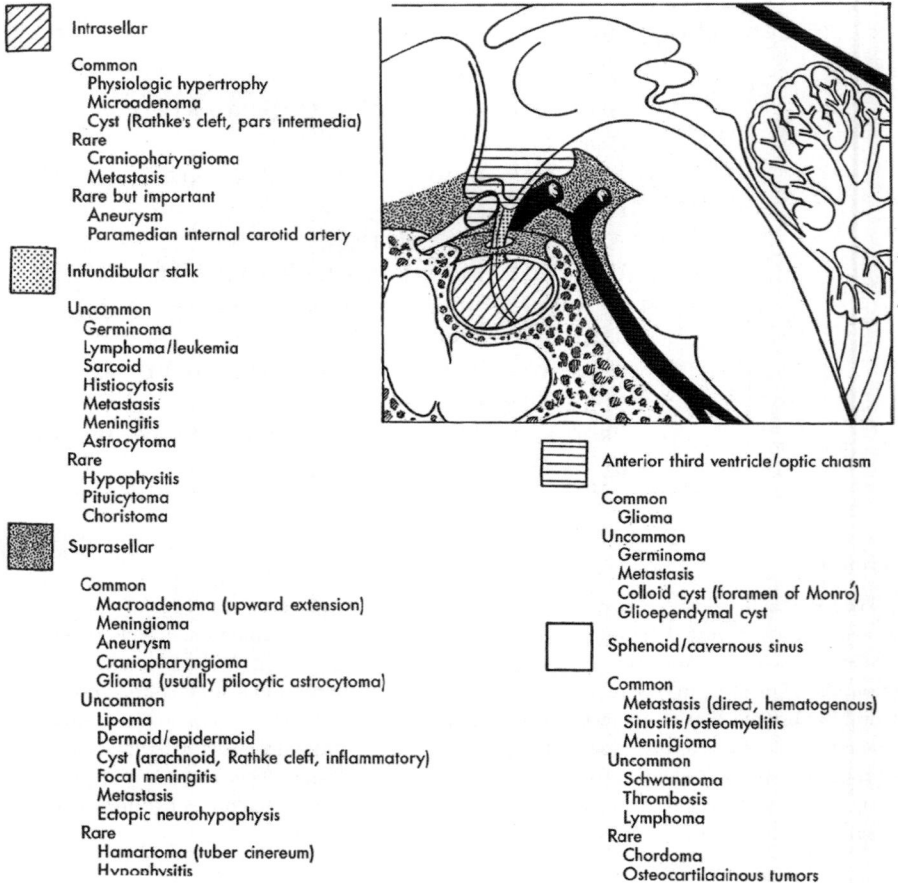

Fig. 1. Anatomic diagram depicts the sella turcica and suprasellar region as seen from the lateral view. Common lesions and their differential diagnosis by location are indicated. (Reproduced with permission from Anne G, Osborn MD. Diagnostic Neuroradiology. St Louis, Mo: Mosby; 1994.)

that develop in this region. The second most common lesion in this area is the craniopharyngioma *(1)*. A large number of other, relatively uncommon lesions that can occasionally arise in this region include meningiomas, Rathke's pouch cysts, lymphoma, teratomas, metastatic lesions, inflammations (i.e., sarcoidosis, histiocytic lesions, lymphocytic adenohypophysisitis), infections (spreading from the paranasal sinuses or subarachnoid space), and vascular lesions (i.e., arteriovenous malformations and aneurysms). This rather broad differential diagnostic list can usually be reconciled to a single diagnosis or two by high-quality neuroimaging. However, the degree to which a patient has been clinically affected by the lesion can be best determined with a neuro-ophthalmic examination, which traditionally includes a detailed historical assessment and physical examination. With lesions in the sellar region, the clinical neuro-ophthalmologic examination often reveals neural dysfunction because several important afferent and efferent visual pathways course near this area. The combination of neuroradiological, neuroendocrinological, and neuro-ophthalmological assessment is needed to properly manage the typical patient with a parasellar lesion.

This chapter will provide an overview of the relevant anatomy and clinical neuro-ophthalmic features of lesions that affect the sellar region.

2. ANATOMY OF THE OPTIC CHIASM AND THE PARASELLAR REGION

The bony indentation within the skull base that is referred to as the sella turcica is open superiorly, where it is covered by a sheet of dura mater known as the diaphragma sella, which is a pain-sensitive structure innervated by branches of the fifth cranial nerve. The pituitary stalk, or infundibulum, passes through an opening in the center of the diaphragma sella to connect the overlying hypothalamus to the pituitary gland. The lateral walls of the sella turcica are formed by the cavernous sinus, which is lined medially and laterally by dura mater and which contains cranial nerves III, IV, V1, V2, and VI, a plexus of sympathetic nerve fibers, and the internal carotid artery (Fig. 2). The sphenoid sinus sits below the sella (Fig. 3). The planum sphenoidale is a flat, bony plane above and just in front of the sella turcica. The anterior and posterior clinoid processes demarcate the gross boundaries of the deformation in the skull base that forms the sella turcica (Fig. 4).

The optic chiasm is an X-shaped structure that is composed of the only afferent fibers from the eye to the brain. The chiasm is tilted forward approximately 45° and lies within the subarachnoid space, just inferior to the hypothalamus and anterior to the pituitary stalk. It measures approximately 12 mm wide, 8 mm in anteroposterior diameter, and 4 mm thick. The chiasm is positioned approximately 10 mm above the pituitary gland, although the

Optic chiasm and cavernous sinuses (coronal section)

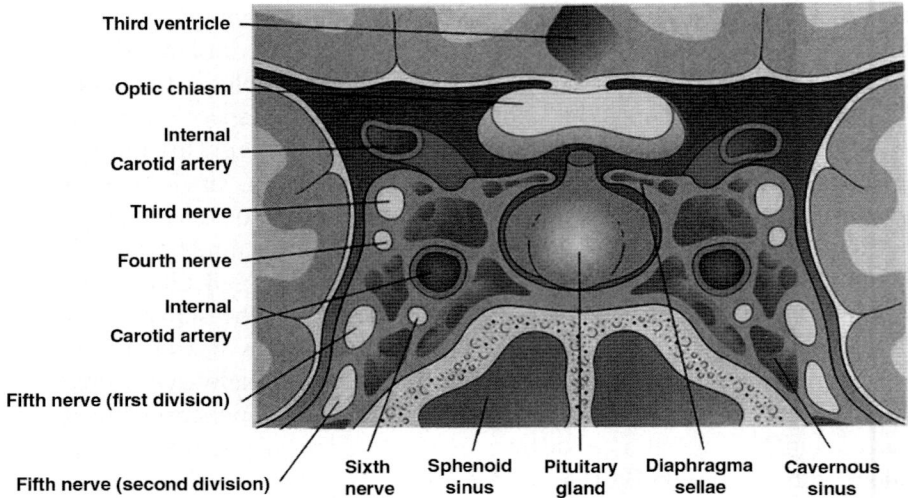

Fig. 2. Coronal section through the optic chiasm and cavernous sinuses. The chiasm is flanked laterally by the supraclinoid segments of the carotid arteries and inferolaterally by the cavernous sinuses through which pass the oculomotor nerves and the first two divisions of the trigeminal nerve. (Reproduced with permission; Yanoff M, Duker JS, editors. Ophthalmology, 2nd ed. St Louis, Mo: Mosby; 2004.)

relative position of the chiasm to the pituitary gland varies from person to person *(2)*. The chiasm lies directly above the pituitary gland in 80% of people, is anterior or "prefixed" and laying over the tuberculum sella in 15% of people, and is posterior or "postfixed" laying over the dorsum sella in 5% of people (Fig. 5) *(3)*.This variability in the position of the chiasm has clinical significance (*see* below).

The X-shaped configuration of the chiasm is the result of the decussation of axons of the retinal ganglion cells that exit from the retinas of both eyes and these axons course toward the brain. Each optic nerve contains approximately 1.2 million axons that transmit visual information from the retina to the brain *(4)*. The retina can be functionally divided into nasal and temporal regions. Light rays that enter the eye from the temporal visual field pass through the pupil and stimulate the nasal retina; conversely, light entering from the nasal visual field stimulates the temporal retina. Axons from the nasal retinae of both eyes cross at the chiasm, whereas fibers from the temporal retinae remain ipsilateral en route to the lateral geniculate body, where all but a small percentage of optic nerve axons synapse. The ratio of crossed to uncrossed fibers is roughly 53:47. The

Relationship of chiasm to neighboring structures (median sagittal section)

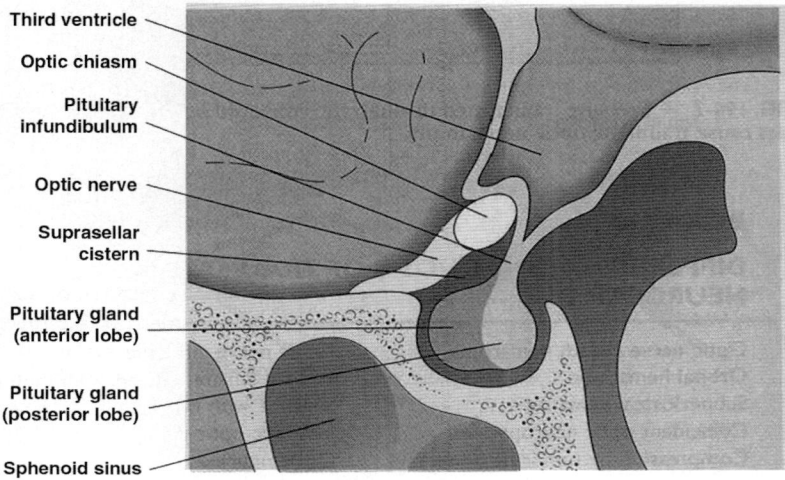

Fig. 3. Median sagittal section through the chiasm and relationship of chiasm to neighboring structures. The optic chiasm is suspended above the pituitary gland and rests in the sella turcica of the sphenoid bone. It is surrounded by cerebrospinal fluid, except posteriorly where it borders the anterior inferior wall of the third ventricle. (Reproduced with permission, Yanoff M, Duker JS, editors. Ophthalmology, 2nd ed. St Louis, Mo: Mosby; 2004.)

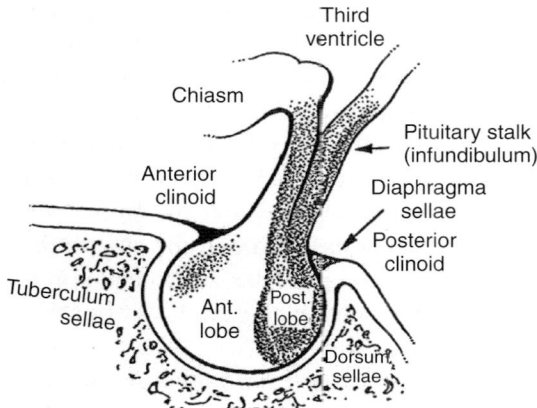

Fig. 4. Drawing, sagittal view, of the chiasm, pituitary gland, and sella. Ant. lobe = anterior lobe of the pituitary gland. Post. lobe = posterior lobe of the pituitary gland. (Reproduced with permission, Liu GT, Volve NJ, Galetta SL. Neuro-ophthalmology Diagnosis and Management. Philadelphia: W.B. Saunders Company; 2001.)

58

Length of optic nerve affects relative position of the chiasm and sellar structures

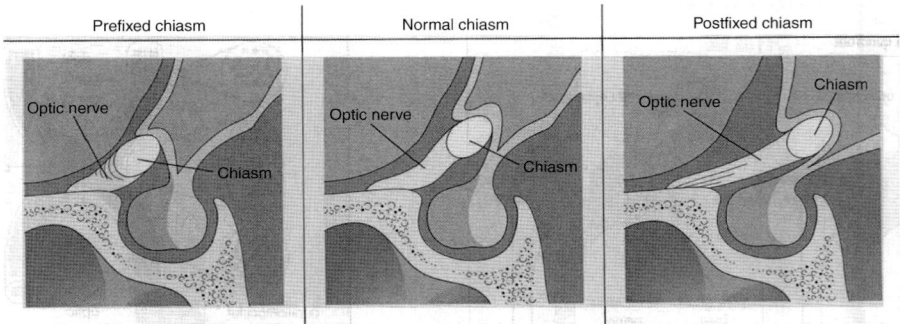

Fig. 5. Variations in the length of the optic nerves alters the relative position of the chiasm to the sellar structures. Prefixed chiasm overlies the chiasmatic sulcus or the tuberculum sellae; normal chiasm overlies the diaphragma sellae; postfixed chiasm lies above the dorsum sellae. (Reproduced with permission, Yanoff M, Duker JS, editors. Ophthalmology, 2nd ed. St Louis, Mo: Mosby, 2004.)

presence of this horizontal decussation of fibers makes it possible for one side of the occipital lobe to receive visual information from both eyes that corresponds to the same side of the visual field. Specifically, the presence of the chiasm makes it possible, for instance, for the right side of the occipital lobe to receive afferent input from the left side of the visual field of both eyes; this input is received from the temporal retina of the ipsilateral eye and the nasal retina of the contralateral (i.e., left) eye (*see* Fig. 6 and Color Plate 9).

The vertical orientation of fibers that emerge from the retina does not change as the axons pass through the chiasm. Axons from the superior retina (i.e., those that subserve the inferior visual field) course through the superior aspect of the chiasm, while axons that originate from the inferior retina (i.e., those that subserve the superior visual field) course through the inferior aspect of the chiasm *(5)*. The majority of fibers in each optic nerve subserve "central" vision, i.e., the region that corresponds to the outflow from the macula. Thus, the majority of all nerve fibers that pass through the chiasm also subserve central vision. This anatomical principle provides an explanation for some characteristics of the visual fields in patients who have lesions of the chiasm (*see* Fig. 7 and Color Plate 10).

Historically, there has been carried forth a notion of an anatomical quirk at the level of the chiasm known as Wilbrand's knee. It had been believed, based on a single anatomical study, that the inferonasal fibers of the posterior optic nerves entered the chiasm and then bent upward approximately 3 mm forward into the contralateral optic nerve before turning posteriorly again. It is now recognized that Wilbrand's knee was an artifact caused by the selective study

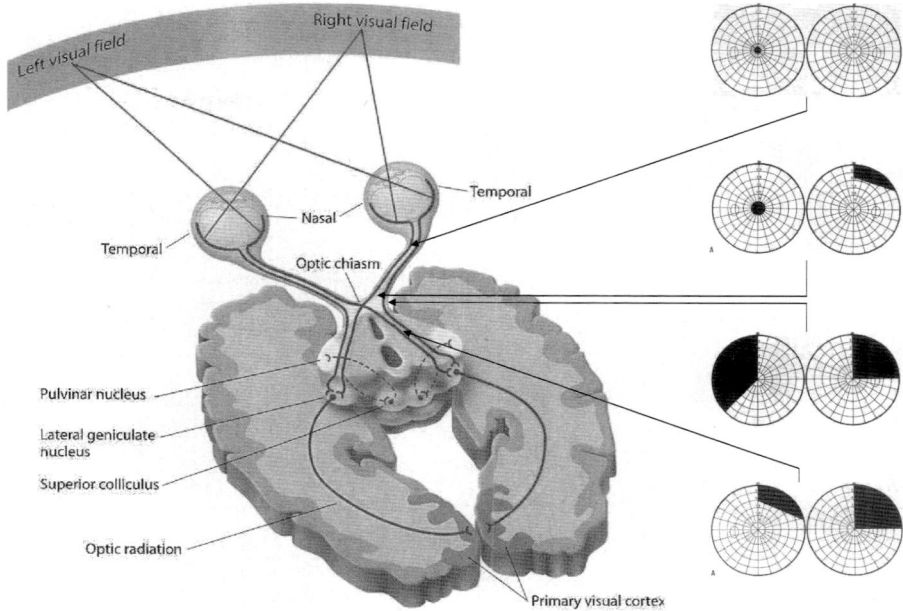

Fig. 6. Horizontal section of the visual pathways. The visual fields demonstrate the correlation of lesion site and field defect. (Reproduced with permission, Yanoff M, Duker JS, editors. Ophthalmology, 2nd ed. St Louis, Mo: Mosby; 2004.) (*See* Color Plate 9.)

of two patients who had each lost one eye *(6,7)*. The gliosis of the residual, posterior segment of the optic nerve in these patients seemingly caused a deformation of the proximal fibers of the optic chiasm. Curiously, clinicians have long recognized a pattern of visual field deficit (i.e., the "junctional" scotoma) that was thought to be explained by the presence of a Wilbrand's knee. This discrepancy cannot be explained, but it is still believed that the finding of a junctional scotoma correlates with lesions that arise at the junction of the optic nerve and chiasm (Fig. 7).

All but a very small number of axons that enter the chiasm leave the chiasm posteriorly to form the left and right optic tracts *(8)*. Each optic tract is composed of the ipsilateral temporal and contralateral nasal retinal fibers. The small number of fibers, perhaps 20,000 or so (out of roughly 2.4 million), that exit the posterior aspect of the chiasm at its interface with the anterior aspect of the hypothalamus synapse directly with several nearby nuclei, including the suprachiasmal nuclei that control circadian rhythms that are regulated by the day versus night cycle via input from this retinohypothalmic tract *(9)*.

The optic chiasm is located between the anterior and posterior aspects of the circle of Willis, which receives its anterior blood supply from the internal

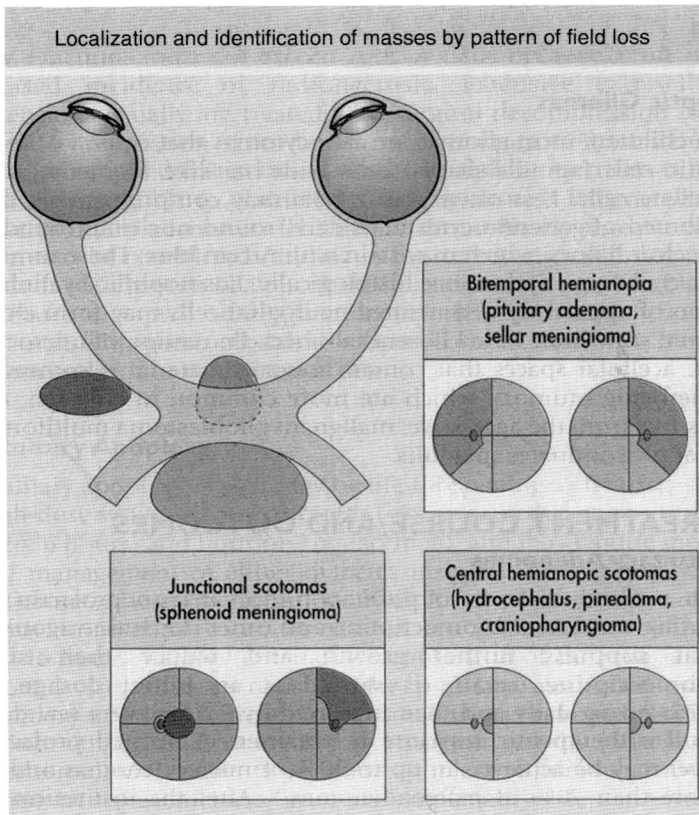

Fig. 7. Localization and probable identification of masses by pattern of field loss. Junctional scotomas occur with compression of the anterior angle of the chiasm (sphenoid meningiomas). Bitemporal hemianopia results from compression of the body of the chiasm from below (e.g., pituitary adenoma, sellar meningiomas). Compression of the posterior chiasm and its decussating nasal fibers may cause central bitemporal scotomas (e.g., hydrocephalus, pinealoma, craniopharyngioma). (Reproduced with permission, Yanoff M, Duker JS, editors. Ophthalmology, 2nd ed. St Louis, Mo: Mosby; 2004.) (*See* Color Plate 10.)

carotid arteries as they emerge from the cavernous sinuses (Fig. 8). These "supraclinoid" segments of the internal carotid arteries ascend lateral to the chiasm. Lying amidst these large blood vessels, the optic chiasm receives a generous blood supply from many small arteries that come off of the anterior cerebral, superior hypophyseal, internal carotid, posterior communicating, and posterior cerebral arteries. This rich suffusion of blood provides nearly foolproof protection of the optic chiasm from ischemia.

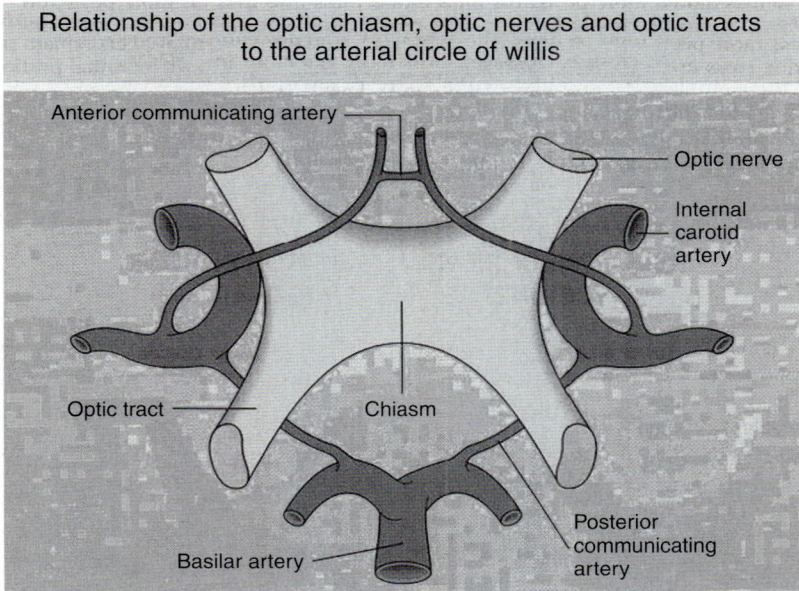

Fig. 8. Relationship of the optic chiasm, optic nerves, and optic tracts to the arterial circle of Willis. The chiasm passes through the circle of Willis and receives its arterial supply from the anterior cerebral and communicating arteries from above and the posterior communicating, posterior cerebral, and basilar arteries from below. (Reproduced with permission, Yanoff M, Duker JS, editors. Ophthalmology, 2nd ed. St Louis, Mo: Mosby; 2004.)

3. SIGNS AND SYMPTOMS OF SELLA AND PARASELLAR LESIONS

The clinical aspects of lesions that involve the chiasm and surrounding nerves can be divided into those that cause a disruption of afferent neuro-ophthalmic function (i.e., loss of visual input to the brain) versus those that cause a disruption of efferent neuro-ophthalmic function (i.e., alteration in eye movement control). Lesions in the parasellar region often cause both afferent and efferent neuro-ophthalmic dysfunction.

4. AFFERENT DYSFUNCTION

The time course or tempo of visual loss is often helpful in determining the etiology of blindness. Acute visual loss usually implies a vascular, inflammatory, infectious, or demyelinating etiology, whereas slow visual deterioration over weeks or months is more consistent with a slowly expanding lesion.

The afferent visual pathway is composed of nerve fibers that transmit visual information to the visual cortex and other areas of the brain. The crossing of optic nerve axons at the chiasm provides a means for the clinician to divide neuro-ophthalmic findings into distinct syndromes of prechiasmal, chiasmal, and postchiasmal disease. These clinical distinctions, which are made with a standard neuro-ophthalmological examination that provides information on central visual acuity, color vision, pupillary function, pattern of visual field loss, and the appearance of the optic nerve heads, quite often correlates with the neuroradiological evidence of the gross relationship between the location of a mass lesion and the location of the optic chiasm. However, the superb resolution of modern magnetic resonance imaging (MRI) scans has revealed frequent mismatches between the neuroradiological interpretation of involvement of the chiasm by a mass lesion and the results of a neuro-ophthalmological examination. In particular, MRI images often show apparent contact between a tumor and the chiasm without clinical evidence of visual loss.

4.1. Central Acuity

The ability to visually resolve fine details of an image is routinely tested by using some characteristic set of letters (i.e., optotypes). The Snellen chart has been the historical standard for such testing, but more recently a modification of this basic testing utilizes an "EDTRS" chart combined with a "log MAR" (log MAR is an expression of visual acuity as the logarithm of the mean visual resolution) stratification of the test lines. This allows an equally detailed measurement of visual function for patients with relatively good and relatively poor vision. The Snellen charts, for instance, provided comparatively little incremental assessment at the lower end of visual function, which thus compromised the ability to judge the relative degree to which vision improved after treatment if a group of patients with good and bad vision were being studied.

A mass lesion that compresses one optic nerve most typically impairs visual acuity from that eye, because as stated above, the majority of fibers from the optic nerve emerge from the macula, which provides the finest level of visual resolution. It is also true that at the level of the chiasm, central visual acuity is usually affected by compressive lesions because the majority of chiasmal fibers subserve central vision. However, for lesions of the retrochiasmal pathway (e.g., the optic tract), central visual acuity is not impaired if there is only unilateral involvement *(10)*. The central most visual projections from the retina, which derive from the fovea (i.e., the center of the macula), are equally distributed to both occipital cortices by the crossing and noncrossing fibers that pass through the chiasm *(11)*. Thus, complete ablation of one retrochiasmal visual structure (e.g., complete loss of one occipital lobe) does not degrade central visual acuity. In practice, lesions that compress the optic chiasm produce a wide range of central acuity *(12)*. Compression at the lateral margin of the chiasm may only impair central acuity in the ipsilateral eye, whereas compression of the chiasm proper, which is the most common scenario, commonly leads to an impairment of central visual acuity in both eyes. Lateral compression of the posterior optic nerve may produce a nasal depression of the visual field *(13)*. Generally, the degree of impairment of central acuity corresponds to the severity of the visual field defect in each eye *(10)*. It is important to note, however, that central visual acuity is not always a sensitive test of optic chiasm function and that it may remain normal in the setting of a compressive lesion that involves the optic chiasm.

4.2. Color Vision

Loss of color vision (i.e., dyschromatopsia) is a very sensitive indicator of optic nerve dysfunction. Asymmetry of color vision is an important clue to the presence of an optic neuropathy or chiasmal lesion, especially with respect to compressive lesions. A relatively easy and rapid screen of color vision is most typically performed with the Ishihara test plates. This test was designed to assess the frequent imperfections in color vision that are present because of genetic influences that alter the protein structure of the chromophores of the cones, which capture the incoming light rays. Approximately 7% of men and 0.1% of women have a congenital deficiency of color vision, which is usually along the red-green color axis *(14)*. The Ishihara plates test color function only along this most commonly affected axis. The Ishihara plates do not check vision along the blue-yellow axis, which is only rarely compromised by genetic factors but which is not uncommonly impaired with acquired lesions of the afferent visual pathway. An alternative test, the Hardy–Rand–Ritter plates, is also easy to use and provides an assessment across the entire color spectrum. Neither test should be considered to be a true quantitative assessment of vision. However, any asymmetry in color vision between the eyes, which would never result from a genetic mutation of the chromophores, is indicative of an acquired lesion of the afferent visual pathway. Even a slowing in the recognition of the color plates in one eye versus the other suggests an asymmetrical disruption in the afferent visual pathway. Highly quantitative measures of color vision (i.e., Farnsworth D-100 panel) are available but are not typically used in clinical practice because they are time-consuming and because the information gained from the additional detail does not impact on clinical decision making.

4.3. Pupil

The response of the pupils to a light stimulus is controlled by a reflex arc of the second (i.e., optic) and third cranial nerves. The afferent limb of this reflex arc is believed to be mediated by a relatively small population of "pupil-lomotor" retinal ganglion cells whose axons enter both optic nerves, course through the chiasm, and decussate in equal proportion to all other chiasmatic fibers that enter the optic tract. These pupillomotor fibers do not synapse at the lateral geniculate body en route to the primary occipital cortex, as do almost all other axons in the optic tract. Rather, the pupillomotor fibers exit the optic tract just before the tract reaches the lateral geniculate body, and course along the brachium of the superior colliculus to enter the midbrain, where they synapse within nuclei that provide the efferent (i.e., motor) drive that is transmitted by the third cranial nerve back out to the eye to cause pupillary constriction in response to a light stimulus (see Fig. 9 and Color Plate 11). The clinical examination of the pupillary responses to light can distinguish disruption along the afferent versus efferent limbs of the pupillomotor reflex pathway.

The assessment of the pupillary response to a light stimulus can be thought of as reflecting the overall amount of afferent input to the midbrain. Given the symmetry in the decussation of the pupillomotor fibers and the retinocal-carine fibers (which mediate conscious vision), it is reasonable to think of any asymmetry in afferent input of the pupillomotor reflex pathway as being

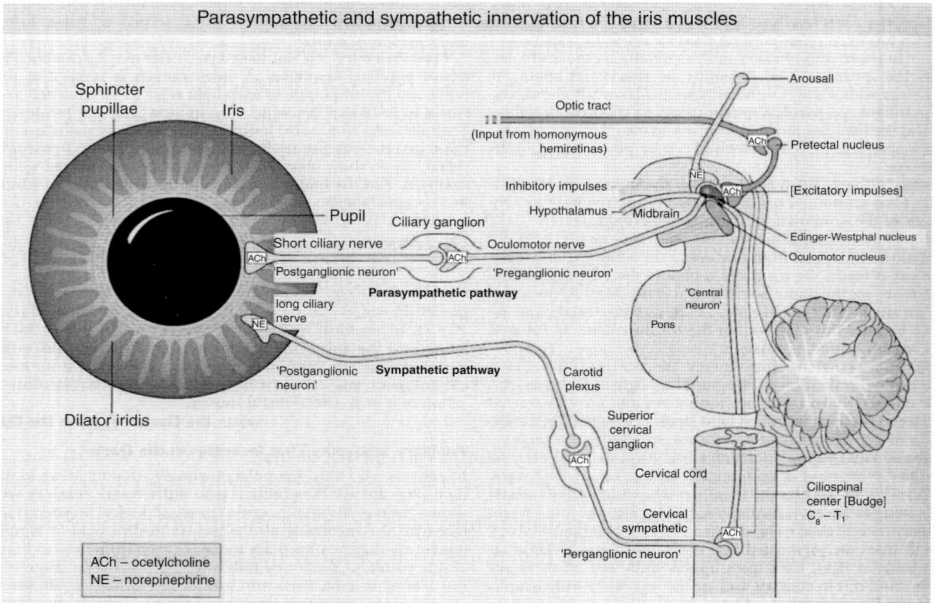

Fig. 9. Parasympathetic and sympathetic innervation of the iris muscles. (Reproduced with permission, Yanoff M, Duker JS, editors. Ophthalmology, 2nd ed. St Louis, Mo: Mosby; 2004.) (See Color Plate 11.)

somewhat reflective of a similar degree of disruption in the afferent input to the primary visual cortex. Indeed, there is a reasonably good correlation between the density of disruption of the pupillary response to light and a patient's perceived sense of the degree of brightness, which is mediated by the retinocalcarine pathway *(15)*.

Any roughly equivalent disruption in transmission between the two optic nerves produces pupillary responses to light that are similar, and thus not clinically useful when attempting to assess afferent visual function. By comparison, any disproportionate disruption in transmission between the optic nerves to the optic tracts produces a very valuable clinical sign of pupillary dysfunction. Such asymmetries in afferent input to the pupillomotor nuclei of the midbrain will produce a "relative afferent pupillary defect" (RAPD) *(16)*. This sign is one of the most sensitive and highly localizing signs in the field of clinical neurology. The relative activity of the pupils in response to light is best discerned by performing the "swinging-flashlight" test, in which a light stimulus is shone into one and then the other eye *(17)*. Care needs to be taken to stimulate both eyes equally. Normally, the pupillary responses to light are roughly identical when the light stimulus is shifted between the eyes. Any asymmetry in response of the pupils to light entering one eye versus the other is prima facie evidence of asymmetrical input to the midbrain pupillomotor nuclei and implies there is either an ipsilateral optic neuropathy, a maculopathy, or rarely a contralateral optic tract lesion.

Care must also be taken in the interpretation of these pupillary responses to light. In the presence of a lesion of one optic nerve, for instance, both pupils will respond relatively poorly to a light stimulus presented to the ipsilateral eye, but conversely both pupils will respond equally and more vigorously to a light stimulus presented to the normal (or better-seeing) eye. Light directed into the abnormal eye causes bilateral pupillary dilation (perhaps after an initial, brief constriction of the pupils) because of the reduced neural input that reaches the pretectal region of the midbrain *(18)*. This pattern of response must be distinguished from a disruption along the *efferent* limb of the pupillomotor reflex arc. An efferent pupillary defect (as is seen with a lesion of the third cranial nerve or more commonly as a manifestation of a tonic, or Adie's, pupillary defect) will produce a dilated pupil on the affected side that responds identically to a light stimulus that is shown into either eye.

A RAPD will usually be present ipsilateral to an optic neuropathy. A pure chiasmal syndrome will generally not cause a RAPD because of the symmetrical involvement of axons that cross in the chiasm. A postchiasmal but pregeniculate body lesion (i.e., an optic tract lesion) will produce a contralateral RAPD because the optic tract is composed of a greater number of crossed versus uncrossed axons from the retinal ganglion cellaxons *(19)*.

4.4. Funduscopy

The appearance of the optic nerve head as viewed in a funduscopic examination is an important part of the assessment of lesions of the afferent visual pathway. In general, the optic nerve may appear to be normal, or it may be swollen and pale or have pathological cupping. Optic nerve head edema is often seen with compressive or infiltrative lesions along the optic nerve, but edema is much less commonly observed with lesions that are as far posterior as the optic chiasm *(20)*. If a parasellar lesion is large enough to produce hydrocephalus (which is not common), then swelling of the optic nerve head would develop. In this case, swelling of the optic nerve head occurs secondary to elevated intracranial pressure, and the term "papilledema" may be applied to convey the finding of elevated optic nerve heads. With either etiology of nerve head swelling (i.e., direct compression/infiltration or elevation of the intracranial pressure), the swelling results from stasis of axoplasmic flow along the retinal ganglion cells axons that comprise the optic nerve and chiasm. Swelling of the optic nerve head, therefore, is a sign of metabolic compromise of these cells (*see* Fig. 10 and Color Plate 12).

A persistently swollen optic nerve head will eventually become pale; in this case, the resolution of the nerve head edema is not a sign of recovery but rather a sign of loss of nerve fibers. Atrophy of the fibers of the optic nerve produces a pale appearance of the optic nerve head. Pallor of the optic nerve will not become evident until 4 or more weeks after the injury to the fibers of the afferent pathway (Fig. 10).

Pathological expansion of the optic nerve cup is most commonly caused by glaucoma, but compressive lesions of the anterior visual pathway can also cause "cupping" *(21)*. Aneurysms located at the junction of the internal carotid and ophthalmic arteries are especially prone to cause pathological cupping of the optic nerves *(22)*. The combination of a pale and pathologically cupped optic nerve is not typically found in patients with glaucoma, and this combination of findings should raise suspicion of "neurogenic" causes of cupping, like compressive lesions in the sphenoid or parasellar region.

Other findings of the optic nerve head may have diagnostic value. Compressive lesions of the optic nerve can cause chronic optic disk swelling that may be associated with "shunt" vessels *(23)*. Infiltrative lesions along the optic nerve, especially optic nerve sheath meningiomas, can elevate the pressure in the central retinal vein and thus impair outflow from the eye. Shunt vessels, which are expansions of normal telangiectatic vessels, develop to permit egress of blood from the retina via the cilliary circulation. Shunt vessels are not found with lesions that originate from the parasellar region, but they may occur in cases of mass lesions that are more proximal along the anterior visual pathway (i.e., closer to the eyeball) and their detection by

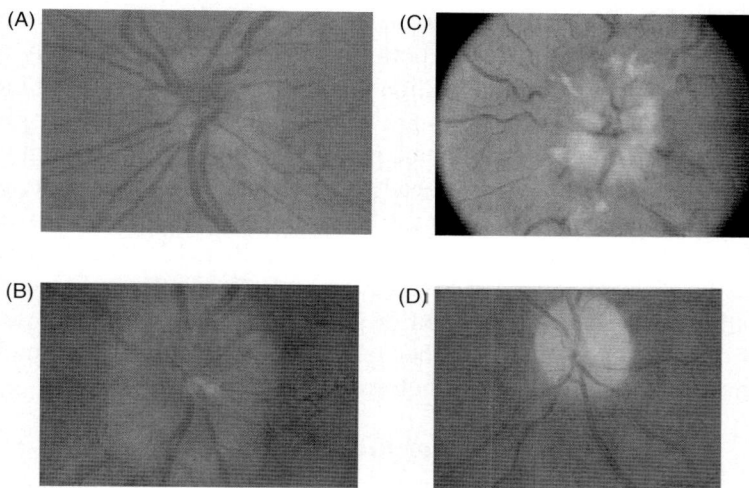

Fig. 10. (A) Early papilledema. The optic disk of an 18-year-old man 2 weeks after he had complained of diplopia arising from sixth cranial nerve palsies caused by increased intracranial pressure. Note the minimal evidence of edema. (Reproduced with permission, Yanoff M, Duker JS, editors. Ophthalmology, 2nd ed. St Louis, Mo: Mosby; 2004.) (B) Developed papilledema. The optic disk of a 36-year-old woman who suffered headache and blurred vision for 2 months. Fully developed disk edema present—note the engorged veins and peripapillary hemorrhages. (Reproduced with permission, Yanoff M, Duker JS, editors. Ophthalmology, 2nd ed. St Louis, Mo: Mosby; 2004.) (C) Chronic papilledema. Severe and chronic disk edema in a 27-year-old very obese woman who has pseudotumor cerebri. Note that the disk cup is obliterated and hard exudates are present. (Reproduced with permission, Yanoff M, Duker JS, editors. Ophthalmology, 2nd ed. St Louis, Mo: Mosby; 2004.) (D) Secondary optic atrophy from chronic papilledema. The same 27-year-old obese female patient 5 months later. Note the secondary optic atrophy has developed fully. The disk margins appear hazy or "dirty." (Reproduced with permission, Yanoff M, Duker JS, editors. Ophthalmology, 2nd ed. St Louis, Mo: Mosby; 2004.) (*See* Color Plate 12.)

clinical examination can help provide an etiological diagnosis in advance of neuroimaging. Pseudo-drusen of the optic nerve head, which can be recognized as small refractile dots, may also be seen in cases of chronically elevated intracranial pressure or optic nerve sheath meningiomas (24).

There is a fine art in interpreting the appearance of the optic nerve head. Accurate interpretation can only be made with a stereoscopic examination of the nerve head, which requires specialized, ophthalmic equipment. In the absence of this specialized equipment, the use of the direct ophthalmoscope alone can be useful in determining if there is pallor of the optic nerve head, but the three-dimensional changes (i.e., swelling or pathological cupping) of the optic nerve head can be grossly misdiagnosed without a stereoscopic view. However, the direct ophthalmoscope can be useful in detecting any significant asymmetries in the optic nerve head appearance between the eyes, which generally reflects some pathological state. Special caution must be taken when viewing the optic nerve of a myopic eye. These nerves are "tilted," which means that they exit the back of the eye at an oblique angle that precludes a full cross-sectional view of the optic nerve head. These nerve heads may thus appear incomplete, and the cup of these nerves tends to be relatively large and tends to slope toward the temporal rim of the optic nerve (*see* Fig. 11 and Color Plate 13). It can be especially difficult, even for an experienced observer, to determine with confidence if there is true pallor of the neuroretinal rim or pathological cupping. In these cases, one must often depend upon the other features of the neuro-ophthalmological examination to determine if true pathology is present.

4.5. Visual Field Testing

Measurement of central acuity reflects the neural function of only a very small fraction (1 % or so) of the visual field, i.e., the foveal outflow pathway that emerges from the center of the macula. Investigation of visual function

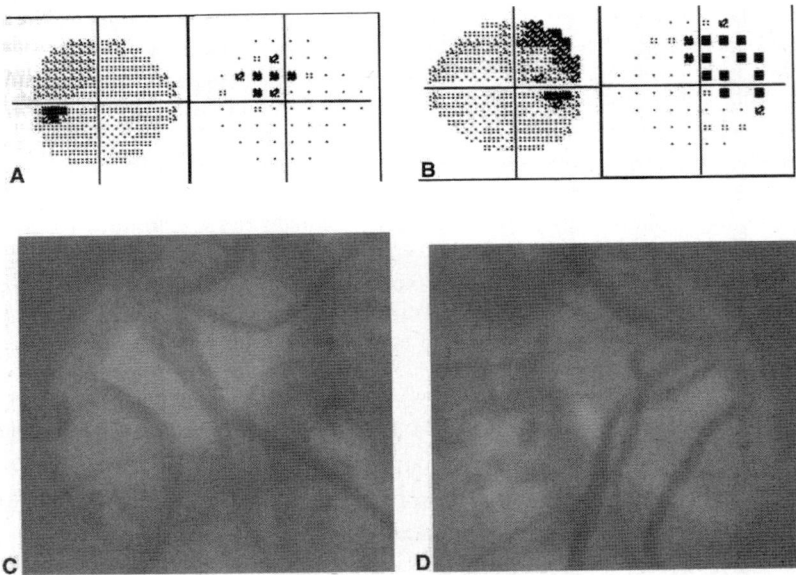

Fig. 11. Optic disk tilting and the resulting visual field defects. (A, B) Visual fields demonstrate bilateral relative superotemporal defects not respecting the vertical midline. (C, D) Fundus photos show bilateral tilted disks, with flattening of the inferonasal disk margins. (Reproduced with permission from The American Academy of Ophthalmology, Basic and Clinical Science Course, Section 5: Neuro-ophthalmology 2005–2006.) (*See* Color Plate 13.)

outside of this foveal outflow zone is most typically performed by testing of the "visual fields." The three most useful methods for obtaining a plot of the topography of the areas of seeing across the visual fields are tangent screens, Goldmann fields, and automated visual fields (Fig. 12). The latter is the most quantitative assessment of the visual field, whereas the former is the least qualitative but does not require expensive equipment. These three testing methods vary in the amount of time they require and the degree of sophistication needed from the patient and the examiner. In all cases, however, the subjective responses of the patient are required to plot the fields. Thus, the examiner is to a large extent limited by the ability and willingness of the patient to cooperate in providing accurate and reproducible responses. In general, the more demanding the test, the more challenging it is to obtain accurate and reproducible results from older, distracted, or poorly cooperative patients. "Confrontation" visual fields, in which the examiner tests the ability of a patient to count fingers or see motion in each quadrant of each eye, can provide a very crude estimate of the visual fields, and it is worthwhile to perform them if no other method is available. One should not expect to detect defects smaller than a quadrantic loss of vision by this method, unless the examiner is being especially rigorous. A relative new electrophysiological test, the multifocal visual evoked potentials (MVEP), is able to record responses from electrodes placed on the skull over the visual cortex to photic stimuli that are presented randomly in small sectors of the visual field. By using signal processing techniques, the test can provide an objective assessment of the visual fields, i.e., one that is not dependent upon the subjective responses to the stimuli. The MVEP requires even more specialized equipment than is used for standard visual field testing, and at present it is only available in a limited number of academic settings.

Any method of visual field testing is performed with each eye individually. Tangent visual field testing is quick and easy to perform, and only requires a relatively inexpensive black felt screen that is hung along a wall. Test stimuli, which are typically white, red, or blue circular disks that range from 1 to 18 mm in diameter, are moved slowly from the periphery to the center of each eye, which thus allows a measurement of the "kinetic" visual field. The patient simply states when they are able to see the stimulus, and thus a map of the contour of the visual field can be plotted. A very good facsimile of this test can be performed by simply shining a handheld laser pointer onto a blank, white wall. In a few minutes, it is possible to detect visual field defects that involve a quadrant of the visual field or less, depending upon the level of scrutiny that is applied. This test has the advantage that it can be performed while a patient is lying in bed.

Goldmann perimetry provides a highly detailed and efficient measurement of the visual fields. Measurement of Goldmann fields requires a special perimetry

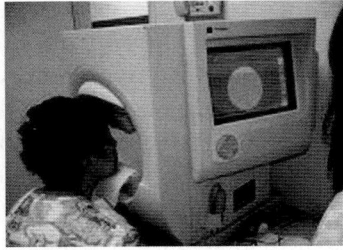

A

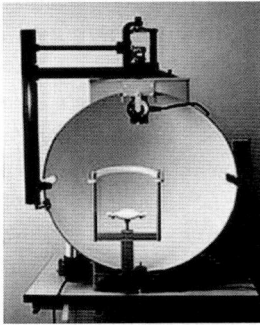

B

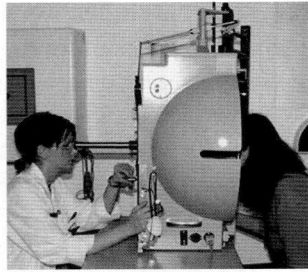

C

Fig. 12. Visual field apparati. (A) Automated Humphrey visual field. (B, C) Goldmann perimeter.

machine that is hand-driven by the examiner. This test requires a moderate level of sophistication of the examiner, who is able to perform both kinetic and static testing rapidly throughout the entire visual field, which ranges from 180° to the temporal periphery and roughly 60° to the nasal periphery of each eye. The examiner can easily adjust the size and intensity of light as the borders (isopters) of the visual field are mapped. This testing method has the distinct advantage that an experienced examiner can quickly screen for and detect defective areas of the visual field. The reliability of the patient's responses can be judged directly by the examiner, who must confront directly any inconsistencies in the responses. This testing method is time-consuming for the examiner, and this technique is now used only at a limited number of neuro-ophthalmic practices. This testing method affords the greatest efficiency when searching for visual field defects when a patient is initially examined. Subsequent comparisons of any visual field defect, however, are best made by the newer, automated visual field testing methods, described below.

Automated visual field testing is now the standard of care. These devices use a computer algorithm to determine the threshold for seeing a light stimulus at prescribed locations within the visual field to yield a "static" visual field. A fixed stimulus size is used, and a "staircase" method of search is used to iteratively approximate the threshold point by varying the intensity of light at fixed points in the visual field. A newer version of the software permits both static and kinetic testing of the visual field. Because automated testing is not dependent upon the examiner and is performed by the computer in the same way each time the test is given clearly makes automated visual field testing the preferred method for following the progression or recovery of known visual field defects, as for instance might occur after surgical removal of a pituitary tumor. This highly reproducible attribute for conducting the test is also a limitation of these devices since this methodical search method can be arduous especially for older patients or those who have difficulty concentrating. Patients not uncommonly begin to move their eyes and produce false-positive and false-negative responses, which confounds the interpretation of the visual fields, even with the numerical values that provide insight into the technical performance of the patients. The time-consuming nature of threshold determination makes it impractical to test the full area of the visual fields, and most typically these tests are used to assess only the 24–30° of visual field to the temporal and nasal side of the central fixation point. This more limited search method is not a significant compromise (versus testing the full extent of the visual field) because there is a disproportionate distribution of afferent visual pathway neurons within the center of the visual fields.

5. DIAGNOSTICALLY USEFUL CHARACTERISTICS OF VISUAL FIELD DEFECTS ASSOCIATED WITH CHIASMAL LESIONS

Deficits in the visual field are described as being either a scotoma or a depression. The term scotoma is derived from the Greek language and literally means "blind spot." The term scotoma is used when there is an area of visual field depression surrounded by an area of better vision, which has been metaphorically described as an "island" of visual deficit, surrounded by a sea of better vision (25). A "depression" of the visual field is more simply a region of decreased visual sensitivity that begins peripherally and extends toward the center. In this case, the outer perimeter of what should be a normal seeing region of vision is pushed inward toward fixation. Within a "depressed" area of vision, patients require brighter or larger stimuli to detect the photic stimuli.

The most straightforward pattern of visual field loss seen in patients with chiasmal lesions is a "bitemporal scotoma" (Fig. 13) (26). Often, the entire temporal field of both eyes is lost, and there is total or at least relative sparing

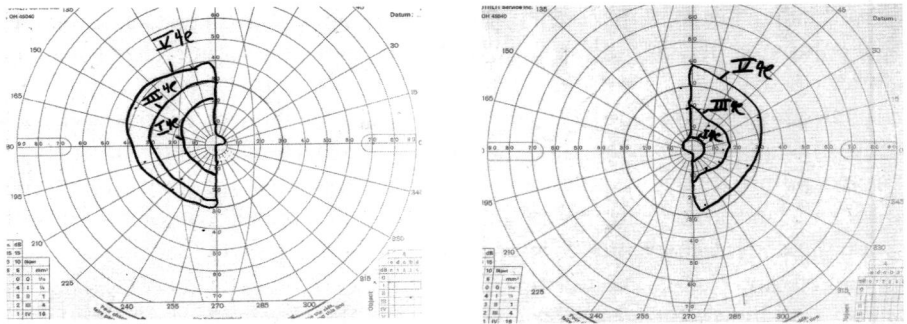

Fig. 13. Bitemporal hemianopia. Goldmann visual field demonstrating a dense bitemporal hemianopia in a patient with a large pituitary adenoma displacing the optic chiasm.

of the nasal visual field of each eye. It can be inferred that this type of visual field defect results from a relatively selective dysfunction of the crossing fibers within the chiasm, which derive from the nasal retinae that subserve the peripheral visual field of each eye. The most diagnostically significant feature of this type of visual field defect is the remarkable degree to which the field defect extends up to but does not cross (obeys) the vertical meridian of the visual field. There has never been a widely accepted explanation as to why these crossing fibers are selectively vulnerable, and the occurrence of this limited but significant pattern of visual field loss seems especially peculiar in situations in which neuroimaging reveals a large pituitary adenoma that severely compresses and flattens the entire chiasm *(27)*. Part of the answer to this clinical conundrum may be related to our testing methods. Nonetheless, there is no doubt that there is a significant disproportion in the tendency for the temporal fields to be compromised with lesions of the chiasm. In some cases, the temporal defect is found only in one eye *(28)*. Such monocular temporal field defects have the same localizing significance as do bitemporal defects. In one study from the Mayo Clinic, 9% of patients with pituitary adenomas had a visual field defect in only one eye, most commonly a superior temporal defect *(29)*.

The "density" of the visual field defect is not typically uniform across the temporal visual field. Almost always, the visual field defect is densest nearer to fixation, presumably because the density of nerve fibers that subserve central vision is substantially greater than the more peripheral region of the visual field *(30)*. On automated visual field testing, this feature of inhomogeneity is revealed by the finding of higher thresholds nearer to fixation on an automated visual field map, which means that relatively brighter lights were required to see the stimuli more centrally. On Goldmann testing, the plot of isopters to varying sizes or intensities of light shows a greater depression of isopters centrally. That is, for a given size and intensity of light that was being moved from the periphery toward the center, the patient would show greater inward bending of the isopters in the more central versus peripheral areas of the temporal visual field. In some cases, the inhomogeneity across the visual field is seen only as small scotomas in the paracentral region only on the temporal side of fixation. Such small scotomas have the same diagnostic significance as complete bitemporal hemianopias. In other cases, an "arcuate" pattern of visual field loss, which by definition involves the visual field zone between roughly 10 and 30? from fixation, can be seen only on the temporal side of the visual field.

Lesions that impinge upon the chiasm from below, which is the most common scenario since pituitary adenomas are by far the most common cause of a chiasmopathy, produce a bitemporal field defect that is usually present only in the superior temporal quadrants of each eye (Fig. 14). Expansion of the tumor can cause the field defect to extend to the inferior quadrant, and thus produce a complete bitemporal hemianopsia *(30)*. Conversely, lesions that impinge upon the chiasm from above. as occurs with some craniopharyngiomas, will produce a bitemporal field defect that initially may only involve the inferior temporal quadrants (Fig. 15) *(29)*. These patterns of visual field loss simply reflect the organization of the afferent visual fibers that preserves the vertical topography of the fibers as they pass through the optic nerve and chiasm. Fibers that emerging from the superior retina, which subserve the inferior visual field, remain in a superior location along the proximal aspect of the afferent visual pathway.

In practice, the pattern of visual field loss seen in patients with chiasmal lesions varies considerably. Lesions in the chiasmal region may produce selective involvement of the optic nerves, chiasm or optic tracts, or any combination thereof. This variability is presumably related to the pattern of tumor growth and the specific anatomy of the patient, i.e., whether the chiasm is prefixed or postfixed, for example (see above). The clinical characteristics of visual deficits is distinctly different for patients with an optic neuropathy, chiasmopathy or optic tract lesion, although these distinctions blur when more than one structure is involved, which commonly occurs.

In brief, an *optic neuropathy* will produce reduced central acuity and color vision, an afferent pupillary defect, and most typically a central scotoma on visual field testing. Other visual field defects that may be seen with an optic neuropathy include a nasal "step," arcuate (Bjerrum) scotoma, altitudinal defect, or temporal "wedge." If both optic nerves are involved to a fairly equal degree, a "relative" afferent pupillary defect would not be present (see above). A *chiasmopathy* will produce a pattern of bitemporal visual field loss, often without compromise of central acuity, color vision, or pupillary responses,

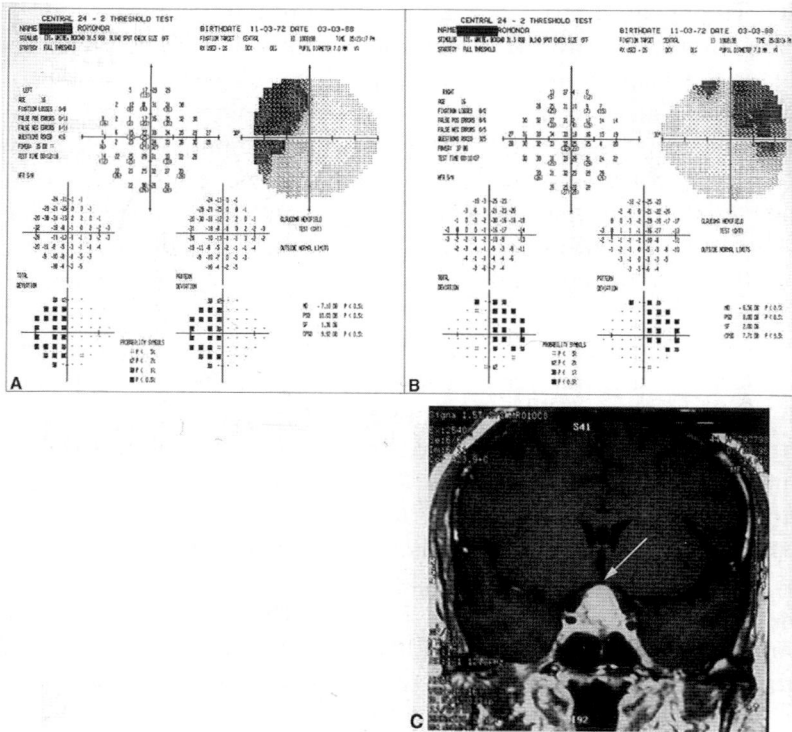

Fig. 14. (A, B) Visual fields in a patient with a pituitary tumor, showing bitemporal depression worse superiorly, with margination along the vertical midline. (C) T1-weighted coronal MRI scan demonstrates intrasellar enhancing mass, with extension into the suprasellar cistern and upward displacement and compression of the chiasm (arrow). (Reproduced with permission from The American Academy of Ophthalmology, Basic and Clinical Science Course, Section 5: Neuro-ophthalmology 2005–2006.)

since a true bitemporal defect spares half of the visual field, including the nasal paracentral region of vision, in each eye, which is sufficient to preserve the fine detail of central visual function in each eye. (N.B. The projection of the foveal outflow pathway from each eye is equally distributed between the crossed and uncrossed chiasmal fibers, hence disruption of only the crossed fibers does not degrade central visual function, at least not as revealed by the standardly used methods of assessing vision.) An *optic tract lesion* will produce a "homonymous" visual field defect, which is typically highly incongruous (i.e., the extent and depth of the visual field defect is fairly asymmetrical between the eyes). In addition, the disproportion of crossed versus uncrossed fibers produces an asymmetry in pupillary responses, which is seen as a RAPD in the

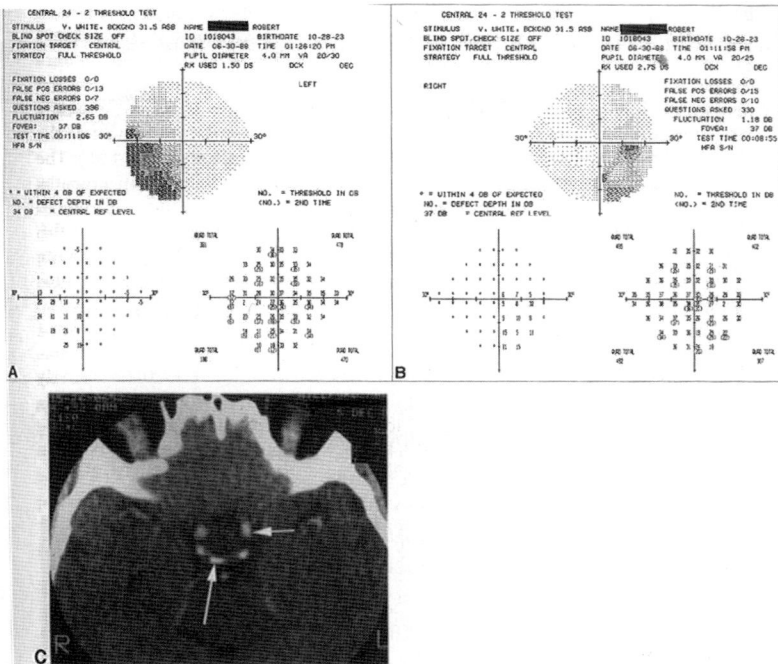

Fig. 15. Patient with craniopharyngioma involving the suprasellar cistern, with compression of the chiasm from above. (A, B) Visual fields show bilateral inferotemporal depression respecting the vertical midline. (C) Axial CT scan shows cystic mass with peripheral calcification within the suprasellar cistern (arrows). (Reproduced with permission from The American Academy of Ophthalmology, Basic and Clinical Science Course, Section 5: Neuro-ophthalmology 2005–2006.)

eye opposite to the side of the optic tract lesion. This afferent pupillary defect is typically quite subtle, owing to the small percentage difference of crossed versus uncrossed fibers within the optic tract *(19)*. Unilateral involvement of the retrochiasmal visual pathway, as occurs with lesions of the optic tract, does not compromise central acuity or color vision. As stated above, chiasmal lesions can produce any combination of clinical deficit of a unilateral or bilateral optic neuropathy, chiasmopathy, or involvement of the optic tracts, on one or both sides (Table 1).

Impingement at the junction of the optic nerve and chiasm produces a "junctional" field defect, which displays two distinct but related findings: in the eye ipsilateral to the lesion there is a field defect that is typical of an optic neuropathy, most commonly a central scotoma; in addition, in the eye contralateral to the lesion there is a depression of the superotemporal field

Table 1
Summary of the Neuro-ophthalmic Findings in Lesions of the Optic Nerve, Chism, and the Optic Tract

	Optic Nerve	Chiasm	Optic Tract
Visual acuity	Decreased	Variable (normal to decreased)	Normal
Color vision	Decreased	Variable (normal to decreased)	Normal
RAPD	Present ipsilaterally	Variable	Present contralaterally
Optic Disk findings	Variable (normal, edematous, atrophic)	Variable; "band" optic atrophy; temporal wedge atrophy, or much less commonly, papilledema	Bilateral optic atrophy with ipsilateral temporal pallor and contralateral "bowtie" atrophy
Field defect	Unilateral and variable	Monocular or binocular bitemporal defect respecting the vertical meridian	Incongruous homonymous hemianopias of variable density with sloping margins

(Fig. 7). As discussed above, the anatomical explanation for this selective involvement of the superotemporal field is not known. Whatever its cause, the discovery of a junctional visual field defect is highly predictive of a mass lesion that is compressing the junction of the optic nerve and chiasm.

6. CORRELATION OF NEUROIMAGING TO VISUAL FIELD DEFECT

Modern-day neuroimaging provides highly detailed representations of the afferent visual pathway around the chiasm and the topography of mass lesions in this area. The fact that the nerve pathways are surrounded by the perichiasmatic cistern filled with cerebrospinal fluid enhances the ability of MRI to provide exceptional detail of this anatomy. Perhaps somewhat surprisingly, mass lesions that appear to contact or even compress the chiasm do not always correlate with the presence of a measurable visual field defect. However, any obvious displacement or stretching of the chiasm is essentially always associated with a characteristic visual field defect of a chiasmopathy.

7. PROGNOSIS OF VISUAL FIELD DEFECTS PRODUCED BY CHIASMAL MASS LESIONS

The degree of displacement or stretching of the chiasm is not a good predictor of the potential for visual recovery after treatment is given to shrink or remove the offending mass lesion *(31–34)*. Some patients will enjoy a remarkable degree of recovery after prolonged compression of the chiasm, even in cases in which bilateral optic nerve pallor has developed. Even more surprising, quite dramatic recovery of vision following surgical removal of mass lesions can occur within a day or two, even after there is good evidence of prolonged compression of the chiasm.

7.1. Pseudo-Bitemporal Visual Field Defect

A visual field defect that presents in a quasi-bitemporal manner occurs with relatively high frequency in patients who are simply near-sighted. Myopia is caused by growth of an eye to a point where its axial length is too long, with the consequence that light rays are focused in front of the retina. Other anatomical anomalies occur as a part of myopia, including a "tilted" optic nerve head (Fig. 11) *(35)*. Such myopic nerves exit the eye at an oblique angle, which does not allow the examiner to appreciate the full cross-sectional area of the nerve on a funduscopic examination. This tilt is also associated with a very slight bowing out of the contour of the back of the eye (i.e., ectasia), but (usually) only in the inferior aspect of the eye. Thus, the light rays that approach the retina tend to be out of focus inferiorly. When performing visual field testing, especially Goldmann kinetic testing with smaller and less intense stimuli, patients often take longer to recognize the moving light entering from their superior visual field, because the image is less well focused in this area of the visual field. The visual field plot, then, shows a relative depression of the superior visual field. This defect is almost always on the temporal side of the field because the ectasia of the back of the eye is very slightly greater to the nasal side.

This myopic-related visual field defect is usually easily distinguished from that caused by a mass lesion. Because the field defect is caused by a retinal factor, the field defect does not "obey" the vertical meridian; rather the defect slopes across the vertical meridian, a feature that can usually be easily appreciated by Goldmann perimetry. Also, the field defect can be easily improved simply by retesting with a myopic correction, which more properly focuses the incident light rays on the ecstatic region of retina. The myopic field defect is generally less evident on automated perimetry, perhaps because this test is normally performed with a relatively large light stimulus, which is less likely to be undetected when only a slight myopic error is present. The degree to which a myopic field defect is present generally correlates with the degree of myopia.

7.2. Ocular Motor Dysfunction in Patients with Chiasmal Lesions

The ocular motor nerves (CN III, IV, and VI) course through the cavernous sinus, which lies just lateral to the sella turcica (Fig. 16). Expansile lesions that arise in the sella can extend into the cavernous sinus and cause an ocular motor palsy, which results in diplopia. In a Mayo Clinic series, single or multiple ocular motor palsies were found in only 46 of 1000 cases (29). Rarely, a pituitary tumor may present as an isolated ocular motor paresis, without loss of vision.

The particular pattern of diplopia caused by lesions that extend into the cavernous sinus varies in accordance to which ocular motor nerves are involved and how severely they are compromised. Despite the fact that a mass lesion may appear to fill the cavernous sinus, it is not uncommon for only the sixth cranial nerve to develop dysfunction, presumably because the other ocular motor cranial nerves course through the cavernous sinus within the protective confines of the lateral wall of the cavernous sinus (Fig. 2). If there is an "isolated" sixth nerve palsy, the patient would report horizontal diplopia, and the degree of horizontal separation of the images would become more obvious as the patient looks further toward the side with the abduction paresis caused by the compromise of the sixth cranial nerve. The eye would tend to be inwardly displaced (i.e., esotropic) on the involved side.

Involvement of the third cranial nerve usually produces a more complex presentation, which includes both vertical and horizontal diplopia, given that

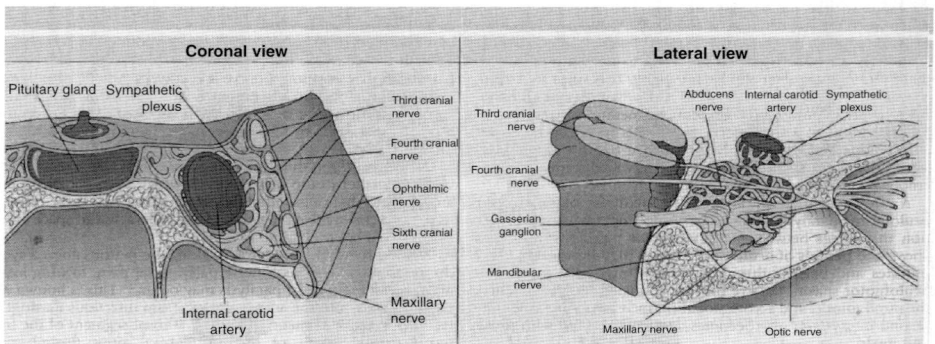

Fig. 16. Anatomy of the cavernous sinus. Coronal and lateral views. (Reproduced with permission, Yanoff M, Duker JS, editors. Ophthalmology, 2nd ed. St Louis, Mo: Mosby; 2004.)

the third cranial nerve innervates four extraocular muscles (superior rectus, inferior rectus, medial rectus, and inferior oblique) that influence both the horizontal and the vertical position of the eye. Usually, involvement of the third cranial nerve causes the eye to be outwardly displaced (i.e., exotropic), and there is generally limitation of the inward, upward, and downward movement of the affected eye. The pupil usually becomes large (i.e., mydriatric) and responds poorly to a light stimulus (i.e., "pupil-involving third nerve palsy"). The mydriasis is caused by disruption of the parasympathetic fibers that travel with the third cranial nerve; this autonomic defect also diminishes the capacity to accommodate to a near target, thus patients will often report blurred vision especially at near. This type of blurriness must be distinguished from true loss of vision, as occurs when the afferent visual pathway is involved. Lastly, the lid will be ptotic, owing to the involvement of the third nerve fibers that innervate the levator palpebrae muscle.

Long-standing compression of the third cranial nerve can lead to regeneration of the compromised axons leading toward the eye. These sprouting axons tend to innervate the wrong muscles, possibly because the embryologic markers that would normally be present during development to direct the innervational pattern of nerves onto muscles are not expressed after development has occurred. The consequence of this poorly orchestrated sprouting is the development of synkinetic phenomena, which produce cocontraction of the eyelids and pupil, and is evidence of "aberrant regeneration of the third cranial nerve." Most typically, aberrant regeneration can be recognized as elevation of the eyelid with attempted downgaze or contraction of the pupil with adduction or depression of the eye.

Dysfunction of the fourth cranial nerve can be difficult to ascertain when there is compromise of the third and fourth cranial nerves because the influence of the fourth cranial nerve over eye movement is more subtle than for the other ocular motor nerves. Diplopia caused by a fourth nerve palsy produces a subtle vertical diplopia that is worse to the side opposite the palsy. This subtle vertical misalignment of the eyes is usually dwarfed by the degree of strabismus caused by involvement of the third cranial nerve.

7.3. See-saw Nystagmus

A rare ocular motor abnormality sometimes associated with parasellar tumors is see-saw nystagmus, in which there is a dyscconjugate vertical oscillation of the eyes that show intorsion of the elevated eye and extorsion of the downgoing eye (36). This phenomenon is not specific to tumors compressing the chiasm; it has been reported in patients with and without bitemporal hemianopia and in patients who have developmental abnormalities affecting the chiasm or upper brainstem or a history of significant head trauma.

7.4. Visual Symptoms Experienced by Patients Who Develop Chiasmal Lesions

Patients with lesions of the perichiasmal region may develop afferent or efferent neuro-ophthalmic problems, or both. Most commonly, patients develop loss of vision, i.e., afferent visual dysfunction. Patients differ considerably in their ability to recognize visual loss, even with significant loss of their peripheral visual field. Even very bright, attentive, and detailed-oriented patients may not recognize the visual loss. Sometimes, patients will report a "haze" or "blur" in the temporal visual field, without recognizing that vision has actually been lost in that area. Rarely, patients report photophobia (37). The visual loss can be severe enough that patients begin to walk into walls or get into automobile accidents, and these untoward events may occur repeatedly before the patient (or their spouse) has the epiphany that something is wrong with their vision. Patients tend to be much better at recognizing loss of central acuity, as occurs when one or both optic nerves are compromised.

One rare but interesting visual experience that occurs in some patients with chiasmal lesions is the "hemifield" slide phenomenon (Fig. 17) (38). This illusory phenomenon occurs in patients who have a dense, bitemporal defect. Patients may report that they intermittently, usually in brief episodes that last only seconds, lose "depth perception," experience episodes of double vision

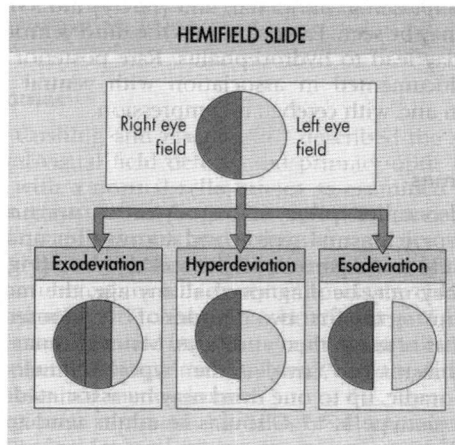

Fig. 17. Phenomenon of "hemifield slide." In patients affected by a complete bitemporal hemianopia, preexisting phorias may result in a separation of the hemifields vertically (hyperdeviation) or horizontally (esodeviation), or in double vision if the intact nasal hemifields overlap (exodeviation). (Reproduced with permission, Yanoff M, Duker JS, editors. Ophthalmology, 2nd ed. St Louis, Mo: Mosby; 2004.)

(without evidence of an ocular motor palsy), or experience a vanishing of detail in the center of an image. The latter phenomenon has been recognized by some of our patients as brief but recurrent loss of the numbers in the center of a license plate as observed when driving a car. The hemifield slide phenomenon probably occurs because of a loss of fusional stabilization between the eyes. In essence, the brain uses afferent input from the entire retina to help maintain binocular alignment of the eyes. This capacity is diminished when there is a complete loss of both temporal visual fields, at least when looking at objects that are not too distant. When looking in the far distance, the two temporal visual fields are in essence looking in different directions. When looking at an object that is relatively close, however, the two temporal fields overlap at any distance behind the near point of fixation (Fig. 6). In this situation, blindness in the temporal fields limits the fusional capacity of the brain, and the eyes can move slightly inward and outward with respect to one another. These movements can produce double vision, or loss of the object of regard if the near point of attention is directed more closely, which thus positions the original object of regard more distantly and within the overlapping zone of the blind hemifields. Rarely, the ocular movement can occur vertically, thus leading to a vertical hemifield slide phenomenon *(39)*.

The presence or absence of pain is not particularly helpful in the diagnosis of a pituitary tumor. It is true, however, that tumors that grow large enough to stretch the diaphragma sella (i.e., the dural covering of the sella turcica) can cause pain that usually is referred to the forehead because the diaphragma sella is innervated by branches of the first division of the fifth cranial nerve. Expansion of tumors into the cavernous sinus is also frequently accompanied by pain, especially if the patient experiences apoplexy (see below). However, many patients, even those with very large pituitary tumors, do not experience any pain or discomfort.

7.5. *Pituitary Apoplexy*

Pituitary apoplexy is typically a dramatic event in which hemorrhage occurs into a preexisting adenoma (*see* Fig. 18 and Color Plate 14). It is described in detail in Chapter 19. Patients may develop blindness from involvement of the afferent visual pathway, diplopia from involvement of the efferent visual pathway, endocrinological dysfunction (sometimes in the absence of any neuro-ophthalmological signs or symptoms), or just pain. A paucity of signs may occur in patients in whom the tumor expands downward into the sphenoid sinus. This condition is considered a neurologic emergency since patients can die from hypotension resulting from adrenal insufficiency, and urgent neurosurgical consultation is required.

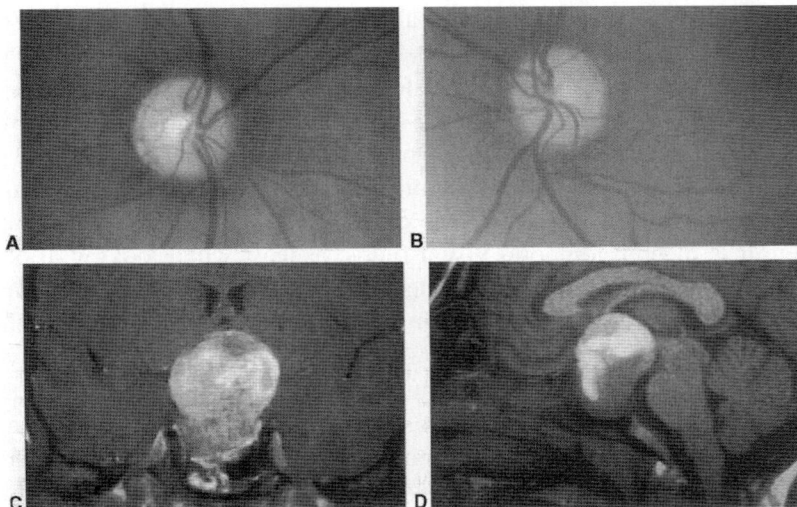

examinations with visual fields. Neuroimaging alone can be deceptive and even lesions displacing the chiasm can cause no detectable visual deficits and can often be observed. Careful serial neuro-ophthalmic examinations can detect the first sign of visual dysfunction indicating the need for surgical intervention.

REFERENCES

1. Deutsch H, Kothbaur K, Persky M, Epstein F, Jallo G. Infrasellar craniopharyngiomas: case report and review of the literature. Skull Base 2001;11:121–8.
2. Hupp S, Kline L. Magnetic resonance imaging of the optic chiasm. Surv Ophthalmol 1991;36:207–16.
3. Bergland R, Ray B, Torack R. Anatomical variations in the pituitary gland and adjacent structures in 225 human autopsy cases. J Neurosurg 1968;28:93–9.
4. Saadati H, Hsu H, Heller K, Sadun A. A histopathologic and morphometric differentiation of nerves in optic nerve hypoplasia and Leber hereditary optic neuropathy. Arch Ophthalmol 1998;116:911–6.
5. Hoyt W, Luis O. The primate chiasm. Details of the visual fiber organization studied by silver impregnation techniques. Arch Ophthamology 1963;70:69–85.
6. Horton J. Wilbrand's knee of the primate optic chiasm is an artifact of monocular enucleation. Am Ophthalmol Soc 1997;95:579–609.
7. Lee J, Tobias S, Kwon J, Sade B, Kosmorsky G. Wilbrand's knee: does it exist? Surg Neurol 2006;66:11–7.
8. Sadun A, Rubin R. The anterior visual pathways – Part II. J Neuro-ophthalmol 1996;16: 212–22.
9. Sadun A, Schaechter J, Smith L. A retinohypothalamic pathway in man: light meditation of circadian rhythms. Brain Res 1984;202:371–7.
10. Frisen L. The neurology of visual acuity. Brain 1980;103:, 639–70.
11. Bunt A, Minckler D. Foveal sparing: New anatomical evidence for bilateral representation of the central retina. Arch Ophthalmol 1977;95:1445–7.
12. Gregorius F, Hepler R, Stern W. Loss and recovery of vision with suprasellar meningiomas. J Neurosurg 1975;42:69–75.
13. Peiris J, Ross Russell R. Giant aneurysms of the carotid system presenting as visual defect. J Neurol Neurosurg Psychiatry 1980;43:1053–64.
14. Swanson W, Cohen J. Color vision. Ophthalmol Clin North Am 2003;16:179–203.
15. Sadun A, Lessell S. Brightness-sense and optic nerve disease. Arch Ophthalmol 1985;103:39–43.
16. Trobe J, Tao A, Schuster J. Perichiasmal tumors: diagnostic and prognostic features. Neurosurgery 1984;15:391–9.
17. Stanley J, Baise G. The swinging flashlight test to detect minimal optic neuropathy. Arch Ophthalmol 1968;80:769–71.
18. Lagreze W-D, Kardon R. Correlation of relative afferent pupillary defect and estimated retinal ganglion cell loss. Graefes Arch Clin Exp Ophthalmol 1998;236:401–4.
19. Kardon R, Kawaski A, Miller N. Origin of the relative pupillary defect in optic tract lesion. Ophthalmology 2006;113:1345–53.
20. Frohman L, Guirgis MT, RE, Bielory L. Sarcoidosis of the anterior visual pathway: 24 new cases. J Neuro-ophthalmol 2003;23:187–9.
21. Bianchi-Marzoli S, Rizzo J, Brancato R, Lessell S. Quantitative analysis of optic disc cupping in compressive optic neuropathy. Ophthalmology 1995;102:436–40.

22. Portney G, Roth A. Optic cupping caused by an intracranial aneurysm. Am J Ophthalmol 1977;84:98–103.
23. Miller N, Solomon S. Retinochoroidal (optocililary) shunt veins, blindness, and optic atrophy: a non-specific sign of chronic optic nerve compression. Aust N Z J Ophthalmol 1991;19:105–9.
24. Sibony P, Kennerdell J, Slamovits T, Lessell S, Krauss H. Intrapapillary refractile bodies in optic nerve sheath meningioma. Arch Ophthalmol 1985;103:383–5.
25. Traquair H. Clinical detection of early changes in the visual field. Trans Am Ophthalmol Soc. 1939;37:158–79.
26. Foroozan R. Chiasmal syndromes. Curr Opin Ophthalmol 2003;14:325–31.
27. Mellwaine G, Carrim Z, Lueck C, Chrisp T. Amechanical theory to account for bitemporal hemianopia from chiasmal compression. J Neuro-ophthalmol 2005;25:40–3.
28. Hershenfeld S, Sharpe J. Monocular temporal hemianopia. Br J Ophthalmol 1993;77:424–7.
29. Schiefer U, Isbert M, Mikolaschek E, et al. Distribution of scotoma pattern related to chiasmal lesions with special reference to anterior junction syndrome. Graefes Arch Clin Exp Ophthalmol 2004;242:468–77.
30. Gittinger J. Ophthalmological evaluation of pituitary adenomas. In: Post K, Jackson I, Reichlin S, editors. The Pituitary Adenoma. New York: Plenum Medical Book Company 1980;259–86.
31. Chiu E, Nichols J. Sellar lesions and visual loss: key concepts in neuro-ophthalmology. Expert Rev Anticancer Ther 2006;6:S23–8.
32. Rosiene J, Liu X, Imielinska C, et al. Structure-function relationships in the human visual system using DTI, fMRI, and visual field testing: pre- and post-operative assessments in patients with anterior visual pathway compression. Stud Health Technol Inform. 2006;119:464–6.
33. Ikeda H, Yoshimoto T. Visual disturbances in patients with pituitary adenoma. Acta Neurol Scand 1995;92:157–60.
34. Eda M, Saeki N, Fujimoto N, Sunami K. Demonstration of the optic pathway in large pituitary adenoma on heavily weighted MR images. Br J Neurosurg 2002;16:21–9.
35. Shikishima K, Kitahara K, Mizobuchi T, Yoshida M. Interpretation of visual field defects respecting the vertical meridian and not related to distinct chiasmal or postchiasmal lesions. J Clin Neurosci 2006;13:923–8.
36. Fein J, Williams R. See-saw nystagmus. J Neurol Neurosurg Psychiatry 1969;32:202.
37. Kawaski A, Purvin V. Photophobia as the presenting visual symptom of chiasmal compression. J Neuro-ophthalmol 2002;22:3–8.
38. Lyle T, Clover P. Ocular symptoms and signs in pituitary tumors. Proc R Soc Med 1961;54:611.
39. Borchert M, Lessell S, Hoyt W. Hemifield slide diplopia from altitudinal field defects. J Neuro-ophthalmol 1996;16:107–9.

6   Prolactinomas: *Diagnosis and Management*

Amal Shibli-Rahhal, MD, and Janet A. Schlechte, MD

CONTENTS

1. INTRODUCTION
2. CLINICAL PRESENTATION
3. OTHER CAUSES OF HYPERPROLACTINEMIA
4. DIAGNOSTIC EVALUATION
5. DOPAMINE AGONIST THERAPY
6. TREATMENT WHEN FERTILITY IS THE GOAL
7. TREATMENT WHEN FERTILITY IS NOT AN ISSUE
8. IS MEDICAL THERAPY THE ONLY OPTION?
9. CAN DOPAMINE AGONIST THERAPY BE DISCONTINUED?

Summary

Prolactin-secreting adenomas account for 40% of all pituitary tumors and are classified as microadenomas (<10mm) and macroadenomas (>10mm). Microprolactinomas are more common in women and most women present with menstrual dysfunction, infertility or galactorrhea. Men commonly present with large tumors and although prolactinomas in men lead to hypogonadism, most men seek medical attention because of headaches or neurologic deficits.

After ruling out secondary causes of hyperprolactinemia, the diagnosis of a prolactinoma is established with an elevated serum prolactin and radiographic evidence of a pituitary tumor. The treatment of choice for all prolactinomas is a dopamine agonist, and the goals of therapy are to normalize prolactin, restore gonadal function and fertility, reduce tumor size and reverse pituitary dysfunction. Bromocriptine and cabergoline are the two dopamine agonists used in the United States for treatment of prolactinomas and both are effective in normalizing prolactin and decreasing tumor size. Cabergoline is more potent, has fewer side effects and can be given twice weekly. Transsphenoidal surgery may be necessary in patients who do not respond to or

From: *Contemporary Endocrinology: Diagnosis and Management of Pituitary Disorders*
Edited by: B. Swearingen and B. M. K. Biller © Humana Press, Totowa, NJ

are intolerant of dopamine agonists. Radiation therapy may be necessary in patients with large tumors who fail to respond to medical or surgical treatment.

Key Words: Prolactinoma, Dopamine agonist, Bromocriptine, Cabergoline.

1. INTRODUCTION

Prolactin-secreting adenomas account for about 40% of all pituitary tumors with an estimated annual incidence of 6–10 cases/million/year. The tumors occur most frequently in women during the second through fifth decades. After the fifth decade, the tumors are more common in men *(1,2)*. Over 90% of prolactinomas are small and do not give rise to mass effects on the pituitary or surrounding structures. Postmortem studies reveal an equal sex distribution of prolactinomas and no preponderance of large tumors *(3)*. Approximately 20% of patients with multiple endocrine neoplasia have prolactinomas *(4)*. Prolactinomas are uncommon in children and malignant prolactinomas are rare.

The pathogenesis of prolactinomas is controversial. Hypothalamic dysregulation may play a role but it is most likely that the tumors arise from clonal proliferation of a single mutated cell *(5,6)*. In some growth hormone-secreting and ACTH-secreting adenomas a *gsp* oncogene has been identified but no precise mutation or rearrangement of a single oncogene has been regularly reported in prolactinomas *(7,8)*.

The regulation of prolactin secretion is mediated primarily through prolactin inhibitory factors arising in the hypothalamus. The most important inhibitory factor is dopamine, which binds to D_2 receptors on the lactotroph cell membrane. Any process that interferes with dopamine receptors, dopamine synthesis, or dopamine transport to the pituitary via the portal vessels leads to hyperprolactinemia. It was the delineation of the regulation of prolactin secretion that led to the development of medical therapy for prolactinomas.

The primary action of prolactin is to promote lactation but it is the effect on the reproductive system that brings patients to clinical attention. In both sexes, hypersecretion of prolactin interferes with the pulsatile secretion of gonadotropin releasing hormone, inhibits LH and FSH secretion, and impairs gonadal steroid production leading to gonadal dysfunction and infertility *(9–11)*. Prolactinomas are classified as microadenomas (< 10 mm), macroadenomas (> 10 mm), or macroadenomas with extrasellar extension.

2. CLINICAL PRESENTATION

2.1. Women

How a prolactinoma presents depends on the sex of the patient and the size of the tumor. In women, the majority of prolactinomas are microadenomas (Fig. 1) and women seek medical attention because of menstrual

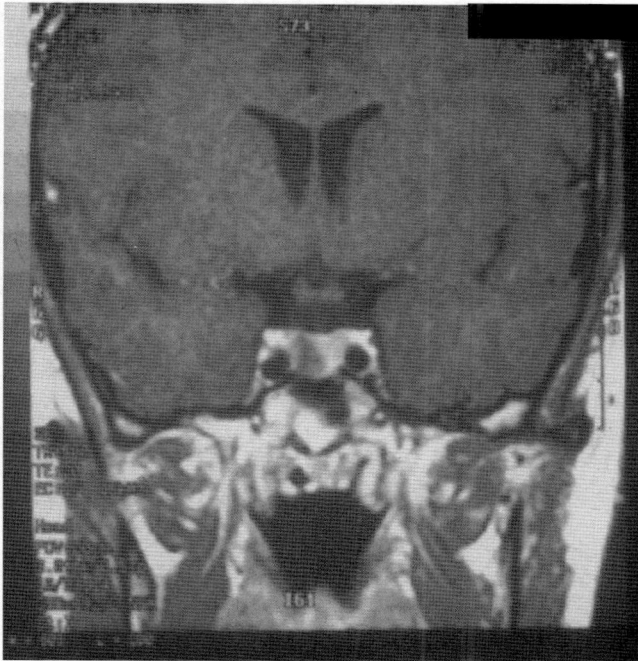

Fig. 1. Coronal view of gadolinium-enhanced pituitary MRI showing hypodense area on the right consistent with microadenoma.

dysfunction and infertility. Amenorrhea or oligomenorrhea occur in more than 90% and galactorrhea occurs in 50–80% *(12–14)*. Galactorrhea may occur with or without menstrual dysfunction, and it is controversial whether the severity of menstrual abnormalities correlates with the level of serum prolactin *(13)*. Hyperprolactinemia is commonly detected during evaluation of "postpill" amenorrhea. Despite a temporal association, case control studies have not shown a relationship between the clinical appearance of a prolactinoma and prior oral contraceptive use *(15)*. Because the tumors are small, women rarely develop visual loss or hypopituitarism.

2.2. Men

In men, 80% of prolactinomas are macroadenomas that are commonly associated with headaches, neurologic deficits, or visual loss *(16–18)* (Fig. 2). Although hypogonadal symptoms are not the usual reason that men with hyperprolactinemia seek medical attention, elevated prolactin leads to impotence, infertility, decreased libido, and oligospermia. Gynecomastia and galactorrhea are uncommon *(19,20)*. Anterior pituitary dysfunction is common and ACTH

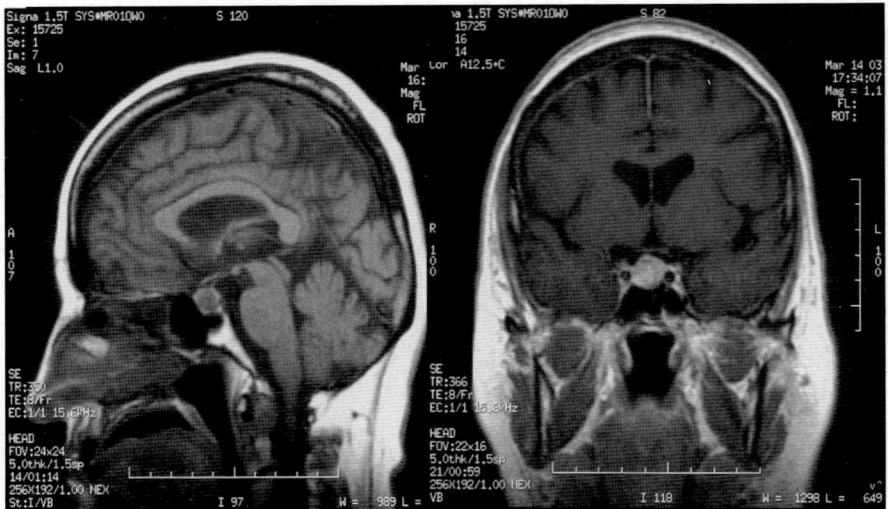

Fig. 2. Sagittal (left) and coronal (right) views of pituitary showing macroadenoma with suprasellar extension sparing the optic chiasm.

and TSH deficiency have been reported in 41 % and 25 %, respectively, of men with macroadenomas *(16,17)*.

The reason for the higher prevalence of macroadenomas in men has not been elucidated. It has been suggested that microadenomas and macroadenomas represent the early and late stages of a single pathologic process and that larger tumors in men represent a delay in diagnosis. Another possibility is that tumors in men have greater proliferative potential but a molecular basis for greater proliferative activity has not been elucidated *(21,22)*.

In both men and women, prolactin-induced decreases in testosterone and estrogen lead to low spinal bone density, although no increase in fracture risk has been reported *(23,24)*.

3. OTHER CAUSES OF HYPERPROLACTINEMIA

Prolactin is secreted episodically and serum levels are usually < 25 μg/l in females and < 20 μg/l in males. Emotional stress, exercise, and chest wall stimulation lead to mild (< 40 μg/l) increases in serum prolactin and during pregnancy levels may exceed 200 μg/l *(25)*. There are a variety of conditions, other than prolactinomas, that can interfere with dopaminergic control of prolactin secretion leading to hyperprolactinemia.

3.1. Medications

Drugs affecting dopamine synthesis or release are a frequent cause of hyperprolactinemia. Several drugs, including metoclopramide, phenothiazines, butyrophenones, and risperidone, block dopamine D_2 receptors and can be associated with prolactin levels > 100 µg/l *(26–29)*. Tricyclic antidepressants and monoamine oxidase inhibitors cause less prominent elevation of serum prolactin, and the selective serotonin reuptake inhibitors rarely lead to prolactin levels outside the normal range *(30,31)*. Verapamil causes hyperprolactinemia and hypogonadism in about 8% of patients taking the drug *(32)* and women receiving oral contraceptives or hormone replacement therapy also develop mild hyperprolactinemia (< 40 µg/l) *(33,34)* Other agents that can lead to hyperprolactinemia are listed in Table 1. In most cases, medication-induced

Table 1
Causes of Hyperprolactinemia

Physiologic Causes	Hypothalamic and Pituitary Conditions	Medical Conditions	Medications
Pregnancy	Severe head trauma	Primary hypothyroidism	Antipsychotics: phenothiazines, thioxanthenes, butyrophenones, dibenzoxazepine, risperidone
Physical and emotional stress	Radiation therapy to the brain	Chronic renal failure	Antidepressants: tricyclic antidepressants, serotonin-reuptake inhibitors, monoamine oxidase inhibitors
Exercise	Infiltrative diseases of the hypothalamus	Liver cirrhosis	Antihypertensives: methyldopa, reserpine, verapamil
Chest wall stimulation	Large functioning and nonfunctioning pituitary tumors		Gastrointestinal: metoclopramide, domperidone, H_2 blockers
	Lymphocytic hypophysitis		Others: cocaine, opiates, estrogen, protease inhibitors

hyperprolactinemia is reversible within days of stopping the potential offending drug. Changing or discontinuing an antipsychotic agent in a patient with hyperprolactinemia should only be considered or undertaken in consultation with a patient's psychiatrist. If a medication cannot be safely discontinued in a patient with sustained hyperprolactinemia, radiographic evaluation of the pituitary should be undertaken.

3.2. Pituitary/Hypothalamic Disorders

Very large nonsecreting pituitary tumors and craniopharyngiomas cause mild elevation in prolactin (< 200 µg/l) by compressing the pituitary stalk and inhibiting dopamine transport to the pituitary. About 30 % of growth hormone-secreting pituitary tumors secrete prolactin *(35)* and hyperprolactinemia has been reported in patients with lymphocytic hypophysitis *(36)*

3.3. Other Disorders

Some patients with end-stage kidney disease and liver cirrhosis develop hyperprolactinemia due to decreased clearance of prolactin. About one-third of patients with polycystic ovarian disease have hyperprolactinemia *(37)* and patients with primary hypothyroidism may develop mild hyperprolactinemia due to stimulation of lactotrophs by thyrotropin releasing hormone *(38)*.

Occasionally, no etiology of hyperprolactinemia is identified and the condition is termed idiopathic hyperprolactinemia. In these cases, a pituitary tumor may be the cause of the elevated prolactin but is too small to be detected. In about one-third of patients with idiopathic hyperprolactinemia, prolactin levels normalize over time and only 10 % eventually develop radiographic evidence of a tumor *(39,40)*.

3.4. Macroprolactin

When a patient does not have the expected clinical symptoms (amenorrhea, galactorrhea, or infertility) of hyperprolactinemia it is important to question the diagnosis and to consider the presence of a biologically inactive hormone. Macroprolactin is a glycosylated form of prolactin that circulates in large aggregates not readily cleared by the kidney. This high molecular weight molecule normally accounts for less than 1 % of circulating prolactin, develops as a consequence of IgG binding to prolactin and is biologically inactive *(41,42)*. Many prolactin immunoassays do not recognize macroprolactin but it can be detected after polyethylene glycol precipitation. We screen all hyperprolactinemic sera for the presence of macroprolactin. While not widely available such screening has been shown to prevent unnecessary radiographic studies and treatment *(43)*.

4. DIAGNOSTIC EVALUATION

The diagnosis of prolactinoma is established by sustained hyperprolactinemia and radiographic evidence of a pituitary tumor. A single measurement of serum prolactin is usually adequate to document hyperprolactinemia, but in cases where the level is only mildly elevated, samples may need to be drawn on different days. A history and physical examination, pregnancy test, and measurement of thyroid, liver, and renal function will elucidate most causes of hyperprolactinemia. When other causes of hyperprolactinemia have been excluded, gadolinium-enhanced magnetic resonance imaging (MRI) should be used to visualize the pituitary gland. Computed tomography with intravenous contrast enhancement is less expensive but is not as effective in delineating extrasellar tumor extension or in identifying very small adenomas. Only patients with macroadenomas that demonstrate extrasellar extension need formal visual field testing and assessment of anterior pituitary function upon diagnosis. Provocative tests utilizing thyrotropin releasing hormone, levodopa, and insulin-induced hypoglycemia are not useful in the diagnosis of a prolactinoma *(44)*.

In general, the serum prolactin level will parallel the size of the tumor. Prolactin-secreting macroadenomas are typically associated with prolactin levels >250 µg/l and levels may exceed 1,000 µg/l. If a patient with a macroadenoma has a prolactin level of <250 µg/l, it is more likely that the hyperprolactinemia is due to compression of the pituitary stalk than to a prolactinoma. When the serum prolactin level is inappropriately low in the presence of a macroadenoma, another potential explanation is an artifact in the prolactin immunoradiometric assay. This artifact, termed the hook effect, is a consequence of extremely high prolactin concentrations saturating the antibody and can be eliminated by performing serial dilution of the samples *(45)*.

5. DOPAMINE AGONIST THERAPY

5.1. General Principles

The goals in treatment of a prolactinoma are to normalize prolactin, restore gonadal function and fertility, reduce tumor size, and reverse pituitary dysfunction. The treatment of choice is a dopamine agonist and prolactinomas are the only pituitary tumor where medical therapy is the primary option. Dopamine agonists bind to D_2 receptors in the anterior pituitary and decrease prolactin synthesis, limit cell multiplication, and reduce tumor size *(46,47)*. Lowering of prolactin occurs within days and tumor shrinkage is usually apparent 3–6 months after therapy. Prolactin lowering usually precedes a decrease in the size of the tumor, and reduction in tumor size is usually accompanied by improvement of visual fields and pituitary function *(48,49)*.

Dramatic improvement can be seen (Fig. 3). Interruption of therapy usually leads to recurrence of hyperprolactinemia and tumor regrowth. Whether therapy with a dopamine agonist can ever be discontinued is discussed below.

5.2. Efficacy

The dopamine agonists approved for use in the United States are bromocriptine and cabergoline, which differ primarily in half-life and affinity for the D2 receptor. Quinagolide is not available in the United States.

With a half life of 8–12 h, bromocriptine must be taken at least twice daily. Cabergoline, with a half-life of over 24 h, can be administered once or twice weekly. Both drugs are available in generic formulation. The usual daily dose of bromocriptine is 5 mg for microadenomas and 7.5 mg for macroadenomas. For cabergoline, the usual dose is 1 mg weekly.

In a multicenter randomized trial, cabergoline induced normal prolactin in 83 % versus 59 % of subjects receiving bromocriptine and was also more effective in restoring ovulatory cycles and pregnancies (49). Cabergoline is also effective in 70 % of patients who do not respond to bromocriptine (50). Bromocriptine normalizes prolactin levels, restores gonadal function, and decreases tumor size in 80–90 % of patients with microadenomas and about 70 % of patients with macroadenomas (48,51). About 10–20 % of patients with microadenomas and 20–30 % with macroadenomas will fail to respond to usual daily doses and are deemed dopamine agonist resistant (48,50).

Both bromocriptine and cabergoline are associated with side effects including nasal stuffiness, nausea, and orthostatic hypotension but fewer women taking cabergoline discontinue therapy due to drug intolerance (49). When compared directly, 68 % of patients taking cabergoline developed gastrointestinal and other side effects compared to 78 % with bromocriptine (49). Symptoms (especially with bromocriptine) usually occur at initiation of therapy and can be minimized by initiating therapy at bedtime and increasing the dose slowly. Intravaginal administration of bromocriptine reduces gastrointestinal side effects but may result in vaginal irritation (52). Depression and digital vasospasm are rare side effects only reported in patients receiving high doses of bromocriptine (31).

In the 1980s pleural thickening and retroperitoneal fibrosis were noted in some patients with Parkinson's disease treated with high doses of bromocriptine (53,54). More recently, an increased risk of cardiac valve regurgitation was reported in patients with Parkinson's disease treated with cabergoline and pergolide (55,56). While never approved for treatment of hyperprolactinemia in the United States, pergolide has now been withdrawn from the market. It should be emphasized that doses of cabergoline used in treatment of Parkinson's disease are substantially higher than those used in standard treatment of prolactinomas (3 mg daily versus 1 mg weekly). While the risk of valvular disease during therapy for hyperprolactinemia is not established, patients receiving cabergoline should be informed of the findings in patients with Parkinson's disease. Decisions about the need for and/or frequency of echocardiographic monitoring of patients taking long-term cabergoline will need to be individualized until more data become available. In all cases administration of cabergoline should always utilize the lowest dose and shortest duration possible.

It remains controversial whether long-term treatment with a dopamine agonist has a detrimental effect on surgical outcome. The development of tumor fibrosis after bromocriptine therapy could become clinically important if surgery becomes necessary in a patient who fails to respond to a dopamine agonist *(57,58)*.

6. TREATMENT WHEN FERTILITY IS THE GOAL

6.1. Microadenoma

Based on an extensive safety record ($\sim$ 6,000 pregnancies) bromocriptine is the treatment of choice when pregnancy is the goal *(59)*. Therapy should be initiated at bedtime with a dose of 0.625 mg. After 1 week, twice daily dosing is begun with the addition of a morning dose of 1.25 mg. The dose should be increased by 1.25 mg at weekly intervals until a daily dose of 5 mg is reached. After the patient has taken 5 mg daily for 6–8 weeks a prolactin level should be repeated.

At initiation of therapy, women should use a mechanical form of contraception until at least two regular menstrual cycles have occurred. Bromocriptine should be discontinued as soon as pregnancy is confirmed. Administered in this fashion, bromocriptine has not been associated with an increased incidence of spontaneous abortion, ectopic pregnancy, or congenital malformation *(59)*. It is not necessary to perform serial measurements of serum prolactin during pregnancy because rising levels of prolactin do not reliably correlate with tumor enlargement *(60)*. While the high estrogen levels associated with pregnancy lead to lactotroph hyperplasia and an increase in the size of the pituitary, the risk of clinically significant tumor enlargement with a microadenoma is only about 1 % *(61)*. It is thus not necessary to perform serial MRI scans or formal visual field testing in women with microadenomas during pregnancy. Breastfeeding is not associated with tumor growth and women wishing to breast-feed should not be given a dopamine agonist as lowering the prolactin level will impair lactation *(62)*.

6.2. Macroadenomas

Treatment of a macroadenoma in anticipation of pregnancy is more complicated. With an intrasellar macroadenoma the risk of clinically significant tumor growth during pregnancy is about 1% *(61)*. In contrast, there is a 15–30% risk of tumor enlargement during pregnancy with a macroadenoma that demonstrates extrasellar extension *(61)*. With these invasive tumors there is no ideal treatment option and treatment must be highly individualized. It may be necessary to surgically debulk the tumor prior to conception and/or to administer bromocriptine throughout pregnancy *(63,64)*. There is minimal information available related to the safety of any dopamine agonist administered *during* pregnancy. While bromocriptine has been used in about 50 pregnancies and no major complications or fetal abnormalities have been identified *(63–66)*, it is *not* approved by the United States Food and Drug Administration for use during pregnancy. There is no information related to the use of cabergoline administered *throughout* pregnancy. With some macroadenomas it may be necessary to consider therapy with cabergoline if bromocriptine is ineffective or if the patient is intolerant to it.

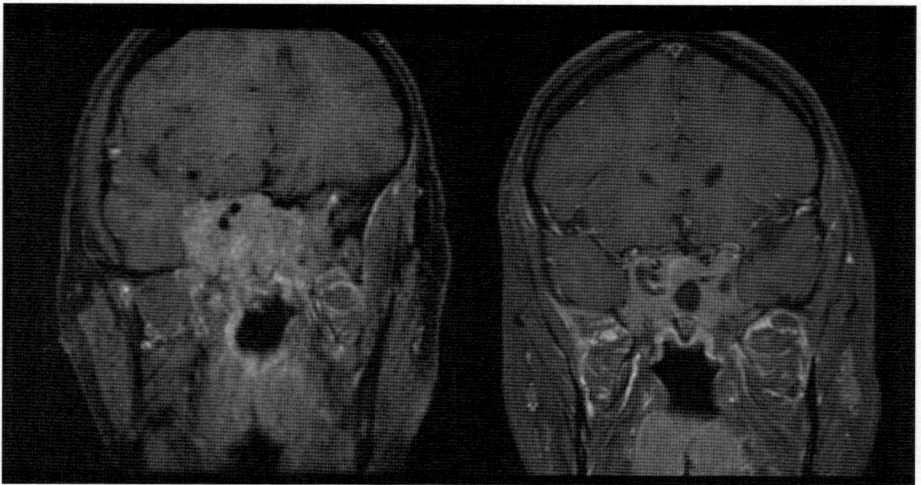

Fig. 3. Coronal view of pituitary MRI showing a giant invasive macro-prolactinoma before (left) and after (right) dopamine agonist treatment.

7. TREATMENT WHEN FERTILITY IS NOT AN ISSUE

7.1. Microadenomas

As 95 % of microadenomas do not progressively increase in size, prevention of tumor growth is not an indication for therapy *(67–69)*. To restore gonadal function, either bromocriptine or cabergoline may be used. Bromocriptine is less expensive but also has more side effects. Treatment may restore gonadal function *without* normalization of serum prolactin and it is not necessary to increase the dose of cabergoline or bromocriptine merely to normalize prolactin once gonadal function has been restored. Prolactin levels should be monitored yearly, even in patients not receiving therapy. Because of the very low growth potential we do not recommend serial MRI scans or formal visual field testing for patients with untreated microadenomas. An MRI scan should be obtained if there is a marked increase in prolactin (> 250 µg/l) or clinical signs of tumor expansion such as headaches or visual changes.

Since both cabergoline and bromocriptine are expensive and have side effects, another option when fertility is not an issue is to treat with estrogen. Oral contraceptives are better tolerated and less expensive than dopamine agonists and the estrogen protects the skeleton. While high levels of estrogen lead to lactotroph hyperplasia, short-term use of oral contraceptive has not been associated with tumor growth *(70,71)*. Hyperprolactinemic women treated with estrogen should undergo annual measurements of serum prolactin. An MRI should be obtained if clinical signs of tumor expansion appear or prolactin levels exceed 250 µg/l. Estrogen should be used with caution in women with macroadenomas as even small changes in tumor size may have significant clinical effects.

In men with prolactinomas, sex hormone replacement is a less attractive therapeutic option. Administration of testosterone has not been reported to lead to tumor growth but testosterone replacement also does not uniformly restore sexual function in hyperprolactinemic men *(18,19)*. It may, however, improve bone density and metabolic function even if sexual function is not restored.

7.2. Macroadenomas

In addition to restoring gonadal function, therapy should decrease tumor size, relieve chiasm compression, and restore pituitary function. The greater potency of cabergoline makes it an obvious first choice but bromocriptine can also be effective. Patients with macroadenomas generally require higher doses of bromocriptine and cabergoline and adenomas resistant to dopamine agonist therapy are more likely to be large tumors. Visual field testing and an MRI scan should be repeated about 3 months after initiation of therapy and yearly until tumor size stabilizes. While restoration of gonadal function and normalization of prolactin may occur *without* a change in tumor size, the dose of a dopamine agonist should be increased until maximum tumor shrinkage has been obtained. In patients presenting with visual field loss, primary medical treatment is still appropriate, but careful monitoring of the visual field examination and tumor size is required. Surgical referral may become necessary in those cases where the chiasm remains compressed and/or visual impairment persists despite maximal medical treatment.

8. IS MEDICAL THERAPY THE ONLY OPTION?

Prior to the development of dopamine agonists the treatment of prolactinomas was transsphenoidal surgery. Even if it is performed by an experienced surgeon, the procedure does not offer a long-term cure especially in patients with invasive macroadenomas. Success rates for microadenomas are around 72% and 30–50% for macroadenomas *(72)*. Better success rates (close to 90%) are achievable in young patients and in those with very small tumors *(72,73)*, but 13–50% of patients develop recurrent hyperprolactinemia after surgery *(74,75)*. Transsphenoidal surgery *should* be considered in patients who do not respond to or are intolerant of dopamine agonists. In addition, some patients may request surgery to avoid protracted medical therapy. Radiation has no role as primary therapy for prolactinomas but may be necessary in patients with large tumors who fail to respond to medical or surgical treatment.

9. CAN DOPAMINE AGONIST THERAPY BE DISCONTINUED?

Because discontinuation of a dopamine agonist is usually associated with tumor regrowth and recurrence of hyperprolactinemia, it has been assumed that therapy must be lifelong *(76)*. Recent analyses suggest that discontinuation of therapy is feasible in a select subgroup of patients *(77–80)*. In a prospective analysis of patients treated with cabergoline, 69% with microadenomas and 64% with macroadenomas had remission of hyperprolactinemia and no tumor growth after drug withdrawal *(77)*. In a smaller study of patients with microadenomas treated with bromocriptine and cabergoline 35% attained remission of hyperprolactinemia *(80)*. Recurrence of hyperprolactinemia was more likely in the presence of a tumor remnant at the time of withdrawal *(77)*, and the majority of subjects who developed recurrent hyperprolactinemia did so within 1 year of discontinuation of therapy *(77,80)*.

The possibility that long-term dopamine agonist therapy may be unnecessary is intriguing but many questions remain. The optimal length of therapy prior to drug withdrawal has not been defined, and the follow-up interval after drug withdrawal has been very short. In addition, there are, as yet, no precise criteria to predict which patients might benefit from drug withdrawal. Prospective long-term studies will be necessary to determine the safety and efficacy of stopping dopamine agonist therapy. It is encouraging that expensive lifelong therapy may not be inevitable in all cases.

REFERENCES

1. Mindermann T, Wilson CB. Age-related and gender-related occurrence of pituitary adenomas. Clin Endocrinol (Oxf) 1994;41:359–64.
2. Ciccarelli A, Daly AF, Beckers A. The epidemiology of prolactinomas. Pituitary 2005;8: 3–6.
3. Scheithauer BW, Kovacs KT, Randall RV, Ryan N. Effects of estrogen on the human pituitary: a clinicopathologic study. Mayo Clinic Proc 1989;64:1077–84.
4. Burgess J R, Shepherd JJ, Parameswaran V, Hoffman L, Greenaway TM. Prolactinomas in a large kindred with multiple endocrine neoplasia type 1: clinical features and inheritance pattern. J Clin Endocrinol Metab 1996;81:1841–5.
5. Herman V, Fagin J, Gonsky R, Kovacs K, Melmed S. Clonal origin of pituitary adenomas. J Clin Endocrinol Metab 1990;71:1427–33.
6. Fine SA, Frohman LA. Loss of central nervous system component of dopaminergic inhibition of prolactin secretion in patients with prolactin-secreting pituitary tumors. J Clin Invest 1978;61:973–80.
7. Clayton RN, Boggild M, Bates AS, Ricknell J, Simpson D, Farrell W. Tumor suppressor genes in the pathogenesis of human pituitary tumors. Horm Res 1997;47:185–93.
8. Spada A, Mantovani G, Lania A. Pathogenesis of prolactinomas. Pituitary 2005;8:7–15.
9. Sauder SE, Frager M, Case GD, Kelch RP, Marshall JC. Abnormal patterns of pulsatile luteinizing hormone secretion in women with hyperprolactinemia and amenorrhea: response to bromocriptine. J Clin Endocrinol Metab 1984;59:941–8.
10. Sartorio A, Pizzocaro A, Liberati D, De Nicolao G, Veldhuis JD, Faglia G. Abnormal LH pulsatility in women with hyperprolactinemic amenorrhea normalizes after bromocriptine treatment: deconvolution-based assessment. Clin Endocrinol (Oxf) 2000;52:703–12.
11. Dorrington J, Gore-Langton RE. Prolactin inhibits oestrogen synthesis in the ovary. Nature 1981;290:600–2.
12. Schlechte J, Sherman B, Halmi N, et al. Prolactin-secreting pituitary tumors in amenorrheic women: a comprehensive study. Endocr Rev 1980;1:295–308.
13. Touraine P, Plu-Bureau G, Beji C, Mauvais-Jarvis P, Kuttenn F. Long-term follow-up of 246 hyperprolactinemic patients. Acta Obstet Gynecol Scand 2001;80:162–8.
14. Corenblum B, Pairaudeau N, Shewchuk AB. Prolactin hypersecretion and short luteal phase defects. Obstet Gynecol 1976;47:486–8.
15. Pituitary Adenoma Study Group. Pituitary adenomas and oral contraceptives: a multicenter case-control study. Fertil Steril 1983;39:753–60.
16. Sibal L, Ugwu P, Kendall-Taylor P, et al. Medical therapy of macroprolactinomas in males: I. prevalence of hypopituitarism at diagnosis. II. Proportion of cases exhibiting recovery of pituitary function. Pituitary 2002;5:243–6.
17. Colao A, Vitale G, Cappabianca P, et al. Outcome of cabergoline treatment in men with prolactinoma: effects of a 24-month treatment on prolactin levels, tumor mass, recovery of pituitary function, and semen analysis. J Clin Endocrinol Metab 2004;89:1704–11.
18. Carter JN, Tyson JE, Tolis G, Van Vliet S, Faiman C, Friesen HG. Prolactin secreting tumors and hypogonadism in 22 men. N Engl J Med 1978;299:847–52.

19. De Rossa M, Zarrilli S, Vitale G, et al. Six months of treatment with cabergoline restores sexual potency in hyperprolactinemic males: an open longitudinal study monitoring nocturnal penile tumescence. J Clin Endocrinol Metab 2004;89:621–5.

20. Segal S, Yaffe H, Laufer N, Ben-David M. Male hyperprolactinemia: effects on fertility. Fertil Steril 1979;32:556–61.

21. Delgrange E, Trouillas J, Maiter D, Donckier J, Tourniaire J. Sex-related difference in the growth of prolactinomas: a clinical and proliferation marker study. J Clin Endocrinol Metab 1997;82:2102–7.

22. Nishioka H, Haraoka J, Akada K. Growth potential of prolactinomas in men: is it really different from women? Surg Neurol 2003;59:386–91.

23. Klibanski A, Biller BM, Rosenthal DI, Schoenfeld DA, Saxe V. Effects of prolactin and estrogen deficiency in amenorrheic bone loss. J Clin Endocrinol Metab 1998;67:124–30.

24. Schlechte J, Walker L, Kathol M. A longitudinal analysis of premenopausal bone loss in healthy women and women with hyperprolactinemia. J Clin Endocrinol Metab 1992;75:698–703.

25. Tyson JE, Ito P, Guyda H, et al. Studies of prolactin in human pregnancy. Am J Obstet Gynecol 1972;113:14–20.

26. McCallum RW, Sowers JR, Hershman JM, Studevant RA. Metoclopramide stimulates prolactin secretion in man. J Clin Endocrinol Metab 1976;42:1148–52.

27. Green AI, Brown WA. Prolactin and neuroleptic drugs. Endocrinol Metab Clin North Am 1988;17:213–23.

28. Langer G, Sachar EJ. Dopaminergic factors in human prolactin regulation: effects of neuroleptics and dopamine Psychoneuroendocrinology 1977;2:373–8.

29. David SR, Taylor CC, Kinon BJ, Breier A. The effects of olanzapine, risperidone, and haloperidol on plasma prolactin levels in patients with schizophrenia. Clin Ther 2000;22:1085–96.

30. Meltzer HY, Fang VS, Tricou BJ, Robertson A. Effect of antidepressants on neuroendocrine axis in humans. In: Costa E, Racagni G, editors. Typical and Atypical Antidepressants: Clinical Practice. New York: Raven Press; 1982. pp. 303–16.

31. Molitch ME. Medication-induced hyperprolactinemia. Mayo Clin Proc 2005;80:1050–7.

32. Kelley SR, Kamal TJ, Molitch ME. Mechanism of verapamil calcium channel blockade-induced hyperprolactinemia. Am J Physiol 1996;270:E96–100.

33. Reyniak JV, Wenof M, Aubert JM, Stangel JJ. Incidence of hyperprolactinemia during oral contraceptive therapy. Obstet Gynecol 1980;55:8–11.

34. Grasso A, Baraghini F, Barbieri C, et al. Endocrinological features and endometrial morphology in climacteric women receiving hormone replacement therapy. Maturitas 1982;4:19–26.

35. Abs R, Verhelst J, Maiter D, et al. Cabergoline in the Treatment of Acromegaly: A Study in 64 Patients. J Clin Endocrinol Metab 1998;83:374–8.

36. Portocarrero CJ, Robinson AG, Taylor AL, Klein I. Lymphoid hypophysitis. An unusual cause of hyperprolactinemia and enlarged sella turcica. JAMA 1981;246:1811–2.

37. Franks S. Polycystic ovary syndrome. N Engl J Med 1995;333:853–61.

38. Grubb MR, Chakeres D, Malarkey WB. Patients with primary hypothyroidism presenting as prolactinoma. Am J Med 1987;83:765–9.

39. Martin TL, Kim M, Malarkey WB. The natural history of idiopathic hyperprolactinemia. J Clin Endocrinol Metab 1985;60:855–8.

40. Sluijmer AV, Lappöhn RE. Clinical history and outcome of 59 patients with idiopathic hyperprolactinemia. Fertil Steril 1992;58:72–7.

41. Vallette-Kasic S, Morange-Ramos I, Selim A, et al. Macroprolactinemia revisited: a study of 106 patients. J Clin Endocrinol Metab 2002;87:581–8.
42. Strachan MW, Teoh WL, Don-Wauchope AC. Seth J, Stoddart M, Beckett GJ. Clinical and radiological features of patients with macroprolactinemia. Clin Endocrinol (Oxf) 2003;59:339–46.
43. Gibney J, Smith TP, McKenna TJ. The impact on clinical practice of routine screening for macroprolactin. J Clin Endocrinol Metab 2005;90:3927–32.
44. Sawers HA, Robb OJ, Walmsley D, Strachan FM, Shaw J, Bevan JS. An audit of the diagnostic usefulness of PRL and TSH responses to domperidone and high resolution magnetic resonance imaging of the pituitary in the evaluation of hyperprolactinemia. Clin Endocrinol 1997;46:321–6.
45. St-Jean E, Blain F, Comtois R. High prolactin levels may be missed by immunoradiometric assay in patients with macroprolactinomas. Clin Endocrinol (Oxf) 1996;44:305–9.
46. MacLeod RM, Lehmeyer JE. Suppression of pituitary tumor growth and function by ergot alkaloids. Cancer Res 1973;33:849–55.
47. Asa SL, Ezzat S. Medical management of pituitary adenomas: structural and ultrastructural changes. Pituitary 2002;5:133–9.
48. Molitch ME, Elton RL, Blackwell RE, et al. Bromocriptine as primary therapy for prolactin-secreting macroadenomas: results of a prospective multicenter study. J Clin Endocrinol Metab 1985;60:698–705.
49. Webster J, Piscitelli G, Polli A, Ferrari CI, Ismail I, Scanlon MF. A comparison of cabergoline and bromocriptine in the treatment of hyperprolactinemic amenorrhea. N Engl J Med 1994;331:904–9.
50. Colao A, Di Sarno A, Sarnacchiaro S, et al. Prolactinomas resistant to standard dopamine agonists respond to chronic cabergoline treatment. J Clin Endocrinol Metab 1997;82:876–83.
51. Bevan JS, Webster J, Burke CW, Scanlon MF. Dopamine agonists and pituitary tumor shrinkage. Endocr Rev 1992;13:220–40.
52. Jasonni VM, Raffeilli R, de March A, Frank G, Flanigni L. Vaginal bromocriptine in hyper-prolactinemic patients and puerperal women. Acta Obstet Gynecol Scand 1991;70:493–5.
53. Demont JF, Rostin M, Dueymes JM, Ioualalen A, Montastruc JL, Rascol A. Retroperitoneal fibrosis and treatment of Parkinson's disease with high doses of bromocriptine. Clin Neuropharmacol 1986;9:200–1.
54. McElvaney NG, Wilcox PG, Churg A, Fleetham JA. Pleuropulmonary disease during bromocriptine treatment of Parkinson's disease. Arch Intern Med 1988;148:2231–6.
55. Schade R, Andersohn F, Suissa S, Haverkamp W, Garbe E. Dopamine agonists and the risk of cardiac-valve regurgitation. N Engl J Med 2007;356:29–38.
56. Zanettini R, Antonini A, Gatto G, Gentile R, Tesei S, Pezzoli G. Valvular Heart Disease and the Use of Dopamine Agonists for Parkinson's Disease. N Engl J Med 2007;356:39–46.
57. Landolt AM, Osterwalder V. Perivascular fibrosis in prolactinomas: is it increased by bromocriptine? J Clin Endocrinol Metab 1984;58:1179–83.
58. Esiri MM, Bevan JS, Burke CW, Adams CB. Effect of bromocriptine treatment on the fibrous tissue content of prolactin-secreting and nonfunctioning macroadenomas of the pituitary gland. J Clin Endocrinol Metab 1986;63:383–8.
59. Krupp P, Monka C. Bromocriptine in pregnancy: safety aspects Klin Wochenschr 1987;65:823–7.
60. Bronstein MD. Prolactinomas and pregnancy. Pituitary 2005;8:31–8.
61. Molitch ME. Pregnancy and the hyperprolactinemic woman. N Engl J Med 1985;312:1365–70.

62. Holmgren U, Bergstrand G, Hagenfeldt K, Werner S. Women with prolactinoma – effect of pregnancy and lactation on serum prolactin and on tumour growth. Acta Endocrinol (Copenh) 1986;111:452–9.

63. Canales ES, Garcia IC, Ruiz JE, Zarate A. Bromocriptine as prophylactic therapy in prolactinoma during pregnancy. Fertil Steril 1986;36:524–6.

64. van Roon E, van der Vijver JCM, Gerretsen G, Hekster REM, Wattendorff RA. Rapid regression of a suprasellar extending prolactinoma after bromocriptine treatment during pregnancy. Fertil Steril 1981;36:173–7.

65. Konopka P, Raymond JP, Merceron RE, Seneze J. Continuous administration of bromocriptine in the prevention of neurological complications in pregnant women with prolactinomas. Am J Obstet Gynecol 1983;146:935–8.

66. Weil C. The safety of bromocriptine in long-term use: a review of the literature. Curr Res Opin 1986;10:25–51.

67. Schlechte J, Dolan K, Sherman B, Chaplet F, Luciano A. The natural history of untreated hyperprolactinemia: a prospective analysis. J Clin Endocrinol Metab 1989;68:412–8.

68. March C, Kletzky O, Davajan V, et al. Longitudinal evaluation of patients with untreated prolactin-secreting pituitary adenomas. Am J Obstet Gynecol 1981;139:835–44.

69. Weiss MH, Teal J, Gott P, et al. Natural history of microprolactinomas: six-year follow-up. Neurosurgery 1983;12:180–3.

70. Fathy UM, Foster PA, Torode HW, Hartog M, Hull MG. The effect of combined estrogen/progesterone treatment in women with hyperprolactinemic amenorrhea. Gynecol Endocrinol 1992;6:183–8.

71. Corenblum B, Donovan L. The safety of physiological estrogen plus progestin replacement therapy with oral contraceptive therapy in women with pathological hyperprolactinemia. Fertil Steril 1993;59:671–3.

72. Jane JA, Jr, Laws ER Jr. The surgical management of pituitary adenomas in a series of 3,093 patients. J Am Coll Surg 2001;193:651–9.

73. Nomikos P, Buchfelder M, Fahlbusch R. Current management of prolactinomas. J Neurooncol 2001;54:139–150.

74. Schlechte JA, Sherman BM, Chapler FK, VanGilder J. Long-term follow-up of women with surgically treated prolactin-secreting pituitary tumors. J Clin Endocrinol Metab 1986;62:1296–301.

75. Serri O, Rasio E, Beauregard H, Hardy J, Somma M. Recurrence of hyperprolactinemia after selective transsphenoidal adenomectomy in women with prolactinoma. N Engl J Med 1983;309:280–3.

76. Faglia G. Should dopamine agonist treatment for prolactinomas be life-long? Clin Endocrinol 1991;34:173–4.

77. Colao A, Di Sarno A, Cappabianca P, Di Somma C, Pivonello R, Lombardi G. Withdrawal of long-term cabergoline therapy for tumoral and nontumoral hyperprolactinemia. N Engl J Med 2003;349:2023–33.

78. Jeffcoate WJ, Pound N, Sturrock ND, Lambourne J. Long-term follow-up of patients with hyperprolactinaemia. Clin Endocrinol (Oxf) 1996;45, 299–303.

79. Passos VQ, Souza JJ, Musolino NR, Bronstein MD. Long-term follow-up of prolactinomas: normoprolactinemia after bromocriptine withdrawal. J Clin Endocrinol Metab 2002;87:3578–82.

80. Biswas M, Smith J, Jadon D, et al. Long-term remission following withdrawal of dopamine agonist therapy in subjects with microprolactinomas. Clin Endocrinol 2005;63:26–31.

7

Acromegaly: *Pathogenesis, Natural History, and Diagnosis*

David R. Clemmons, MD

Summary

Acromegaly is usually caused by somatotroph adenomas of the pituitary gland that secrete excess growth hormone (GH). This state of GH excess stimulates IGF-I, a peptide hormone that stimulates cell growth. This chronic stimulation of tissue growth leads to multiple symptoms and signs that comprise the acromegalic condition, characterized by tissue overgrowth leading to significant morbidity. The diagnosis can be confirmed by measuring GH suppression following oral glucose administration and measurement of serum IGF-I concentration. Early diagnosis is facilitated by an awareness of the presenting features of the disease and the availability of high-quality, specific, and sensitive diagnostic tests.

Key Words: Pituitary tumor, Insulin-like growth factor-I, Somatotropin, Growth hormone releasing hormone, Somatostatin, IGF-I, IGFBP-3, Acid labile subunit.

From: *Contemporary Endocrinology: Diagnosis and Management of Pituitary Disorders*
Edited by: B. Swearingen and B. M. K. Biller © Humana Press, Totowa, NJ

1. INTRODUCTION

Acromegaly results from the somatic response to chronic growth hormone (GH) excess. In almost all cases, GH excess results from unrestrained hypersecretion by the somatotroph cells of the pituitary. Under normal conditions GH secretion is regulated by GHRH, which is synthesized and released in the hypothalamus in response to a variety of stimuli, and somatostatin, a GH release inhibitory factor that is also synthesized in the hypothalamus. Other variables that control pituitary somatotroph function include circulating insulin-like growth factor-I concentrations, which exert negative feedback regulation, and ghrelin, a gut-derived peptide that binds to the GHS receptor and acts to induce GH secretion *(1)*.

2. CAUSES OF GH HYPERSCRETION

Pituitary tumors usually arise as a result of clonal expansion of somatotrophs *(2)*. These include both pure somatotroph tumors and mixed somatomammotroph tumors that secrete both GH and prolactin. Patients with McCune Albright syndrome, which occurs as a result of a G protein-activating mutation, may have acromegaly and in these patients somatotroph hyperplasia, as well as somatotroph adenomas, may be encountered *(3)*. Rarely, acromegaly may occur as a result of excessive GHRH secretion, resulting in somatotroph hyperplasia and GH hypersecretion. Excessive GHRH secretion may be due to primary hypothalamic lesions such as hamartomas or gangliocytomas. Ectopic GHRH production can occur at other anatomic sites, such as in carcinoid syndrome or islet cell tumors, small cell lung cancer, adrenal adenoma, medullarly thyroid carcinoma, and pheochromocytoma *(4)*. Excessive GHRH production may play a role in the generation of somatotroph adenomas in some cases where there are activating mutations of guanosine triphosphosphatase (GTPase), resulting in ligand-independent activation of GHRH signaling *(5)*. Likewise, a mutation in the cyclic AMP response binding protein can activate GHRH signaling.

Because almost all cases of acromegaly result from clonal expansion of the adenomatous cells, several candidate genes that could account for this have been examined in animal models. These include the retinoblastoma tumor suppression gene and p27 *(6)*. Disruption of the MENIN gene, resulting in MEN-I syndrome, can be associated with somatotroph adenomas *(7)*. Ras mutations have been reported to activate GH secretion in experimental animal models, as have mutations of a pituitary tumor transforming gene. Recently a common mutation in a tumor suppressor gene (arylhydrocarbon receptor interacting protein) in a Finnish population was reported to account for over 40% of cases in acromegaly in patients diagnosed at age less than 30 years *(8)*.

In spite of all of these reports, there is as yet no genetic screening test that has been utilized to routinely screen subjects at high risk for acromegaly. There are also familial syndromes that are associated with acromegaly. These include MEN-I, as previously mentioned, involving the MENIN gene *(7)*, and the Carney complex *(9)*, which presents with myxomas, spotty skin pigmentation, and testicular, adrenal, and pituitary tumors.

3. NATURAL HISTORY

Because acromegaly is a rare disease (750–900 new cases annually in the United States) and because the rate of change of symptoms and signs is slow and insidious, the disease has generally been present for several years before diagnosis. Often, patients will have complained to their primary care physician of symptoms that are highly suggestive of acromegaly, and in many cases will have received specific medical or surgical care for a known comorbidity, such as orthodontia or carpal tunnel release. In spite of improvements in diagnostic testing, the usual period from earliest onset of symptoms and signs (usually identified by photographs) to diagnosis is 8–10 years *(10)*. The clinical manifestations of expression of the adenoma itself are usually confined to headaches. When the tumor enlarges greatly in size, a bitemporal heminopsia or cranial nerve palsies may occur, but these are less common symptoms at presentation.

4. CLINICAL CHARACTERISTICS

Due to the generalized effects of GH and IGF-I on tissue growth, multiple organs and tissues are involved during the period of disease progression *(11)*. Characteristic findings include enlargement of the bones in the hands and feet, as well as several facial bones, the most prominent being the mandible. There is also excessive sodium and water retention, resulting in further swelling of the enlarged hands. Historical evaluation reveals that patients have changed shoe or glove size and required ring enlargement in many cases. Altered facial features include enlargement of the nose and frontal bones as well as the mandible, resulting in significant orthodontia. Multiple joints may be involved, with the development of progressive osteoarthritis, although this is age dependent. Arthralgias are a common symptom even in the absence of arthritic changes. Skeletal changes often lead to back pain and kyphosis, which can result in significant disability. Skin thickening is generally present and multiple skin tags appear over time. Hyperhydrosis at rest is common and it is due to sweat gland hypertrophy. Moderate hirsutism can present in some females. Major clinical manifestations can occur as a result of soft tissue enlargement in the oropharynx. There is often a deepening of the voice, but, more importantly, macroglossia and palette enlargement can result in sleep apnea, with airway obstruction in up to 50% of patients in some series (12). Thyroid enlargement occurs in most patients. This is usually manifested as a symmetric, smooth, enlarged goiter that does not result in a change in thyroid function. Cardiac enlargement can occur; this is generally manifested as increased ventricular mass and wall thickening (13). Hypertension is also common and cardiomyopathy appears in patients with disease of long-standing duration. However, it is rare for these patients to present with overt heart failure. Due to GH's direct antagonistic effects on insulin action, glucose intolerance and/or diabetes can present in a significant percentage of patients. When carefully analyzed only 25% of patients have completely normal insulin and glucose dynamics. The most common presentation is either insulin resistance or mild hyperglycemia that does not require specific glucose lowering therapy; however, overt diabetes mellitus can present in up to 25% of patients. Abnormalities of gonadal function are common in acromegaly. Women may present with amenorrhea and signs of estrogen insufficiency (11). Men may present with impotence, loss of libido, and testicular atrophy. Hypogonadism in men or women may be accompanied by hyperprolactinemia but this is seen only in a minority of cases. Neuromuscular manifestations are also common. Unexplained weakness occurs in a high percentage of cases; however, peripheral neuropathies and paresthesias, as well as discrete syndromes such as carpal tunnel syndrome, clearly occur. Other nerve entrapment syndromes are unusual. There has been a great deal of concern regarding the increased risk of developing neoplasms, but malignancies have not been demonstrated to account for the known increase in mortality, and only colon cancer has an increased relative risk ratio of 2.4:1 (14).

In general a careful history and physical examination will reveal several of the manifestations listed previously. A constellation of findings of commonly appreciated symptoms such as headache, weakness, acral enlargement, arthralgias, swelling of the hands and feet, and typical facial changes should be strongly suggestive of a positive diagnosis. Physical examination demonstrating thickening of the skin, enlargement of the hands and feet, and typical facial features will often be confirmatory and suggest an immediate need for laboratory evaluation to establish the diagnosis. Occasional patients who do not have acromegaly do present with this constellation of physical findings. These patients will not have a history of progressive hand and foot enlargement and examination of photographs will usually not reveal serial changes. However, if physical findings are suggestive, laboratory testing should be undertaken to exclude the diagnosis.

5. LABORATORY CONFIRMATION USING GH AND IGF-I MEASUREMENTS

At the time of diagnosis, significant abnormalities exist in both regulation of GH secretion and the ambient level of IGF-I. Measurement of both peptides is important in the initial diagnostic evaluation and should be performed in all cases. This is because analysis of GH secretion provides direct information regarding the secretory output of the tumor, and measurement of IGF-I confirms that the level of secretory activity of tumor is such that it has resulted in significant morbidity and, importantly, provides a baseline from which to evaluate the success of various therapeutic options. The degree of change in IGF-I often correlates better with symptomatic improvement than does the change in GH secretion. Therefore, measurement of both these peptides provides qualitatively different types of information that are helpful in the management of patients with this disease. The majority of patients who have not received therapy will have significant abnormalities of GH secretion, such that obtaining a random GH will often show an abnormal value. However, since GH secretion is controlled in normal individuals by stress, exercise, fasting, and other variables that can result in substantial increases, the recommended measurement for establishing the diagnosis of acromegaly is a glucose suppression test. Following ingestion of 75 g of glucose there should be suppression of GH to less than 1 ng/ml if assessed by a conventional radioimmunoassay, and to less than 0.3 ng/ml if an ultrasensitive, immunoradioimmetric, or chemiluminescent test is used *(15,16)*. In general, following administration of glucose, patients with somatotroph adenomas will have minimal suppression of GH, show no change, or show paradoxical increase in GH secretion. Any of these three patterns will establish the diagnosis. Occasionally, (<2–3%) patients will present with very subtle abnormalities of GH secretion. Frequent 24-h GH sampling in these patients has shown that they rarely suppress GH to undetectable levels and rarely achieve levels greater than 1–2 ng/ml throughout a 24-h cycle *(17,18)*. Most patients that exhibit this pattern of GH secretion have symptoms and signs of acromegaly, and the persistent tonic low level of GH secretion results in abnormal pathophysiologic consequences that can often be illustrated by elevation of serum IGF-I. In such patients, glucose suppression testing can be helpful, although occasional patients have been reported in whom there is adequate suppression of GH following glucose administration *(18)*. In these patients, measurement of IGF-I is mandatory as it may show a value that is diagnostic of acromegaly. In rare cases, such as differentiating children with gigantism from normal tall adolescents, other provocative tests may be required. Approximately 60% of patients with acromegaly respond to thyrotrophin releasing hormone with an increase in GH. Similarly, about 50% of patients will suppress GH in response to acute administration of a dopaminergic agonist, whereas normal subjects increase GH; this may be helpful in difficult diagnostic situations (19).

Unlike GH, IGF-I has an extremely stable half-life of 16 h. Therefore, minute to minute fluctuations and changes in exercise, meal, stress, etc., do not perturb IGF-I concentrations. Although multiple variables such as thyroxine, cortisol, sex steroids, and nutrient intake determine IGF-I in normal subjects, in acromegaly GH hypersecretion is the principal determinant of IGF-I. Therefore IGF-I provides a very specific and sensitive index of excessive GH secretion (19). IGF-I can be obtained randomly and does not require fasting. Under such conditions, ambient IGF-I total concentrations are increased in greater than 99% of subjects with proven acromegaly, and it is a very rare individual that has clear-cut manifestations of GH hypersecretion with a normal IGF-I. The exception to this would be subjects who are markedly restricting nutrient intake or subjects with severe, poorly controlled, type I diabetes. This is due to the fact that a relatively normal caloric intake and/or response to insulin is required to synthesize and secrete IGF-I in response to GH. These situations will rarely confound the diagnosis of acromegaly. Two significant clinical situations will complicate the use of IGF-I measurements in acromegaly. The first is the known age-related variation that occurs in GH secretion in normal subjects. GH secretion is 3–4 times higher in adolescence than in adulthood. This results in substantial increases in IGF-I, and the upper limit of normal for 13-year-olds to 15-year-olds is so high that it clearly overlaps the range of values in acromegaly (19). Therefore, patients who potentially have gigantism should receive both glucose suppression testing and IGF-I measurements, as IGF-I may not always be unequivocally elevated in such patients. Because of this known age-related change in GH secretion, adequate normative data are required for all age ranges (21). It is recommended that reference laboratories divide their normal values into intervals of no less than 10 years for subjects greater than 30 years and 5-year intervals for subjects less than 30 years, and that at least 50 normal male and female values for each age-related interval be obtained. This type of age stratification results in much more precise utilization of IGF-I assays as a diagnostic test in acromegaly.

A second problem that derives from using IGF-I as a diagnostic test is that the abnormal range is defined statistically. That is, 2.5% of all normal subjects will have an elevated IGF-I by definition because their values will be greater than the 95% confidence interval. Because acromegaly is such a rare disease, random screening of the normal population will reveal many more elevated IGF-Is than actual subjects with acromegaly. Therefore the appropriate use of an IGF-I value is in a patient with signs and symptoms of acromegaly and abnormal GH suppression following glucose. If a high IGF-I value is obtained prior to performing GH suppression testing, GH suppression testing should still be performed to confirm the diagnosis.

6. ROLE OF OTHER DIAGNOSTIC TESTS

Unlike most peptide hormones, IGF-I circulates bound to high-affinity binding proteins. Although there are six binding proteins in serum, the majority of IGF-I (greater than 80%) is bound to a protein termed IGFBP-3. IGFBP-3 concentrations in serum are GH dependent and therefore there has been interest in determining whether direct measurement of IGFBP-3 would also be of aid in the diagnosis of acromegaly *(22)*. Although direct measurement of IGFBP-3 in untreated acromegalic subjects has shown that it is significantly elevated above the normal range in greater than 85% of such subjects, comparison studies have shown that measurement of IGFBP-3 offers no enhanced benefit as compared to measuring total IGF-I, and therefore it is not recommended as a diagnostic test. However, in subjects where there is a discrepancy between clinical findings and GH suppression testing or GH suppression testing and total IGF-I, measurement of IGFBP-3 may help to confirm or exclude the diagnosis.

A third protein, termed acid labile subunit or ALS, is a GH-dependent peptide that binds to the complex of IGFBP-3 and IGF-I. ALS functions to further stabilize this complex, prolonging its half-life to 16 h. Because synthesis of ALS is dependent upon GH secretion, there has been interest in determining its utility in diagnosing acromegaly. The sensitivity and specificity of ALS measurements have been reported to be greater than 90%; however, ALS concentrations are also partially determined by total IGFBP-3 concentrations. Since IGF-II is not elevated in acromegaly and acts as a restraining influence on IGFBP-3, it also acts as a restraining influence on ALS; therefore the degree of change in ALS is less than for IGF-I, i.e., the mean values are increased 3.5-fold *(23)*. Therefore the clinical utility of measuring ALS is similar to that of IGFBP-3, and it can be of help in diagnostic situations where IGF-I concentrations and GH suppression are discordant, but it is not useful as a primary diagnostic test.

Free IGF-I measurement has also been advocated as a superior measurement. However, when free IGF-I is compared to total IGF-I, total IGF-I is a superior measurement *(24)*. This probably derives from the fact that there are less normative data available for estimating free IGF-I concentrations in the normal population and the fact that free IGF-I is a technically difficult measurement. For these reasons, it is not advocated as a primary diagnostic test.

In summary, the total IGF-I measurement remains the diagnostic gold standard in acromegaly. Because it correlates well with the severity of disease at the time of diagnosis in terms of both symptomatic activity and soft tissue enlargement *(19)*, it provides information that is not provided by GH suppression testing. For these reasons, it should be utilized to confirm the diagnosis and establish the degree of disease severity at the time of initiation of treatment.

7. OTHER LABORATORY ABNORMALITIES AT DIAGNOSIS

Frequently, other laboratory tests may be abnormal at the time of diagnosis. These include an elevated fasting serum phosphorus, elevated fasting blood glucose, and hyperprolactinemia. Glucose and prolactin should be measured during the initial evaluation as changes in these tests may help to choose among various therapeutic alternatives. To localize the source of GH hypersecretion, MRI is recommended in all subjects. Since most of these patients will have a macroadenoma, the MRI provides definitive identification of a pituitary mass and may provide helpful information to the surgeon regarding invasion into the cavernous sinus or suprasellar extension *(11,19)*. Absence of a distinct mass lesion on MRI will necessitate further radiologic evaluation to look for ectopic sources of GH and/or GHRH. This should include imaging of the chest or abdomen. Some ectopic tumors may be located on head MRI. However, if no mass lesion is detected in the face of clinical signs and abnormal biochemical measures, then imaging of the chest or abdomen followed by catheterization techniques should be performed in order to localize the tumor. If such studies are undertaken, biochemical measurements should be made for both GH and GHRH.

8. FURTHER DIAGNOSTIC EVALUATION

Diagnostic evaluation of comorbidities should be undertaken if symptoms and/or signs suggest that these may be present. If symptoms suggest that sleep apnea is present, a detailed sleep study is indicated, since reversal of this abnormality may require specific therapeutic interventions over and above those necessary to cure the acromegalic disease state. Echocardiography should be undertaken if evidence of severe ventricular dysfunction is present. Radiographic evaluation of arthropathy is rarely indicated since it is unlikely to change the therapeutic approach. Nerve conduction studies may be of help in confirming the presence of a nerve entrapment syndrome such as carpal tunnel syndrome. A screening colonoscopy is recommended at diagnosis for all patients.

9. SUMMARY

Confirmation of the diagnosis of acromegaly does not represent a problematic endeavor since sensitive and specific tests are available to definitively establish the diagnosis. By far the most common problem in diagnosis is failure to recognize the slow and insidious progression of symptoms and signs in a given patient by a primary care provider, thus leading to a significant delay in diagnosis, which increases morbidity and mortality as well as limits the treatment options. Awareness of the commonly associated comorbidities as well as the typical presenting signs and symptoms is likely to lead to greater recognition.

REFERENCES

1. Melmed S, Jameson JS. Disorders of the Anterior Pituitary and Hypothalamus. In: Kasper DL, Fauci AS, Hauser SL, et al., editors. Harrison's Principles of Internal Medicine, 26th ed. New York: McGraw-Hill; 2005. pp. 2976–2097.
2. Herman V, Fagin J, Gonsky R, Kovacs K, Melmed S. Clonal origin of pituitary adenomas. J Clin Endocrinol Metab 1990;71:1427–33.
3. Weinstein LS, Shenker A, Gejman PV, Merino MJ, Friedman E, Spiegel AM. Activating mutations of the stimulatory G protein in the McCune-Albright syndrome. N Engl J Med 1991;325:1688–95.
4. Thorner MO, Perryman RL, Cronin MJ, et al. Somatotroph hyperplasia. Successful treatment of acromegaly by removal of a pancreatic islet tumor secreting a growth hormone-releasing factor. J Clin Invest 1982;70:965–77.
5. Melmed S, Ho K, Klibanski A, Reichlin S, Thorner M. Clinical review 75: Recent advances in pathogenesis, diagnosis, and management of acromegaly. J Clin Endocrinol Metab 1995;80:3395–402.
6. Herman V, Drazin NZ, Gonsky R, Melmed S. Molecular screening of pituitary adenomas for gene mutations and rearrangements. J Clin Endocrinol Metab 1993;77:50–5.
7. Prezant TR, Levine J, Melmed S. Molecular characterization of the men1 tumor suppressor gene in sporadic pituitary tumors. J Clin Endocrinol Metab 1998;83:1388–91.
8. Vierimaa O, Georgitsi M, Lehtonen R, et al. Pituitary adenoma predisposition caused by germline mutations in the AIP gene. Science 2006;312:1228–30.
9. Stratakis CA, Carney JA, Lin JP, et al. Carney complex, a familial multiple neoplasia and lentiginosis syndrome. Analysis of 11 kindreds and linkage to the short arm of chromosome 2. J Clin Invest 1996;97:699–705.
10. Nabarro JD. Acromegaly. Clin Endocrinol (Oxf) 1987;26:481–512.
11. Molitch ME. Clinical manifestations of acromegaly. Endocrinol Metab Clin North Am 1992;21:597–614.
12. Grunstein RR, Ho KY, Sullivan CE. Sleep apnea in acromegaly. Ann Intern Med 1991;115:527–32.
13. Colao A, Cuocolo A, Marzullo P, et al. Effects of 1-year treatment with octreotide on cardiac performance in patients with acromegaly. J Clin Endocrinol Metab 1999;84:17–23.
14. Renehan AG, Bhaskar P, Painter JE, et al. The prevalence and characteristics of colorectal neoplasia in acromegaly. J Clin Endocrinol Metab 2000;85:3417–24.
15. Giustina A, Barkan A, Casanueva FF, et al. Criteria for cure of acromegaly: a consensus statement. J Clin Endocrinol Metab 2000;85:526–9.
16. Freda PU. Current concepts in the biochemical assessment of the patient with acromegaly. Growth Horm IGF Res 2003;13:171–84.
17. Dimaraki EV, Jaffe CA, DeMott-Friberg R, Chandler WF, and Barkan AL. Acromegaly with apparently normal GH secretion: implications for diagnosis and follow-up. J Clin Endocrinol Metab 2002;87:3537–4218.

18. Barkan AL. Acromegaly. Diagnosis and therapy. Endocrinol Metab Clin North Am 1989;18:277–310.
19. Clemmons DR, Van Wyk JJ, Ridgway EC, Kliman B, Kjellberg RN, and Underwood LE. Evaluation of acromegaly by radioimmunoassay of somatomedin-C. N Engl J Med 1979;301:1138–42.
20. Juul A, Dalgaard P, Blum WF, et al. Serum levels of insulin-like growth factor (IGF)-binding protein-3 (IGFBP-3) in healthy infants, children, and adolescents: the relation to IGF-I, IGF-II, IGFBP-1, IGFBP-2, age, sex, body mass index, and pubertal maturation. J Clin Endocrinol Metab 1995;80:2534–42.
21. Brabant G, von zur Muhlen A, and Wuster C, et al. Serum insulin-like growth factor I reference values for an automated chemiluminescence immunoassay system: results from a multicenter study. Horm Res 2003;60:53–60.
22. Grinspoon S, Clemmons D, Swearingen B, and Klibanski A. Serum insulin-like growth factor-binding protein-3 levels in the diagnosis of acromegaly. J Clin Endocrinol Metab 1995;80, 927–32.
23. Fukuda I, Hizuka N, Itoh E, et al. Acid-labile subunit in growth hormone excess and deficiency in adults: evaluation of its diagnostic value in comparison with insulin-like growth factor (IGF)-I and IGF-binding protein-3. Endocr J 2002;49:379–86.
24. van der Lely AJ, de Herder WW, Janssen JA, and Lamberts SW. Acromegaly: the significance of serum total and free IGF-I and IGF-binding protein-3 in diagnosis. J Endocrinol 2001; 155 Suppl:1S9–13; discussion S15–16.

8 Acromegaly: *Medical Management*

Pamela U. Freda, MD

CONTENTS

1. INTRODUCTION
2. DOPAMINE AGONISTS
3. SOMATOSTATIN ANALOGS
4. GH RECEPTOR ANTAGONIST: PEGVISOMANT
5. CONCLUSION

Summary

In recent years, significant advances in the pharmacological options for therapy of acromegaly have been made and thus medical management has a major role in the care of patients with this disease. Disease-specific medical therapies are directed at controlling the excessive hormone secretion i.e. normalizing serum levels of GH and IGF-I. These medical therapies are used predominantly after surgical therapy that was not curative, in some cases also after radiotherapy and in others as primary therapy.

Three classes of medication are now available, dopamine agonists, somatostatin analogs and a GH receptor antagonist, pegvisomant. These medications work at different targets along the GH-IGF-I axis and thus treat acromegaly by different mechanisms. Dopamine agonists inhibit pituitary GH secretion by unclear mechanisms, somatostatin analogs activate somatostatin receptors that suppress tumoral GH secretion with the subsequent fall in serum IGF-I levels and pegvisomant blocks peripheral GH action leading to the fall in IGF-I levels. Dopamine agonists are orally active, but have a low rate of success and do not produce significant tumor shrinkage in patients with acromegaly. The clinically available long acting somatostatin analogs, octreotide LAR and lanreotide autogel, comparably normalize IGF-I levels in up to two-thirds of patients. The extent of biochemical control achieved with somatostatin analogs is similar when used as adjunctive or primary therapy. Signs and symptoms of acromegaly and other clinical sequelae of the disease generally improve with somatostatin analog therapy, but their effects on glucose tolerance and insulin resistance are variable. Long-acting somatostatin analog use is can be associated with tumor shrinkage, which is greater when they are given as primary therapy. Gastrointestinal complaints are the most common side effects of somatostatin analogs, but do

From: *Contemporary Endocrinology: Diagnosis and Management of Pituitary Disorders*
Edited by: B. Swearingen and B. M. K. Biller © Humana Press, Totowa, NJ

not typically limit their clinical use. Pegvisomant, the GH receptor antagonist, was found, in clinical trials, to normalize IGF-I levels in nearly all patients. Pegvisomant therapy improves the signs and symptoms of acromegaly, reduces insulin resistance and lowers insulin and/or oral agent requirements in patients with diabetes. Liver enzyme elevations, which occur in a small percentage of patients, need to be monitored for, but only rarely limit therapy. In general, tumor size does not change on pegvisomant therapy, but it does not reduce their size and 2–3% of tumors continue to grow while on this therapy.

Treatment of acromegaly often requires use of multiple modalities in order to achieve adequate control of the disease. The approach to medical therapy should be individualized considering disease severity, symptoms, tumor size and location, co-morbid conditions and patient preferences. Recent advances in the options for medical management of acromegaly have now made disease control achievable in all patients with acromegaly.

Key Words: Acromegaly, Dopamine agonists, Somatostatin analogs, Octreotide, Growth hormone receptor antagonist, Pegvisomant.

1. INTRODUCTION

Medical management of acromegaly plays a major role in the care of patients with this disease. It includes use of disease-directed pharmacotherapies as well as the management of comorbid conditions that result from acromegaly such as hypertension, heart disease, diabetes mellitus, sleep apnea, articular damage, and other pituitary hormone deficiencies (1,2). Disease-specific medical therapies are directed at controlling excessive hormone secretion by normalizing serum levels of growth hormone (GH) and IGF-I. These medical therapies are used predominantly after surgical therapy that was not curative and/or after radiotherapy, but may also be used in some cases as primary therapy. Surgical therapy remains preferred as initial therapy, because in many patients it can rapidly normalize the hormonal excesses obviating the need for any further therapy and it relieves the compressive effects of the tumor mass. Radiotherapy is now often a third-line therapy and medical treatment is still needed to lower GH and IGF-I levels, often for years afterwards, until radiation therapy takes effect. A significant percentage of patients, however, still require further therapy. Medical therapies have now taken on an increasingly important role as adjunctive therapy of acromegaly (3).

In recent years, significant advances in the pharmacological options for therapy of acromegaly have been made. Three classes of medication are now available: dopamine agonists, somatostatin analogs, and a growth hormone (GH) receptor antagonist, pegvisomant. These medications work at different targets along the GH–IGF-I axis and thus treat acromegaly by different mechanisms. Dopamine agonists inhibit pituitary GH secretion by unclear mechanisms, somatostatin analogs activate somatostatin receptors that suppress tumoral GH secretion with the subsequent fall in serum IGF-I levels, and pegvisomant blocks peripheral GH action leading to the fall in IGF-I levels.

In this chapter, the efficacy and uses of each of these therapies for acromegaly are discussed individually followed by a summary of their role in the medical management of acromegaly.

2. DOPAMINE AGONISTS

Although dopamine agonists have been used for many years to treat acromegaly, they have a limited role in the current medical management of this disease. By binding to pituitary dopamine receptors, dopamine agonists may paradoxically suppress GH secretion in acromegaly (4), but the extent of clinical and biochemical response to these drugs in these patients is heterogeneous. Bromocriptine, the first dopamine agonist to be introduced for therapy of acromegaly, is effective in only a minority of patients, suppressing GH levels in about 20% and normalizing IGF-I levels in 10% of patients (4). Cabergoline, a newer and more potent dopamine agonist, may be more effective for the treatment of acromegaly than bromocriptine (5). In one study, cabergoline therapy normalized IGF-I levels in 35% and suppressed GH levels to less than 2 µg/l in 44% of 48 patients with pure GH-secreting tumors. In other smaller studies, however, cabergoline therapy normalized IGF-I levels overall in only 22% (range 0–27%) of such patients (6–9). In another study, IGF-I levels normalized initially in 57% of patients, but the efficacy waned with time as only 21% had a persistently normal IGF-I with up to 18 months of cabergoline therapy (10). Prolactin cosecretion has been variably predictive of an improved response to dopamine agonists (5,10). A rare patient with a true mixed tumor, who has significantly elevated levels of both prolactin and GH, may be very responsive to dopamine agonist therapy alone (10). Response to cabergoline may to be more favorable among patients with lower pretherapy GH and IGF-I levels (5).

In general, dopamine agonists do not produce significant shrinkage of GH-secreting tumors. In 62 patients treated with bromocriptine, most with coexistent hyperprolactinemia, 29% had some tumor shrinkage (4). With cabergoline therapy, five of the nine macroadenomas had some shrinkage of <50%; shrinkage was reported to be greater for patients with mixed GH-secreting and prolactin-secreting tumors (5).

Side effects of dopamine agonists when used in patients with acromegaly most frequently include nausea, constipation, headache, mood disturbances, nasal stuffiness, and dizziness (4,5,10). When used to treat prolactinomas, cabergoline seems to be associated with fewer side effects (11), but as larger doses are required to treat acromegaly, side effects necessitating drug withdrawal do occur in 3% (5) to 21% (10) of patients with acromegaly. Typically, bromocriptine doses up to 20 mg/day or cabergoline 1–2 mg/week are necessary, but the use of cabergoline up to 3.5 mg/week has been reported *(5)*. Slow escalation of the dose can help to minimize side effects. In addition, two recent studies reported an increased risk of valvular heart disease in patients with Parkinson's disease treated with cabergoline at much higher doses than those used to treat acromegaly *(12,13)*. Although there are no data to support an association of cabergoline use with valvular disease in acromegaly, given that these patients are at increased baseline risk for cardiac disease, consideration should be given to assessment of their valvular function before and periodically during treatment until further safety data become available.

In most studies, dopamine agonists have been employed as monotherapy for acromegaly, but they may also be used in combination with somatostatin analogs. Overall, about 10–20% of somatostatin analog-resistant patients seemed to benefit from the addition of bromocriptine to the somatostatin analog *(14–17)*. In two reports of patients who were partial somatostatin analog responders, the addition of cabergoline decreased GH levels in 21% and normalized IGF-I in 42% *(18)* and cabergoline and bromocriptine reduced GH levels by 36.1% and IGF-I levels by 35.2% *(19)*.

Dopamine agonists provide the advantages of being orally administered as well as being less expensive than other therapies. Dopamine agonists are not FDA approved for the therapy of acromegaly. Overall, although a trial of cabergoline may be considered as adjunctive therapy alone or in addition to somatostatin analogs in select patients with mild disease and small tumor residuals, the expectation for biochemical control in these patients needs to be kept low, even for tumors that cosecrete GH and prolactin.

3. SOMATOSTATIN ANALOGS

Since their introduction into clinical use more than two decades ago, analogs of somatostatin have been the most widely used medical therapy for acromegaly. The two clinically available analogs, octreotide and lanreotide have greatest affinity for somatostatin receptor subtypes 2 and 5. Although these are the subtypes most commonly found in GH-secreting pituitary tumors *(20)*, receptor specificity renders their efficacy dependent on and potentially limited by tumoral characteristics *(21)*. Importantly, however, in somatostatin analog-responsive patients, tachyphylaxis to the inhibition of GH secretion does not occur *(20)*. Octreotide was first available in a short-acting form administered subcutaneously thrice daily and is now available in a long-acting-release (LAR) preparation *(22)* that can be administered at doses of 10–30 mg by intramuscular injection every month or at more widely spaced intervals in some patients *(23–25)*. Lanreotide is available as a slow-release (SR) preparation administered by injection every 10–14 days, and as a newer autogel preparation that is given by a subcutaneous injection every 28 days at doses of

60, 90, or 120 mg *(26,27)*. The depot analogs, octreotide LAR and lanreotide autogel, are likely to be the forms chosen in clinical practice because of better patient acceptance.

3.1. Efficacy: GH and IGF-I Levels

Long-acting somatostatin analogs are used most often as adjunctive therapy in patients unsuccessfully treated by surgery and/or radiotherapy. A recent meta-analysis found that, overall, when used in this setting, GH efficacy criteria (typically GH suppression to <2.0 or 2.5 µg/l), were met in 57% of octreotide LAR-treated patients and 48% of lanreotide SR-treated patients *(28)*. IGF-I normalization was achieved in 67% of octreotide LAR-treated and 47% of lanreotide SR-treated patients. It is important to recognize that the reported efficacy of somatostatin analogs varies considerably from study to study in large part because of heterogeneity of study populations and study designs. A statistically combined synthesis of these data provides useful information, but it is necessary to recognize the potential limitations of combining these data *(28)*. In recent studies, lanreotide autogel therapy suppressed GH levels in 33% *(27)* to 46% *(29)* of patients and normalized IGF-I levels in 39% *(27)*, 46% *(29)*, and 54% with up to 4 years of therapy *(30)*. In a group of seven octreotide LAR-responsive patients switched to lanreotide autogel, efficacy of both drugs was comparable *(31)*. Overall, the rate of IGF-I normalization is somewhat better among subjects selected for study inclusion based on prior somatostatin analog responsiveness, a factor that may explain some interstudy variability of responses to somatostatin analogs *(28)*. The GH level at the start of somatostatin analog therapy is also a determinant of efficacy; higher GH levels predict less of a chance of achieving adequate biochemical efficacy criteria *(28)*.

When used as primary therapy, the extent of biochemical control achieved with somatostatin analogs is similar to that achieved in patients who have had other prior therapy *(28,32)*. In part, these data could be confounded by the fact that baseline hormone levels are generally higher in newly diagnosed patients (a negative predictor of somatostatin analog efficacy), yet posttherapy levels are similar, suggesting greater lowering of GH levels in newly diagnosed patients *(28)*. Overall, in data combined from a number of studies, primary therapy with subcutaneously administered octreotide normalized IGF-I levels in 54% of patients and suppressed GH levels in 53% of patients *(28)*. Similarly, in one individual study, primary therapy with octreotide followed by octreotide LAR normalized IGF-I levels in 53% *(33)*. In a recent study, primary therapy with either octreotide LAR or lanreotide autogel, 60–90 mg, controlled GH levels in 57.6%, normalized IGF-I levels in 45.5%, and achieved both criteria in 42.4% of 99 patients *(34)*. In another recent study, IGF-I levels normalized in 70.1% of 67 consecutive newly diagnosed patients with acromegaly treated with octreotide LAR *(35)*. Efficacy of primary somatostatin analog therapy may be somewhat dependent on pretherapy tumor size as octreotide LAR therapy suppressed GH levels in 84.6% versus 45% and normalized IGF-I levels in 61.5% versus 35% of microadenomas versus macroadenomas, respectively *(36)*. Lower pretreatment GH levels also predict a more favorable response to primary somatostatin analog therapy *(33)*.

Even though the evidence suggests that the rate of hormone normalization is higher in newly diagnosed patients, in a given patient, the efficacy of somato- statin analog therapy may also be enhanced if therapy is administered after surgical debulking has been carried out. It has been proposed that because some invasive GH-secreting pituitary adenomas are rarely cured by surgery, such patients should be treated only with somatostatin analog therapy. However, it may be that surgical debulking of these tumors should be undertaken anyway, because this seems to improve the response to medical therapy *(37)*. Data in support of this come from two retrospective studies in which somatostatin analog administration normalized IGF-I levels in 45.8% versus 78.3% *(38)* and 10% versus 55% of patients treated preoperatively versus postoperatively, respectively *(39)*.

The impact of preoperative somatostatin analog administration on periop- erative morbidity and surgical outcome has also been studied. Some clinical conditions may improve preoperatively with somatostatin analog therapy, in particular soft tissue swelling of the upper airway may be lessened, reducing intubation-related complications *(40)*. Among pretreated patients, one study found improvements in blood pressure and a reduction in the length of hospital stay *(41)*, but another found no significantly reduced perioperative morbidity *(42)*. Most studies have demonstrated no statistically significant differences in surgical outcome in patients pretreated with somatostatin analogs versus outcome in untreated patients *(42–45)*. In a review of 14 studies that examined the effect of preoperative somatostatin analog therapy on surgical remission rates, 37.5–89% of macroadenomas were found to achieve disease control *(40)*. Given the long half-life of somatostatin analogs, months off this therapy may be required to make a true assessment of the presence or absence of residual disease. Overall, data are insufficient to support use of preoperative somatostatin analogs to improve operative outcome

3.2. Clinical and Metabolic Effects

Signs and symptoms of acromegaly, including headache, soft tissue swelling, arthralgia, carpal tunnel syndrome, snoring, hyperhidrosis, and fatigue, improve overall in 64–74% of patients treated with depot somatostatin analog therapy *(46)*. Primary somatostatin analog therapy can also improve these symptoms

(34). Improvements may occur upon the lowering of GH and IGF-I levels even without their complete normalization. In particular, headaches, a prominent symptom in acromegaly, can often be successfully managed with octreotide, most likely because of an analgesic effect of the somatostatin analog *(47,48)*.

Somatostatin analog therapy can also improve other clinical sequelae of acromegaly. Suppression of GH and IGF-I levels with lanreotide therapy can lessen articular and periarticular soft tissue hypertrophy of various joints *(49)*. Sleep apnea, a prominent, but often unrecognized manifestation of acromegaly, can also be improved along with hormonal control by octreotide sc or sandostatin LAR *(50,51)* and is likely due to a reduction in tongue volume *(52)*. The cardiovascular disease of acromegaly also improves with somatostatin analog therapy *(2)*. Normalization of biochemical parameters with these drugs can reduce left ventricular hypertrophy, improve left ventricular mass index *(53–55)*, and improve cardiac performance as demonstrated by increase left ventricular ejection fraction at rest and exercise *(56,57)*.

Somatostatin analogs have variable effects on glucose tolerance and insulin resistance, which are common metabolic abnormalities in acromegaly *(58)*. While octreotide suppresses insulin secretion, the lowering of GH levels can reduce insulin resistance *(58)*. Most patients have improvements in insulin resistance in conjunction with normalization of GH and IGF-I levels *(59–61)*, but some have no change in glucose tolerance or insulin resistance *(62,63)*, and others develop glucose intolerance with octreotide treatment *(58,62)*. Peripheral insulin resistance may also improve on depot somatostatin analogs *(64,65)*, but some patients develop impaired insulin secretion *(64)* and deterioration of glucose tolerance *(65)*. Overall, these changes do not typically limit therapy, but may require the adjustment of diabetes therapies in some patients.

3.3. Effects on Pituitary Tumor Size

Another important aspect of the use long-acting somatostatin analogs is their effect on pituitary tumor size; their use is associated with tumor shrinkage in a significant percentage of patients with acromegaly. In data from a number of studies in which somatostatin analogs were used as adjunctive therapy, tumor shrinkage occurred in about 47% of octreotide LAR-treated and 21% of lanreotide SR-treated patients *(28)*; in most cases tumor size was reduced by 20–50%. The likelihood of tumor shrinkage was greater among subjects who had demonstrated somatostatin analog responsive prior to entry into the individual studies *(28)*. In another review, when used as adjuvant therapy, somatostatin analogs resulted in tumor shrinkage in 21% of patients *(66)*. The biochemical responsive to adjuvant or primary somatostatin analog therapy does not necessarily seem to be predictive of whether or not tumor shrinkage will occur *(66)*.

Shrinkage of GH-secreting tumors is greater when somatostatin analogs are given as primary therapy than as adjunctive therapy. Among subjects who received somatostatin analog as primary therapy, tumor shrinkage ≥10% occurred in 88% of octreotide LAR-treated, 51% of lanreotide-treated and 41% of octreotide sc-treated patients *(28)*. In another review, primary somatostatin analog therapy resulted, overall, in tumor shrinkage in 52% of patients, which was on average a 50% reduction in tumor size *(66)*. In another recent review of 14 studies, 36.6% of patients receiving primary somatostatin analog therapy for acromegaly experienced a significant reduction, >50%, in tumor size *(67)*. A number of recent studies have provided important information with regard to tumor shrinkage with depot somatostatin analog therapy. In one study, 75.5% of 99 newly diagnosed patients who were treated with octreotide LAR or lanreotide autogel had a ≥25% reduction in tumor size *(34)*; the percentage decrease in IGF-I and GH levels significantly predicted tumor volume reduction *(34)*. Of 67 consecutive newly diagnosed acromegaly patients, 82% had a mean reduction in tumor size of 62±31% with octreotide LAR therapy *(35)*. Primary octreotide followed by LAR therapy produced ≥30% tumor shrinkage in 73% of patients *(33)*. Some, but not all, studies have reported that macroadenomas are more likely to demonstrate shrinkage than microadenomas *(28,36,66)*.

An increase in pituitary tumor size during somatostatin analog therapy is very rare, being reported, overall, in approximately 2% of patients *(28)*. Similarly, in one individual study, 2 of 99 patients receiving primary octreotide LAR or lanreotide but who were poorly responsive had mild tumor size increases (34% and 31.2%, respectively) *(34)*. Thus, data suggest that somatostatin analogs may have some effect in preventing further tumor growth even in patients who do not experience tumor shrinkage *(66)*.

3.4. Side Effects

Gastrointestinal complaints are the most common side effects of depot somatostatin analog therapy *(46)*, but do not typically limit their clinical use. About 50% of patients initially experience abdominal discomfort, frequent stools, and nausea, but these symptoms improve in most. Similar side effects were reported in 44% of patients receiving primary somatostatin analog therapy *(34)*. New gallstones develop in about 15% of patients, most often within the first year of therapy *(46)*, but it is not felt to be necessary to routinely screen for these. Many patients experience some transient discomfort at the injection site for 1–2 days after depot analog administration. Transient hair loss, hypothyroidism, and vitamin B12 deficiency have also been reported.

3.5. Somatostatin Analogs in Clinical Development

Early clinical studies in acromegaly with SOM 230, a somatostatin analog with a more universal somatostatin receptor binding profile, look promising. SOM 230 has the highest affinity for SSTR 5, but also for SSTR subtypes 1, 2, and 3 *(68)*. An early clinical study in 47 patients found suppression of GH or normalization of IGF-I in 63.8% of patients and a >20% tumor volume reduction in 42% of patients with acromegaly treated with SOM 230 *(69)*. Also being studied are chimeric compounds that possess both somatostatin and dopamine receptor binding; these drugs have been demonstrated to suppress GH secretion from GH-secreting tumors in vitro *(70,71)*. The place of these newer compounds in the therapy of acromegaly remains to be determined.

4. GH RECEPTOR ANTAGONIST: PEGVISOMANT

Pegvisomant, the latest option for the medical therapy of acromegaly *(3)*, is a genetically engineered analog of human GH and contains nine mutations that render the molecule a functional antagonist at the GH receptor *(72)*. Each GH analog molecule is covalently linked to 4–5 polyethylene moieties that prolong its circulating half-life *(73)* and potentially reduce its immunogenicity *(74)*. In peripheral tissues, pegvisomant blocks GH receptor-mediated functions and thus as a therapy for acromegaly it blocks GH-mediated IGF-I production and lowers serum IGF-I levels *(72)*. The efficacy of therapy with pegvisomant is monitored by serum IGF-I levels, since GH levels are expected to increase after GH receptor blockade.

4.1. Efficacy: Normalization of IGF-I Levels

In the first large study in 112 patients with acromegaly, pegvisomant was demonstrated to be highly efficacious, normalizing serum IGF-I levels in 54%, 81%, and 89% of patients treated with 10, 15, and 20 mg of pegvisomant daily for 12 weeks *(74)*. Other GH-dependent proteins, IGFBP-3, and acid labile subunit (ALS), and free IGF-I levels also fell with pegvisomant therapy. In a longer-term study, 10 to 40 mg per day of pegvisomant for 12 to 18 months normalized IGF-I levels in 87 of 90 (97%) patients *(75)*. Most patients studied in clinical trials had failed prior multimodality therapy *(75)*. Pegvisomant has been shown to normalize IGF-I levels in patients previously resistant to somatostatin analogs *(76,77)*.

4.2. Clinical, Metabolic, and Other Endocrine Effects

Pegvisomant therapy improves the signs and symptoms of acromegaly such as soft tissue swelling, excessive perspiration, and fatigue and may decrease ring size, a marker of soft tissue swelling *(74)*. Pegvisomant therapy can reduce insulin resistance and lower insulin and/or oral agent requirements in patients with diabetes *(78,79)*. In the largest clinical trial, significant reductions in fasting serum insulin and glucose concentrations were sustained with up to 18 months of pegvisomant therapy *(75)*. Glycemic control also improved after patients resistant to somatostatin analogs were switched from the analogs to pegvisomant therapy *(80)*. Lipid levels, specifically total and LDL cholesterol, generally do not change *(75)*, but may rise somewhat from low levels to the normal range during pegvisomant therapy *(81)*. Pegvisomant therapy has also been shown to reduce the increased rate of bone turnover characteristic of acromegaly *(82,83)*. Pegvisomant was also reported to bring cortisol metabolism to normal in patients with acromegaly *(84)*.

The effects of pegvisomant and somatostatin analog cotreatment of patients with acromegaly have been investigated recently. In one study, combined pegvisomant and somatostatin analog therapy administered to 11 partial somatostatin analog responders was more effective than either therapy alone at normalizing IGF-I levels *(85)*. Coadministration of large doses of pegvisomant (40–80 mg) once weekly and octreotide LAR or lanreotide normalized IGF-I levels in 95% of 26 somatostatin analog-resistant patients *(86)*. Cotreatment has also been reported to control pituitary tumor growth in a patient whose tumor had increased in size on pegvisomant alone *(87)*.

Pegvisomant is typically administered as daily subcutaneous injections of 10, 15, or 20 mg *(88)*, but because of the drug's long half-life *(89,90)* less frequent dosing may be sufficient to maintain normal IGF-I levels in some patients with modest degrees of GH excess *(91)*. Less frequent dosing has potential advantages with regard to improved patient compliance and cost. Dose requirements of pegvisomant vary among patients in part because of the need for larger doses in patients with higher baseline GH and IGF-I levels *(77,92)* and greater weight *(91,92)* and in women *(92)*. Individualized dosing regimens may also be necessary in order to achieve amelioration in symptoms as well as effectively control comorbidities such as diabetes mellitus *(91)*.

4.3. Safety and Tolerability

Pegvisomant is generally well tolerated. Injection site reactions, generally mild and self-limited, occur in 3.7% *(80)* to 11% *(75)* of patients. Liver enzyme elevations do occur in a small percentage of patients, generally within the first few months of therapy. Overall, mild, transient, and reversible elevations in liver transaminases occurred in 1.2% of patients in preclinical studies and in subsequent studies in 4% *(93)* to 5.6% *(80)* of pegvisomant-treated and 38% of pegvisomant/octreotide LAR-cotreated patients *(86)*. In initial studies, two patients, 0.8%, had marked elevations of liver transaminases to greater than 10 times the upper limit of normal that subsequently resolved on drug withdrawal

(74,75,94). In another report, 4% of patients had liver transaminases increased that necessitated drug withdrawal *(93).* Liver function tests should be assessed at regular intervals during therapy *(95).*

Native GH levels rise to approximately twice the baseline level within the first few weeks of pegvisomant therapy and then plateau in patients with acromegaly *(74,75).* This does not appear to be related to any accelerated rate of tumor growth. It is not necessary to monitor endogenous serum GH levels during pegvisomant therapy, but as native human GH and pegvisomant share so much homology, some commercially available GH assays cannot distinguish between the two and measurement of serum GH level in a patient on pegvisomant could be misleading. In clinical studies, anti-GH antibodies developed in 10–16.9% of patients, but these were not found to be neutralizing and no tachyphylaxis to the effects of pegvisomant have been reported *(74,75).* During pegvisomant therapy it is prudent to maintain serum IGF-I levels in the midnormal range because of the potential for inadvertent overtreatment suppressing IGF-I level below the age-adjusted normal range *(75),* which could signify GH deficiency *(96).*

4.4. Effects on Tumor Size

Pegvisomant therapy does not reduce tumor size, but in general, tumor size does not change on this therapy *(75).* However, some tumors already prone to rapid growth do continue to grow on pegvisomant; overall, significant tumor enlargement has occurred in 2–3% of pegvisomant-treated patients *(97).* Clinically, significant increases were reported in two patients with large, globular tumors who had not received radiotherapy *(75,87).* In 2 of 53 patients who were switched from somatostatin analog to pegvisomant, tumor size initially increased, but stabilized with continued therapy *(80).* Similarly, of 313 pegvisomant-treated patients, tumor enlargement occurred in seven (none of whom had RT) and in four of these, the initial increase in tumor size, which then stabilized, also occurred after somatostatin analog withdrawal *(97).* In two studies, combined pegvisomant and somatostatin analog was not associated with tumor increases *(85,86).* Prior to the start of pegvisomant therapy an MRI should be done and tumor size should be monitored every 6 months for the first year and yearly thereafter. All patients on any medical therapy for acromegaly should have tumor size followed yearly.

5. CONCLUSION

Treatment of acromegaly often requires use of multiple modalities in order to achieve adequate control of the disease. The approach to medical management can be individualized considering disease severity, symptoms, tumor size and location, comorbid conditions, and patient preferences. Medical therapy is guided primarily by the biochemical goals of therapy, which are to achieve strict biochemical control, normalization of IGF-I, and suppression of GH after oral glucose to <1 μg/l *(98)*. Disease control should be able to arrest the progression of, although not eliminate, the physical changes, improve the associated morbidities, and normalize mortality to expected rates *(99)*. Management of acromegaly also requires attention to diagnosis and treatment of other pituitary insufficiencies and comorbidities including hypertension, diabetes mellitus, and sleep apnea and arthropathy.

In our center primary therapy is almost always transsphenoidal surgery. Primary somatostatin analog therapy should not be considered in patients with visual or neurological compromise because somatostatin analog therapy does not consistently provide adequate tumor shrinkage to relieve these signs of tumor mass effect *(100)*. Primary somatostatin analog therapy may be considered in patients whose tumor is clearly not resectable, such as cavernous sinus lesions, yet not threatening other structures. Preoperative somatostatin analog therapy may improve perioperative morbidity in some patients, but is not universally of significant benefit *(40)*. Although it has been argued that invasive macroadenomas, as not likely to be cured surgically, should be considered for somatostatin analog therapy alone, this is not supported by evidence that the response to somatostatin analogs is improved after surgical debulking. In addition, surgical debulking, even if not curative, lessens the likelihood of tumor size concerns during pegvisomant therapy or radiotherapy should these be needed.

The choice of therapy, if surgery has not been curative, can be individualized. Factors to consider in this choice include the tumor size, comorbidities such as diabetes mellitus, and the patient's preference. Most patients begin depot somatostatin analog therapy and some pegvisomant. Factors favoring the use of somatostatin analogs include the potential to arrest or shrink residual pituitary tumor and patient preference for monthly injections. Prominence of headaches would favor somatostatin analog use. Drawbacks to the use of somatostatin analogs include gastrointestinal side effects and the realization that one-third of patients will need additional therapy. If hormone levels are not normalized with somatostatin analogs a dopamine agonist can be added or the patient can be switched to pegvisomant. As cabergoline is oral, some patients with mild residual disease will undergo a 3-month to 6-month trial of this alone despite the low likelihood of complete efficacy. Some patients may begin pegvisomant as initial adjunctive therapy. The greater chance of IGF-I normalization and the greater efficacy in reducing insulin resistance and diabetes mellitus than somatostatin analogs may favor pegvisomant's use. Daily injections may be a drawback for some patients although options for alternative dosing regimens may improve patient acceptance of this therapy. Other potential advantages to pegvisomant are its uniform effectiveness, independent of tumoral receptor characteristics. However, as a trade-off for this, tumor size becomes a potential limitation of this therapy. Caution needs to be exercised when administering pegvisomant alone in patients with significant tumor mass, especially in patients who have not had RT or those whose tumor is near the chiasm. In determining the appropriateness of pegvisomant for patients with tumors of significant size it is important to recognize that although most GH-secreting tumors appear to be very slow growing, some are not and in this latter group, a minority of will have continued tumor growth whether on or off pegvisomant therapy *(75)*. A rationale exists for combined use of somatostatin analogs, known to shrink or retard tumor growth in acromegaly, and pegvisomant for its IGF-I lowering. Early studies suggest that this may be promising in selected patients, but additional data on this are required. The great expense of such therapy also needs to be considered.

Radiotherapy, traditionally the principal adjunctive therapy for those patients who were not cured by surgery, is generally now reserved for patients resistant to or intolerant of medical therapy and those with a clinically significant tumor mass in spite of other therapies. The long lag time till effect of RT and the high rate of hypopituitarism are its main drawbacks *(101)*. Some patients opt for radiotherapy initially after failed transsphenoidal surgery even if tumor size and growth do not suggest the need for radiotherapy because of their desire to not be committed to lifelong injectable medical therapies; medical therapy is still needed, usually for years.

In conclusion, recent years have seen major advances to the medical therapy of acromegaly; now with multimodality therapy all patients should be able to be effectively treated. The principles guiding medical therapy include consideration of the advantages as well as the limitations of each of the currently available medical therapies and individualization of therapy to the patient.

REFERENCES

1. Ezzat S, Forster MJ, Berchtold P, Redelmeier DA, Boerlin V, Harris AG. Acromegaly. Clinical and biochemical features in 500 patients. Medicine (Baltimore) 1994;73:233–40.
2. Colao A, Ferone D, Marzullo P, Lombardi G. Systemic complications of acromegaly: epidemiology, pathogenesis, and management. Endocr Rev 2004;25:102–52.
3. Clemmons DR, Chihara K, Freda PU, et al. Optimizing control of acromegaly: integrating a growth hormone receptor antagonist into the treatment algorithm. J Clin Endocrinol Metab 2003;88:4759–67.
4. Jaffe CA, Barkan AL. Treatment of acromegaly with dopamine agonists Endocrinol Metab Clin North Am 1992;21:713–35.

5. Abs R, Verhelst J, Maiter D, et al. Cabergoline in the treatment of acromegaly: a study in 64 patients. J Clin Endocrinol Metab 1998;83:374–8.
6. Ferrari C, Paracchi A, Romano C, et al. Long-lasting lowering of serum growth hormone and prolactin levels by single and repetitive cabergoline administration in dopamine-responsive acromegalic patients. Clin Endocrinol (Oxf) 1988;29:467–76.
7. Cozzi R, Attanasio R, Barausse M, et al. Cabergoline in acromegaly: a renewed role for dopamine agonist treatment? Eur J Endocrinol 1998;139:516–21.
8. Colao A, Ferone D, Marzullo P, et al. Effect of different dopaminergic agents in the treatment of acromegaly. J Clin Endocrinol Metab 1997;82:518–23.
9. Jackson SN, Fowler J, Howlett TA. Cabergoline treatment of acromegaly: a preliminary dose finding study. Clin Endocrinol (Oxf) 1997;46:745–9.
10. Freda PU, Reyes CM, Nuruzzaman AT, Sundeen RE, Khandji AG, Post KD. Cabergoline therapy of growth hormone & growth hormone/prolactin secreting pituitary tumors. Pituitary 2004;7:21–30.
11. Webster J, Piscitelli G, Polli A, Ferrari CI, Ismail I, Scanlon MF. A comparison of cabergoline and bromocriptine in the treatment of hyperprolactinemic amenorrhea. Cabergoline Comparative Study Group [see comments] N Engl J Med 1994;331:904–9.
12. Zanettini R, Antonini A, Gatto G, Gentile R, Tesei S, Pezzoli G. Valvular heart disease and the use of dopamine agonists for Parkinson's disease. N Engl J Med 2007;356: 39–46.
13. Schade R, Andersohn F, Suissa S, Haverkamp W, Garbe E. Dopamine agonists and the risk of cardiac-valve regurgitation. N Engl J Med 2007; 356:29–38.
14. Flogstad AK, Halse J, Grass P, et al. A comparison of octreotide, bromocriptine, or a combination of both drugs in acromegaly. J Clin Endocrinol Metab 1994;79:461–5.
15. Marzullo P, Ferone D, Di Somma C, et al. Efficacy of combined treatment with lanreotide and cabergoline in selected therapy-resistant acromegalic patients. Pituitary 1999;1: 115–20.
16. Lamberts SW, Zweens M, Verschoor L, del Pozo E. A comparison among the growth hormone-lowering effects in acromegaly of the somatostatin analog SMS 201–995, bromocriptine, and the combination of both drugs. J Clin Endocrinol Metab 1986;63: 16–19.
17. Minniti G, Jaffrain-Rea ML, Baldelli R, et al. Acute effects of octreotide, cabergoline and a combination of both drugs on GH secretion in acromegalic patients. Clin Ter 1997;148:601–7.
18. Cozzi R, Attanasio R, Lodrini S, Lasio G. Cabergoline addition to depot somatostatin analogues in resistant acromegalic patients: efficacy and lack of predictive value of prolactin status. Clin Endocrinol (Oxf) 2004;61:209–15.
19. Selvarajah D, Webster J, Ross R, Newell-Price J. Effectiveness of adding dopamine agonist therapy to long-acting somatostatin analogues in the management of acromegaly. Eur J Endocrinol 2005;152:569–74.
20. Lamberts SW, van der Lely AJ, de Herder WW, Hofland LJ. Octreotide N Engl J Med 1996;334:246–54.
21. Reubi JC, Landolt AM. The growth hormone responses to octreotide in acromegaly correlate with adenoma somatostatin receptor status. J Clin Endocrinol Metab 1989;68:844–50.
22. Lancranjan I, Bruns C, Grass P, et al. Sandostatin LAR: a promising therapeutic tool in the management of acromegalic patients. Metabolism 1996;45:67–71.
23. Jenkins PJ, Akker S, Chew SL, Besser GM, Monson JP, Grossman AB. Optimal dosage interval for depot somatostatin analogue therapy in acromegaly requires individual titration. Clin Endocrinol (Oxf) 2000;53:719–24.

24. Stewart PM, Kane KF, Stewart SE, Lancranjan I, Sheppard MC. Depot long-acting somatostatin analog (Sandostatin-LAR) is an effective treatment for acromegaly. J Clin Endocrinol Metab 1995;80:3267–72.

25. Biermasz NR, van den Oever NC, Frolich M, et al. Sandostatin LAR in acromegaly: a 6-week injection interval suppresses GH secretion as effectively as a 4-week interval. Clin Endocrinol (Oxf) 2003;58:288–95.

26. Heron I, Thomas F, Dero M, et al. Pharmacokinetics and efficacy of a long-acting formulation of the new somatostatin analog BIM 23014 in patients with acromegaly. J Clin Endocrinol Metab 1993;76:721–7.

27. Caron P, Beckers A, Cullen DR, et al. Efficacy of the new long-acting formulation of lanreotide (lanreotide autogel) in the management of acromegaly. J Clin Endocrinol Metab 2002;87:99–104.

28. Freda PU, Katznelson L, van der Lely AJ, Reyes CM, Zhao S, Rabinowitz D. Long-acting somatostatin analog therapy of acromegaly a meta-analysis. J Clin Endocrinol Metab 2005;90:4465–73.

29. Caron P, Cogne M, Raingeard I, Bex-Bachellerie V, Kuhn JM. Effectiveness and tolerability of 3-year lanreotide Autogel treatment in patients with acromegaly. Clin Endocrinol (Oxf) 2006;64:209–14.

30. Gutt B, Bidlingmaier M, Kretschmar K, Dieterle C, Steffin B, Schopohl J. Four-year follow-up of acromegalic patients treated with the new long-acting formulation of Lanreotide (Lanreotide Autogel). Exp Clin Endocrinol Diabetes 2005;113:139–44.

31. van Thiel SW, Romijn JA, Biermasz NR, et al. Octreotide long-acting repeatable and lanreotide Autogel are equally effective in controlling growth hormone secretion in acromegalic patients. Eur J Endocrinol 2004;150:489–95.

32. Newman CB, Melmed S, George A, et al. Octreotide as primary therapy for acromegaly. J Clin Endocrinol Metab 1998;83:3034–40.

33. Bevan JS, Atkin SL, Atkinson AB, et al. Primary medical therapy for acromegaly: an open, prospective, multicenter study of the effects of subcutaneous and intramuscular slow-release octreotide on growth hormone. insulin-like growth factor-I, and tumor size. J Clin Endocrinol Metab 2002;87:4554–63.

34. Colao A, Pivonello R, Auriemma RS, et al. Predictors of tumor shrinkage after primary therapy with somatostatin analogs in acromegaly: a prospective study in 99 patients. J Clin Endocrinol Metab 2006;91:2112–18.

35. Cozzi R, Montini M, Attanasio R, et al. Primary treatment of acromegaly with octreotide LAR: a long-term (up to nine years) prospective study of its efficacy in the control of disease activity and tumor shrinkage. J Clin Endocrinol Metab 2006;91:1397–403.

36. Colao A, Pivonello R, Rosato F, et al. First-line octreotide-LAR therapy induces tumour shrinkage and controls hormone excess in patients with acromegaly: results from an open, prospective, multicentre trial. Clin Endocrinol (Oxf) 2006;64:342–51.

37. Wass J. Debulking of pituitary adenomas improves hormonal control of acromegaly by somatostatin analogues. Eur J Endocrinol 2005;152:693–4.

38. Petrossians P, Borges-Martins L, Espinoza C, et al. Gross total resection or debulking of pituitary adenomas improves hormonal control of acromegaly by somatostatin analogs. Eur J Endocrinol 2005;152:61–6.

39. Colao A, Attanasio R, Pivonello R, et al. Partial surgical removal of growth hormone-secreting pituitary tumors enhances the response to somatostatin analogs in acromegaly. J Clin Endocrinol Metab 2006;91:85–92.

40. Ben-Shlomo A, Melmed S. Clinical review 154: The role of pharmacotherapy in perioperative management of patients with acromegaly. J Clin Endocrinol Metab 2003;88: 963–8.

41. Colao A, Ferone D, Cappabianca P, et al. Effect of octreotide pretreatment on surgical outcome in acromegaly. J Clin Endocrinol Metab 1997;82:3308–14.
42. Losa M, Mortini P, Urbaz L, Ribotto P, Castrignano T, Giovanelli M. Presurgical treatment with somatostatin analogs in patients with acromegaly: effects on the remission and complication rates. J Neurosurg 2006;104:899–906.
43. Biermasz NR, van Dulken H, Roelfsema F. Direct postoperative and follow-up results of transsphenoidal surgery in 19 acromegalic patients pretreated with octreotide compared to those in untreated matched controls. J Clin Endocrinol Metab 1999;84:3551–5.
44. Kristof RA, Stoffel-Wagner B, Klingmuller D, Schramm J. Does octreotide treatment improve the surgical results of macro-adenomas in acromegaly? A randomized study. Acta Neurochir (Wien) 1999;141:399–405.
45. Abe T, Ludecke DK. Effects of preoperative octreotide treatment on different subtypes of 90 GH-secreting pituitary adenomas and outcome in one surgical centre. Eur J Endocrinol 2001;145:137–45.
46. Freda PU. Somatostatin analogs in acromegaly. J Clin Endocrinol Metab 2002;87:3013–18.
47. Musolino NR, Marino Jr, R, Bronstein MD. Headache in acromegaly: dramatic improvement with the somatostatin analogue SMS 201–995. Clin J Pain 1990;6:243–5.
48. Williams G, Ball JA, Lawson RA, Joplin GF, Bloom SR, Maskill MR. Analgesic effect of somatostatin analogue (octreotide) in headache associated with pituitary tumours. Br Med J (Clin Res Ed) 1987;295:247–8.
49. Colao A, Marzullo P, Vallone G, et al. Ultrasonographic evidence of joint thickening reversibility in acromegalic patients treated with lanreotide for 12 months. Clin Endocrinol (Oxf) 1999;51:611–8.
50. Ip MS, Tan KC, Peh WC, Lam KS. Effect of Sandostatin LAR on sleep apnoea in acromegaly: correlation with computerized tomographic cephalometry and hormonal activity. Clin Endocrinol (Oxf) 2001;55:477–83.
51. Grunstein RR, Ho KK, Sullivan CE. Effect of octreotide, a somatostatin analog, on sleep apnea in patients with acromegaly. Ann Intern Med 1994;121:478–83.
52. Herrmann BL, Wessendorf TE, Ajaj W, Kahlke S, Teschler H, Mann K. Effects of octreotide on sleep apnoea and tongue volume (magnetic resonance imaging) in patients with acromegaly. Eur J Endocrinol 2004;151:309–15.
53. Giustina A, Boni E, Romanelli G, Grassi V, Giustina G. Cardiopulmonary performance during exercise in acromegaly, and the effects of acute suppression of growth hormone hypersecretion with octreotide. Am J Cardiol 1995;75:1042–7.
54. Baldelli R, Ferretti E, Jaffrain-Rea ML, et al. Cardiac effects of slow-release lanreotide, a slow-release somatostatin analog, in acromegalic patients. J Clin Endocrinol Metab 1999;84:527–32.
55. Hradec J, Kral J, Janota T, Krsek M, Hana V, Marek J, Malik M. Regression of acromegalic left ventricular hypertrophy after lanreotide (a slow-release somatostatin analog). Am J Cardiol 1999;83:1506–19, A8.
56. Colao A, Marzullo P, Ferone D, et al. Cardiovascular effects of depot long-acting somatostatin analog Sandostatin LAR in acromegaly. J Clin Endocrinol Metab 2000;85:3132–40.
57. Colao A, Cuocolo A, Marzullo P, et al. Is the acromegalic cardiomyopathy reversible? Effect of 5-year normalization of growth hormone and insulin-like growth factor I levels on cardiac performance. J Clin Endocrinol Metab 2001;86:1551–7.
58. Ho KK, Jenkins AB, Furler SM, Borkman M, Chisholm DJ. Impact of octreotide, a long-acting somatostatin analogue, on glucose tolerance and insulin sensitivity in acromegaly. Clin Endocrinol (Oxf) 1992;36:271–9.

59. Sassolas G, Harris AG, James-Deidier A. Long term effect of incremental doses of the somatostatin analog SMS 201–995 in 58 acromegalic patients. French SMS 201–995 approximately equal to Acromegaly Study Group. J Clin Endocrinol Metab 1990;71: 391–7.

60. Sato K, Takamatsu K, Hashimoto K. Short-term effects of octreotide on glucose tolerance in patients with acromegaly. Endocr J 1995;42:739–45.

61. James RA, Moller N, Chatterjee S, White M, Kendall-Taylor P. Carbohydrate tolerance and serum lipids in acromegaly before and during treatment with high dose octreotide. Diabet Med 1991;8:517–23.

62. Koop BL, Harris AG, Ezzat S. Effect of octreotide on glucose tolerance in acromegaly. Eur J Endocrinol 1994;130:581–6.

63. Breidert M, Pinzer T, Wildbrett J, Bornstein SR, Hanefeld M. Long-term effect of octreotide in acromegaly on insulin resistance. Horm Metab Res 1995;27:226–230.

64. Baldelli R, Battista C, Leonetti F, et al. Glucose homeostasis in acromegaly: effects of long-acting somatostatin analogues treatment. Clin Endocrinol (Oxf) 2003;59: 492–9.

65. Ronchi C, Epaminonda P, Cappiello V, Beck-Peccoz P, Arosio M. Effects of two different somatostatin analogs on glucose tolerance in acromegaly. J Endocrinol Invest 2002;25:502–507.

66. Bevan JS. Clinical review: The antitumoral effects of somatostatin analog therapy in acromegaly. J Clin Endocrinol Metab 2005;90:1856–63.

67. Melmed S, Sternberg R, Cook D, et al. A critical analysis of pituitary tumor shrinkage during primary medical therapy in acromegaly. J Clin Endocrinol Metab 2005;90: 4405–10.

68. van der Hoek J, van der Lelij AJ, Feelders RA, et al. The somatostatin analogue SOM230, compared with octreotide, induces differential effects in several metabolic pathways in acromegalic patients. Clin Endocrinol (Oxf) 2005;63m:176–84.

69. Petersenn S, Glusman JE, Schopohl J, et al. The novel multi-ligand somatostatin analogue pasireotide (SOM230) is a potential new therapy for patients with acromegaly; preliminary results of a Phase II safety and efficacy study in active acromegaly. Proceedings of the 88th Annual Meeting of the Endocrine Society OR9–5.2006.

70. Jaquet P, Gunz G, Saveanu A, et al. Efficacy of chimeric molecules directed towards multiple somatostatin and dopamine receptors on inhibition of GH and prolactin secretion from GH-secreting pituitary adenomas classified as partially responsive to somatostatin analog therapy. Eur J Endocrinol 2005;153:135–41.

71. Jaquet P, Gunz G, Saveanu A, et al. BIM-23A760, a chimeric molecule directed towards somatostatin and dopamine receptors, vs universal somatostatin receptors ligands in GH-secreting pituitary adenomas partial responders to octreotide. J Endocrinol Invest 2005;28:21–7.

72. Muller AF, Kopchick JJ, Flyvbjerg A, van der Lely AJ. Clinical review 66: Growth hormone receptor antagonists. J Clin Endocrinol Metab 2004;89:1503–11.

73. Clark R, Olson K, Fuh G, et al. Long-acting growth hormones produced by conjugation with polyethylene glycol. J Biol Chem 1996;271:21969–77.

74. Trainer PJ, Drake WM, Katznelson L, et al. Treatment of acromegaly with the growth hormone-receptor antagonist pegvisomant [see comments] N Engl J Med 2000;342: 1171–7.

75. van der Lely AJ, Hutson RK, Trainer PJ, et al. Long-term treatment of acromegaly with pegvisomant, a growth hormone receptor antagonist. Lancet 2001;358:1754–9.

76. Herman-Bonert VS, Zib K, Scarlett JA, Melmed S. Growth hormone receptor antagonist therapy in acromegalic patients resistant to somatostatin analogs. J Clin Endocrinol Metab 2000;85:2958–61.

77. Drake WM, Parkinson C, Akker SA, Monson JP, Besser GM, Trainer PJ. Successful treatment of resistant acromegaly with a growth hormone receptor antagonist. Eur J Endocrinol 2001;145:451–6.

78. Rose DR, Clemmons DR. Growth hormone receptor antagonist improves insulin resistance in acromegaly. Growth Horm IGF Res 2002;12:418–24.

79. Drake WM, Rowles SV, Roberts ME, et al.. Insulin sensitivity and glucose tolerance improve in patients with acromegaly converted from depot octreotide to pegvisomant. Eur J Endocrinol 2003;149:521–7.

80. Barkan AL, Burman P, Clemmons DR, et al. Glucose homeostasis and safety in patients with acromegaly converted from long-acting octreotide to pegvisomant. J Clin Endocrinol Metab 2005;90:5684–91.

81. Parkinson C, Drake WM, Wieringa G, Yates AP, Besser GM, Trainer PJ. Serum lipoprotein changes following IGF-I normalization using a growth hormone receptor antagonist in acromegaly. Clin Endocrinol (Oxf) 2002;56:303–11.

82. Fairfield WP, Sesmilo G, Katznelson L, et al. Effects of a growth hormone receptor antagonist on bone markers in acromegaly. Clin Endocrinol (Oxf) 2002;57:385–90.

83. Parkinson C, Kassem M, Heickendorff L, Flyvbjerg A, Trainer PJ. Pegvisomant-induced serum insulin-like growth factor-I normalization in patients with acromegaly returns elevated markers of bone turnover to normal. J Clin Endocrinol Metab 2003;88:5650–5.

84. Trainer PJ, Drake WM, Perry LA, Taylor NF, Besser GM, Monson JP. Modulation of cortisol metabolism by the growth hormone receptor antagonist pegvisomant in patients with acromegaly. J Clin Endocrinol Metab 2001;86:2989–92.

85. Jorgensen JO, Feldt-Rasmussen U, Frystyk J, et al. Cotreatment of acromegaly with a somatostatin analog and a growth hormone receptor antagonist. J Clin Endocrinol Metab 2005;90:5627–31.

86. Feenstra J, de Herder WW, ten Have SM, et al. Combined therapy with somatostatin analogues and weekly pegvisomant in active acromegaly. Lancet 2005;365:1644–6.

87. van der Lely AJ, Muller A, Janssen JA, et al. Control of tumor size and disease activity during cotreatment with octreotide and the growth hormone receptor antagonist pegvisomant in an acromegalic patient. J Clin Endocrinol Metab 2001;86:478–81.

88. Somavert. Pegvisomant for Injection. Package Insert. December 2005. Pfizer Inc., New York, NY.

89. Rodvold KA, van der Lely AJ. Pharmacokinetics and pharmacodynamics of B2036-PEG, a novel growth hormone receptor antagonist, in acromegalic subjects. Proceedings of the 81st Annual Endocrine Society Meeting, June 12–15, 1999. San Diego, CA.

90. Rodvold KA, Bennett WF, Zib KA. Single-dose safety and pharmacokinetics of B2036-PEG (Somavert) after subcutaneous administration in healthy volunteers. J Clin Pharmacol 1997;37:869.

91. Jehle S, Reyes CM, Sundeen RE, Freda PU. COMMENT: Alternate day administration of pegvisomant maintains normal serum insulin like growth factor-I (IGF-I) levels in patients with acromegaly. J Clin Endocrinol Metab. 2005;90:1566–93.

92. Parkinson C, Burman P, Messig M, Trainer PJ. The influence of gender and weight on the dose of pegvisomant required to normalize serum IGF-1 in patients with active acromegaly. Proceedings of the 85th Annual Endocrine Society Meeting OR40–6, June 16–19, 2004. New Orleans, LA.

93. Biering H, Saller B, Bauditz J, et al. Elevated transaminases during medical treatment of acromegaly: a review of the German pegvisomant surveillance experience and a report of a patient with histologically proven chronic mild active hepatitis. Eur J Endocrinol 2006;154:213–20.

94. Drake WM, Trainer PJ. Clinical use of pegvisomant for the treatment of acromegaly. Treat Endocrinol 2003;2:369–74.

95. Freda P. Pegvisomant therapy for acromegaly. Expert Rev Endocrinol Metab 2006;1: 489–98.

96. Ho KK. Place of pegvisomant in acromegaly. Lancet 2001;358:1743–4.

97. Besser GM, Burman P, Daly AF. Predictors and rates of treatment-resistant tumor growth in acromegaly. Eur J Endocrinol 2005;153:187–93.

98. Freda PU. Current concepts in the biochemical assessment of the patient with acromegaly. Growth Hormone & IGF Research 2003;13:171–84.

99. Swearingen B, Barker FG, 2nd, Katznelson L, et al. Long-term mortality after transsphenoidal surgery and adjunctive therapy for acromegaly [see comments] J Clin Endocrinol Metab 1998;83:3419–26.

100. Baldelli R, Colao A, Razzore P, et al. Two-year follow-up of acromegalic patients treated with slow release lanreotide (30 mg). J Clin Endocrinol Metab 2000;85:4099–103.

101. Freda PU. How effective are current therapies for acromegaly? Growth Horm IGF Res 2003;13 Suppl A:S144–51.

9 Acromegaly: *Surgical Management*

Michael Buchfelder, MD, PhD, and Panagiotis Nomikos, MD

Contents

Summary

Although medical alternatives now exist, transsphenoidal surgery remains the primary therapy in the management of acromegaly. This chapter describes the indications for surgery, techniques, and complications, as well as management strategies for persistent and recurrent disease.

Key Words: Acromegaly, Transsphenoidal surgery.

1. INTRODUCTION

Acromegaly is a rare but serious disease, almost always caused by a growth hormone (GH)-producing pituitary adenoma. Ectopic GH or GH-releasing hormone production or a pituitary carcinoma may very infrequently also cause acromegaly. Several retrospective cohort studies suggest that mortality in acromegaly is at least twice of that of the general population *(1–3)*. The cause of death is most commonly cardiac or vascular. These studies also demonstrated that a reduction of GH levels significantly lowered mortality

From: *Contemporary Endocrinology: Diagnosis and Management of Pituitary Disorders*
Edited by: B. Swearingen and B. M. K. Biller © Humana Press, Totowa, NJ

risk *(4)*. Thus, aggressive management to lower serum GH levels is justified once the diagnosis has been confirmed. For the majority of patients the generally accepted first-line therapy is surgery, either alone or in combination with medical treatment and/or radiotherapy. The goals of surgical therapy in acromegaly include the normalization of dynamic GH secretion pattern as well as normalization of IGF-I, preservation of normal pituitary function, and elimination of mass effect. The definition of disease remission has changed over time as GH assays have improved. A modern definition of cure was formulated by International Consensus Conferences *(5–7)*. Most of the recently published surgical results refer to the criteria of early remission as defined in Cortina d'Ampezzo *(5)*. In this consensus, random GH levels below 2.5 μg/l, in combination with suppression of GH to below 1 μg/l following an oral glucose load, and a normal age-adjusted IGF-1 were defined as criteria for remission of the disease, based on hormone determinations with commercially available standardized assays. Usually, the endocrinological evaluation upon which the decision is made is performed within 2 to 6 months after surgery.

2. INDICATIONS FOR SURGERY

Until the advent of medical treatment, surgery was almost always considered to be the primary treatment for this disease. However, with the recent availability of various pharmacologic agents, alternatives now exist for those patients who are poor surgical candidates, and for those whose invasive tumors may be surgically unresectable. Generally, tumors that are deemed to be totally resectable remain excellent candidates for primary surgical therapy. Whether debulking of an invasive tumor prior to medical treatment or irradiation improves long-term remission rates is currently under investigation. Recent data suggest that debulking improves the results of medical therapy even in tumors that could not be completely resected *(8)*.

3. PREOPERATIVE EVALUATION

Generally, the best preoperative imaging technique is a high field strength magnetic resonance imaging (MRI) scan that depicts the tumor in T1-weighted images before and after the injection of contrast medium in at least the sagittal and coronal planes. Other sequences may provide additional information. In selected cases a coronal CT scan is useful since it provides valuable information about the structure and segmentation of paranasal sinuses. Endocrinological investigation should provide information about the magnitude of GH oversecretion and the potential presence of hypopituitarism. The preoperative evaluation of the patient with acromegaly is described in Chapter 7. Hypopituitarism requires adequate perioperative substitution therapy. In all lesions with suprasellar extension, an ophthalmological evaluation should be performed, with testing of visual perimetry and acuity. Particularly with acromegaly, the patient requires assessment for associated comorbidities that may affect operative risk (cardiac disease, hypertension, glucose intolerance, and respiratory disease), as well as a careful evaluation by the anesthesiologist for possible airway difficulties.

4. SURGICAL TECHNIQUES

Although a number of approaches to the sella have been described historically, the transsphenoidal approach is commonly employed today, and can be used in more than 90% of pituitary cases. A general approach to the surgical management of pituitary disease is described in Chapters 15 and 16. A number of variations in the transsphenoidal route are possible. While some surgeons prefer to operate on a patient in supine position with the head slightly extended *(9)*, others favor a semi-sitting position. Radiofluoroscopic control is a commonly used procedure for navigation and intraoperative imaging, although neuronavigational techniques are also useful. This surgery can be performed with or without dissection of the septal mucosa. Creation of a submucous tunnel, as in septal corrective surgeries, can be performed through either a sublabial or a medial nasal incision. Then, the medial nasal mucosa is unilaterally detached from the cartilaginous and osseous nasal septae, respectively. A nasal speculum is inserted to keep the mucosal tunnel open. At this stage the operating microscope is usually brought into place. The vomer, which serves as an excellent midline orientation, is exposed and opened with forceps and drill. The septations of the sphenoid sinus are resected. Usually, at this stage the sellar floor is visualized through the sphenoid sinus. Incomplete pneumatization of the sphenoid requires extensive drilling to approach the floor of the sella. Once the sellar floor is opened, the basal dura of the pituitary fossa is incised, allowing a soft tumor to protrude through this opening. Variously shaped curettes and microforceps are used to resect the tumor. The compressed normal pituitary is identified by its yellowish color, firmer consistency, and vascular surface structure, and is preserved. The extent of tumor resection can be estimated by inspection and palpation of the tumor cavity, visualization of the cavernous sinus bilaterally, and, in larger tumors with suprasellar extension, by the arachnoid herniation that descends into the intrasellar space. Intraoperative MRI, where available, is sometimes useful. The size of the tumor is not the only factor determining the extent of resection. A wide connection between intrasellar and extrasellar tumor portions permits a more extensive resection of a large adenoma. Even with invasive tumors extensive and sometimes total resection can be achieved. Invaded mucosa of the sphenoid sinus can be resected, invaded bone of the skull base can be drilled away, and tumor portions with invasion into the cavernous sinus can be traced gently, once the perforation site has been identified. Clearly, if there is tumor in the MRI that extends lateral from the carotid artery, residual adenoma tissue will persist after transsphenoidal surgery. In small microadenomas the gland will need to be sectioned. The term "enlarged adenomectomy" refers to a portion of normal gland (periadenoma) resected around the adenoma. The normal size of the gland, the vascularization of the basal dura, and the proximity of the cavernous sinus and carotid arteries, respectively, make it a technically demanding enterprise. In the past, tumor extension to the planum sphenoidale was considered a contraindication for transsphenoidal surgery. This is no longer the case. With the extended transsphenoidal approach, opening of the tuberculum sellae from below can allow even subfrontal tumors to be removed through the nasal route. The additional use of the endoscope opens new avenues for the visualization of such lesions, and the indications for transcranial surgery have become progressively more restrictive. A suprasellar tumor with little or no intrasellar component continues to require a craniotomy in the hands of the most expert neurosurgeons (10).

5. SURGICAL OUTCOME

As a result of the changes in criteria over the years for postoperative endocrinological remission, and the variations in criteria used by different investigators (5–7), the reported remission rates vary significantly in published series from different institutions (Table 1).

In early series, the criterion for remission was a postoperative random GH level below 5 µg/l. Ross et al. (11) in 1998 analyzed the results of 30 published series and yielded an overall "cure" rate of 56% in 153 cases. In another multicenter review published by Zervas et al. (12) in 1987, the overall "cure" rate was 66% in 1,256 cases. Using the more restrictive criterion of GH suppression after an oral glucose load, rates of endocrinological remission were found to be lower, as in our early series from 1992 (13). In this report, the remission rate was 71% with a basal GH level below 5 µg/l as the criterion, but decreased to 57% when a glucose-suppressed GH level below 2 µg/l was used. Similar results were found in other series published by Losa et al. (14) and Valdemarsson et al. (15,16). The use of all three criteria, including normalization of basal IGF-I, does not further change the previously reported remission rates, as shown by Tindall et al. (1993) (17), Laws et al. (2000) (18), Kreutzer et al. (2001) (19), and Nomikos et al. (2005) (20). The role of postoperative IGF-I levels in the long-term outcome of the disease has not been fully elucidated, since the assays used to determine IGF-1 changed over time. Normalization of IGF-I and clinical improvement are significantly correlated, but in clinical practice discrepancies between these criteria were observed. In

Table 1
Results of Primary Transsphenoidal Surgery for GH-Secreting Pituitary Adenomas

Series	No. Cases	Total Remission Rate (%)	Microadenomas	Macroadenomas	Definition of Remission
Ross and Wilson (1988) [11]	153	56	N/A	N/A	GH <5 µg/l
Losa et al. (1989) [14]	29	55	N/A	N/A	GH <1 µg/l and normal IGF-I level
Fahlbusch et al. (1992) [13]	222	57	72	49	GH < 2 µg/l OGT GH <5 µg/l
Tindall et al. (1993) [17]	91	82	81	65	GH <5 µg/l and/or normal IGF-I level
Davis et al. (1993) [39]	174	52	N/A	N/A	GH ≤2 µg/l (basal or OGT)
Sheaves et al. (1996) [27]	100	42	61	23	GH ≤2.5 µg/l
Abosch et al. (1998) [53]	254	76	75	71	GH <5 µg/l
Freda et al. (1998) [54]	115	61	88	53	GH <2 µg/l OGT or normal IGF-I level
Laws et al. (2000) [18]	117	67	87	50.5	GH ≤2.5 µg/l, GH ≤1 µg/l, normal IGF-I level
Kreutzer et al. (2001) [19]	57	70	N/A	N/A	Normal IGF-I level
Nomikos et al. (2005) [20]	490	56	78	50	Basal GH ≤5 µg/l, GH ≤2 µg/l (OGT), normal IGF-I level

individual patients, elevated levels of IGF-I could still be found even if GH levels could be suppressed to below 1 µg/l. Despite the persistent elevation of IGF-I, many of these patients had a favorable long-term outcome with clinical remission of disease. Based on our personal experience in the treatment of acromegalic patients, we feel that even when the most stringent criteria are satisfied, no definite "cure" of the disease can be claimed. Even following "successful" surgical treatment, GH levels remain detectable and pulses of GH secretion are not normal in frequency and size *(21)*. In acromegaly the goal is normalization of GH secretion, with relief of symptoms and restoration of normal life expectancy. The relationship between IGF-1 and GH in predicting these outcomes continues to be under investigation. Together with the development of more sensitive enzyme-linked immunoabsorbent assays and the evaluation of further markers of disease activity such as acid-labile subunits (ALSs) *(22)*, we might hopefully be better enabled to define a "cure" in acromegalic patients. Certainly, GH and IGF-1 are more sensitive parameters than even sophisticated MRI. Thus, an apparently normal postoperative MRI (Fig. 1) can be seen with normalized GH and IGF-1 secretion, or sometimes in cases of persistent disease. In contrast, depictions of residual tumor such as parasellar portions lateral of the carotid artery are always indicative of active acromegaly (Fig. 2).

The overall rate for endocrinological remission with respect to normalization of basal GH (below 2.5 µg/l) and to normalization of IGF-I and to GH levels below 1 µg/l during OGTT was found to vary between 10% and 75.3%. Several factors related to the tumor could be detected as predictors of the surgical result, such as tumor size, invasiveness, extrasellar growth, and secretory activity. Depending on the degree and direction of extrasellar expansion, GH-secreting adenomas are classified as microadenomas (tumor diameter ≤10 mm), macroadenomas (with a tumor diameter >10 mm), and giant adenomas (with an extension of >40 mm at least in one plane) *(23)*. Microadenomas have a more favorable surgical outcome than macroadenomas, particularly those with extrasellar extension. In microadenomas, a remission rate as high as 88% could be achieved. With increasing tumor diameter and extrasellar extension, remission drops stepwise to 0% for giant adenomas. Similar results were found in other published series, as in the outcome analysis of Tindall et al. *(17)* and Ross et al. *(11)*. The main reason for this drop is the increasing invasiveness seen in larger adenomas. Pituitary adenomas are considered invasive if they have infiltrated or perforated the normal anatomical confines of the pituitary gland, namely the sellar diaphragm, basal dura, clivus, or sphenoidal and cavernous sinuses. Although invasion tends to be more common with increasing tumor size, microadenomas may also have an invasive character and, conversely, large tumors may reach a considerable size by

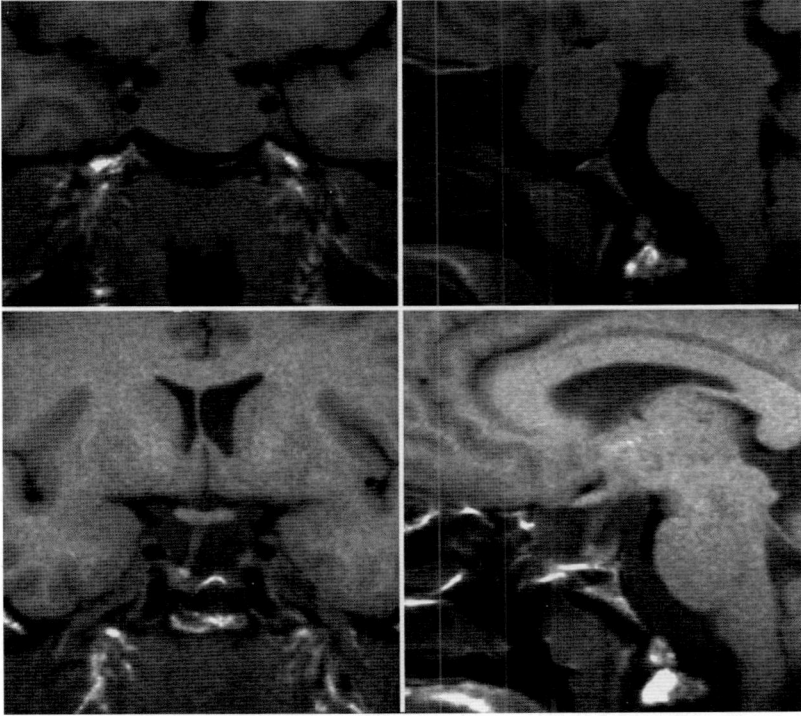

Fig. 1. Intrasellar and suprasellar pituitary enclosed adenoma with GH levels around 110 ng/ml. Postoperatively, there are no obvious tumor remnants visible. However, GH oversecretion persisted with mean GH levels around 7 ng/ml and an elevated IGF-1.

simply displacing the adjacent anatomical structures without actually invading them. Localized or generalized invasion, however, should not be equated with malignancy of the tumor. The diagnosis of pituitary carcinoma is only justified when subarachnoid dissemination and brain or distant metastases are documented. Pituitary carcinomas associated with acromegaly are extremely rare *(24)*. Invasion can be documented by intraoperative findings, neuroradiological investigations, and/or histological examination. Surgical invasion describes the invasive nature of the tumor as recognized during operation, while histological invasion, although more frequent, can only be demonstrated by investigating the anatomical structures in the vicinity of the tumor. In up to 80% of the cases, dural invasion can be detected, when the basal dura is thoroughly investigated *(25,26)*. In our series, the overall remission rate of noninvasive adenomas was 76% and decreased to 24% for invasive tumors. Similarly, for transcranial surgery increased invasiveness of the tumor is the

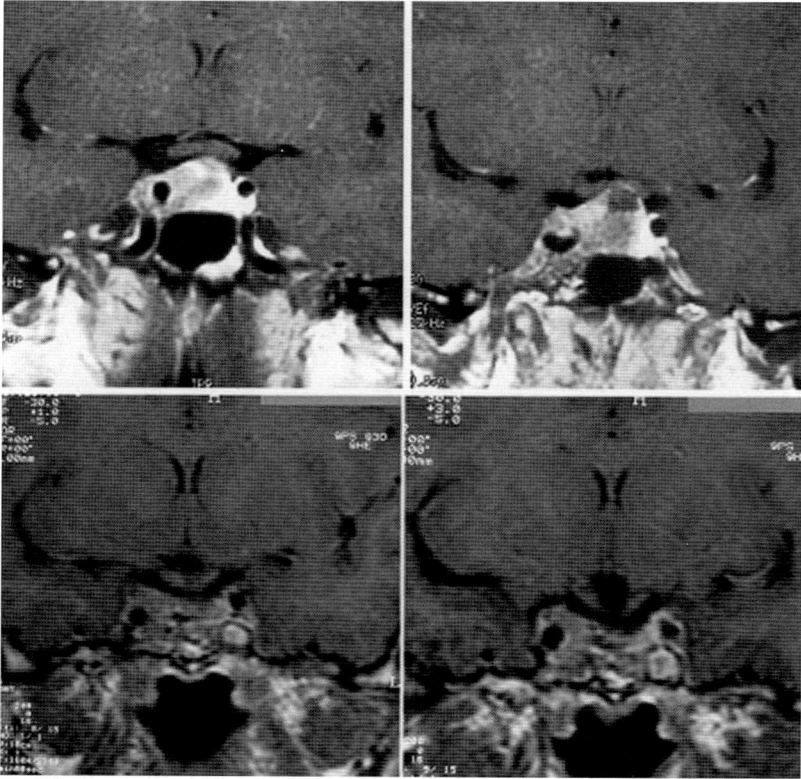

Fig. 2. Intrasellar, suprasellar, and parasellar pituitary adenoma with encasement of the intracavernous part of the right carotid artery. During surgery the intrasellar and suprasellar part of the tumor could be totally removed. Tumor remnant is seen within the cavernous sinus and there was abnormal GH secretion on postoperative testing.

main reason for incomplete tumor resection. Following transcranial surgery, we thus observed a remission rate of only 5.2% *(20)*.

The secretory activity of the adenoma also seems to influence the response to surgical therapy, as observed in several published series *(11,17,27)*. Various thresholds of preoperative basal GH levels between 40 and 70 µg/l have been proposed. Preoperative GH levels above these values are inversely related with the likelihood of postoperative biochemical remission. Years ago, we reported that this inverse relationship has an almost linear character *(13)* and recently confirmed it with updated figures *(20)*. If a basal GH level of 50 µg/l is defined as an arbitrary threshold for the secretory activity of an adenoma, then the overall cure rate drops from 74% in cases with preoperative GH levels below this threshold to 25% in cases with preoperative GH levels above this threshold *(20)*. It has not yet been convincingly demonstrated that presurgical treatment with somatostatin analogs significantly improves the surgical results in acromegaly *(28–30)*.

Another factor that correlates with surgical success is independent from the characteristics of the tumor and relates to the surgeon's experience. It has been reported that increased experience at an individual center over time is correlated with an increase in the surgical success rate *(31)*. With a designated pituitary surgeon, more individual experience can be gained and the surgical success rate is dramatically increased *(32)*. Moreover, as Barker et al. have demonstrated, experienced surgeons have fewer complications *(33)*.

6. COMPLICATIONS

To date, the complication rate of both transsphenoidal and transcranial surgery is relatively low, and appears to be related to the experience of the surgeon and the case load of the service. Barker et al. have shown that the total number of pituitary surgeries performed by an individual surgeon and the annual number of cases done within one service correlates with both mortality and complication rate, and found an inverse relationship of complications to both hospital and surgeon volume *(33)*. Although these data were derived from all types of pituitary adenomas, they are clearly applicable to GH-secreting tumors. Ross and Wilson reviewed the operative complications in 30 published surgical series and estimated an operative mortality rate of 1.04% *(11)*. In our own series of acromegalic patients, one patient died (0.1%) from the postoperative hemorrhage of the suprasellar parts of an incompletely removed giant adenoma *(20)*. Morbidity in our series was relatively low: meningitis and CSF fistula occurred in 1.8% and 0.8% of the cases, respectively. Due to specific precautions taken in the high-risk group of acromegalic patients, the complication rate is comparable to that of nonacromegalic patients undergoing transsphenoidal surgery for other types of pituitary adenomas. Deterioration of pituitary function was rarely found following primary transsphenoidal surgery *(20)*. In 16 cases, additional endocrine deficits required permanent replacement therapy (3.2%). Preoperative evaluation included assessment of the cardiac function, blood pressure, respiratory function, and metabolic disturbances. Morphological abnormalities, such as macroglossia and prognathism, may hinder endotracheal intubation *(34)*. In some cases, fiberoptic endotracheal intubation is necessary. Patients with severe sleep apnea should be monitored with pulse oximetry, and may require observation in an intensive care unit. The multiple medical comorbidities seen in acromegaly require careful postoperative management in order to keep the complication rate as low as possible. In case of markedly reduced general condition, preoperative short-term medical treatment with somatostatin analogs should be considered, which may be helpful in improving the anesthetic and surgical risks.

7. RECURRENCES

Success or failure following surgical treatment of secreting tumors needs to be clearly defined (35). Failure to achieve the current normalization criteria implies persistent disease. Ideally, within several hours after successful transsphenoidal surgery, a rapid decrease of GH can be documented. Normalization of GH secretion as defined by individual investigators and consensus conferences (5) is usually accompanied by a normal (delayed postoperative) MRI investigation without radiographic evidence of residual disease. However, biochemical remission and radiological findings are not necessarily congruent, particularly in the early postoperative period, since in several instances normal GH and IGF-1 levels have been measured in patients with clearly visible persistent tumor.

The medical literature provides us with conflicting estimates of recurrence after transsphenoidal surgery within various follow-up periods. Remission criteria, however, have changed over time and are not always congruent with today's standards. Reported recurrences rates vary from 0% to 16% (36), even when basal GH levels were just below 5 µg/l within 5–10 years after surgery. Thus, these data certainly do not reflect remission according to current criteria, and by modern criteria, patients with persistent disease are incorporated in this group. In the past, several investigators reported that the likelihood of recurrence was low when the postoperative GH could be suppressed to below 2 µg/l following an oral glucose load (35,36). However, even when the more stringent criteria of the consensus conference on normalization of acromegaly after treatment (5) are used, recurrence rates between 0% (14,37) and 8.4% (38) have been reported (Table 2). In a recent reevaluation of our series, we found 0.4% real recurrences in 368 patients followed up for a mean of 10 years (20). Thus, in general, real recurrences are rare events in acromegaly, once currently used criteria of normalization are utilized. However, in other published series with less stringent criteria of surgical remission, recurrences rates up to 17.8% are encountered (39).

Recurrent acromegaly may develop early or late, and latencies of 10 years and more have been described (40). Recurrence of acromegaly is frequently not associated with the appearance of tumor on MRI. A rough estimation would suggest that visible tumor may be found in slightly less than 50% of cases with true recurrence (41). Biochemical parameters remain the most sensitive measure of active disease.

Several investigators suggest that very low postoperative basal GH levels, very low GH levels during postoperative OGTT, and a lack of GH increase after TRH or other stimulating agents (e.g., arginine) following surgery indicate

Table 2
True Recurrences Following Surgery for GH-Secreting Pituitary Adenomas in Series Using Current Cure Criteria of the Disease: a Literature Survey

Author	OP/cured	Follow-up (yrs)Mean (range)	Recurrence Abs/%	Criteria for Remission GH/OGTT/IGF-1
Freda et al. (1998) (54)	115/70		5/4.3	<2.0 + <2 + normal IGF-1
Ahmed et al. (1999) (31)	139/94	5.0 (0.1–17)	7/7.4	<2.5 + <1 ± normal IGF-1
Laws et al. (2000) (18)	117/78		1/1.3	<2.5 ± <1 ± normal IGF-1
Kreutzer et al. (2001) (19)	57/40	3.1 (1–7.3)	1/2.5	<2.5 ± <1 ± normal IGF-1
De et al. (2003) (55)	90/57	11 (0.5–20)	0/0	<2.5 + <1 ± normal IGF-1
Beauregard et al. (2003) (38)	56/99	12 (1–30)	4/8.3	<2.5 + <1 ± normal IGF-1
Nomikos et al. (2005) (20)	368	10 (1.3–17.5)	1/0.4	<2.5 + <1 ± normal IGF-1

the most favorable prognosis for long-term remission, and strongly predict against later recurrence. Using a highly sensitive GH assay, Freda et al. (42) differentiated their patients in remission into two groups, one with low GH matching levels of normal controls and patients with somewhat higher suppressed levels. Those with very low GH levels had persistent long-term remission, while 5 of the 19 patients with suppressed GH levels between 0.14 and 1 μg/l developed recurrences. In a further study (43), they showed that the groups also had different mean hourly GH levels and a different response to arginine stimulation. Likewise, Biermasz et al. (44) emphasize the persistent postoperative GH increase after TRH as a prognostic indicator for potential later recurrence. These findings would suggest that very low postoperative basal, stimulated, and suppressed GH levels after surgery indicate a low risk of recurrence. It seems that higher, although still "normal," levels might be indicators of a small tumor residual, which may later progress to recurrent disease. However, in a recent study, Ronchi et al. (37) also grouped their postoperative patients into those with very low GH levels (matching normal controls) and others with slightly higher levels, although still below 1 μg/l after glucose. On follow-up, both groups behaved similarly, demonstrating the same clinical parameters and absence of signs of disease activity, and in neither of the groups were recurrences observed. Postoperative radiotherapy may prevent late recurrences. While Biermasz et al. *(40)* observed 5 recurrences in 27 patients who did not undergo postoperative radiotherapy, there was no recurrence observed in the 9 patients who were irradiated. In general, however, routine postoperative radiotherapy is not recommended.

Management options for recurrent disease include repeat surgery, medical treatment, or irradiation. There are little data on the benefits of repeat surgery for recurrent disease. However, if the results of repeat transsphenoidal surgery for residual and recurrent tumor are considered together, a remission rate of slightly below 20% can be anticipated, irrespective of radiological findings *(45)*. Only Kurosaki et al. *(46)* reported considerably better results after transsphenoidal reoperations. Although there is little experience with the medical management of recurrent acromegaly, in general medical treatment or radiotherapy may be better options.

7.1. Persistent Disease

The management of patients with persistent acromegaly after initial surgery is a matter of ongoing discussion. Several attempts have been made to achieve a consensus about as to how these patients should be treated. Many of these patients might be candidates for repeat surgery. We found reexploration to be particularly successful in those cases in which neither surgical nor histological invasion could be demonstrated during the first surgery. In our own series, reexplorations have been performed in 156 cases, mainly in patients with MRI studies that demonstrated residual adenomatous tissue. As expected, the overall remission rate was worse than in the primary surgery group, at 21.3%. Nevertheless, a remission rate of 37.3% could be achieved in patients with noninvasive tumors and an initial GH level below 40 µg/l prior to the first surgical approach *(20)*. To evaluate the effectiveness of secondary transnasal microsurgery 28 patients with persistent or recurrent acromegaly were analyzed by Abe et al. (1998) *(47)*. The overall endocrinological remission rate was found to be 57.1% (16 of 28 patients) without serious morbidity and no mortality. The absence of major surgical complications and the significant endocrinological deterioration of other pituitary functions combined with the possibility of long-term control of the disease support reexploration as a treatment option in a number of selected patients with persistent acromegaly.

7.2. New Technologies

New surgical techniques have recently been applied to the surgical management of acromegaly *(48)*. The use of an endoscope, with its main advantage of panoramic visualization of the anatomical structures through the wide angle of view and powerful light devices, makes the extended transsphenoidal approach to parasellar lesions safer. Additionally, the direct nasal approach, without paraseptal dissection, may frequently avoid the need for postoperative nasal tamponades and may therefore lead to a better subjective result from the patient's perspective. Intraoperative blood sampling and determination of GH levels have been suggested as a means of improving surgical results by identifying residual tumor *(49)*. Neuronavigation is helpful for the localization of anatomic structures intraoperatively. This method allows virtual surgery with three-dimensional reconstruction of the tumor and its adjacent structures, and therefore allows a safe approach to the sella even in cases with vascular anomalies, narrow sellar floors, poor pneumatization of the paranasal sinuses, and loss of anatomical landmarks in reoperations *(50)*. Intraoperative MRI, until recently only available in a few centers, allows neurosurgeons to perform surgery interactively using MRI guidance and, more importantly, allows a resection control, particularly in large intrasellar, suprasellar, and parasellar tumors. From a morphological consideration, intraoperative MRI is the ideal quality control to immediately determine the extent of adenoma resection and identify residual tumor tissue *(51,52)*. Its application during transsphenoidal surgery of acromegalic patients with large adenomas has been strongly recommended *(52)*.

REFERENCES

1. Rajasoorya C, Holdaway IM, Wrightson P, Scott DJ, Ibbertson HK. Determinants of clinical outcome and survival in acromegaly. Clin Endocrinol (Oxf) 1994;41:95–102.
2. Orme SM, McNally RJ, Cartwright RA, Belchetz PE. Mortality and cancer incidence in acromegaly: a retrospective cohort study. United Kingdom Acromegaly Study Group. J Clin Endocrinol Metab 1998;83:2730–4.
3. Swearingen B, Barker FG, II, Katznelson L, et al. Long-term mortality after transsphenoidal surgery and adjunctive therapy for acromegaly. J Clin Endocrinol Metab 1998;83:3419–26.
4. Bates AS, Van't Hoff W, Jones JM, Clayton RN. An audit of outcome of treatment in acromegaly. Q J Med 1993;86:293–9.
5. Giustina A, Barkan A, Casanueva FF, et al. Criteria for cure of acromegaly: a consensus statement. J Clin Endocrinol Metab 2000;85:526–9.
6. Bonadonna S, Doga M, Gola M, Mazziotti G, Giustina A. Diagnosis and treatment of acromegaly and its complications: consensus guidelines. J Endocrinol Invest 2005;28:43–7.
7. Melmed S, Casanueva F, Cavagnini F, et al. Consensus statement: medical management of acromegaly. Eur J Endocrinol 2005;153:737–40.
8. Colao A, Attanasio R, Pivonello R, et al. Partial surgical removal of growth hormone-secreting pituitary tumors enhances the response to somatostatin analogs in acromegaly. J Clin Endocrinol Metab 2006;91:85–92.
9. Buchfelder M, Fahlbusch R. The "classic" transsphenoidal approach for resection of pituitary tumors. Operat Techn Neurosurg 2002;4:210–17.

10. Couldwell WT. Transsphenoidal and transcranial surgery for pituitary adenomas. J Neurooncol 2004;69:237–56.
11. Ross DA, Wilson CB. Results of transsphenoidal microsurgery for growth hormone-secreting pituitary adenoma in a series of 214 patients. J Neurosurg 1988;68:854–67.
12. Zervas NT. Multicenter surgical results in acromegaly. In: Ludecke D, Tolis G, editors. Growth Hormone, Growth Factors, and Acromegaly. New York: Raven Press; 1987. pp. 253–7.
13. Fahlbusch R, Honegger J, Buchfelder M. Surgical management of acromegaly. Endocrinol Metab Clin North Am 1992;21:669–92.
14. Losa M, Oeckler R, Schopohl J, Muller OA, Alba-Lopez J, von Werder K. Evaluation of selective transsphenoidal adenomectomy by endocrinological testing and somatomedin-C measurement in acromegaly. J Neurosurg 1989;70:561–7.
15. Valdemarsson S, Bramnert M, Cronquist S, et al. Early postoperative basal serum GH level and the GH response to TRH in relation to the long-term outcome of surgical treatment for acromegaly: a report on 39 patients. J Intern Med 1991;230:49–54.
16. Valdemarsson S, Ljunggren S, Bramnert M, Norrhamn O, Nordstrom CH. Early postoperative growth hormone levels: high predictive value for long-term outcome after surgery for acromegaly. J Intern Med 2000;247:640–50.
17. Tindall GT, Oyesiku NM, Watts NB, Clark RV, Christy JH, Adams DA. Transsphenoidal adenomectomy for growth hormone-secreting pituitary adenomas in acromegaly: outcome analysis and determinants of failure. J Neurosurg 1993;78:205–15.
18. Laws ER, Vance ML, Thapar K. Pituitary surgery for the management of acromegaly. Horm Res 2000;53:71–5.
19. Kreutzer J, Vance ML, Lopes MB, Laws ER, Jr. Surgical management of GH-secreting pituitary adenomas: an outcome study using modern remission criteria. J Clin Endocrinol Metab 2001;86:4072–7.
20. Nomikos P, Buchfelder M, Fahlbusch R. The outcome of surgery in 668 patients with acromegaly using current criteria of biochemical "cure." Eur J Endocrinol 2005;152:379–87.
21. Peacey SR, Toogood AA, Veldhuis JD, Thorner MO, Shalet SM. The relationship between 24-hour growth hormone secretion and insulin- like growth factor I in patients with successfully treated acromegaly: impact of surgery or radiotherapy. J Clin Endocrinol Metab 2001;86:259–66.
22. Morrison KM, Wu Z, Bidlingmaier M, Strasburger CJ. Findings and theoretical considerations on the usefulness of the acid-labile subunit in the monitoring of acromegaly. Growth Horm IGF Res 2001;11(Suppl A):S61–3.
23. Hardy J. Transsphenoidal microsurgery of the pathological and normal pituitary. Clin Neurosurg 1969;16:185–217.
24. Kaltsas GA, Nomikos P, Kontogeorgos G, Buchfelder M, Grossman AB. Clinical review: Diagnosis and management of pituitary carcinomas. J Clin Endocrinol Metab 2005;90:3089–99.
25. Ahmadi J, North CM, Segall HD, Zee CS, Weiss MH. Cavernous sinus invasion by pituitary adenomas. AJR Am J Roentgenol 1986;146:257–62.
26. Buchfelder M, Fahlbusch R, Adams EF, Kiesewetter F, Thierauf P. Proliferation parameters for pituitary adenomas. Acta Neurochir Suppl 1996;65:18–21.
27. Sheaves R, Jenkins P, Blackburn P, et al. Outcome of transsphenoidal surgery for acromegaly using strict criteria for surgical cure. Clin Endocrinol (Oxf) 1996;45:407–13.
28. Colao A, Ferone D, Cappabianca P, et al. Effect of octreotide pretreatment on surgical outcome in acromegaly. J Clin Endocrinol Metab 1997;82:3308–14.

29. Kristof RA, Stoffel-Wagner B, Klingmuller D, Schramm J. Does octreotide treatment improve the surgical results of macro- adenomas in acromegaly? A randomized study. Acta Neurochir 1999;141:399–405.
30. Plockinger U, Quabbe HJ. Presurgical octreotide treatment in acromegaly: no improvement of final growth hormone (GH) concentration and pituitary function. A long-term case-control study. Acta Neurochir (Wien) 2005;147:485–93; discussion 493.
31. Ahmed S, Elsheikh M, Stratton IM, Page RC, Adams CB, Wass JA. Outcome of transsphenoidal surgery for acromegaly and its relationship to surgical experience. Clin Endocrinol (Oxf) 1999;50:561–7.
32. Clayton RN, Stewart PM, Shalet SM, Wass JA. Pituitary surgery for acromegaly. Should be done by specialists. BMJ 1999;319:588–9.
33. Barker FG, II, Klibanski A, Swearingen B. Transsphenoidal surgery for pituitary tumors in the United States, 1996–2000: mortality, morbidity, and the effects of hospital and surgeon volume. J Clin Endocrinol Metab 2003;88:4709–19.
34. Schmitt H, Buchfelder M, Radespiel-Troger M, Fahlbusch R. Difficult intubation in acromegalic patients: incidence and predictability. Anesthesiology 2000;93:110–14.
35. Buchfelder M, Brockmeier S, Fahlbusch R, Honegger J, Pichl J, Manzl M. Recurrence following transsphenoidal surgery for acromegaly. Horm Res 1991;35:113–18.
36. Arafah BM, Rosenzweig JL, Fenstermaker R, Salazar R, McBride CE, Selman W. Value of growth hormone dynamics and somatomedin C (insulin-like growth factor I) levels in predicting the long-term benefit after transsphenoidal surgery for acromegaly. J Lab Clin Med 1987;109:346–54.
37. Ronchi CL, Varca V, Giavoli C, et al. Long-term evaluation of postoperative acromegalic patients in remission with previous and newly proposed criteria. J Clin Endocrinol Metab 2005;90:1377–82.
38. Beauregard C, Truong U, Hardy J, Serri O. Long-term outcome and mortality after transsphenoidal adenomectomy for acromegaly. Clin Endocrinol (Oxf) 2003;58:86–91.
39. Davis DH, Laws ER, Jr, Ilstrup DM, et al. Results of surgical treatment for growth hormone-secreting pituitary adenomas. J Neurosurg 1993;79:70–5.
40. Biermasz NR, van Dulken H, Roelfsema F. Ten-year follow-up results of transsphenoidal microsurgery in acromegaly. J Clin Endocrinol Metab 2000;85:4596–602.
41. Zirkzee EJ, Corssmit EP, Biermasz NR, et al. Pituitary magnetic resonance imaging is not required in the postoperative follow-up of acromegalic patients with long-term biochemical cure after transsphenoidal surgery. J Clin Endocrinol Metab 2004;89:4320–4.
42. Freda PU, Post KD, Powell JS, Wardlaw SL. Evaluation of disease status with sensitive measures of growth hormone secretion in 60 postoperative patients with acromegaly. J Clin Endocrinol Metab 1998;83:3808–16.
43. Freda PU, Nuruzzaman AT, Reyes CM, et al. Significance of "abnormal" nadir growth hormone levels after oral glucose in postoperative patients with acromegaly in remission with normal insulin-like growth factor-I levels. J Clin Endocrinol Metab 2004;89:495–500.
44. Biermasz NR, Smit JW, van Dulken H, Roelfsema F. Postoperative persistent thyrotrophin releasing hormone-induced growth hormone release predicts recurrence in patients with acromegaly. Clin Endocrinol (Oxf) 2002;56:313–9.
45. Long H, Beauregard H, Somma M, Comtois R, Serri O, Hardy J. Surgical outcome after repeated transsphenoidal surgery in acromegaly. J Neurosurg 1996;85:239–47.
46. Kurosaki M, Luedecke DK, Abe T. Effectiveness of secondary transnasal surgery in GH-secreting pituitary macroadenomas. Endocr J 2003;50:635–42.
47. Abe T, Ludecke DK. Recent results of secondary transnasal surgery for residual or recurring acromegaly. Neurosurgery 1998;42:1013–21; discussion 1021–2.

48. Fahlbusch R. Future avenues in treatment of pituitary adenomas. Pituitary 1999;2:113–15.
49. Abe T, Ludecke DK. Recent primary transnasal surgical outcomes associated with intra-operative growth hormone measurement in acromegaly. Clin Endocrinol (Oxf) 1999;50: 27–35.
50. Buchfelder M. Treatment of pituitary tumors: surgery. Endocrine 2005;28:67–75.
51. Fahlbusch R, Ganslandt O, Buchfelder M, Schott W, Nimsky C. Intraoperative magnetic resonance imaging during transsphenoidal surgery. J Neurosurg 2001;95:381–90.
52. Fahlbusch R, Keller B, Ganslandt O, Kreutzer J, Nimsky C. Transsphenoidal surgery in acromegaly investigated by intraoperative high-field magnetic resonance imaging. Eur J Endocrinol 2005;153:239–48.
53. Abosch A, Tyrrell JB, Lamborn KR, Hannegan LT, Applebury CB, Wilson CB. Transsphe-noidal microsurgery for growth hormone-secreting pituitary adenomas: initial outcome and long-term results. J Clin Endocrinol Metab 1998;83:3411–18.
54. Freda PU, Wardlaw SL, Post KD. Long-term endocrinological follow-up evaluation in 115 patients who underwent transsphenoidal surgery for acromegaly. J Neurosurg 1998;89: 353–8.
55. De P, Rees DA, Davies N, et al. Transsphenoidal surgery for acromegaly in Wales: results based on stringent criteria of remission. J Clin Endocrinol Metab 2003;88:3567–72.

10 Cushing's Disease: *Diagnostic Evaluation*

James W. Findling, MD, and Hershel Raff, PhD

CONTENTS

1. INTRODUCTION
2. SCREENING FOR CUSHING'S SYNDROME
3. DIAGNOSTIC TESTS
4. DIFFERENTIAL DIAGNOSIS

Summary

The diagnosis and differential diagnosis of Cushing's syndrome continues to be a challenging problem for clinical endocrinologists. The use of nocturnal salivary cortisol testing now provides a sensitive and specific means to screen patients with suspected hypercortisolism. The overnight 1 mg dexamethasone suppression test and the 24-h urine free cortisol (UFC) test are complementary and may help to provide confirmation of the diagnosis of Cushing's syndrome. Discrimination of patients with pathologic hypercortisolism from those with physiologic activation of the hypothalamic–pituitary–adrenal axis is probably best done clinically and with repeat biochemical testing. A specific and sensitive immunometric assay for ACTH, CRH stimulation testing, pituitary imaging with MRI, and inferior petrosal ACTH sampling with CRH stimulation provides the means for an accurate differential diagnosis of Cushing's syndrome so that appropriate and effective therapy can be recommended.

Key Words: Cushing's disease, ACTH, Inferior petrosal sinus sampling, Pituitary tumor.

1. INTRODUCTION

… how can we expect to detect the mildest forms of the disorder by data (i.e., the dexamethasone suppression and the ACTH response tests) obtained only from florid instances of the disease? It is already apparent that not all instances of florid Cushing's syndrome hyperrespond to the administration

From: *Contemporary Endocrinology: Diagnosis and Management of Pituitary Disorders*
Edited by: B. Swearingen and B. M. K. Biller © Humana Press, Totowa, NJ

of ACTH and it has also become evident, as one might have predicted, a priori, that the suppression test is not infallible. Accordingly, the tests may fail particularly in those instances when we are uncertain as to the presence or absence of the disease. J. Lester Gabrilove, 1965 *(1)*.

This prophetic statement, despite being over 40 years old, still elegantly describes the current diagnostic dilemma and challenges in the evaluation of patients with suspected endogenous hypercortisolism. The clinical manifestations of excessive glucocorticoid exposure—endogenous or exogenous—are protean, often quite subtle, and frequently overlooked even by skilled clinicians. Recognition that patients with mild or subclinical hypercortisolism frequently have improvement in their diabetes, hypertension, and obesity after its surgical correction *(2,3)* increases the importance of establishing the diagnosis of even mild Cushing's syndrome.

2. SCREENING FOR CUSHING'S SYNDROME

Screening studies for Cushing's syndrome should be performed in subjects who have relatively specific signs and symptoms of hypercortisolism or in patients who have clinical diagnoses that may be caused or aggravated by endogenous hypercortisolism. Recent studies performed in high-risk populations have demonstrated an unexpectedly high incidence of unrecognized Cushing's syndrome. Approximately 2–5% of patients with poorly controlled diabetes mellitus may have occult Cushing's syndrome as a contributing factor in their poorly controlled diabetes *(4,5)* and women with polycystic ovary syndrome may have unappreciated endogenous hypercortisolism. A recent study has also demonstrated that 5% of patients with idiopathic osteoporosis actually have unsuspected Cushing's syndrome *(6)*. Moreover, subclinical hypercortisolism may be present in up to 10% of patients with adrenal incidentalomas *(7)*, which are present in at least 2% of the adult population *(8)*. One can surmise, then, that spontaneous Cushing's syndrome is more common than previously thought.

2.1. Specific Signs and Symptoms

Table 1 lists some of the clinical signs and symptoms that mandate screening evaluation for possible hypercortisolism. Weight gain, particularly in a central distribution, is a common finding. Unfortunately, this type of weight gain is difficult to distinguish from patients with the dysmetabolic syndrome (syndrome of insulin resistance) *(9)*. Old photographs may help appreciate these changes. Other findings that mandate evaluation for hypercortisolism include a marked increase in supraclavicular fullness and dorsocervical fat. Facial rounding with plethora is also common, but may be subtle. The catabolic effects of excessive cortisol excess also result in cutaneous wasting with ecchymoses, and wide violaceous striae (≥ 1 cm) may be observed in younger patients. These catabolic effects also result in proximal myopathy that may be the most prominent symptom, particularly in older adults. Hyperandrogenism may be present and may result in facial hirsutism, although glucocorticoid-dependent vellus hypertrichosis (lanugo hair) may be more common in women with spontaneous Cushing's syndrome. Decreased linear growth velocity with generalized obesity is the hallmark of Cushing's syndrome in children *(10)*.

2.2. Clinical Diagnoses Associated with Hypercortisolism

Table 1 also summarizes clinical disorders whose presence should at least stimulate the consideration of Cushing's syndrome. Endogenous hypercortisolism results in the entire clinical spectrum of the dysmetabolic syndrome including obesity, diabetes, hypertension, and gonadal dysfunction that are

Table 1
Who Should be Screened for Cushing's Syndrome?

Signs and symptoms
Central obesity with:
- Facial rounding with plethora
- Increased supraclavicular and dorsocervical fat
- Cutaneous wasting with ecchymoses
- Wide violaceous striae (greater than 1 cm)
- Proximal myopathy
- Increased lanugo hair
- Growth retardation (in children)

Clinical diagnosis
Metabolic syndrome X/dysmetabolic syndrome
- Diabetes mellitus (HgbA1C $>8\%$)
- Hypertension
- Hyperlipidemia
- Polycystic ovary syndrome (PCOS)

Hypogonadotropic hypogonadism
- Oligomenorrhea/amenorrhea/infertility
- Decreased libido and impotence

Osteoporosis (especially with rib fractures)
- Patients aged <65 years

Incidental adrenal mass

relatively common findings in the population. Nonetheless, patients with the dysmetabolic syndrome should be considered for screening particularly if they demonstrate any of the signs or symptoms described above. Women with oligomenorrhea/amenorrhea or the polycystic ovary syndrome should be evaluated for possible endogenous hypercortisolism if other causes are not apparent *(11,12)*. In addition, men with unexplained hypogonadotropic hypogonadism should probably be screened. The devastating effects of glucocorticoid excess on bone are well appreciated *(13)*. In light of the recent study mentioned previously *(6)* and from our experience, patients with unexplained osteoporosis should undergo a screening test for possible Cushing's syndrome. The high prevalence of mild hypercortisolism in patients with adrenal nodules (≥ 2 cm) should also mandate a screening test.

3. DIAGNOSTIC TESTS

Currently, there are three diagnostic tests used in the United States for the evaluation of patients with suspected endogenous hypercorticosolism. These three tests are complementary and all of them have liabilities. As Dr Gabrilove predicted 40 years ago, all or some of these tests may be normal in patients with mild hypercortisolism. All three tests have been employed as screening tests as well as diagnostic tests.

3.1. Urine Free Cortisol

The measurement of free cortisol in a 24-h urine collection has been the gold standard for the diagnosis of endogenous hypercortisolism. The concept is that as the daily production of cortisol is increased, the free cortisol filtered and not reabsorbed or metabolized in the kidneys will be increased. However, it is now clear that many patients with mild Cushing's syndrome do not have elevations of urine free cortisol (UFC), making it a poor screening test for this condition *(14)*. Patients with mild hypercortisolism may have only small but significant increases in nighttime cortisol secretion. Since most of the cortisol secreted during a 24-h period is usually between 4 a.m. and 4 p.m., subtle increases in nighttime secretion may not be detected in the standard 24-h urine collection. In addition, even modest decreases in renal function may obfuscate the reliability of UFC collections *(15)*.

Another problem with UFC is the different measurement methods used. Some reference laboratories continue to use direct immunoassays of cortisol without chromographic separation. This type of assay lacks specificity, but may be useful in the patient excreting an unusual pattern of cortisol metabolites that cross-react with the cortisol antibody. Many reference laboratories now use some type of chromographic separation (usually high performance liquid chromatography), and many laboratories now use tandem mass spectrometry as a means of detection. Despite the increased sophistication of measurement of free cortisol in the urine, many problems still arise. Substances that would interfere with some of the chromatographic methods, including carbamazepine and fenofibrate, may cause false elevations of UFC and provoke significant confusion in the evaluation of these patients *(16,17)*. Finally, the sensitivity of UFC for Cushing's syndrome is only 45–71% at 100% specificity *(12)*. The measurement of UFC is probably most useful when clearly elevated; if severalfold above the upper limit of normal, it may exclude pseudo-Cushing's syndrome.

3.2. Low-Dose Dexamethasone Suppression Test

The low-dose dexamethasone suppression test relies on the concept that the correct dose of dexamethasone will suppress ACTH, and hence, cortisol release in normal subjects, while patients with ACTH-secreting tumors will not suppress below a specified cutoff. Obviously, ACTH-independent (adrenal) Cushing's syndrome should be unaffected by dexamethasone administration. Nonetheless, because of the significant variability of the biological behavior of corticotroph adenomas, neither the overnight 1 mg dexamethasone suppression test nor the more traditional 2-day low-dose dexamethasone suppression test appears to be reliable using standard cutoffs for serum cortisol *(18,19,20)*. It remains controversial as to what the cutoff should be; however, a consensus of experts in the field have proposed that the cutoff for serum cortisol following the overnight 1 mg dexamethasone suppression test should be < 1.8 mcg/dl ($\leq$50 nmol/l) *(21)*. Although this criterion improves sensitivity to greater than 95%, there is a substantial reduction in specificity. Moreover, we have recently reported that up to 8% of patients with Cushing's disease may have false-negative results (serum cortisol $\leq$2 mcg/dl [55 nmol/l]), indicating that no cutoff reliably excludes Cushing's syndrome *(18)*. Adding to this problem is that, at low levels of serum cortisol, differences in assay performance may add significant error to the testing *(22)*. Despite these limitations, the low-dose overnight 1 mg dexamethasone suppression test is a simple and useful diagnostic test. The more traditional 2-day low-dose dexamethasone suppression test may also be a useful diagnostic tool particularly if serum cortisol is used as the criterion for normalcy. In our experience, the measurement of urine steroids in response to this test is unreliable and obviously cumbersome. It is not clear what the cutoff should be in the setting of medications that increase cortisol-binding globulin levels (e.g., estrogen), and therefore increase total serum cortisol.

3.3. Nocturnal Salivary Cortisol

The earliest biochemical abnormality in patients with mild Cushing's syndrome is a failure to decrease cortisol secretion to its nadir at night. This observation has been exploited for the diagnosis of Cushing's syndrome using several different approaches. Initially, serum cortisol at midnight was found to have a very high sensitivity and specificity for spontaneous Cushing's syndrome (23,24); patients with true Cushing's syndrome had midnight serum cortisol levels greater than 3–7 mcg/dl (83–193 nmol/l). In Europe, this approach is still used, but patients need to be hospitalized overnight with an indwelling catheter and should be sleeping to obtain a reliable specimen. This approach is not satisfactory for clinicians in the United States and a more simple (and reliable) method has been developed.

The measurement of a late-night salivary cortisol—a surrogate for serum free cortisol—has proven to be a sensitive and specific means of determining the presence or absence of endogenous hypercortisolism (25). There have been several studies validating this approach to screen for Cushing's syndrome, and the test is now widely available from several reference laboratories in the United States (26). There is a salivary cortisol enzyme immunoassay that has been FDA-cleared for the diagnosis of Cushing's syndrome (27). Nocturnal salivary cortisol measurements yield a remarkable 93 % sensitivity at 100 % specificity. Currently, there is no diagnostic test used in the evaluation of Cushing's syndrome that performs better (26).

Nonetheless, the measurement of nocturnal salivary cortisol has limitations. Many factors may falsely elevate nocturnal cortisol secretion including proximal stress, sleep disturbances, psycho-neuroendocrine factors, and contamination of the saliva sample (28). Subjects who do not have a normal sleep-wake cycle will not have a nadir of cortisol secretion late at night obfuscating the clinical utility of the test.

Our diagnostic approach currently includes the measurement of two 11 p.m. and midnight salivary cortisol measurements in patients with suspected hypercortisolism (26). If the nocturnal salivary cortisol levels are consistently < 4.0 nmol/l, the diagnosis of significant Cushing's syndrome is very unlikely. If the index of suspicion is high or intermittent or cyclical Cushing's syndrome is considered, repeat measurements are needed. Nonetheless, repeatedly normal salivary cortisol measurements at 11 p.m. and midnight make the diagnosis of pathological Cushing's syndrome remote. If the two measurements are discordant, we simply repeat the measurements. There are no data on the outcome of patients with internally discordant results, but it seems likely that most of them are probably normal and do not have endogenous hypercortisolism. Nocturnal salivary cortisol levels consistently greater than 7–8 nmol/l are clearly abnormal and the diagnosis of Cushing's syndrome is likely. The overnight 1 mg dexamethasone suppression test is usually employed at this point and we also collect a 24-h UFC. If two of these three tests are abnormal and the nocturnal salivary cortisol test is already abnormal, the diagnosis of endogenous hypercortisolism is likely. Rarely, there are patients with true spontaneous Cushing's syndrome who may have only elevations of nocturnal salivary cortisol particularly early in the course of the disease process. As more clinicians use nocturnal salivary cortisol in the diagnosis of Cushing's syndrome, many of these issues may be resolved.

4. DIFFERENTIAL DIAGNOSIS

4.1. Pathologic Hypercortisolism versus Physiologic Hypercortisolism

After the biochemical diagnosis of endogenous hypercortisolism has been established, the clinician must differentiate pathologic Cushing's syndrome from physiologic activation of the hypothalamic–pituitary–adrenal axis (Table 2). Although this discrimination can usually be based on clinical grounds, many of the disorders that activate the hypothalamic–pituitary–adrenal (HPA) axis may also have some clinical features of pathologic Cushing's

Table 2
Differential Diagnosis of Endogenous Hypercortisolism

Pathologic
    ACTH-dependent
        Pituitary tumor (Cushing's disease)
        Nonpituitary tumor (ectopic ACTH)
    ACTH-independent
        Adrenal neoplasm (adenoma/carcinoma)
        Bilateral nodular adrenal hyperplasia
            Carney complex (e.g., protein kinase A mutation)
            Aberrant adrenal receptor expression (e.g., GIP, vasopressin)
            McCune–Albright syndrome (mutations of $G_{S\alpha}$)
Physiologic
    ACTH-dependent
        Alcoholism
        Eating disorders/starvation
        Severe neuropsychiatric illness
        Multiple sclerosis
        Pregnancy
        Poorly controlled diabetes mellitus
        Critical illness (acute, subacute)

syndrome. This group of disorders has been referred to as "pseudo-Cushing's syndrome." This is somewhat of a misnomer since the majority of patients with endogenous activation of the HPA axis do not have clinical Cushing's syndrome and, of course, some patients with true pathologic Cushing's syndrome do not have many of the classic features of the Cushing's phenotype.

The best-appreciated disorder that activates the hypothalamic pituitary adrenal axis is alcoholism (29). Many of these patients are quite Cushingoid and usually have some degree of alcoholic liver disease. The pathophysiology of this hypercortisolism is not well understood and may include direct activation of the HPA axis as well as possible alterations in cortisol metabolism in the liver. The diagnosis can usually be established with a good history and the hypercortisolism usually remits promptly following discontinuation of alcohol consumption. Eating disorders, particularly anorexia nervosa, has also been shown to cause endogenous hypercortisolism. These subjects often have abnormal dexamethasone suppression, elevations of late-night salivary cortisol, and elevations of 24-h UFC (30). Although it is rare that these patients would be difficult to distinguish from a patient with true Cushing's syndrome, it should be appreciated that anorexia may be a rare neuropsychiatric manifestation of Cushing's disease (31). Severe endogenous depression, which is also a common feature of true Cushing's syndrome, may be characterized by abnormalities in the HPA axis. These subjects have abnormal low-dose dexamethasone suppression that, in fact, was formerly used as a diagnostic test for depression (32). Dysregulation of the HPA axis has also been observed in multiple sclerosis and the magnitude of cortisol secretion may correlate with the severity and stage of this inflammatory demyelinating process (33). Hypercortisolism is observed in the third trimester of pregnancy possibly as the result of excessive secretion of CRH from the placenta (34).

Biochemical differentiation of physiologic hypercortisolism from true pathologic Cushing's syndrome is not simple. Some investigators have advocated the use of a low-dose dexamethasone suppression test in combination with CRH stimulation (35). The theory is that only abnormal corticotrophs will respond to CRH during suppression with dexamethasone. Starting at noon, dexamethasone (0.5 mg) is administered every 6 h for a total of eight doses, with the last given at 6 a.m. before dynamic studies (CRH 1 mcg/kg) is then administered intravenously at 8 a.m., with measurement of cortisol and ACTH every 15 min for 1 h. A serum cortisol greater than 1.4 mcg/dl (38.6 nmol/l) is considered abnormal. There are currently no accepted criteria for abnormal plasma ACTH response to this test. Although the initial studies with the low-dose dexamethasone suppression CRH test were promising, this test may not provide adequate discriminatory power (36,37). Patients with anorexia nervosa frequently have an abnormal test and we have observed patients with false-positive and false-negative low-dose dexamethasone suppression CRH testing. The measurement of serum cortisol late at night has also been proposed as a means of distinguishing true pathologic Cushing's syndrome from the so-called "pseudo-Cushing" conditions; however, even patients with anorexia nervosa may have elevations of nocturnal salivary cortisol *(38)*. Therefore, no single biochemical test can distinguish mild spontaneous Cushing's syndrome from patients with chronic physiologic hypercortisolism.

Theoretically, the use of a DDAVP stimulation test might distinguish patients with a true ACTH-dependent Cushing's syndrome from those with physiologic hypercortisolism in that patients with ACTH-secreting pituitary tumors display an exaggerated ACTH response to DDAVP *(36,39)*. Unfortunately, this test has not been well studied in patients with the disorders known to activate the HPA axis. In addition, 15% of normal obese subjects have an ACTH and cortisol response to DDAVP *(39)*.

4.2. ACTH-Dependent versus ACTH-Independent Cushing's Syndrome

Once the diagnosis of pathologic Cushing's syndrome is firmly established, differential diagnosis is crucial in order that appropriate therapy can be offered to the patient (Fig. 1). Approximately 80% of patients with Cushing's syndrome have an ACTH-secreting neoplasm (ACTH-dependent Cushing's syndrome) from a pituitary tumor (Cushing's disease) or a nonpituitary neoplasm (ectopic ACTH) (Table 2). Many patients with ectopic ACTH-secreting neoplasms (particularly those with neuroendocrine tumors such as bronchial carcinoids) may present with hypercortisolism many years before there is radiographic evidence of the tumor (occult ectopic ACTH syndrome). These forms of ACTH-dependent Cushing's syndrome are often clinically and biochemically indistinguishable from each other and careful testing is often required for an appropriate diagnosis.

ACTH-independent Cushing's syndrome is due to either autonomous adrenal production of cortisol or by prolonged glucocorticoid therapy. Most patients with spontaneous ACTH-independent Cushing's syndrome have a solitary benign adrenocortical neoplasm. A minority have bilateral nodular adrenal hyperplasia. There are several mechanisms known for bilateral nodular adrenal hyperplasia including mutations in protein kinase A (Carney complex), aberrant regulation of cortisol production by the abnormal expression of hormone receptors such as those for glucose-dependent insulinotropic polypeptide, vasopressin, beta-human chorionic gonadotropin/luteinizing hormone, or activating mutations of the receptor subunit Gs-alpha in McCune–Albright syndrome *(40)*.

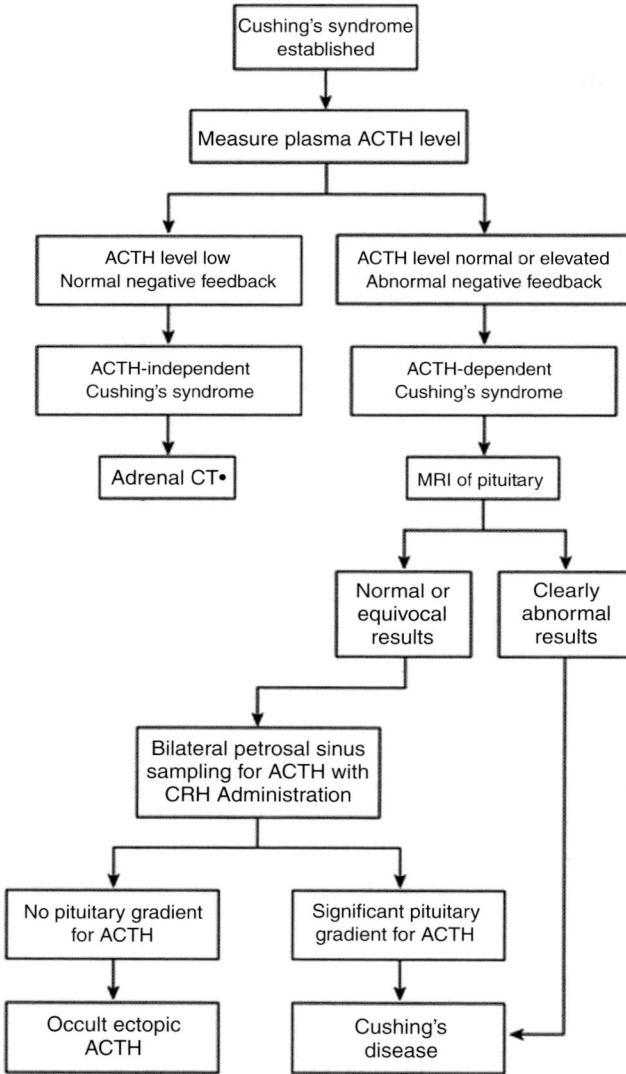

Fig. 1. The differential diagnosis of Cushing's syndrome. MRI, magnetic resonance imaging; ACTH, adrenocorticotropic hormone; CT, computed tomography; CRH, corticotrophin-releasing hormone. (•) for a more thorough listing of different types of adrenal Cushing's disease, see Table 1. Reprinted with permission from the Annals of Internal Medicine *(9)*.

The development of a two-site immunometric assay for ACTH has simplified the initial differential diagnostic step. If the morning plasma ACTH is suppressed below 5 pg/ml (1.1 pmol/l), the patients most likely have adrenal-dependent Cushing's syndrome, and computed tomography of the adrenal glands should be performed. It is often needed to measure plasma ACTH on multiple occasions to ensure diagnostic accuracy, and appropriate collection of plasma samples is important. Plasma ACTH levels between 5 and 20 pg/ml (1.1–4.4 pmol/l) may be consistent with either ACTH-dependent or ACTH-independent Cushing's syndrome and it is often necessary to perform a CRH stimulation test to identify patients with ACTH-secreting tumors with a low range of basal plasma ACTH *(41)*. The ACTH response to CRH should be blunted in adrenal Cushing's syndrome due to negative feedback and is usually exaggerated in Cushing's disease if the pituitary tumor expresses the CRH receptor.

4.3. Differentiation of the Pituitary and Ectopic ACTH-Dependent Cushing's Syndrome

The vast majority (90–95%) of patients with ACTH-dependent Cushing's syndrome harbor a pituitary corticotroph microadenoma. Since the pretest probability of Cushing's disease is very high, differential diagnostic testing must be very accurate. Simple clinical measures actually have a good predictive value for establishing the presence of Cushing's disease *(42)*. A woman with mild hypercortisolism, a normal or slightly elevated plasma ACTH, and normokalemia has an approximately 95% likelihood of having Cushing's disease before any differential diagnostic testing is performed. In contrast, a male patient with prodigious hypercortisolism of rapid onset, hypokalemia, and marked elevations of plasma ACTH may be more likely to have an occult ectopic ACTH-secreting tumor.

The initial diagnostic study should be a pituitary MRI. Unfortunately, 50% of patients with ACTH-secreting microadenomas will have a normal study *(43)*. The use of dynamic MRI with intravenous gadolinium and spoiled gradient sequences may increase the sensitivity *(44)*. Nonetheless, this must be weighed against the 10% rate of pituitary incidentalomas in the normal population *(45)*. The presence of an unequivocal pituitary lesion (greater than 6 mm) with MRI in a patient without clinical features suggesting an ectopic ACTH-secreting tumor is probably adequate to proceed with pituitary microsurgery *(21)*.

High-dose dexamethasone suppression testing has also been used to discriminate pituitary from ectopic ACTH-dependent Cushing's syndrome. However, it has been established that many patients with neuroendocrine, nonpituitary ACTH-secreting tumors (particularly bronchial carcinoids) may have dexamethasone suppression of cortisol that is indistinguishable from those in patients with Cushing's disease *(42)*. This diagnostic test is no longer recommended.

Inferior petrosal sinus ACTH sampling (IPSS) with CRH stimulation is really the only study with the potential to yield a diagnostic sensitivity and specificity for Cushing's disease higher than its pretest probability *(46,47)*. The study should be performed at an experienced center dedicated to performing it safely and correctly. In the presence of documented hypercortisolism (we collect a nocturnal salivary cortisol before the procedure), the presence of an unequivocal pituitary ACTH gradient (dominant inferior petrosal sinus to peripheral ACTH ratio > 2.0 in the basal state and/or > 3.0 after CRH) yields a diagnostic sensitivity of nearly 100%. Although the absence of a pituitary ACTH gradient usually represents an occult ectopic ACTH-secreting neoplasm, it has recently been shown that there are several patients with proven Cushing's disease who usually have false-negative IPSS due to technical problems with the procedure or anomalous venous drainage *(48)*. Recently, it has been shown that the measurement of inferior petrosal sinus prolactin as an index of the fidelity of pituitary venous effluent may help to identify patients with Cushing's disease even in the absence of a pituitary ACTH gradient during IPSS *(49)*. Consequently, patients without a significant pituitary ACTH gradient during IPSS should have samples evaluated retrospectively for a prolactin gradient in order to ensure that adequate pituitary venous effluent was secured.

In summary, the differential diagnosis of ACTH-dependent Cushing's syndrome relies on inferior petrosal sinus sampling for ACTH after CRH administration, particularly when there is no definitive pituitary lesion on imaging. The lack of an inferior petrosal sinus to peripheral vein gradient for ACTH does not prove ectopic ACTH; adequacy of sampling should be confirmed by the measurement of prolactin gradients before the search for an ectopic tumor is started.

4.4. Search for the Occult Ectopic ACTH-Secreting Tumor

The majority of occult ectopic ACTH-secreting tumors are either bronchial or thymic carcinoids or other neuroendocrine tumors such as islet cell pancreas tumors, medullary carcinoma of the thyroid, or pheochromocytoma *(50)*.

Imaging of the thorax and the abdomen with computed tomography will yield the highest detection rate in searching for an occult ectopic ACTH-secreting neoplasm. MRI of the chest may also provide some additional benefit since some bronchial carcinoids have a central location and may be mistaken on computed tomography for a blood vessel *(51)*.

If these studies are inconclusive, somatostain receptors scintigraphy (SRS) may be used since many of these neuroendocrine tumors express somatostatin receptors. However, many of these tumors are quite small and the resolution of SRS may not be adequate to find them *(52,53)*. Although the low metabolic activity of the occult ectopic ACTH-secreting neoplasms usually render a positron emission tomography (PET) with 18-flurodioxyglucose inadequate *(54)*, recent improvements in camera techniques may help to find these small lesions *(55)*. Measurement of other neuropeptides such as plasma calcitonin, gastrin, glucagon, and somatostain may be elevated but are usually not helpful in identifying the source of the occult neoplasm. Multiorgan venous sampling for ACTH is rarely helpful.

REFERENCES

1. Gabrilove, JL. The continuum of adrenocortical disease: a thesis and its lesson to medicine. J Mount Sinai Hospital 1965;32:634–6.
2. Terzolo M, Pia A, Ali A, et al. Adrenal incidentaloma: a new cause of the metabolic syndrome? J Clin Endocrinol Metab 2002;87:998–1003.
3. Reincke M, Nieke J, Krestin GP, Saeger W, Allolio B, Winkelmann W. Preclinical Cushing's syndrome in adrenal "incidentalomas": comparison with adrenal Cushing's syndrome. J Clin Endocrinol Metab 1992;75:826–32.
4. Leibowitz G, Tsur A, Chayen SD, et al. Pre-clinical Cushing's syndrome: an unexpected frequent cause of poor glycaemic control in obese diabetic patients. Clin Endocrinol 1996;44:717–22.
5. Catargi B, Rigalleau V, Poussin A, et al. Occult Cushing's syndrome in type-2 diabetes. J Clin Endocrinol Metab 2003;88:5808–13.
6. Chiodini I, Mascia ML, Muscarella S, et al. Subclinical hypercortisolism among outpatients referred for osteoporosis. Ann Intern Med 2007;147:541–548.
7. Terzolo M, Bovio S, Reimondo G, et al. Subclinical Cushing's syndrome in adrenal incidentalomas. Endocrinol Metab Clin N Am 2005;34:423–39.
8. Mansmann G, Lau J, Balk E, Rothberg M, Miyachi Y, Bornstein SR. The clinically inapparent adrenal mass: update in diagnosis and management. Endocr Rev 2004;25: 309–40.
9. Raff H, Finding JW. A physiologic approach to diagnosis of Cushing syndrome. Ann Intern Med 2003;138:980–91.
10. Lebrethon MC. Grossman AB. Afshar F. Plowman PN. Besser GM. Savage MO. Linear growth and final height after treatment for Cushing's disease in childhood. J Clin Endocrinol Metab 2000;85:3262–5.
11. Kaltsas GA, Korbonits M, Isidori AM, et al. How common are polycystic ovaries and the polycystic ovarian syndrome in women with Cushing's syndrome? Clin Endocrinol 2000; 53:493–500.
12. Findling JW, Raff H. Screening and diagnosis of Cushing's syndrome. Endocrinol Metab Clin N Am 2005;34:385–402.
13. Shaker JL, Lukert BP. Osteoporosis associated with excess glucocorticoids. Endocrinol Metab Clin N Am 2005;34:341–56.
14. Kidambi S, Raff H, Findling JW. Limitations of nocturnal salivary cortisol and urine free cortisol in the diagnosis of mild Cushing's syndrome. Eur J Endocrinol 2007;157: 725–731.

15. Murphy BEP. Urinary free cortisol determinations: what they measure. The Endocrinologist 2002;12:143–50.
16. Findling JW, Pinkstaff SM, Shaker JL, Raff H, Nelson JC. Pseudohypercortisoluria: spurious elevation of urinary cortisol due to carbamazepine. The Endocrinologist 1998;8:51–4.
17. Meikle AW, Findling J, Kushnir MM, Rockwood AL, Nelson GJ, Terry AH. Pseudo-Cushing's syndrome caused by fenofibrate interference with urinary cortisol assayed by high-performance liquid chromatography. J Clin Endocrinol Metab. 2003;88:3521–4.
18. Findling JW, Raff H, Aron DC. The low-dose dexamethasone suppression test: a re-evaluation in patients with Cushing's syndrome. J. Clin Endocrinol Metab 2004;89:1222–6.
19. Isidori AM, Kaltsas GA, Mohammed S, Morris DG, Jenkins P, Chew SL. Discriminatory value of the low-dose dexamethasone suppression test in establishing the diagnosis and differential diagnosis of Cushing's syndrome. J Clin Endocrinol Metab 2003;88:5299–5306.
20. Friedman TC. An update on the overnight dexamethasone suppression test for the diagnosis of Cushing's syndrome: limitations in patients with mild and/or episodic hypercortisolism. Exp Clin Endocrinol Diabetes 2006;114:356–60.
21. Arnaldi G, Angeli A, Atkinson AB, et al. Diagnosis and complications of Cushing's syndrome: a consensus statement. J Clin Endocrinol Metab 2003;88:5593–602.
22. Odagiri E, Naruse M, Terasaki K, et al. The diagnostic standard of preclinical Cushing's syndrome: evaluation of the dexamethasone suppression test using various cortisol kits. Endocrine J 2004;51:295–302.
23. Newell-Price J, Trainer P, Perry L, Wass J, Grossman A, Besser M. A single sleeping midnight cortisol has 100% sensitivity for the diagnosis of Cushing's syndrome. Clin Endocrinol 1995;43:545–50.
24. Papanicolaou DA, Yanovski JA, Cutler GB, Chrousos GP, Nieman LK. A single midnight cortisol measurement distinguishes Cushing's syndrome from pseudo-Cushing's states. J Clin Endocrinol Metab 1998;83:1163–7.
25. Raff H, Raff JL, Findling JW. Late-night salivary cortisol as a screening test for Cushing's syndrome. J Clin Endocrinol Metab 1998;83:2681–6.
26. Findling JW, Raff H. Cushing's syndrome: important issues in diagnosis and management. J Clin Endocrinol Metab 2006;91:3746–53.
27. Raff H, Homar PJ, Skoner DP. A new enzyme immunoassay for salivary cortisol. Clin Chem 2003;49:203–4.
28. Raff H. Salivary cortisol: a useful measurement in the diagnosis of Cushing's syndrome and the evaluation of the hypothalamic-pituitary-adrenal axis. The Endocrinologist 2000;10: 9–17.
29. Wand GS, Dobs AS. Alterations in the hypothalamic-pituitary-adrenal axis in actively drinking alcoholics. J Clin Endocrinol Metab. 1991;72:1290–5.
30. Gold PW, Gwirtsman H, Avgerinos PC, et al. Abnormal hypothalamic-pituitary-adrenal function in anorexia nervosa. Pathophysiologic mechanisms in underweight and weight-corrected patients. New Engl J Med 1986;314:1335–42.
31. Kontula K, Mustajoki P, Paetau A, Pelkonen R. Development of Cushing's disease in a patient with anorexia nervosa. J Endocrinol Invest 1984;7:35–40.
32. Carroll BJ, Feinberg M, Greden JF, et al. A specific laboratory test for the diagnosis of melancholia. Standardization, validation, and clinical utility. Arch Gen Psychiat 1981;38:15–22.
33. Then Bergh F, Kumpfel T, Trenkwalder C, Rupprecht R, Holsboer F, Dysregulation of the hypothalamo-pituitary-adrenal axis is related to the clinical course of MS. Neurology 1999;53:772–7.

34. Goland RS, Conwell IM, Warren WB, Wardlaw SL. Placental corticotropin-releasing hormone and pituitary-adrenal function during pregnancy. Neuroendocrinology 1992;56: 742–9.
35. Yanovski JA, Cutler GB Jr., Chrousos GP, Nieman LK. Corticotropin-releasing hormone stimulation following low-dose dexamethasone administration. JAMA 1993;269:2232–8.
36. Pecori GF, Pivonello R, Ambrogio AG, et al. The dexamethasone-suppressed corticotropin-releasing hormone stimulation test and the desmopressin test to distinguish Cushing's syndrome from pseudo-Cushing's states. Clin Endocrinol (Oxf) 2007;66:251–7.
37. Martin NM, Dhillo WS, Banerjee A, et al. Comparison of the dexamethasone-suppressed corticotropin-releasing hormone test and low-dose dexamethasone suppression test in the diagnosis of Cushing's syndrome. J Clin Endocrinol Metab 2006;91:2582–6.
38. Putignano P, Dubini A, Toja P, et al. Salivary cortisol measurement in normal-weight, obese and anorexic women: comparison with plasma cortisol. Eur J Endocrinol 2001;145:165–71.
39. Tsagarakis S, Vasiliou V, Kokkoris P, Stavropoulos G, Thalassinos N. Assessment of cortisol and ACTH responses to the desmopressin test in patients with Cushing's syndrome and simple obesity. Clin Endocrinol 1999;51:473–7.
40. Lacroix A, Bourdeau I. Bilateral adrenal Cushing's syndrome: macronodular adrenal hyperplasia and primary pigmented nodular adrenocortical disease. Endocrinol Metab Clin N Am 2005;34:441–8.
41. Trainer PJ, Faria M, Newell-Price J, et al. A comparison of the effects of human and ovine corticotropin-releasing hormone on the pituitary-adrenal axis. J Clin Endocrinol Metab 1995;80:412–7.
42. Aron DC, Raff H, Findling JW. Effectiveness versus efficacy: The limited value in clinical practice of high dose dexamethasone suppression testing in the differential diagnosis of adrenocorticotrophin-dependent Cushing's syndrome. J Clin Endocrinol Metab 1997;82:1780–5.
43. Tabarin A, Laurent F, Catargi B, et al. Comparative evaluation of conventional and dynamic magnetic resonance imaging of the pituitary gland for the diagnosis of Cushing's disease. Clin Endocrinol (Oxf) 1998;49:293–300.
44. Patonas N, Bulakbasi N, Stratakis CA, et al. Spoiled gradient recalled acquisition in the steady state technique is superior to conventional postcontrast spin echo technique for magnetic resonance imaging detection of adrenocorticotrophin-secreting pituitary tumors. J Clin Endocrinol Metab 2003;88:1565–9.
45. Hall WA, Luciano MG, Doppman JL, Patronas NJ, Oldfield EH. Pituitary magnetic resonance imaging in normal human volunteers: occult adenomas in the general population. Ann Intern Med 1994;120:817–20.
46. Findling JW, Kehoe ME, Shaker JL, Raff H. Routine inferior petrosal sinus sampling in the differential diagnosis of ACTH-dependent Cushing's syndrome; early recognition of the occult ectopic ACTH syndrome. J Clin Endocrinol Metab 1991;73:408–13.
47. Oldfield EH, Doppman JL, Nieman LK, et al. Petrosal sinus sampling with and without corticotrophin-releasing hormone for the differential diagnosis of Cushing's syndrome. N Engl J Med 1991;325:897–905.
48. Swearingen B, Katznelson L, Miller K, et al. Diagnostic errors after inferior petrosal sinus sampling. J Clin Endocrinol Metab 2004;89:3752–63.
49. Findling JW, Kehoe ME, Raff H. Identification of patients with Cushing's disease with negative pituitary adrenocorticotropin gradients during inferior petrosal sinus sampling: prolactin as an index of pituitary venous effluent. J Clin Endocrinol Metab 2004;89:6005–9.
50. Lindsay JR, Nieman LK. Differential diagnosis and imaging in Cushing's syndrome. Endocrinol Metab Clin N Am 2005;34:403–21.

51. Doppman JL, Pass HI, Nieman LK, et al. The detection of ACTH-producing bronchial carcinoid tumors; comparison of MR imaging with CT. Am J Roentgenol. 1991;15:39–43.
52. Tabarin A, Valli N, Chanson P, et al. Usefulness of somatostatin receptor scintigraphy in patients with occult ectopic adrenocorticotropin syndrome. J Clin Endocrinol Metab 1999;84:1193–202.
53. Tsagarakis S, Christoforaki M, Giannopoulou H, et al. A reappraisal of the utility of somatostatin receptor scintigraphy in patients with ectopic adrenocorticotropin Cushing's syndrome. J Clin Endocrinol Metab. 2003;88:4754–8.
54. Pacak K, Ilias I, Chen CC, Corrasqvillo JA, Whatley M, Nieman LK. The role of [(18)F]fluorodeoxyglucose positron emission tomography and [(111)In]-diethylenetriaminepentaacetate-D-Phe-pentetreotide scintigraphy in the localization of ectopic adrenocorticotropin-secreting tumors causing Cushing's syndrome. J Clin Endocrinol Metab. 2004;89:2214–21.
55. Kumar J, Spring M, Carroll PV, Barrington SF, Powrie JK. 18Flurodeoxyglucose positron emission tomography in the localization of ectopic ACTH-secreting neuroendocrine tumors. Clin Endocrinol 2006;64:371–4.

11 Cushing's Disease: *Surgical Management*

Daniel F. Kelly, MD

CONTENTS

1. INTRODUCTION
2. SUCCESS RATE OF TRANSSPHENOIDAL SURGERY FOR CUSHING'S DISEASE
3. ENDONASAL TRANSSPHENOIDAL SURGICAL TECHNIQUE
4. PREDICTING LONG-TERM REMISSION AFTER TRANSSPHENOIDAL SURGERY
5. MANAGEMENT OF CUSHING'S DISEASE AFTER FAILED TRANSSPHENOIDAL SURGERY
6. NELSON'S SYNDROME—TREATMENT
7. SUMMARY

Summary

Cushing's disease is a serious endocrinopathy that if untreated greatly increases morbidity and carries a fourfold increase in mortality, largely related to associated cardiovascular complications and abnormal glucose metabolism. This chapter discusses the surgical management of Cushing's disease, including surgical techniques, complications, and outcomes, as well as the management of residual or recurrent disease.

Key Words: Cushing's disease, Transsphenoidal surgery.

1. INTRODUCTION

1.1. Incidence and Rationale for Treatment

Endogenous Cushing's syndrome is caused by an ACTH-secreting pituitary adenoma (Cushing's disease) in approximately 70% of cases *(1–4)*. Cushing's

From: *Contemporary Endocrinology: Diagnosis and Management of Pituitary Disorders*
Edited by: B. Swearingen and B. M. K. Biller © Humana Press, Totowa, NJ

disease is relatively rare, with new cases estimated to occur in 0.7 to 2.4 individuals per million per year *(5–7)*. There is a strong female preponderance, with women accounting for 68% to 87% of patients; the mean age at diagnosis ranges from 35 to 39 years although the disease may develop in children and the elderly *(5,8–14)*. Cushing's disease is a serious endocrinopathy that if untreated greatly increases morbidity and carries a fourfold increase in mortality, largely related to associated cardiovascular complications and abnormal glucose metabolism *(6,15,7,16,17)* . In addition to hypertension and diabetes mellitus, other problems of cortisol excess including hyperlipidemia, metabolic syndrome, coagulopathy, osteoporosis, depression, anxiety, and cognitive impairment may further debilitate patients *(1,4)*. Given the multiple deleterious effects, treatment to achieve eucortisolemia is indicated for all patients with CD. Effective treatment decreases morbidity (e.g., hypertension and diabetes mellitus) and mortality, and typically results in age-adjusted and sex-adjusted survival rates similar to the general population *(18,15,19,17,20)*.

1.2. Diagnosis of Cushing's Disease and Pituitary Imaging

As discussed in the previous chapter, the diagnosis of CD is based on clinical findings and laboratory criteria including loss of diurnal variation in serum cortisol levels, inappropriately normal or elevated ACTH levels, failure of cortisol suppression after low-dose (1 mg) dexamethasone test; and/or elevated 24-h urinary free cortisol concentrations and midnight salivary cortisol levels *(21,4)*. After establishing a patient has ACTH-dependent Cushing's syndrome, a determination must be made as to whether the patient has ectopic Cushing's or CD. The diagnosis of CD can be confirmed by demonstrating suppression of cortisol after a high-dose dexamethasone suppression test; however, a substantial minority of patients with CD may not suppress with high-dose dexamethasone *(22,23)*. The definitive test for distinguishing CD versus ectopic Cushing's disease is bilateral inferior petrosal sinus sampling (IPSS) with corticotropin releasing hormone (CRH) administration; a central to peripheral serum ACTH gradient after CRH ≥ 3 is typically considered confirmatory of CD *(24)*. However, IPSS is an invasive test that requires an experienced interventional neuroradiology team to obtain safe and reliable results. Therefore, it is generally reasonable to not perform IPSS in patients who meet all the following criteria:

(i) biochemically proven ACTH-dependent Cushing's disease in a patient with a history of clinical changes for at least 1 to 2 years,
(ii) younger age,
(iii) female gender, and
(iv) a well-defined adenoma seen on a pituitary MRI *(22)*.

In patients who do not meet these criteria, IPSS with CRH stimulation is warranted. Some centers would advocate IPSS in all patients with MRI evidence of a lesion smaller than 1 cm, since it is conceivable that a patient with an ectopic source could also have an incidental pituitary adenoma.

1.3. Imaging

A high-resolution (1.5 tesla) spin-echo MRI of the pituitary–hypothalamic region, before and after intravenous administration of gadolinium–DTPA, is indicated in all patients prior to undergoing transsphenoidal surgery. Approximately 70% to 95% of patients with CD have microadenomas while only 5% to 25% have a macroadenoma. However, 25% to 40% of patients with CD will have microadenomas that are too small to be seen on a high-quality conventional spin-echo contrast-enhanced MRI *(25,8,26,11,27,12,20,14)*. The newer technique of dynamic MRI (spoiled gradient recalled acquisition in the steady state—SPGR) with gadolinium enhancement has been shown to be superior to conventional spin-echo contrast-enhanced MRIs for detecting small microadenomas and appears to be more reliable in finding an area of hypoenhancement consistent with a microadenoma *(28,26,29 29,31)*. A dynamic post-gadolinium MRI is recommended in all patients with a presumed diagnosis of CD based on biochemical data but who have a normal-appearing pituitary gland or equivocal findings on a conventional pituitary MRI.

1.4. Preoperative Medical Evaluation

Given the frequent presence of hypertension, diabetes mellitus, obesity, and poor wound healing in patients with CD, a thorough preoperative evaluation is needed to reduce the risk of intraoperative and postoperative complications. It is reasonable and perhaps warranted in most patients with CD to have a preoperative evaluation by a cardiologist with a stress test. Hypertension and diabetes mellitus should be well controlled, and active infections should be treated with appropriate antibiotic therapy. In patients who are American Society of Anesthesiologists (ASA) physical status category IV or V, surgery should generally be postponed until their risk status can be improved. Use of oral ketoconazole or intravenous etomidate (as detailed in Chapter 12) is a relatively effective pharmacological means for rapidly but transiently lowering cortisol levels in such cases *(32–38)*. For patients with far advanced CD and multiple associated complications, use of these agents for up to several weeks can markedly improve a patient's medical status and reduce the risk of complications.

2. SUCCESS RATE OF TRANSSPHENOIDAL SURGERY FOR CUSHING'S DISEASE

2.1. Introduction

For more than two decades, evidence indicates that transsphenoidal adenomectomy offers the best chance for a sustained remission of CD. Adenomectomy for CD was first performed by Hardy in the early 1960s *(39–42)*. In the 1970s, other groups including Salassa and Laws *(43)* and Tyrrell and Wilson *(44)* also began to adopt this approach for CD with similarly encouraging results. In considering these three reports of transsphenoidal microsurgery for CD totaling 63 patients, the clinical remission rate ranged from 68% to 89% with no mortalities *(42–44)*. During the same period, hypophysectomy as an effective treatment for patients with CD was reported by Ludecke in 1976 and Carmalt in 1977 with remission rates of 50% and 85%, respectively *(45,46)*. Over the subsequent decades, there have been numerous reports describing outcomes after transsphenoidal surgery for CD performed by the sublabial route, the transseptal endonasal route and the direct endonasal route using the operating microscope; more recently, the purely endonasal endoscopic approach *(47)* or the microscopic approach with endoscopic assistance have been employed.

2.2. Long-term Outcome in Contemporary Transsphenoidal Microsurgical Series for Cushing's Disease

In 18 retrospective reports published since 1995 for over 3,000 patients, all with a minimum of 40 patients and a minimum 6-month follow-up period, the long-term remission rate ranged from 69% to 98% (simple unweighted average 79%), the recurrence rate from 3% to 17% (simple unweighted average 10%), and the acute surgical mortality rate from 0% to 1.9% (Table 1). Of single-center series, the smallest had 40 patients and the largest had 310 patients *(48,49)*. Of studies addressing transsphenoidal surgery as the primary treatment, long-term remission rates ranged from 69% to 98% (simple unweighted average 83%), the recurrence rate from 5% to 11.5% (unweighted average 8%), and the mortality rate from 0% to 1.9% *(50,9,15,46,51,49,12,20,14)*. The best long-term remission rates, ranging from 86% to 98%, are seen in patients with noninvasive microadenomas treated with primary transsphenoidal tumor removal *(25,52,53,50,9,15,51,12,20)*. In contrast, lower remission rates are seen in patients with macroadenomas (range 31% to 83%) or invasive adenomas (22% to 65%) *(25,52,15,51,12,20)*. Long-term postoperative surveillance of successfully treated patients with CD is important given that late recurrences occur with the median interval from 2.3 to 7.2 years after surgery and as late as 10 years after surgery *(8,15,11,20)*. Similar rates of remission (56–98%)

Table 1
Cushing's Disease—Outcomes after Transsphenoidal Microsurgery

Author (year)	Evidence Class	N	Mean Age (range) Percent Female	Follow-up (years)	Remission rate (%)	Recurrence Time to Recur	Mortality
Hofmann (2006)	III	100	N/A	N/A	75	4.8%	0
Esposito (2006)	III	40	39 (21–70 years) 93%	2.7 years (mean)	79.5—all 93—primary 45—secondary	3% 1.7 years (one patient)	0% (n = 1)
Hammer (2004)	III	289	37 (18–72 years) 83%	11.1 years (median)	82—all primary 86—micro 83—macro 65—invasive	9% of 1504.9 years (median)1–11 years (range)	1%
Rollin[a,b] (2004)	II	41	38 (12–62 years) 73%	4.8 years (mean)	87.5—all primary	5%	N/A
Chen[b] (2003)	III	174	8–57 years	≥ 5 years (min)	74 (primary versus secondary N/A)	7% 2.3 years (median)	0%
Flitch (2003)	III	147	35 years 68% 76%	5.1 years (mean)	98—all primary	5.5%	0%

(Continued)

Table 1
(Continued)

Author (year)	Evidence Class	N	Mean Age (range) Percent Female	Follow-up (years)	Remission rate (%)	Recurrence Time to Recur	Mortality
Pereira[a,b] (2003)	III	78	37 (12–81 years)	7 years (median)	72—primary and secondary	9%7.2 years (median) 2–20 years (range)	1.2%
Shimon[a,b] (2002)	III	82	39 (8–72 years) 80%	4.2 years (mean)	78—primary 62—secondary 79—micro 33—macro	5%	0%
Rees[b] (2002)	III	54	41 (14–73 years) 87%	6 years (median)	77—all primary 86—intrasellar 40—extrasellar	5%1.1–3 years (range)	1.9%
Yap[b] (2002)	III	97	39 (14–82 years) 78%	7.7 years (mean)	69—all primary	11.5% 0.7–6 years (range)	1%
Cavagnini (2001)	III	300	N/A 80%	N/A	70 (primary versus secondary N/A)	15%	N/A
Chee[a,b] (2001)	III	61	37 (12–69 years) 83%	7.3 years (median)	79—primary and secondary	14.6% 1.8–13 years (range)	0%

Study							
Invitti (1999)	III	236	36 (11–72 years) 83%	2.3 years (median)	69 (primary versus secondary N/A)	17%	N/A
Swearingen[a,b] (1999)	III	161	38 (8–76 years)	8 years (median)	85—primary and secondary 90—primary micro 65—primary macro	7% 4 years (median) 1–11 years (range)	0%
Blevins (1998)	III	106	N/A 80% 38 years	5.2 years (mean)	91—micro 67—macro (primary versus secondary N/A)	12%—micro 36%—macro	N/A
Sonino[b] (1996)	II	103	37 (11–71 years) 77%	7 years (median)	77—all primary	19% at 5 years 26% at 10 years	N/A
Knappe (1996)	III	310	N/A N/A	3.6 years (mean)	85—all primary	11% within 10 years	0.6%
Bochicchio[a,b] (1995)	III	668	38 (8–84 years) 77%	2 years (mean)	76—primary and secondary	13% 0.5–8.7 years (range)	1.9%

[a] In six series including patients treated with surgery both as primary and as secondary therapy (re-do transsphenoidal surgery), the percent of patients undergoing a second procedure ranged from 4% to 26%

[b] In ten series, pediatric patients were included (5,6,13,14,15,27,31,38,43,70,75,76,83,87,87,88,98).

have been seen for pediatric CD patients treated by transsphenoidal surgery *(54–62)*. However, the recurrence rate may be somewhat higher as shown in several series *(55,58,59,61)*.

2.3. Selective Adenomectomy versus Hypophysectomy

In all of the series cited above, the initial goal generally was to selectively remove an adenoma. If no adenoma was found, in most instances a partial or total hypophysectomy was performed. In these series, the type of operation performed (selective adenomectomy, partial hypophysectomy versus total hypophysectomy) does not appear to have a significant bearing on the long-term remission rate *(5,8,15,51)*. However, with increasing removal of pituitary gland tissue, there is an increased rate of anterior and posterior pituitary failure *(15,51)*. In two earlier series in which total hypophysectomy was the goal, new pituitary failure was seen in 79% to 95%; however, with hemihypophysectomy, the rate of new failure is considerably lower *(63,8,64)*.

2.4. New Pituitary Failure and Other Complications

The overall rate of anterior pituitary failure in the 18 series cited in Table 1 and published since 1995 ranged from 2% to 41% but was typically less than 20% in most series and permanent diabetes insipidus ranged from 3% to 9%. This relatively high rate of hypopituitarism associated with adenomectomy appears directly related to the use of partial or complete hypophysectomy required in a substantial minority of patients to maximize the chance of remission. Other surgical complications are generally uncommon, including CSF leaks (0–8%), meningitis (0–3%), new neurological deficits (0–2%), postoperative hematomas (0–6%, generally less than 1%), thromboembolic events (0–4%), and wound or nasoseptal complications (0–4%) *(8,50,15,65)*.

2.5. Early Reoperations for Persistent Cushing's Disease

After an unsuccessful initial operation, early reoperation within 60 days after the original surgery can result in a sustained remission in 38–67% patients *(66,48,67,68)*. If obvious adenoma was left behind within the gland at the first operation, this tumor may be visible on a postoperative MRI; however, in most instances there is little utility of repeat MRI in these patients. In contrast, petrosal sinus sampling with CRH stimulation appears useful in confirming the need for repeat surgery, if not done prior to the initial procedure *(67)*. In most reports a hemihypophysectomy or total hypophysectomy was performed after a more limited first operation. However, repeat operations are associated with a higher rate of postoperative CSF leaks and hypopituitarism *(66,48,67,68)*. Thus, it is reasonable to consider early reoperation only if residual adenoma is thought to reside in the gland and not within the cavernous sinus or skull base bone, which are factors that reduce the likelihood of achieving remission to under 50% *(25,52,53,15)*.

3. ENDONASAL TRANSSPHENOIDAL SURGICAL TECHNIQUE

3.1. Introduction

Transsphenoidal surgery for CD is currently performed by a variety of approaches including the traditional sublabial route, the transseptal endonasal route, and the direct endonasal route using the operating microscope, as well as the purely endoscopic approach or endoscope-assisted technique *(50,15,69,70, 47,71)*. Described here is a technique now commonly used at many pituitary centers worldwide, known as the direct endonasal transsphenoidal route as originally described by Griffith and Veerapen and more recently by our group *(72,71)*.

3.2. Endonasal Approach, Sphenoidotomy and Sellar Bone Removal

Following induction of general anesthesia, patients are placed in the supine, semi-slouch position, with the head resting freely in the horseshoe head-holder angled approximately 30 degrees toward the left shoulder. The nostrils are swabbed with betadiene and the abdomen is prepped for a possible fat graft. Perioperative antibiotics (cefazolin) are given for 24 h. The nostril chosen for the approach is based on tumor location as defined by the patient's preoperative MRI. In general, for tumors projecting more to one side, the contralateral nostril is used given that exposure across the midline is typically better than to the ipsilateral side. In patients with normal size sellas and relatively central microadenomas, as is often the case in patients with Cushing's disease, the right nostril is chosen given the surgeon stands on the patient's right side.

The procedure is performed with the operating microscope and intermittent fluoroscopy for trajectory guidance. A handheld speculum is inserted into the nostril in a trajectory along the middle turbinate. In the posterior nasal cavity, a vertical mucosal incision is made at the junction of the keel of the sphenoid and the posterior nasal septum. The septum, with its mucosa intact, is then pushed off the midline by the medial blade of the speculum. Bilateral mucosal flaps over the keel of the sphenoid are elevated and reflected laterally with identification of the sphenoid ostia. The handheld speculum is then replaced by a thin Hardy-type speculum that is placed up to the sphenoid keel. Rongeurs are then used to make a large sphenoidotomy extending beyond the sphenoid ostia to provide adequate sellar exposure. Next, the bony sellar floor is opened widely in standard fashion with Kerrison rongeurs or a high-speed drill. It is critical in the patient with CD that the exposure extend from cavernous sinus to cavernous sinus and that the sellar dura from the sellar floor to the tuberculum sella be exposed. This wide and tall exposure is especially critical in patients with a normal sellar MRI in which no obvious adenoma is seen.

3.3. Dural Opening and Tumor Removal

The sellar dura is opened in a low curvilinear U-shaped incision and extended superiorly. After a wide dural opening, the anterior, inferior, and lateral surfaces of the gland should be carefully inspected to look for adenoma. In patients with visible tumor on preoperative MRI, selective adenomectomy is performed in standard fashion with microdissectors and ring curettes. Taking advantage of the tumor pseudocapsule as described by Oldfield is helpful and recommended to ensure a complete tumor removal *(73)*. When no tumor is visible on preoperative MRI but IPSS demonstrates a large side-to-side gradient (> 1.4), the first exploratory incisions can be made in the paramedian adenohypophysis on the side of the high ACTH gradient. A series of parallel vertical incisions are made within the gland separated by several millimeters and explored. If this initial exploration is negative, the central and contralateral hemihypophysis should be similarly explored through multiple vertical incisions. If no tumor is found from exploring the gland, then a partial hemihypophysectomy should be performed on the side with the higher ACTH gradient from IPSS or the side with more "suspicious"-appearing tissue based on the pathologists' intraoperative assessment; total hypophysectomy is generally not performed even if no tumor was found. After tumor removal, full-strength hydrogen peroxide, which has been shown to be tumoricidal, is placed in the resection cavity for approximately 5 min then irrigated away with saline *(74)*.

3.4. CSF Leak Repair and Closure

As previously described, when an intraoperative CSF leak occurs, the repair is based on the size of the leak *(75,71)*. Small leaks are repaired with a two-layered collagen sponge and buttress technique; if it is a larger leak, it is repaired with a fat graft and collagen sponge followed by a buttress of the sellar floor with either titanium mesh or an absorbable plate and additional fat placed in the sphenoid sinus. BioGlue tissue sealant is placed in the sphenoid sinus over the last layer of the repair as a reinforcing layer. After speculum removal, the nasal septum is returned to the midline and the ipsilateral middle turbinate is medialized to prevent a maxillary sinus mucocele. Nasal packing is not placed.

3.5. General Postoperative Care and Discharge

Deep vein thrombosis and pulmonary emboli are relatively common in the postoperative period, occurring in 4% and 6% of patients from two recent series

(51,65). Pulsatile stockings placed in the operating room and subcutaneous heparin twice daily are recommended in the postoperative period. Patients are typically discharged home on postoperative day 2.

3.6. Postoperative Endocrine Management and Follow-up

Blood sampling for serum cortisol and ACTH are performed twice daily beginning the morning of postoperative day 1 at 6 a.m. and 6 p.m. and continued on postoperative day 2. Glucocorticoids are not given in the perioperative period until biochemical evidence of hypocortisolemia is documented or until clinical evidence of adrenal insufficiency (e.g., nausea, anorexia, headache, arthralgias) is evident. A patient is deemed to be in *early remission* if the morning cortisol level is ≤ 5 mcg/dl on either postoperative day 1 or day 2, necessitating glucocorticoid replacement. Subsequent assessments of corticotroph function are performed at a minimum of 3, 6, and 12 months after surgery. Criteria for sustained remission include need for glucocorticoid replacement for at least 6 months and clinical and biochemical evidence of eucortisolemia (serum a.m. cortisol 8 to 25 mcg/dl and normal 24-hour urinary free cortisol) thereafter. Patients with successful surgery are generally not able to be weaned off of glucocorticoid replacement for at least 6–12 months after surgery. Return of normal corticotroph function earlier than 6 months after surgery suggests an early recurrence of CD. Additional biochemical assessments of anterior pituitary function are taken within 3 months of the operation including thyrotroph, gonadotroph, and somatotroph function.

4. PREDICTING LONG-TERM REMISSION AFTER TRANSSPHENOIDAL SURGERY

Several methods for assessing early remission have been used to predict long-term remission from CD. Provocative tests include the overnight low-dose dexamethasone suppression test and the CRH stimulation test. Nonprovocative tests include assessment of serum cortisol and ACTH levels and 24-h urinary free cortisol concentrations within the early postoperative period. Recent studies indicate that both provocative and nonprovocative tests have a similar high rate of predicting remission. For example, Chen et al. showed that a morning cortisol level on post-operative day 3 of ≤ 3 mcg/dl after an overnight 1 mg dexamethasone suppression test was predictive of sustained remission in 93% of patients. In the subset of 116 patients with microadenomas, the remission rate at 5 years after surgery was 96.5% *(8)*.

In contrast, in three recent reports in which glucocorticoids were withheld in the early postoperative period until hypocortisolemia was evident, subnormal but not necessarily undetectable serum cortisol levels within 72 h of surgery were highly predictive of sustained remission *(50,49,76)*. In the report by Simmons et al., cortisol levels were drawn every 6 h for up to 3 days after surgery, with a "low serum cortisol" cutoff of 10 mcg/dl (275.9 nmol/l); 21 patients (78%) met this cutoff criterion and 100% of these 21 patients were in remission at a mean follow-up of 27 months *(76)*. In the report by Rollin et al., cortisol levels were drawn at 6, 12, and 24 h postoperatively. Of 21 patients (81%) in remission at a median follow-up of 34 months, serum cortisol levels 24 h after surgery averaged 4.7 ± 6.8 mcg/dl (range 0.5–30 mcg/dl) *(49)*. In our recent series, in the 32 patients achieving early remission, the average a.m. cortisol nadir was 2.05 ± 1.2 mcg/dl. An A.M. cortisol level of ≤ 5 mcg/dl on postoperative day 1 or 2 was predictive of sustained remission in 97% of patients *(50)*.

Regarding the absolute cortisol criterion establishing early remission, it appears that use of a more traditional value of a nondetectable serum cortisol (< 50 nmol/l [< 1.8 mcg/dl]) is excessively stringent given that over 50% of patients that achieved remission in these three studies had a nadir cortisol above this threshold within 3 days of surgery *(50,49,76)*. It should be noted that these studies also show that up to 4.5% of patients who achieve remission will not be identified within the first 72 postoperative h and instead will have a delayed decrease in their cortisol values *(50,49,76)*. Regarding the predictive value of early ACTH levels, only one-third of the patients in our recent series had a subnormal ACTH level during this early postoperative period, indicating that the absolute ACTH level is a poor predictor of sustained remission *(50)*.

The advantages of using early postoperative serum cortisol levels to assess early remission are several. First, this method requires no provocative testing and it gives an early and relatively reliable answer as to whether the patient is in remission, typically within 48 h of surgery and prior to the patient being discharged home. Second, although patients with a successful operation without glucocorticoid replacement often develop symptoms of hypocorti-solemia, manifestations of an adrenal crisis have not been reported. Finally, this paradigm allows early identification of patients who initially had an unsuc-cessful first surgery, that may be candidates for an reoperation within days of the first operation *(50,67)*.

5. MANAGEMENT OF CUSHING'S DISEASE AFTER FAILED TRANSSPHENOIDAL SURGERY

After a failed transsphenoidal surgery for CD, treatment options include *(1)* repeat transsphenoidal surgery, *(2)* bilateral adrenalectomies, *(3)* radiotherapy, *(4)* pharmacological therapy, or *(5)* a combination of these measures. The treatment options of bilateral adrenalectomy and radiotherapy are discussed below.

Bilateral adrenalectomy for the treatment of CD became popular in the 1950s. As perioperative management and steroid replacement became widely available, the mortality and immediate morbidity of the operation was greatly reduced. Primary or secondary bilateral adrenalectomy for CD has a very high success rate in reversing hypercortisolism ranging from 88% to 100%. However, over time there is a significant risk of patients developing Nelson's syndrome. Of series published since 1983 with adequate follow-up, the rate of Nelson's syndrome ranged from 15% to 46% *(77–84,13)*. Only one study that addressed the role of radiotherapy showed that prior radiation reduced the risk and delayed the onset of developing Nelson's syndrome; however, this potential beneficial effect of radiotherapy remains understudied *(83)*. The average interval between bilateral adrenalectomy and development of Nelson's syndrome is approximately 5 to 10 years but may be as short as 6 months and as long as 24 years *(80,81,83)*. Given that the long-term risk of developing Nelson's syndrome after bilateral adrenalectomy is at least 25% to 30% and there is a significant risk of major pituitary tumor enlargement, particularly in those with visible adenomas on MRI or CT, use of bilateral adrenalectomy as a first-line therapy is generally contraindicated *(13)*. Furthermore, as described below, the ACTH-secreting adenomas associated with Nelson's syndrome tend to be invasive and relatively aggressive in their growth pattern, further complicating their management.

5.1. Radiotherapy

Although radiotherapy was widely used as first-line therapy for CD from the 1940s to the early 1980s, now it is typically used as a secondary treatment after failed transsphenoidal surgery. In the largest series of secondary external radiotherapy after failed surgery, remission rates have ranged from 53% to 83%, with recurrence rates ranging from 0% to 17% *(85–87)*. The study by Sonino indicates that prior unsuccessful surgery is a predictor of long-term success for external radiotherapy. In their study, all 9 patients (100%) with prior transsphenoidal surgery had sustained remission after external radiotherapy while only 7 of 14 patients (50%) with radiation as a primary treatment had sustained remission *(13)*.

In the two largest series of secondary radiosurgery with gamma knife (single-fraction therapy) remission rates were 63% and 73% and the recurrence rate was 11% in the series by Sheehan *(88,89)*, giving a control rate of 52% *(89)*. Both external beam and stereotactic radiotherapy appear to have similar rates of radiation-induced pituitary failure, ranging from 16% to 57%, with the rates of hypopituitarism increasing with longer follow-up *(90,85,91–93,89)*.

Overall, these studies indicate that radiotherapy is an effective secondary treatment for patients with CD who have failed surgery. Currently, however, given the relatively higher long-term remission rates with transsphenoidal adenomectomy, radiotherapy should be considered first-line therapy only in cases of uncontrolled CD with severe medical complications. In such patients who are medically unstable and who pose very high anesthetic risks, radiotherapy is a reasonable treatment option when performed in conjunction with adrenolytic medical therapy to achieve a relatively rapid lowering of cortisol levels.

6. NELSON'S SYNDROME—TREATMENT

The neurosurgical management of Nelson's syndrome is challenging given the aggressive growth pattern typically seen in these adenomas. In five published series from 1982 to 2002, surgery was effective in improving or restoring vision and reducing the degree of hyperpigmentation in the great majority of patients. However, ACTH levels normalized in less than 50% of patients and additional radiation therapy was required in 20–30% of such patients to help control tumor growth *(94–99)*.

7. SUMMARY

Cushing's disease is a serious endocrinopathy that if left untreated is associated with high morbidity and mortality. After a definitive diagnostic confirmation of Cushing's disease, transsphenoidal adenomectomy is the treatment of choice. When performed at experienced transsphenoidal surgery centers, long-term remission rates overall average 80%, surgical morbidity is low, and mortality is typically under 1%; in patients with well-defined noninvasive microadenomas, the long-term remission rate averages 90%. For patients who fail primary surgery, the treatment options of bilateral adrenalectomy, radiotherapy, total hypophysectomy, or adrenolytic medical therapy need to be carefully considered, ideally in a multidisciplinary setting.

REFERENCES

1. Arnaldi G, Angeli A, Atkinson AB, et al. Diagnosis and complications of Cushing's syndrome: a consensus statement. J Clin Endocrinol Metab 2003;88:5593–602.
2. Boscaro M, Barzon L, Fallo F, et al. Cushing's syndrome. Lancet 2001;357:783–91.
3. Newell-Price J. Transsphenoidal surgery for Cushing's disease: defining cure and following outcome. Clin Endocrinol (Oxf) 2002;56:19–21.
4. Orth DN. Cushing's syndrome. N Engl J Med 1995;332:791–803.
5. Bochicchio D, Losa M, Buchfelder M. Factors influencing the immediate and late outcome of Cushing's disease treated by transsphenoidal surgery: a retrospective study by the European Cushing's Disease Survey Group. J Clin Endocrinol Metab 1995;80:3114–20.
6. Etxabe J, Vazquez JA. Morbidity and mortality in Cushing's disease: an epidemiological approach. Clin Endocrinol (Oxf) 1994;40:479–84.

7. Lindholm J, Juul S, Jorgensen JO, et al. Incidence and late prognosis of Cushing's syndrome: a population-based study. J Clin Endocrinol Metab 2001;86:117–23.
8. Chen JC, Amar AP, Choi S, et al. Transsphenoidal microsurgical treatment of Cushing disease: postoperative assessment of surgical efficacy by application of an overnight low-dose dexamethasone suppression test. J Neurosurg 2003;98:967–73.
9. Flitsch J, Knappe UJ, Ludecke DK. The use of postoperative ACTH levels as a marker for successful transsphenoidal microsurgery in Cushing's disease. Zentralbl Neurochir 2003;64:6–11.
10. Mampalam TJ, Tyrrell JB, Wilson CB. Transsphenoidal microsurgery for Cushing disease. A report of 216 cases. Ann Intern Med 1988;109:487–93.
11. Pereira AM, van Aken MO, van Dulken H, et al. Long-term predictive value of postsurgical cortisol concentrations for cure and risk of recurrence in Cushing's disease. J Clin Endocrinol Metab 2003;88:5858–64.
12. Shimon I, Ram Z, Cohen ZR, et al. Transsphenoidal surgery for Cushing's disease: endocrinological follow-up monitoring of 82 patients. Neurosurgery 2002;51:57–61; discussion 61–52.
13. Sonino N, Zielezny M, Fava GA, et al. Risk factors and long-term outcome in pituitary-dependent Cushing's disease. J Clin Endocrinol Metab 1996;81:2647–52.
14. Yap LB, Turner HE, Adams CB, et al. Undetectable postoperative cortisol does not always predict long-term remission in Cushing's disease: a single centre audit. Clin Endocrinol (Oxf) 2002;56:25–31.
15. Hammer GD, Tyrrell JB, Lamborn KR, et al. Transsphenoidal Microsurgery for Cushing's Disease: Initial Outcome and Long-Term Results. J Clin Endocrinol Metab 2004;89: 6348–57.
16. Mancini T, Kola B, Mantero F, et al. High cardiovascular risk in patients with Cushing's syndrome according to 1999 WHO/ISH guidelines. Clin Endocrinol (Oxf) 2004;61:768–77.
17. Pikkarainen L, Sane T, Reunanen A. The survival and well-being of patients treated for Cushing's syndrome. J Intern Med 1999;245:463–8.
18. Grabner P, Hauer-Jensen M, Jervell J, et al. Long-term results of treatment of Cushing's disease by adrenalectomy. Eur J Surg 1991;157:461–4.
19. Ludecke DK, Niedworok G. Results of microsurgery in Cushing's disease and effect on hypertension. Cardiology 1985;72 Suppl 1:91–4.
20. Swearingen B, Biller BM, Barker FG 2nd, et al. Long-term mortality after transsphenoidal surgery for Cushing disease. Ann Intern Med 1999;130:821–4.
21. Findling JW, Raff H. Newer diagnostic techniques and problems in Cushing's disease. Endocrinol Metab Clin North Am 1999;28:191–210.
22. Aron DC, Raff H, Findling JW. Effectiveness versus efficacy: the limited value in clinical practice of high dose dexamethasone suppression testing in the differential diagnosis of adrenocorticotropin-dependent Cushing's syndrome. J Clin Endocrinol Metab 1997;82:1780–5.
23. Wiggam MI, Heaney AP, McIlrath EM, et al. Bilateral inferior petrosal sinus sampling in the differential diagnosis of adrenocorticotropin-dependent Cushing's syndrome: a comparison with other diagnostic tests. J Clin Endocrinol Metab 2000;85:1525–32.
24. Oldfield EH, Doppman JL, Nieman LK, et al. Petrosal sinus sampling with and without corticotropin-releasing hormone for the differential diagnosis of Cushing's syndrome. N Engl J Med 1991;325:897–905.
25. Blevins LS Jr, Christy JH, Khajavi M, et al. Outcomes of therapy for Cushing's disease due to adrenocorticotropin-secreting pituitary macroadenomas. J Clin Endocrinol Metab 1998;83:63–7.

26. Patronas N, Bulakbasi N, Stratakis CA, et al. Spoiled gradient recalled acquisition in the steady state technique is superior to conventional postcontrast spin echo technique for magnetic resonance imaging detection of adrenocorticotropin-secreting pituitary tumors. J Clin Endocrinol Metab 2003;88:1565–9.

27. Semple CG. Transsphenoidal surgery for Cushing's disease: outcome in patients with a normal magnetic resonance imaging scan. Neurosurgery 2000;46:553–8; discussion 558–9.

28. Gao R, Isoda H, Tanaka T, et al. Dynamic gadolinium-enhanced MR imaging of pituitary adenomas: usefulness of sequential sagittal and coronal plane images. Eur J Radiol 2001;39:139–46.

29. Smallridge RC, Czervionke LF, Fellows DW, et al. Corticotropin- and thyrotropin-secreting pituitary microadenomas: detection by dynamic magnetic resonance imaging. Mayo Clin Proc 2000;75:521–8.

30. Tabarin A, Laurent F, Catargi B, et al. Comparative evaluation of conventional and dynamic magnetic resonance imaging of the pituitary gland for the diagnosis of Cushing's disease. Clin Endocrinol (Oxf) 1998;49:293–300.

31. Tomczak R, Merkle E, Fiala S, et al. [Value of dynamic MRI in the diagnosis of hypophyseal microadenomas]. Rofo 1998;168:488–92.

32. Drake WM, Perry LA, Hinds CJ, et al. Emergency and prolonged use of intravenous etomidate to control hypercortisolemia in a patient with Cushing's syndrome and peritonitis. J Clin Endocrinol Metab 1998;83:3542–4.

33. Krakoff J, Koch CA, Calis KA, et al. Use of a parenteral propylene glycol-containing etomidate preparation for the long-term management of ectopic Cushing's syndrome. J Clin Endocrinol Metab 2001;86:4104–8.

34. Nieman LK. Medical therapy of Cushing's disease. Pituitary 2002;5:77–82.

35. Schulte HM, Benker G, Reinwein D, et al. Infusion of low dose etomidate: correction of hypercortisolemia in patients with Cushing's syndrome and dose-response relationship in normal subjects. J Clin Endocrinol Metab 1990;70:1426–30.

36. Hofmann BM, Fahlbusch R. Treatment of Cushing's disease: a retrospective clinical study of the latest 100 cases. Front Horm Res 2006;34:158–184.

37. Sonino N, Boscaro M, Paoletta A, et al. Ketoconazole treatment in Cushing's syndrome: experience in 34 patients. Clin Endocrinol (Oxf) 1991;35:347–52.

38. Tabarin A, Navarranne A, Guerin J, et al. Use of ketoconazole in the treatment of Cushing's disease and ectopic ACTH syndrome. Clin Endocrinol (Oxf) 1991;34:63–9.

39. Bigos ST, Robert F, Pelletier G, et al. Cure of Cushing's disease by transsphenoidal removal of a microadenoma from a pituitary gland despite a radiographically normal sella turcica. J Clin Endocrinol Metab 1977;45:1251–60.

40. Bigos ST, Somma M, Rasio E, et al. Cushing's disease: management by transsphenoidal pituitary microsurgery. J Clin Endocrinol Metab 1980;50:348–54.

41. Hardy J. Presidential address: XVII Canadian Congress of Neurological Sciences. Cushing's disease: 50 years later. Can J Neurol Sci 1982;9:375–80.

42. Hardy J. The transsphenoidal surgical approach to the pituitary. Hosp Pract 1979;14:81–9.

43. Salassa RM, Laws ER Jr, Carpenter PC, et al. Transsphenoidal removal of pituitary microadenoma in Cushing's disease. Mayo Clin Proc 1978;53:24–8.

44. Tyrrell JB, Brooks RM, Fitzgerald PA, et al. Cushing's disease. Selective trans-sphenoidal resection of pituitary microadenomas. N Engl J Med 1978;298:753–8.

45. Carmalt MH, Dalton GA, Fletcher RF, et al. The treatment of Cushing's disease by transsphenoidal hypophysectomy. Q J Med 1977;46:119–34.

46. Ludecke D, Kautzky R, Saeger W, et al. Selective removal of hypersecreting pituitary adenomas? An analysis of endocrine function, operative and microscopical findings in 101 cases. Acta Neurochir (Wien) 1976;35:27–42.

47. Netea-Maier RT, van Lindert EJ, den Heijer M, et al. Transsphenoidal pituitary surgery via the endoscopic technique: results in 35 consecutive patients with Cushing's disease. Eur J Endocrinol 2006;154:675–84.
48. Knappe UJ, Ludecke DK. Persistent and recurrent hypercortisolism after transsphenoidal surgery for Cushing's disease. Acta Neurochir Suppl 1996;65:31–4.
49. Rollin GA, Ferreira NP, Junges M, et al. Dynamics of serum cortisol levels after transsphenoidal surgery in a cohort of patients with Cushing's disease. J Clin Endocrinol Metab 2004;89:1131–9.
50. Esposito F, Dusick JR, Cohan P, et al. Clinical review: Early morning cortisol levels as a predictor of remission after transsphenoidal surgery for Cushing's disease. J Clin Endocrinol Metab 2006;91:7–13.
51. Rees DA, Hanna FW, Davies JS, et al. Long-term follow-up results of transsphenoidal surgery for Cushing's disease in a single centre using strict criteria for remission. Clin Endocrinol (Oxf) 2002;56:541–51.
52. Cannavo S, Almoto B, Dall'Asta C, et al. Long-term results of treatment in patients with ACTH-secreting pituitary macroadenomas. Eur J Endocrinol 2003;149:195–200.
53. Damiani D, Aguiar CH, Crivellaro CE, et al. Pituitary macroadenoma and Cushing's disease in pediatric patients: patient report and review of the literature. J Pediatr Endocrinol Metab 1998;11:665–9.
54. Buchfelder M, Fahlbusch R. Neurosurgical treatment of Cushing's disease in children and adolescents. Acta Neurochir Suppl (Wien) 1985;35:101–5.
55. Devoe DJ, Miller WL, Conte FA, et al. Long-term outcome in children and adolescents after transsphenoidal surgery for Cushing's disease. J Clin Endocrinol Metab 1997;82:3196–202.
56. Dyer EH, Civit T, Visot A, et al. Transsphenoidal surgery for pituitary adenomas in children. Neurosurgery 1994;34:207–12; discussion 212.
57. Kanter AS, Diallo AO, Jane JA Jr, et al. Single-center experience with pediatric Cushing's disease. J Neurosurg 2005;103:413–20.
58. Knappe UJ, Ludecke DK. Transnasal microsurgery in children and adolescents with Cushing's disease. Neurosurgery 1996;39:484–92; discussion 492–83.
59. Leinung MC, Kane LA, Scheithauer BW, et al. Long term follow-up of transsphenoidal surgery for the treatment of Cushing's disease in childhood. J Clin Endocrinol Metab 1995;80:2475–9.
60. Magiakou MA, Mastorakos G, Oldfield EH, et al. Cushing's syndrome in children and adolescents. Presentation, diagnosis, and therapy. N Engl J Med 1994;331:629–36.
61. Partington MD, Davis DH, Laws ER Jr, et al. Pituitary adenomas in childhood and adolescence. Results of transsphenoidal surgery. J Neurosurg 1994;80:209–16.
62. Savage MO, Lienhardt A, Lebrethon MC, et al. Cushing's disease in childhood: presentation, investigation, treatment and long-term outcome. Horm Res 2001;55 Suppl 1:24–30.
63. Brand IR, Dalton GA, Fletcher RF. Long-term follow up of trans-sphenoidal hypophysectomy for Cushing's disease. J R Soc Med 1985;78:291–3.
64. Thomas JP, Richards SH. Long term results of radical hypophysectomy for Cushing's disease. Clin Endocrinol (Oxf) 1983;19:629–36.
65. Semple PL, Laws ER, Jr. Complications in a contemporary series of patients who underwent transsphenoidal surgery for Cushing's disease. J Neurosurg 1999;91:175–9.
66. Chee GH, Mathias DB, James RA, et al. Transsphenoidal pituitary surgery in Cushing's disease: can we predict outcome? Clin Endocrinol (Oxf) 2001;54:617–26.
67. Locatelli M, Vance ML, Laws ER. Clinical review: the strategy of immediate reoperation for transsphenoidal surgery for Cushing's disease. J Clin Endocrinol Metab 2005;90:5478–82.

68. Ram Z, Nieman LK, Cutler GB Jr, et al. Early repeat surgery for persistent Cushing's disease. J Neurosurg 1994;80:37–45.
69. Hardy J. Cushing's disease: pituitary microsurgery. Curr Ther Endocrinol Metab 1997;6:63–5.
70. Ludecke DK, Flitsch J, Knappe UJ, et al. Cushing's disease: a surgical view. J Neurooncol 54:151–66.
71. Zada G, Kelly DF, Cohan P, et al. Endonasal transsphenoidal approach for pituitary adenomas and other sellar lesions: an assessment of efficacy, safety, and patient impressions. J Neurosurg 2003;98:350–8.
72. Griffith HB, Veerapen R. A direct transnasal approach to the sphenoid sinus. Technical note. J Neurosurg 1987;66:140–2.
73. Oldfield EH, Vortmeyer AO. Development of a histological pseudocapsule and its use as a surgical capsule in the excision of pituitary tumors. J Neurosurg 2006;104:7–19.
74. Mesiwala AH, Farrell L, Santiago P, et al. The effects of hydrogen peroxide on brain and brain tumors. Surg Neurol 2003;59:398–407; discussion 407.
75. Dusick JR, Mattozo CA, Esposito F, et al. BioGlue for prevention of postoperative cerebrospinal fluid leaks in transsphenoidal surgery: A case series. Surg Neurol 2006;66:371–376; discussion 376.
76. Simmons NE, Alden TD, Thorner MO, et al. Serum cortisol response to transsphenoidal surgery for Cushing disease. J Neurosurg 2001;95:1–8.
77. Brunicardi FC, Rosman PM, Lesser KL, et al. Current status of adrenalectomy for Cushing's disease. Surgery 1985;98:1127–34.
78. Favia G, Boscaro M, Lumachi F, et al. Role of bilateral adrenalectomy in Cushing's disease. World J Surg 1994;18:462–6.
79. Hardy JD, Moore DO, Langford HG. Cushing's disease today. Late follow-up of 17 adrenalectomy patients with emphasis on eight with adrenal autotransplants. Ann Surg 1985;201:595–603.
80. Invitti C, Giraldi FP, de Martin M, et al. Diagnosis and management of Cushing's syndrome: results of an Italian multicentre study. Study Group of the Italian Society of Endocrinology on the Pathophysiology of the Hypothalamic-Pituitary-Adrenal Axis. J Clin Endocrinol Metab 1999;84:440–8.
81. Kasperlik-Zaluska AA, Nielubowicz J, Wislawski J, et al. Nelson's syndrome: incidence and prognosis. Clin Endocrinol (Oxf) 1983;19:693–8.
82. McCance DR, Russell CF, Kennedy TL, et al. Bilateral adrenalectomy: low mortality and morbidity in Cushing's disease. Clin Endocrinol (Oxf) 1993;39:315–21.
83. Nagesser SK, van Seters AP, Kievit J, et al. Long-term results of total adrenalectomy for Cushing's disease. World J Surg 2000;24:108–13.
84. Pereira MA, Halpern A, Salgado LR, et al: A study of patients with Nelson's syndrome. Clin Endocrinol (Oxf) 1998;49:533–9.
85. Estrada J, Boronat M, Mielgo M, et al. The long-term outcome of pituitary irradiation after unsuccessful transsphenoidal surgery in Cushing's disease. N Engl J Med 1997;336:172–7.
86. Imaki T, Tsushima T, Hizuka N, et al. Postoperative plasma cortisol levels predict long-term outcome in patients with Cushing's disease and determine which patients should be treated with pituitary irradiation after surgery. Endocr J 2001;48:53–62.
87. Vicente A, Estrada J, de la Cuerda C, et al. Results of external pituitary irradiation after unsuccessful transsphenoidal surgery in Cushing's disease. Acta Endocrinol (Copenh) 1991;125:470–4.
88. Pollock BE, Kondziolka D, Lunsford LD, et al. Stereotactic radiosurgery for pituitary adenomas: imaging, visual and endocrine results. Acta Neurochir Suppl 1994;62:33–8.

89. Sheehan JM, Vance ML, Sheehan JP, et al. Radiosurgery for Cushing's disease after failed transsphenoidal surgery. J Neurosurg 2000;93:738–42.
90. Degerblad M, Rahn T, Bergstrand G, et al. Long-term results of stereotactic radiosurgery to the pituitary gland in Cushing's disease. Acta Endocrinol (Copenh) 1986;112:310–14.
91. Littley MD, Shalet SM, Beardwell CG, et al. Long-term follow-up of low-dose external pituitary irradiation for Cushing's disease. Clin Endocrinol (Oxf) 1990;33:445–55.
92. Murayama M, Yasuda K, Minamori Y, et al. Long term follow-up of Cushing's disease treated with reserpine and pituitary irradiation. J Clin Endocrinol Metab 1992;75:935–42.
93. Nagesser SK, van Seters AP, Kievit J, et al. Treatment of pituitary-dependent Cushing's syndrome: long-term results of unilateral adrenalectomy followed by external pituitary irradiation compared to transsphenoidal pituitary surgery. Clin Endocrinol (Oxf) 2000;52:427–35.
94. Kelly PA, Samandouras G, Grossman AB, et al. Neurosurgical treatment of Nelson's syndrome. J Clin Endocrinol Metab 2002;87:5465–9.
95. Kemink SA, Grotenhuis JA, De Vries J, et al. Management of Nelson's syndrome: observations in fifteen patients. Clin Endocrinol (Oxf) 2001;54:45–52.
96. Ludecke DK, Breustedt HJ, Bramswig J, et al. Evaluation of surgically treated Nelson's syndrome. Acta Neurochir (Wien) 1982;65:3–13.
97. Wislawski J, Kasperlik-Zaluska AA, Jeske W, et al. Results of neurosurgical treatment by a transsphenoidal approach in 10 patients with Nelson's syndrome. J Neurosurg 1985;62:68–71.
98. Xing B, Ren Z, Su C, et al. Microsurgical treatment of Nelson's syndrome. Chin Med J (Engl) 2002;115:1150–2.
99. Cavagnini F, Pecori Giraldi F. Epidemiology and follow-up of Cushing's disease. Ann Endocrinol (Paris) 2001;62:168–72.

12 Cushing's Disease: *Medical Management*

John R. Lindsay and Lynnette K. Nieman

CONTENTS

1. INTRODUCTION
2. ESTABLISHED TREATMENTS AND CHRONOLOGY
3. INHIBITORS OF STEROIDOGENESIS
4. NEUROMODULATORY AGENTS
5. PPARγ LIGANDS
6. OTHER NEUROMODULATORY AGENTS
7. SUMMARY AND CONCLUSION

Summary

Transsphenoidal surgery, the optimal treatment for Cushing's disease, achieves remission in 70–90% of patients. Subsequent treatment of patients who remain hypercortisolemic includes radiation therapy or adrenalectomy. However, there is a role for shortterm primary medical therapy and for adjunctive treatment while awaiting the effects of radiotherapy. The well-studied available agents inhibit cortisol production by the adrenal gland. It would be ideal to inhibit ACTH production or secretion from the tumor; however, such neuromodulatory agents are either ineffective or have not been studied extensively. This chapter will review existing agents, their mechanism of action, efficacy, and clinical application.

Key Words: Cushing's disease, Steroidogenesis inhibitors, Glucocorticoid receptor blockers.

1. INTRODUCTION

Transsphenoidal pituitary surgery is the first-line treatment for Cushing's disease and achieves remission in 70–90% of cases *(1)*. When hypercortisolism persists, pituitary irradiation or bilateral adrenalectomy usually effect

From: *Contemporary Endocrinology: Diagnosis and Management of Pituitary Disorders*
Edited by: B. Swearingen and B. M. K. Biller © Humana Press, Totowa, NJ

eucortisolism, but at the expense of surgical morbidity, hypopituitarism, and/or long-term corticosteroid replacement therapy. In this context, an extensive search has been made over the last four decades to identify medical therapeutic agents. Ideally, such agents should reduce tumor growth and ACTH secretion, or act at the adrenal to reduce cortisol production, and could be given long-term as monotherapy. The current options include neuromodulatory drugs that control ACTH secretion, steroidogenesis inhibitors, and glucocorticoid receptor blocking drugs. This chapter will review existing agents, their mechanism of action, efficacy, and clinical application. Recent developments, including the application of peroxisome-proliferator activating receptor-gamma (PPARγ) agonists and the somatostatin analog SOM-230, will be discussed.

2. ESTABLISHED TREATMENTS AND CHRONOLOGY

Adrenal steroidogenesis inhibitors, the first medical agents used to reduce hypercortisolism in Cushing's disease, were introduced after the discovery of the adrenolytic effect of mitotane in the 1950s. Table 1 shows the characteristics of the drug class, mechanism of action, dosing, and side effects of the major agents (aminoglutethimide, mitotane, metyrapone, and ketoconazole). Although there is substantial evidence for the utility of these agents, only aminoglutethimide has FDA-approved labeling for steroidogenesis inhibition. Unfortunately, in the United States, aminoglutethimide has been discontinued by the manufacturer. Subsequently, neuromodulatory drugs that may influence hypothalamic or pituitary control of ACTH release (bromocriptine, octreotide, cabergoline, and cyproheptadine) were evaluated. None of this class of compounds has FDA-approved labeling for modulation of ACTH release.

There are two approaches to medical treatment of Cushing's syndrome: full cortisol blockade with corticosteroid replacement (block and replace) or a titration regimen whereby the lowest dose of drug achieving eucortisolism is used. These options are analogous to strategies used to treat hyperthyroidism. Titration regimens require regular clinical and biochemical monitoring of eucortisolism while the "block and replace" approach requires monitoring for drug toxicity and the adequacy of corticosteroid dosing. Education regarding adrenal insufficiency is critical and precautions such as medic alert tags and "sick day rules" should be followed. Agents may be used alone or in combination. The advantages of the latter approach may be to use lower doses and thereby minimize toxicity. Presently, primary medical therapy for Cushing's disease is generally not recommended because of the need for lifelong therapy, the potential for escape from efficacy, and adverse side effects.

Table 1
Summary of Established Steroidogenesis Inhibitors and Neuromodulatory Agents

Drug	Discovery	Drug class	Mechanism	Dosing	Efficacy/Remission	Side-effect profile	Treatment Duration
Mitotane	1950s	Adrenolytic developed after DDD (dichloro-diphenyl-dichloroethane)	SCC, 11-α and 18-hydroxylase, 3β-HSD blockade	1.2–12 g/day	80% remission (monotherapy)-100% combined with pituitary XRT	GI upset, dizziness, neurological disturbance, rash, deranged LFTs/lipids, hypoad-renalism	8–37 months
Metyrapone	1950s	Pyridine derivative	11β-hydroxylase, 17α, 18- and 19-hydroxylase blockade	2 g	75% (monotherapy) 67–100% with aminoglutethimide	Edema, rash, lethargy, malaise	12 months
Aminoglute-thimide	1960s	Glutarimide derivative	SCC, 21-hydroxylase, 17α-hydroxylase, 11β-hydroxylase, aromatase, C17–20 lyase, 18 hydroxylase blockade	0.75–2 g/day	46% (monotherapy) 80% combined with pituitary XRT	Sedation, nausea, anorexia, rash	36 months

(Continued)

Table 1
(Continued)

Drug	Discovery	Drug class	Mechanism	Dosing	Efficacy/Remission	Side-effect profile	Treatment Duration
Ketoconazole	1970s	Imidazole derivative	SCC, 17,20-lyase, 11β-hydroxylase, 17α-hydroxylase blockade	200–1200 mg/day	Up to 81%	Elevated transaminases, gynecomastia, GI upset, edema, rash	38 months
Bromocriptine	1970s	Dopamine agonist	D2-receptor agonist	3.75–30 mg	25–40%	Nausea, postural hypotension, dry mouth, nasal congestion	6 years
Cyproheptadine	1970s	Serotonin and histamine antagonist, anticholinergic	Presumed via serotonin receptors	4–24 mg	<10%	Sleepiness, weight gain, increased appetite	3–6 months
Octreotide	1990s	Somatostatin analog	Sst 2 agonist	400–1,200 mcg	Ineffective	GI intolerance, gallstones	24 months

XRT: radiotherapy, GI: gastrointestinal, SCC: side-chain cleavage
Adapted from Miller and Crapo (1993) (10)

3. INHIBITORS OF STEROIDOGENESIS

3.1. Mitotane

Mitotane, which inhibits CYP11A, CYP11B1, CYP11B2, and 3beta HSD enzymes, was demonstrated to cause adrenolytic effects in dogs around 1950 *(2)*. Its o,p′DDD isomer, the active component, was initially shown to reduce tumor bulk and corticosteroid levels in patients with adrenocortical cancer *(3)*. In early studies in five patients with Cushing's disease, remission was reported at daily doses of 1–6 g *(4,5)*. Because mitotane increases the metabolism of some medications, such as hydrocortisone, an increased dosage may be required. Urine, rather than serum cortisol levels, should be used to monitor treatment effects, as mitotane increases corticosteroid-binding globulin production and hence total cortisol levels *(6)*. The daily dosage is usually gradually titrated from 0.5–1 g by 0.5–1 g increments every 1–4 weeks. In one of the largest series, 83 % of 62 patients with Cushing's disease achieved remission at a dose of 12 g/day *(7)*. Of 46 who received mitotane alone for up to 8 months, 38 normalized urine 17-hydroxysteroid values *(7)*. Some advocate lower doses (4 g/day) together with metyrapone to minimize poor compliance due to adverse side effects *(8)*. In general, side effects limit use of mitotane as sole therapy, and it has often been used in conjunction with radiation *(7)*.

Mitotane is relatively contraindicated in women planning for pregnancy within 5 years due to teratogenic effects and prolonged release from adipose tissue *(9)*. Limiting side effects include dizziness, neurological impairment, and nausea or diarrhea *(10)*. Other adverse effects include fatigue, rash, hyperlipidemia, and hepatic enzyme disturbance. A no-cost plasma mitotane testing service in Europe (www.lysodren-europe.com) facilitates dose adjustments to achieve plasma levels within 14–20 mg/l in adrenal cancer, to minimize side effects *(11)*. To our knowledge this strategy has not been evaluated in patients with Cushing's disease.

3.2. Metyrapone

Metyrapone, introduced in 1959, reduces corticosteroid production by inhibition of the enzyme CYP11B1, which converts 11-deoxycortisol to cortisol. It has been used to treat ectopic ACTH syndrome, adrenocortical tumors, and Cushing's disease. In one study of 1 to 16 weeks of treatment of Cushing's disease *(12)*, 75 % of 53 patients normalized mean serum cortisol levels at an average daily dose of 2,250 mg/day (overall dose range of 750–6,000 mg). Inhibition of steroidogenesis occurred by 72 h and a full effect was not achieved for 4–6 weeks. A test dose of 750 mg, with hourly monitoring of cortisol for 4 h may help to define whether patients will respond *(8)*.

In a longer-term series the same group examined responses in 24 patients with Cushing's disease after pituitary irradiation *(12)*. Eighty-three percent achieved normal urine free cortisol (UFC) and none required corticosteroid replacement, suggesting that a titration regimen is feasible. The drug has been used for combination treatment with irradiation *(13)*, aminoglutethimide *(14)*, or sodium valproate *(15)*. Metyrapone is generally well tolerated except for temporary reversible symptoms of hypoadrenalism, rash, dizziness, and minor gastrointestinal upset. Hirsutism and acne accompany the associated elevation in adrenal androgens, thereby limiting the acceptability of the drug for use in women. Metyrapone has been successfully used in pregnancy *(16,17,18)*. Although metyrapone is currently not widely available in the United States, it may be possible to negotiate a supply from the manufacturer on a named patient basis.

3.3. Trilostane

Trilostane is a relatively weak inhibitor of 3beta HSD. While an early report showed significant reductions in mean UFC of six patients with Cushing's disease treated for up to 7 months *(19)*, a later study showed that none of five patients achieved remission with daily doses up to 1440 mg *(20)*. Its poor efficacy and toxicity of gastrointestinal disturbance and parethesias limit its use *(6)*.

3.4. Ketoconazole

Ketoconazole is an imidazole derivative that was originally developed as an antifungal agent. The development of hypoadrenalism in patients treated for fungal infections led to the discovery of its inhibitory effects on adrenal steroidogenesis *(21)*. The drug inhibits activity of a range of adrenal enzymes including CYP11A and CYP11B1. Ketoconazole has successfully treated adrenal rest tumor *(22)* and ACTH-dependent cases and is currently the preferred agent for control of hypercortisolism in the United States. It is effective as monotherapy and in combination with pituitary irradiation or other medical agents. Daily doses range between 400 and 1,200 mg; side effects, especially acute hepatic toxicity, limit the maximally tolerated dose *(23)*.

The largest series of 28 patients with Cushing's disease *(24)* showed about 80% decrease in UFC levels, without change in plasma ACTH values, at a daily ketoconazole dose of 400–800 mg for up to 3 years *(24)*. Eucortisolism can be achieved within 4–6 weeks *(25,26)*. In women, the agent has beneficial antiandrogen effects by inhibiting CYP17-lyase. The related side effect of gynecomastia may limit its use in men *(24)*. Other adverse effects include gastrointestinal upset and rash. While mild reversible disturbance in liver function has been observed in 5–10 % of cases, severe hepatic injury is much less common (~1 in 15,000 cases) *(26)*.

3.5. Etomidate

Etomidate, a substituted imidazole derivative, was developed as an anesthesia induction agent. Its inhibitory effect on steroidogenesis was noted due to increased mortality compared with other anesthetic agents *(27)*. Etomidate inhibits CYP11B1 as evidenced by increases in 11-deoxycortisol, DHEAS, and androstenedione during treatment. Parenteral etomidate has been used successfully in rare adult and pediatric cases with severe life-threatening hypercortisolism, without significant adverse effects *(28,29)*. It can be given in a titration or "block and replace" regimen. Schulte determined that a dose of 0.1 mg/kg/h or lower reduced cortisol levels in adults *(30)*. A dosage of 1–3 mg/h was safe and without hypnotic effect in children *(28)*. Eucortisolism may be achieved within 11–48 h by using a continuous infusion *(29)*. The European formulation includes ethyl alcohol. We successfully used the propylene glycol formulation that is available in the United States for up to 5.5 months in a patient with ectopic ACTH secretion and renal failure *(31)*, controlling hypercortisolism with a short (80 mg, 3 h) rather than continuous infusion *(31)*. A higher dosage (200 mg/day) was required upon recovery of renal function. Serum cortisol values should be monitored after discontinuation of the agent, as we observed cortisol suppression for 2 weeks. Etomidate is recommended in life-threatening situations with severe hypercortisolism resistant to conventional therapy, or when oral dosing is contraindicated. In this context it will usually be used for cases with ectopic disease.

4. NEUROMODULATORY AGENTS

4.1. Dopamine Agonists

An early report that bromocriptine, 2.5 mg, reduced plasma ACTH in five of six patients with Cushing's disease was not later confirmed consistently *(32)*. However, it was associated with a 6-year remission in one patient *(33)*. Interpretation of results has been hindered by inadequate randomization or blinding, or short duration of follow-up.

Recent studies evaluated the long-acting dopamine agonist cabergoline *(34)*. In vitro, when tumors expressed the D-2 receptor, ACTH secretion decreased in 60 % and normalized in 40 % *(35)*. At a dose of 0.5 to 1 mg twice weekly, two patients with Nelson's syndrome had improved clinical symptoms, tumor regression, and reduction of ACTH levels *(34)*. A recent report of cardiac valvular abnormalities in patients with Parkinson's disease taking higher levels of this agent may mitigate against use of this agent (36).

4.2. Somatostatin Analogs

Sec 4.2. Normal pituitary tissue contains five somatostatin receptor subtypes (sst 1–5); sst 2 and sst 5 are important for function. As a result, somatostatin analogs can control growth hormone secretion in acromegaly. While octreotide may reduce ACTH concentrations in corticotropinomas in vitro and in Nelson's syndrome in vivo, octreotide, 100–1,200 µg/day, given subcutaneously has not consistently controlled hypercortisolism in Cushing's disease (37–39), although addition of ketoconazole could normalize UFC levels (40). Van der Hoek et al. have speculated that octreotide inhibits ACTH release from corticotrope adenomas only in the absence of peripheral feedback regulation of glucocorticoids, based on the finding that DTPA octreotide imaging is typically negative in Cushing's disease, but positive in Nelson's syndrome (41).

Ongoing studies evaluate pasireotide (SOM-230) as a novel medical therapy for Cushing's disease (42). This agent binds to sst 1–3 and sst 5, and has a 40-fold greater affinity to sst 5 than octreotide. A recent phase II trial studied 14 patients with persistent or recurrent Cushing's disease treated with 600 µg twice daily subcutaneously for 15 days. Of ten patients with substantial reductions in UFC, two normalized UFC and the others had at least 40 % decrease (42). We await further long-term studies in Cushing's disease and Nelson's syndrome.

4.3. Glucocorticoid Receptor Antagonists

Mifepristone is an effective glucocorticoid receptor antagonist (43). It has been used for control of severe hypercortisolism in at least six patients with pituitary-dependent Cushing's syndrome as well as in ectopic and adrenal cases (44). Mifepristone's efficacy in ectopic ACTH syndrome was first reported in 1985 (45). The initial dosing regimen was based on titration increments of 5 mg/kg every 1 to 2 weeks, starting at a baseline dose of 5 mg/kg up to a maximum of 20 mg/kg per day (45). In that report, reversal of clinical features was observed in association with improved glucocorticoid-dependent biochemical measures, but in the absence of normalization of UFC, cortisol or plasma ACTH during 10 weeks of treatment (45). These observations were replicated by other small series in which 400 mg of mifepristone was given daily for 3 days in five patients with Cushing's disease (46). While acute dosing had no effect compared to placebo, longer-term administration in Cushing's disease caused activation of the HPA axis with increases in UFC and plasma cortisol (46). In a more recent report, doses of up to 25 mg/kg/day normalized plasma cortisol and ACTH values for 8 months in a patient with an

ACTH-secreting macroadenoma who was intolerant of other therapies, pending the onset of effects of pituitary irradiation *(44)*. As it is not possible to monitor effects of glucocorticoid action on ACTH or cortisol, titration of dosing can be difficult, necessitating careful monitoring for hypoadrenalism. Some have advocated that mifepristone is best reserved for ectopic ACTH syndrome *(43)*.

5. PPARγ LIGANDS

There has been recent interest in the use of the PPARγ ligands for therapy in Cushing's disease after Heaney et al. demonstrated that PPARγ receptors are present in normal corticotrophs and have increased expression in ACTH-secreting human pituitary tumors *(47,48)*. In vitro, thiazolidinedione (TZD) increased apoptosis of murine corticotroph cell lines and decreased entry into S-phase. In vivo, it prevented the development of ACTH-secreting tumors in nude mice. In the largest human series, 8 of 14 patients with Cushing's disease who received rosiglitazone 8 mg daily did not respond; in the others a 30-day to 60-day treatment normalized UFC and reduced ACTH levels *(49)*. Effects were more modest in another study of two patients *(50)*. Cotreatment with metyrapone *(50)* and ketoconazole *(51)* has been needed in some cases.

While TZDs may improve glucose control, their effects upon hypercortisolism have been modest. Larger doses may be needed to achieve the results seen in the animal models, which used rosiglitazone 150 mg/kg/day, well in excess of licensed human treatment schedules. It is also possible that TZD effects are distinct within each of the drug classes. Pioglitazone 45 mg/day for 30 days did not decrease ACTH or cortisol values in five patients with Cushing's disease *(52)*.

In general, the effect of rosiglitazone, 8 mg daily, in patients with Cushing's disease after bilateral adrenalectomy has been disappointing. Andreassen reported a 40 % decrease in ACTH values in two of three patients with Nelson's syndrome after 5 months *(53)*, with escape of control after 11 months in one and no change in tumor size. In another study, 12 weeks of treatment did not reduce plasma ACTH levels in seven patients *(54)*.

6. OTHER NEUROMODULATORY AGENTS

A suppressive effect of sodium valproate on ACTH release was first observed in patients with epilepsy *(55)*. However, while case reports suggested a response in Cushing's disease, larger long-term series showed no clinically relevant benefits *(56)*, as no patient normalized serum cortisol, UFC, or ACTH levels. Thus, this agent is not an effective treatment *(57)*.

Krieger tested the concept of central neurotransmitter regulation of ACTH release using the serotonin antagonist cyproheptadine. Administration of 24 mg for 3–6 months led to clinical and biochemical remission in the first patient and to reductions in ACTH and prolactin in three subsequent patients with Nelson's syndrome *(58).* In contrast, most later case reports concluded that the drug was ineffective in Cushing's disease *(59).* The predominant side effect is sedation and due to its relatively low efficacy the drug is not widely used.

Ketanserin selectively blocks type 2 serotonin receptors. Demonstration of a 30% reduction in ACTH response to insulin induced hypoglycemia in healthy men, led to trials in Nelson's syndrome *(60).* In a double-blind placebo-controlled study, Prescott et al. demonstrated that ketanserin, 40 mg twice daily, given for 2 months, did not reduce ACTH levels in these patients *(61).* More recently in a small 12-month study, neither ritanserin, a long-acting piperidine derivative, nor ketanserin had efficacy in Cushing's disease *(62).* Additional placebo-controlled randomized trials are needed to evaluate the efficacy of selective serotonergic antagonists.

7. SUMMARY AND CONCLUSION

In conclusion, although a variety of medical therapies are available for control of hypercortisolism in Cushing's disease, no single agent induces disease remission. Adrenal steroidogenesis inhibitors, the most commonly used and efficacious agents for control of hypercortisolism, do not inhibit tumor growth or reduce ACTH production. Their tolerability is often limited by adverse side effects. The available neuromodulatory agents only modestly inhibit ACTH secretion and rarely effect tumor regression. The low prevalence of Cushing's disease limits the opportunity to study new agents. Future agents for medical treatment of Cushing's disease should be tested in multicenter randomized placebo-controlled trials.

ACKNOWLEDGMENT

A portion of this work was supported by the intramural program of the National Institute of Child Health and Human Development

REFERENCES

1. Utz AL, Swearingen B, Biller BM. Pituitary surgery and postoperative management in Cushing's disease. Endocrinol Metab Clin North Am 2005;34:459–78, xi.
2. Nelson AA, Woodard G. Severe adrenal cortical atrophy (cytotoxic) and hepatic damage produced in dogs by feeding 2,2-bis (parachlorophenyl)-1,1-dichloroethane (DDD or TDE). Arch Path (Chicago) 1949;48:387–94.
3. Bergenstal DM, Hertz R, Lipsett MB. Chemotherapy of adrenocortical cancer with o,p'DDD. Ann Intern Med 1960;53:672–82.

4. Temple TE, Jones DJ, Liddle G, Dexter RN. Treatment of Cushing's disease. Correction of hypercortisolism by o,p'DDD without induction of aldosterone deficiency. N Engl J Med 1969;281:801–5.

5. Southren AL, Weisenfeld S, Laufer A. Effect of o,p'DDD in a patient with Cushing's syndrome. J Clin Endocrinol Metab 1961;21:201–8.

6. Nieman LK. Medical therapy of Cushing's disease. Pituitary 2002;5:77–82.

7. Luton JP, Mahoudeau JA, Bouchard P, et al. Treatment of Cushing's disease by O,p'DDD. Survey of 62 cases. N Engl J Med 1979;300:459–64.

8. Morris D, Grossman A. The medical management of Cushing's syndrome. Ann N Y Acad Sci 2002;970:119–33.

9. Leiba S, Weinstein R, Shindel B, et al. The protracted effect of o,p'-DDD in Cushing's disease and its impact on adrenal morphogenesis of young human embryo. Ann Endocrinol (Paris) 1989;50:49–53.

10. Miller JW, Crapo L. The medical treatment of Cushing's syndrome. Endocr Rev 1993;14:443–58.

11. Baudin E, Pellegriti G, Bonnay M, et al. Impact of monitoring plasma 1, 1-dichlorodiphenildichloroethane (o,p'DDD) levels on the treatment of patients with adrenocortical carcinoma. Cancer 2001;92:1385–92.

12. Verhelst JA, Trainer PJ, Howlett TA, et al. Short and long-term responses to metyrapone in the medical management of 91 patients with Cushing's syndrome. Clin Endocrinol (Oxf) 1991;35:169–78.

13. Jeffcoate WJ, Rees LH, Tomlin S, Jones AE, Edwards CR, Besser GM. Metyrapone in long-term management of Cushing's disease. Br Med J 1977;2:215–17.

14. Child DF, Burke CW, Burley DM, Rees LH, Fraser TR. Drug controlled of Cushing's syndrome. Combined aminoglutethimide and metyrapone therapy. Acta Endocrinol (Copenh) 1976;82:330–41.

15. Nussey SS, Price P, Jenkins JS, Altaher AR, Gillham B, Jones MT. The combined use of sodium valproate and metyrapone in the treatment of Cushing's syndrome. Clin Endocrinol (Oxf) 1988;28:373–80.

16. Close CF, Mann MC, Watts JF, Taylor KG. ACTH-independent Cushing's syndrome in pregnancy with spontaneous resolution after delivery: control of the hypercortisolism with metyrapone. Clin Endocrinol (Oxf) 1993;39:375–9.

17. Gormley MJ, Hadden DR, Kennedy TL, Montgomery DA, Murnaghan GA, Sheridan B. Cushing's syndrome in pregnancy–treatment with metyrapone. Clin Endocrinol (Oxf) 1982;16:283–93.

18. Shaw JA, Pearson DW, Krukowski ZH, Fisher PM, Bevan JS, Cushing's syndrome during pregnancy: curative adrenalectomy at 31 weeks gestation. Eur J Obstet Gynecol Reprod Biol 2002;105:189–91.

19. Komanicky P, Spark RF, Melby JC. Treatment of Cushing's syndrome with trilostane (WIN 24,540), an inhibitor of adrenal steroid biosynthesis. J Clin Endocrinol Metab 1978;47:1042–51.

20. Dewis P, Anderson DC, Bu'lock DE, Earnshaw R, Kelly WF. Experience with trilostane in the treatment of Cushing's syndrome. Clin Endocrinol (Oxf) 1983;18:533–40.

21. Tucker WS, Jr, Snell BB, Island DP, Gregg CR. Reversible adrenal insufficiency induced by ketoconazole. JAMA 1985;253:2413–14.

22. Contreras P, Altieri E, Liberman C, et al. Adrenal rest tumor of the liver causing Cushing's syndrome: treatment with ketoconazole preceding an apparent surgical cure. J Clin Endocrinol Metab 1985;60:21–8.

23. McCance DR, Ritchie CM, Sheridan B, Atkinson AB. Acute hypoadrenalism and hepato-toxicity after treatment with ketoconazole. Lancet 1987;1:573.
24. Sonino N, Boscaro M, Paoletta A, Mantero F, Ziliotto D. Ketoconazole treatment in Cushing's syndrome: experience in 34 patients. Clin Endocrinol (Oxf) 1991;35: 347–52.
25. Sonino N, Boscaro M, Merola G, Mantero F. Prolonged treatment of Cushing's disease by ketoconazole. J Clin Endocrinol Metab 61:718–22
26. Tabarin A, Navarranne A, Guerin J, Corcuff JB, Parneix M, Roger P. Use of ketoconazole in the treatment of Cushing's disease and ectopic ACTH syndrome. Clin Endocrinol (Oxf) 1991;34:63–9.
27. Ledingham IM, Watt I. Influence of sedation on mortality in critically ill multiple trauma patients. Lancet 1983;1:1270.
28. Greening JE, Brain CE, Perry LA, et al. Efficient short-term control of hypercortiso-laemia by low-dose etomidate in severe paediatric Cushing's disease. Horm Res 2005;64: 140–3.
29. Allolio B, Schulte HM, Kaulen D, Reincke M, Jaursch-Hancke C, Winkelmann W. Nonhyp-notic low-dose etomidate for rapid correction of hypercortisolaemia in Cushing's syndrome. Klin Wochenschr 1988;66:361–4.
30. Schulte HM, Benker G, Reinwein D, Sippell WG, Allolio B. Infusion of low dose etomidate: correction of hypercortisolemia in patients with Cushing's syndrome and dose-response relationship in normal subjects. J Clin Endocrinol Metab 1990;70:1426–30.
31. Krakoff J, Koch CA, Calis KA, Alexander RH, Nieman LK. Use of a parenteral propylene glycol-containing etomidate preparation for the long-term management of ectopic Cushing's syndrome. J Clin Endocrinol Metab 2001;86:4104–8.
32. Lamberts SW, Birkenhager JC. Effect of bromocriptine in pituitary-dependent Cushing's syndrome. J Endocrinol 1976;70:315–16.
33. Atkinson AB, Kennedy AL, Sheridan B. Six year remission of ACTH-dependent Cushing's syndrome using bromocriptine. Postgrad Med J 1985;61:239–42.
34. Casulari LA, Naves LA, Mello PA, Pereira Neto A, Papadia C. Nelson's syndrome: complete remission with cabergoline but not with bromocriptine or cyproheptadine treatment. Horm Res 2004;62:300–5.
35. Pivonello R, Ferone D, de Herder WW, et al. Dopamine receptor expression and function in corticotroph pituitary tumors. J Clin Endocrinol Metab 2004;89:2452–62.
36. Zanettini R, Antonini A, Gatto G, Gentile R, Tesei S, Pezzoli G. Valvular heart disease and the use of dopamine agonists for Parkinson's disease. N Engl J Med. 2007;356:39–46.
37. Invitti C, de Martin M, Brunani A, Piolini M, Cavagnini F. Treatment of Cushing's syndrome with the long-acting somatostatin analogue SMS 201–995 (sandostatin). Clin Endocrinol (Oxf) 1990;32:275–81.
38. Lamberts SW, Uitterlinden P, Klijn JM. The effect of the long-acting somatostatin analogue SMS 201–995 on ACTH secretion in Nelson's syndrome and Cushing's disease. Acta Endocrinol (Copenh) 1989;120:760–6.
39. Ambrosi B, Bochicchio D, Fadin C, Colombo P, Faglia G. Failure of somatostatin and octreotide to acutely affect the hypothalamic-pituitary-adrenal function in patients with corticotropin hypersecretion. J Endocrinol Invest 1990;13:257–61.
40. Vignati F, Loli P. Additive effect of ketoconazole and octreotide in the treatment of severe adrenocorticotropin-dependent hypercortisolism. J Clin Endocrinol Metab 1996;81: 2885–90.
41. van der Hoek J, Lamberts SW, Hofland LJ. The role of somatostatin analogs in Cushing's disease. Pituitary 2004;7:257–64.

42. Boscaro M, Petersenn S, Atkinson AB, et al. Pasireotide (SOM230), the Novel Multi-Ligand Somatostatin Analogue, is a Promising Medical Therapy for Patients with Cushing's Disease: Preliminary Safety and Efficacy Results of a Phase II Study. Endo 2006 Abstract OR 9–1, 2006

43. Sartor O, Cutler GB, Jr. Mifepristone: treatment of Cushing' syndrome. Clin Obstet Gynecol 1996;39:506–10.

44. Chu JW, Matthias DF, Belanoff J, Schatzberg A, Hoffman AR, Feldman D. Successful long-term treatment of refractory Cushing's disease with high-dose mifepristone (RU 486). J Clin Endocrinol Metab 2001;86:3568–73.

45. Nieman LK, Chrousos GP, Kellner C, et al. Successful treatment of Cushing's syndrome with the glucocorticoid antagonist RU 486. J Clin Endocrinol Metab 1985;61:536–40.

46. Bertagna X, Bertagna C, Laudat MH, Husson JM, Girard F, Luton JP. Pituitary-adrenal response to the antiglucocorticoid action of RU 486 in Cushing's syndrome. J Clin Endocrinol Metab 1986;63:639–43.

47. Heaney AP. PPAR-gamma in Cushing's disease. Pituitary 2004;7:265–9.

48. Heaney AP. Novel medical approaches for the treatment of Cushing's disease. J Endocrinol Invest 2004;27:591–5.

49. Ambrosi B, Dall'Asta C, Cannavo S, et al. Effects of chronic administration of PPAR-gamma ligand rosiglitazone in Cushing's disease. Eur J Endocrinol 2004;151:173–8.

50. Hull SS, Sheridan B, Atkinson AB. Pre-operative medical therapy with rosiglitazone in two patients with newly diagnosed pituitary-dependent Cushing's syndrome. Clin Endocrinol (Oxf) 2005;62:259–61.

51. Heaney AP, Fernando M, Yong WH, Melmed S. Functional PPAR-gamma receptor is a novel therapeutic target for ACTH-secreting pituitary adenomas. Nat Med. 2002;8: 1281–7.

52. Suri D, Weiss RE. Effect of pioglitazone on adrenocorticotropic hormone and cortisol secretion in Cushing's disease. J Clin Endocrinol Metab 2005;90:1340–6.

53. Andreassen M, Kristensen LO. Rosiglitazone for prevention or adjuvant treatment of Nelson's syndrome after bilateral adrenalectomy. Eur J Endocrinol 2005;153:503–5.

54. Mullan KR, Leslie H, McCance DR, Sheridan B, Atkinson AB. The PPAR-gamma activator rosiglitazone fails to lower plasma ACTH levels in patients with Nelson's syndrome. Clin Endocrinol (Oxf) 2006;64:519–22.

55. Kritzler RK, Vining EP, Plotnick LP. Sodium valproate and corticotropin suppression in the child treated for seizures. J Pediatr 1983;102:142–3.

56. Koppeschaar HP, Croughs RJ, van't Verlaat JW, et al. Successful treatment with sodium valproate of a patient with Cushing's disease and gross enlargement of the pituitary. Acta Endocrinol (Copenh) 1984;107:471–5.

57. Loli P, Berselli ME, Frascatani F, Muratori F, Tagliaferri M. Lack of ACTH lowering effect of sodium valproate in patients with ACTH hypersecretion. J Endocrinol Invest 1984;7:93–6.

58. Krieger DT, Amorosa L, Linick F. Cyproheptadine-induced remission of Cushing's disease. N Engl J Med 1975;293:893–6.

59. Scott R, Espiner EA, Donald RA. Cyproheptadine for Cushing's disease (cont.). N Engl J Med 1977;296:57–8.

60. Prescott RW, Kendall-Taylor P, Weightman DR, Watson MJ, Ratcliffe WA. The effect of ketanserin, a specific serotonin antagonist on the PRL, GH, ACTH and cortisol responses to hypoglycaemia in normal subjects. Clin Endocrinol (Oxf) 1984;20: 137–42.

61. Prescott RW, Ratcliffe WA, Taylor PK. Effect of an oral serotonin antagonist, ketanserin, on plasma ACTH concentrations in Nelson's syndrome. Br Med J (Clin Res Ed) 1984;289:787–8.
62. Sonino N, Fava GA, Fallo F, Franceschetto A, Belluardo P, Boscaro M. Effect of the serotonin antagonists ritanserin and ketanserin in Cushing's disease. Pituitary 2000;3:55–9.

13 Thyrotropin-secreting Pituitary Adenomas

Marina S. Zemskova, MD, and Monica C. Skarulis, MD

CONTENTS

1. EPIDEMIOLOGY
2. MOLECULAR PATHOPHYSIOLOGY
3. CLINICAL PRESENTATION
4. CLINICAL EVALUATION
5. LABORATORY EVALUATION
6. RADIOGRAPHIC FEATURES
7. TREATMENT
8. CRITERIA FOR CURE
9. CLINICAL OUTCOMES
10. CONCLUSION

Summary

Thyrotropin (TSH)-secreting pituitary adenomas are rare pituitary tumors that cause central hyperthyroidism by the release of TSH refractory to negative feedback regulation of thyroid hormones. The frequency of this diagnosis has increased because of the widespread availability of ultrasensitive immunometric assays for TSH and the growing awareness by clinicians of the states of inappropriate TSH secretion. The clinical presentation is varied and has been confused with more common causes of thyrotoxicosis or the syndrome of resistance to thyroid hormone. Some patients, especially those previously misdiagnosed and treated with thyroid ablation, present with signs and symptoms resulting from compression of the surrounding nervous structures by growing tumor.

Failure to recognize the inappropriate secretion of TSH caused by the tumor may result in dramatic consequences, such as unnecessary thyroid ablation. In contrast, early diagnosis and correct treatment of pituitary adenomas prevent the development of complications and improve the rate of cure.

From: *Contemporary Endocrinology: Diagnosis and Management of Pituitary Disorders*
Edited by: B. Swearingen and B. M. K. Biller © Humana Press, Totowa, NJ

Key Words: TSH, Thyrotropin-secreting hormone, TSH-omas.

1. EPIDEMIOLOGY

Thyrotropin (TSH)-secreting pituitary adenomas (TSH-omas) are rare tumors that result in central hyperthyroidism *(1)*. The hallmark of this tumor is the autonomous release of TSH refractory to negative feedback regulation of thyroid hormones and is referred to as a state of "inappropriate secretion of TSH." The first case was clinically described in 1960 *(2)* and since that time approximately 350 cases have been reported *(3)*. The clinical presentation is varied and has been confused with more common causes of thyrotoxicosis or the syndrome of resistance to thyroid hormone, a condition associated with mutation of the thyroid hormone receptor.

Representing 0.5–2.8% of pituitary adenomas *(4–6)*, the prevalence of TSH-secreting tumors in the general population is estimated to be one to two cases per million. The frequency of this diagnosis increased during the 1990s, a phenomenon attributed to the widespread availability of ultrasensitive immuno-metric assays for TSH and the growing awareness by clinicians of the states of inappropriate TSH secretion *(6–9)*

2. MOLECULAR PATHOPHYSIOLOGY

Despite advances in techniques to study the pathogenesis and genetics of pituitary tumors, little is known of the molecular mechanisms leading to the formation of TSH-omas. Like most pituitary tumors, TSH-secreting tumors are thought to arise from a single cell mutation followed by clonal expansion *(10–12)*; however, attempts to identify the oncogenes or tumor suppressor genes involved have been unrewarding. Activating mutations of the Gs alpha-subunit (gsp) gene commonly found in somatotropinomas or other G protein subunits have not been found in TSH-secreting tumors *(13)*. Allelic loss of the tumor suppressor gene *Menin*, responsible for multiple endocrine neoplasia type 1 (MEN-1) *(14)*, is found in a minority (3–30%) of sporadic pituitary adenomas *(15,16)* and somatic mutations are rarely found *(17)*. TSH-oma is a rare but recognized feature of MEN-1 syndrome *(18–20)*; however, *Menin* plays little if any role in the primary pathogenesis of sporadic TSH-secreting tumors. Evaluation of the role of various transcription factors in thyrotrope adeno-matous cell proliferation has demonstrated overexpression but no mutations in pituitary-specific transcription factor-1 (Pit-1) *(21,22)* or GATA-2 *(23)*. The significance of these findings is unknown.

The search for somatic mutation of thyroid receptor genes has revealed conflicting results. Ando et al. demonstrated mutation in the thyroid receptor beta (TRβ) gene *(24,25)* in six TSH-omas and both TRα and TRβ mutations were found in two tumors studied *(26)*. The resulting mutant thyroid receptors failed to bind thyroid hormone and interfered with the function of the normal receptor. Defective TR function is a plausible explanation for the loss of negative feedback regulation and nonsuppressible TSH secretion. However, not all studies implicate TR in the molecular pathophysiology of the tumor. A study of nine TSH-omas failed to uncover any mutation in TR genes (27) suggesting that some degree of negative feedback is possible. These data are interesting considering invasive macroadenomas are found two times more frequently in patients treated with thyroid ablation compared with those with intact thyroid (28). Weintraub et al. (29) observed that previous thyroid ablation may induce aggressive transformation of the tumor, resembling Nelson's syndrome seen after adrenalectomy in Cushing's disease. The role of TR in the pathogenesis and clinical behavior of these tumors is still controversial.

Many studies have described molecular features that help explain the observed clinical behavior of TSH-omas. A few small studies have failed to identify either thyrotropin-releasing hormone (TRH) receptor binding (30) or variable in vivo and in vitro response to TRH (31–35). Likewise, variable numbers of both dopamine and somatostatin receptors (SSTR1,2,3,5) have been found (36,37) with the highest numbers of SSTRs identified in mixed GH/TSH pituitary tumors (37,38). Medical treatment with somatostatin analogs inhibits TSH secretion in most cases by inducing changes in membrane polarization and intracellular calcium concentrations (37,39).

2.1. Histopathology

Sometimes referred to as "pituitary stones" (40,41), TSH-omas tend to be highly fibrotic. Ezzat et al. associated tumoral expression of basic fibroblast growth factor and elevated levels in the circulation of two patients with TSH-oma with marked interstitial fibrosis (42). By light microscopy, tumoral cells are often arranged in cords, appearing polymorphous with large nuclei and prominent nucleoli (Fig. 1 and Color Plate 15). The cells are usually chromophobic with occasional mitotic figures raising concerns of malignancy; however, only two cases of TSH-secreting carcinoma have been described in the literature (43,44).

Immunohistochemical studies demonstrate TSH staining in most TSH-secreting adenomas (Fig. 2 and Color Plate 16). The presence of two different cell types, one secreting α-subunit alone and another cosecreting α-subunit and intact TSH molecule (mixed TSH /α-subunit adenomas), has been documented (1,45). Cells from adenomas cosecreting TSH and other pituitary hormones are monomorphus by electron microscopy. The presence of TSH and other pituitary hormones in the same cell or the same secretory granule can be detected by double-gold immunolabeling (32,46).

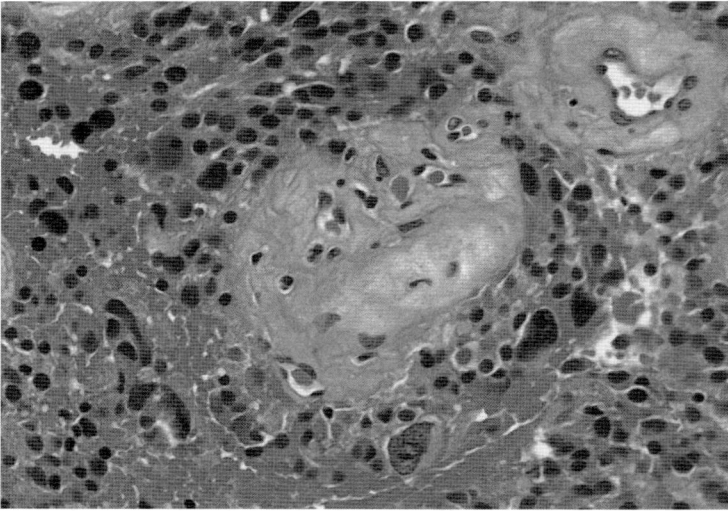

Fig. 1. TSH-oma cells by light microscopy (40× magnification). H&E stain shows significant cytological and nuclear pleomorphism of tumor cells (*see* Color Plate 15).

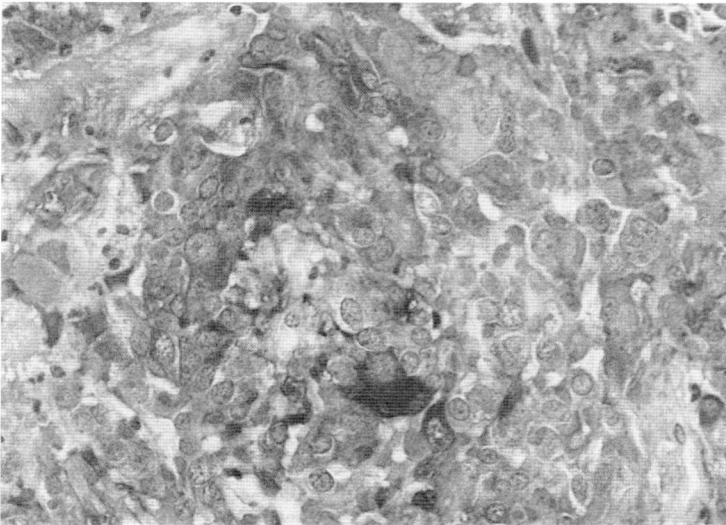

Fig. 2. Immunohistochemical staining of TSH-oma (40× magnification). Tumor cells show positive reaction for TSH. The intensity of staining is variable from cell to cell (*see* Color Plate 16).

3. CLINICAL PRESENTATION

In a review of 236 patients with TSH-oma, men and women were affected equally and the diagnosis was made most commonly early in the fifth decade of life (mean age 42 years) although a wide age range was seen (11–84 years) *(28)*. Familial cases of TSH-oma have been reported only as a part of the MEN-1 syndrome *(19)*. Patients present with a variety of symptoms that can be divided into those predominantly related to excessive thyroid hormone production or those related to the mechanical effects of the expanding tumor within the pituitary sella.

The majority of patients have symptoms and signs of hyperthyroidism similar to other forms of thyroid hyperfunction such as toxic goiter or Graves' disease. The most common findings are thyrotoxicosis (70% of patients) *(47)* and diffuse goiter (up to 80% of patients) *(9)*. Fatigue, tremor, heat intolerance, weight loss, and diarrhea were presenting symptoms in approximately half of the patients in the NIH series. Cardiac symptoms including palpitations, tachycardia, chest pain, and dyspnea predominated in up to 20% of patients. Rarely, patients have presented with memory loss and signs of dementia *(47)*. Thyrotoxic periodic paralysis has been reported in three Asian patients *(48–50)*.

Up to two-thirds of patients, often those with the largest goiters causing compressive symptoms, were misdiagnosed and treated for Graves' disease. Despite prior thyroid-specific treatments, patients are usually biochemically and clinically hyperthyroid at the time of diagnosis of the TSH-secreting tumor.

Some patients, usually males, have extremely mild or no symptoms of thyrotoxicosis *(9,47,51)*. In asymptomatic patients (one-fifth of the NIH series), the diagnosis is made incidentally by blood work or findings of a pituitary mass on computed tomography (CT) or magnetic resonance imaging (MRI) obtained for other indications *(9)*. It is thought that the secretion of tumoral TSH with diminished biological activity may explain these silent TSH-omas.

Another interesting clinical presentation is the TSH-oma that arises in the setting of primary thyroid failure. Failure to achieve normal TSH levels despite increasing doses of levothyroxine should raise suspicions. The most likely diagnosis in this situation is noncompliance with replacement therapy; however, several cases of TSH-oma with concomitant primary hypothyroidism have been reported *(52–54)*.

Approximately 25% of TSH-omas secrete more than one pituitary hormone. Growth hormone (GH) secretion, reported in 15% of cases, presents with typical features of acromegaly. Hyperthyroid symptoms can be overlooked in those cases in which acromegalic features predominate, underscoring the importance of evaluating thyroid function in all patients with pituitary tumors *(1,46,55)*. Hyperprolactinemia, identified in 10% of cases, is due either to the tumor cosecreting prolactin or to compression of the pituitary stalk and interruption of hypothalamic inhibition. Prolactin secretion may be accompanied by galactorrhea and amenorrhea. Rarely, TSH-omas may secrete gonadotropins (1%) *(4,56)*. No reports of cosecretion of corticotropin (ACTH) and TSH are yet found in the literature.

Symptoms related to an expanding pituitary mass are not unusual. Since most of the tumors reported are macroadenomas that invade surrounding structures and extend into the suprasellar area (approximately 70% of all tumors) *(1,8)*, it is generally agreed that TSH-omas exhibit an aggressive growth pattern. The most prevalent symptoms include visual field defects seen in 36–50% of patients and headache in 17–40% of reported cases *(9,28)*.

Many factors contribute to the apparent aggressiveness of these tumors. Many TSH-secreting tumors are large and invasive at the time of diagnosis due to delay of proper diagnosis and time lost to inappropriate thyroid specific treatment. As shown by Brucker-Davis et al., patients who received thyroid-specific therapy suffered from symptoms longer and had a high rate of visual field abnormalities than those patients with intact thyroids *(9)*. These data emphasize the importance of the recognition of TSH-secreting tumors early and withholding thyro-ablative therapy if possible.

4. CLINICAL EVALUATION

4.1. Differential Diagnosis

Several clinical conditions may present with hyperthyroidism and detectable TSH levels and must be considered and eliminated as diagnostic possibilities. Clarification of the clinical and family history, physical findings, and laboratory evaluation including repeat measurement of TSH and free T4 measurement by dialysis are critical to the evaluation. The presence of detectable TSH and elevated free thyroid hormone levels, in general, excludes primary hyperthyroidism due to Graves' disease or other forms of thyrotoxicosis. However, TSH-oma and coexistent Graves' disease has been reported in five cases *(57–61)*. Extrathyroidal manifestations of Graves' disease are rare, although exophthalmos has been described in one of these patients *(62)*. Elevation of thyroid hormone level in the presence of detectable TSH in patients on thyroid hormone replacement therapy may be due the consumption of large L-T4 dose before blood sampling *(63)*. Inaccurate TSH measurements can result from methodological interference, such as in the case of heterophilic antibodies or in autoimmunity *(4)*.

Euthyroid hyperthyroxinemia, characterized by normal TSH and elevated total but usually normal free thyroid hormone levels can easily be excluded prior to considering an extensive workup for inappropriate TSH secretion *(64)*. Among these conditions are elevations in serum thyroxine-binding globulin concentrations and familial dysalbuminemic hyperthyroxinemia. Binding proteins exhibiting increased affinity for thyroid hormone will result in false elevations in free T4 measured by analog but not equilibrium dialysis or other direct methods justifying its use in these cases.

After inappropriate secretion of TSH is confirmed, hyperthyroidism from a tumor must be distinguished from resistance to thyroid hormone (RTH). The thyroid hormone resistance syndrome first described by Refetoff et al. in 1967 *(65)* is characterized by a defect in TR-β. Because of this defect, patients exhibit variable tissue resistance to thyroid hormone action. Despite the resistance, some patients have signs and symptoms of hyperthyroidism. No significant difference in age, sex, TSH levels, or free thyroid hormone concentrations have been found between patients with TSH-oma and with RTH (Table 1) *(9,66)*. There is one TSH-secreting adenoma in a patient with RTH described in the literature *(67)*.Others have reported the findings of pituitary adenomas in RTH, raising the question of whether these patients have a predisposition to the development of pituitary neoplasms *(68,69)*. Advancing directly to pituitary imaging without solid evidence supporting TSH-oma (neuro-ophthalmologic signs or other mass effects) is costly and may lead to confusion.

A positive family history is very important in identifying RTH cases; however, the lack of a family history does not conclusively rule out RTH since sporadic or de novo mutations in TR-β are well recognized. In the absence of a

Table 1
Thyroid Function Testing in Patients with TSH-oma (n=14) versus Resistance to Thyroid Hormone (RTH) (n=34)

	TSH-secreting Tumor	*RTH*
Age (years)	48 ± 4	32 ± 2
T$_4$ [µg/dl]	15.8 ± 0.7	16.5 ± 0.5
Free T$_4$ [ng/dl]	3.5 ± 0.3	3.2 ± 0.1
T$_3$ [ng/dl]	223 ± 18	216 ± 8
TSH [mU/l]	6.2 ± 1.9	3.0 ± 0.3
Stimulated TSH [mU/l]	10.1 ± 2.1	27.7 ± 2.2
% Increase in TSH	189 ± 32	985 ± 68
α-Subunit [µg/l]	16.2 ± 9.4	1.01 ± 0.06
α-Subunit/TSH	28.2 ± 16.5	3.9 ± 0.6

All data are shown as the mean ± SE. Stimulated TSH, peak TSH after stimulation by TRH; % increase in TSH (peak TSH after TRH stimulation divided by baseline TSH) ×100. Normal values are T4, 5–10 µg/dl; free T4, 1–1.9 ng/dl; T3, 75–153 ng/dl; TSH, 0.4–4.4 mU/l; α-subunit, less than 3 µg/l in males and before menopause, less than 5 µg/l after menopause *(9)*.

clear hereditary pattern, the laboratory evaluation can help distinguish between the two entities.

5. LABORATORY EVALUATION

5.1. Thyrotropin

The characteristic biochemical abnormalities in patients with TSH-oma resemble those of hyperthyroidism, with high serum total and free thyroxine and triiodothyronine concentrations. In contrast, TSH concentrations are normal or high but never suppressed. In the largest series reported by a single institution, TSH values varied from 1 to 393 mU/l *(9)*. The highest TSH levels were found in athyreotic patients who failed to exhibit expected suppression of TSH with thyroid hormone therapy. Tumoral TSH has altered biological activity and fails to exhibit a diurnal variation, which may account for clinical observations in patients with TSH-oma.

5.1.1. BIOACTIVITY

The severity of hyperthyroid symptoms varies widely in patients with similar TSH levels. Moreover, 30% of patients who had not received thyroid ablation had serum TSH values within the normal range for the assay but resulted in high T4 and T3 concentrations *(4)*. The variability observed in the thyroid response can be explained in part by considerable variations in the biological activity of the secreted TSH *(4,46)*. The presence of TSH with altered bioactivity is suspected when discrepancies between the clinical features or the biochemical findings and the immunoreactive levels of TSH are found.

Thyrotropin is composed of an α-subunit common to all glycoprotein hormones and the β-subunit, which imparts unique biological and immuno-logical specificity to each hormone *(70)*. Pituitary glycoprotein hormone molecules are heterogeneous and exist as a mixture of isoforms resulting from variant glycosylation during posttranslational processing of two asparagine *N*-linked oligosaccharide chains on the α-subunit and one on the β-subunit *(71–74)*. The different degrees of terminal glycosylation (sialylation, fucosy-lation, and sulfation) of the isoforms impact the hormone bioactivity *(70,72,73,75,76)* through alterations in metabolic clearance rate *(75,77)* and signal transduction.

The biological activity of immunopurified TSH reflects the sum of the biopotency of each individual TSH isoform to induce adenylate cyclase in cell culture *(46,75)*. The ratio of bioactivity (B) and immunoreactivity (I) serves as an index of the overall potency of TSH. The TSH B/I ratio is higher in patients with TSH-omas than in controls *(75,78)* thus explaining the clinical observation of normal TSH levels resulting in goiter and thyroid hormone hypersecretion.

5.1.2. DIURNAL VARIABILITY

Loss of the normal circadian pattern of TSH has been observed in patients with TSH-oma. The normal pattern of thyrotropin secretion is characterized by a nocturnal surge, which begins in the late afternoon after 17:00 hours and peaks between 1:00 and 4:00 hours (79–81). Gesundheit et al. (78) demonstrated that the TSH fluctuations were sporadic and peak values did not occur in the evening in patients with TSH-oma. Later, Beckers et al. (82) described two patterns of abnormal TSH and α-subunit circadian rhythms in patients with TSH-secreting tumors: an inverted rhythm with an acrophase in the middle of the day and a nadir during the night and the complete absence of the circadian variation.

5.1.3. ALPHA-SUBUNIT

An important biochemical abnormality observed in TSH-oma is elevated baseline serum concentration of the α-subunit of glycoprotein hormones. Under most circumstances, α-subunit is synthesized in excess and the β-subunit limits the biosynthesis of the intact hormone, a finding exaggerated in TSH-oma (83). The discordance between α-subunit and TSH can be explained either by unbalanced secretion of the subunit or by the presence of different cells within the tumor that secret specific subunits (45,78,84–86). The latter explanation is supported by immunohistochemical studies demonstrating two populations of cells, one secreting α-subunit alone and another cosecreting α-subunit and TSH (46,87). It is hypothesized that molecular alterations secondary to the inciting event that resulted in monoclonal expansion impairs TSHβ production capability without affecting α-subunit synthesis. The exact mechanism is unknown, but a similar process has been demonstrated in tumor cell cultures where cells retain the ability to make Pit-1 mRNA but fail to make Pit-1 protein required for transcription of TSHβ, but not the TSHα gene (1). In general, in any given tumor there are more cells that stain for the α-subunit than for the β-subunit, which is responsible for the disproportional increase of the α-subunit (21,88).

The absolute level of the α-subunit is increased more frequently in macroadenomas than in microadenomas (8). Generally, the α-subunit is lower in patients with TSH-oma with normal or low gonadotropin levels. Postmenopausal patients with high gonadotropin levels have higher α-subunit levels (9) and this must be taken into consideration when evaluating the specificity of this test.

5.1.4. MOLAR RATIO: α-SUBUNIT/TSH

The increase in the serum α-subunit is greater than that of serum intact TSH, resulting in a high molar ratio of the serum α-subunit to TSH. The molar ratio is calculated using the following formula: (α-subunit in mcg/l divided by TSH in mU/l) times 10 *(89)*. The originally accepted normal cutoff value of one *(89)* is not adequate in many patients. An overlap exists between patients with TSH-oma and normal persons. Findings of ratios as high as 5.7 in normal subjects and 29.1 in hypergonadtropic patients have been reported in the literature *(9,90)*. The molar ratio has significant limitations in its use; individual values have to be compared to the values in control groups matched for TSH and gonadotropin levels *(90)*.

5.2. Thyroid Hormone Action: Clinical Endpoints

As expected, thyroid hormone levels correlate with indices of thyroid hormone action *(9)*, reflecting the absence of acquired resistance to thyroid hormone in patients with TSH-oma. Peripheral parameters of thyroid hormone action, such as sex hormone binding globulin (SHBG) and bone turnover markers, should not be relied on for diagnosis but rather further clinical confirmation of TSH-oma from resistance to thyroid hormone (RTH) because of the tissue variability exhibited in RTH. SHBG concentrations are normal in most patients with RTH and most TSH-oma patients have elevated SHBG *(91)*. Normal SHBG levels are found in patients with mixed GH/TSH tumors due to inhibitory action of GH on SHBG secretion *(63,91)*. In this situation, markers of bone resorption such as carboxyterminal cross-linked telopeptide of type I collagen have been used *(92)*.

5.3. Dynamic Testing of Thyroid Axis

5.3.1. TRH TEST

Stimulatory and inhibitory dynamic test can be used for diagnosis of the TSH-secreting tumor. Of these, the TRH test is the most useful test to evaluate TSH secretion. Serum TSH concentrations do not increase or are much lower in response to TRH in the majority of patients *(9,45,93)*. An absent response is defined as a TSH increment of less than 2 mU/l and a normal response is > 200% of baseline or > 5 mU/l *(9)*. The TRH test has good sensitivity and great specificity in patients with intact thyroid, with slight decrease in sensitivity after thyroidectomy *(9)*.

5.3.2. T3 SUPPRESSION TEST

The T3 suppression test has been used to differentiate the causes of inappropriate secretion of TSH. In normal and hypothyroid individuals, high-dose T3 results in suppression of serum TSH to levels $\leq 10\%$ of baseline. TSH-oma is characterized by absence of complete inhibition of both basal and TRH-stimulated TSH levels *(9,94)*. In contrast, significant suppression of basal TSH concentration is observed in up to 90% of patients with RTH *(93)*. Although the test is easy to perform and generally well tolerated in a highly selected population (young patients with no evidence of heart disease) *(94)*, this test has not been studied well in patients with TSH-oma where it may be useful to determine cure *(9)*.

T3 suppression has also been used as a test to distinguish TSH-oma from thyrotrope hyperplasia from long-standing hypothyroidism. Sarlis et al. *(95)* showed a rapid (within 1 week) shrinkage of a large pituitary mass caused by pituitary hyperplasia in a patient with primary hypothyroidism after administration of a single large dose of T3 (300 mcg) as part of suppression test followed by thyroxine therapy.

5.3.3. OCTREOTIDE SUPPRESSION

A short period of administration of octreotide has been given preoperatively to identify patients with tumors responsive to the somatostatin analog and will benefit from therapy if surgery is not curative. The degree of TSH suppression after octreotide has been used to differentiate patients with a tumor from patients with resistance to thyroid hormone as little TSH decrease is found in patients with resistance *(9,96)*. However, this test has not been fully validated and should be used rarely, if ever, in patients with atypical features at presentation, patients with prior thyroid treatment, hypergonadotropic patients, or when other diagnostic test are inconclusive.

5.4. Summary of Diagnostic Tests

In conclusion, the combination of TRH test, α-subunit, and α-subunit/ TSH ratio is diagnostic in almost all patients and can distinguish between the causes of inappropriate secretion of TSH (Table 2). TRH test has the best combined sensitivity and specificity in patients with intact thyroids (71% and 96%). In

Table 2
Value of Diagnostic Testing to Differentiate TSH-Secreting Tumors from Resistance to Thyroid Hormone in Patients with Intact Thyroid

	Sensitivity (%)	*Specificity (%)*
Elevated baseline TSH	43	88
Flat TRH	50	100
Abnormal response of TSH during TRH test	96	71
Elevated α-subunit	75	90
Elevated α-subunit/TSH	83	65

Abnormal response of TSH during TRH test; flat or decreased response of TSH during TRH test *(9)*.

contrast, α-subunit (90 and 82%) and the α-subunit/TSH ratio (90 and 73%) have the best combined sensitivity and specificity in patients with prior thyroid ablative therapy *(9)*. Unfortunately, TRH is no longer easily commercially available in the United States although it is still used at research centers such as the NIH. The positive predictive value of a flat or decreased TSH response to TRH is ~90% in patients with an intact thyroid.

6. RADIOGRAPHIC FEATURES

Evidence of a pituitary tumor by MRI or computed tomography (CT) in a person with high or inappropriately normal TSH is highly suggestive, but not diagnostic of a functional adenoma, since incidental pituitary tumors are detected on MRI in 10–20% of normal persons *(97,98)*. MRI is the method of choice for the initial evaluation of pituitary tumors because of its superior contrast resolution *(97)* particularly when performed before and after gadolinium injections. Before contrast enhancement, the normal pituitary gland is isointense with brain on T1-weighted images (Fig. 3A). After gadolinium, the appearance of focal hypointensity in the sellar area is the most common appearance of pituitary adenoma *(97)* (Fig. 3B). Moreover, MRI can best determine the relationship of the tumor to surrounding structures. Most TSH-omas are macroadenomas at the time of diagnosis and readily detectable by imaging. Invasion of or extension into the cavernous sinus, the sphenoid sinus, or chiasmatic compression are often present *(9)* (Fig. 4A–C).

A rare but distinguishing feature of TSH-oma is extensive, dense calcifications leading to the descriptive title "pituitary stones" *(40)*. Ectopic TSH-secreting tumors are also extremely rare with three cases reported to date. In two cases the thyrotroph tumor was located in the nasopharyngeal area *(99,100)* and one was found in the vemerosphenoidal junction *(101)*. In such cases, it is proposed that octreotide scanning may be helpful in locating the ectopic tumor *(102)*.

Thyrotroph cell hyperplasia with increased volume of the sella turcica may possibly be confused with TSH-oma *(103)*. In most cases this should not be difficult to elucidate; however, one striking case is reported in the literature in which erratic compliance with thyroid hormone replacement resulted in thyrotroph hyperplasia with a gadolinium-enhancing rim suggestive of a TSH-oma (Fig. 5A). Normalization of pituitary findings and appropriate TSH suppression after T3 administration excluded the diagnosis *(95)* (Fig. 5B). The co-occurrence of hyperplasia and TSH-oma has been reported *(53)*, giving credence to the theory that long-standing hypothyroidism can lead to adenoma formation.

The radiographic features of TSH-oma are useful in determining operative strategy and predicting clinical outcome of surgery. The main prognostic features are the size of the tumor and its invasiveness. Based on size alone, patients in the NIH series who presented with mean tumor diameter of 13 mm or less were cured in comparison with patients with larger tumors *(9)*. In an attempt to develop a detailed MRI staging system to predict outcomes, a cumulative score based on the degree of tumor invasion in the cavernous sinus, sphenoid sinus, and suprasellar extension was analyzed *(41)*. Investigators showed that patients with a score less than 2 (maximal score 9) had no residual tumoral TSH hypersecretion; patients scoring greater or equal to 6 continued to have evidence of tumoral hypersecretion. Patients with intermediate scores had favorable prognosis, but had persistent biochemical indices or abnormal dynamic tests after surgery.

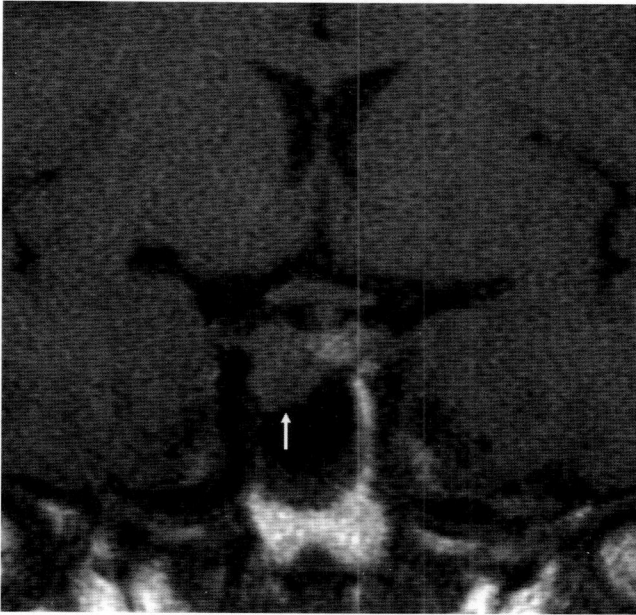

(A)

Fig. 3. (A–C). MRI of pituitary in a 54-year-old female with elevated serum thyroxine and triiodothyronine levels and normal TSH concentration (3.81 mcIU/ml). (A) Precontrast coronal T1-weighted image showing an adenoma in the right half of the pituitary gland. There is erosion and slanting of the floor of the sella turcica (arrow). The mass abuts the medial wall of the right internal carotid artery and possibly invades the right cavernous sinus. (B) Postcontrast coronal T1-weighted image of the pituitary showing homogenous enhancement of the adenoma. Note the degree of enhancement is slightly less intense when compared to normal pituitary parenchyma. (C) Postcontrast right parasagittal image of the pituitary. The homogenously enhancing adenoma is again identified and is shown to extend beyond the anatomical borders of the sella turcica (arrows).

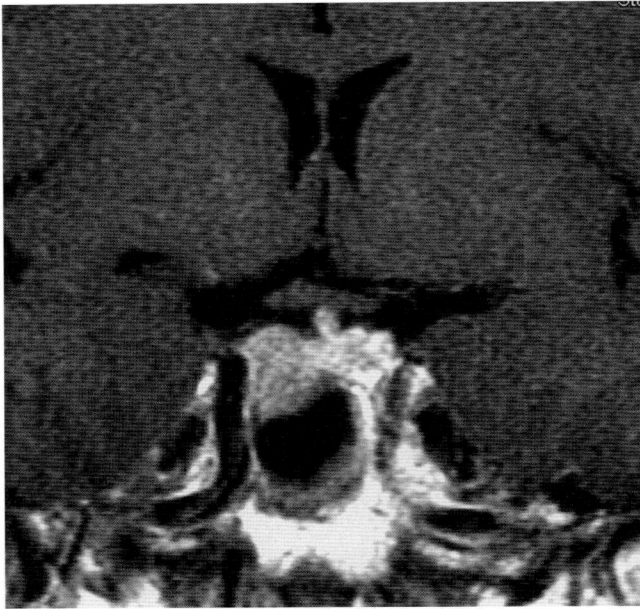

(B)

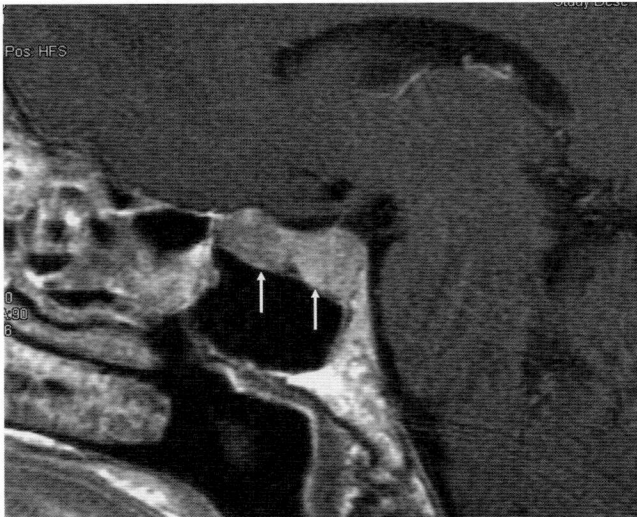

(C)

Fig. 3. (Continued)

With improved diagnostic techniques and awareness of the disease, TSH-secreting tumors are increasingly being diagnosed as microadenomas *(8)*. Currently, microadenomas account for 13–15% of all recorded cases in both clinical and surgical series *(3,63)*. Sensitivity in radiographic detection of the adenoma has not been a problem of clinical significance in TSH-oma; however, greater resolution to detect the extent of invasion would be helpful. As yet there is no published experience with MRI using magnets such as 3 tesla,

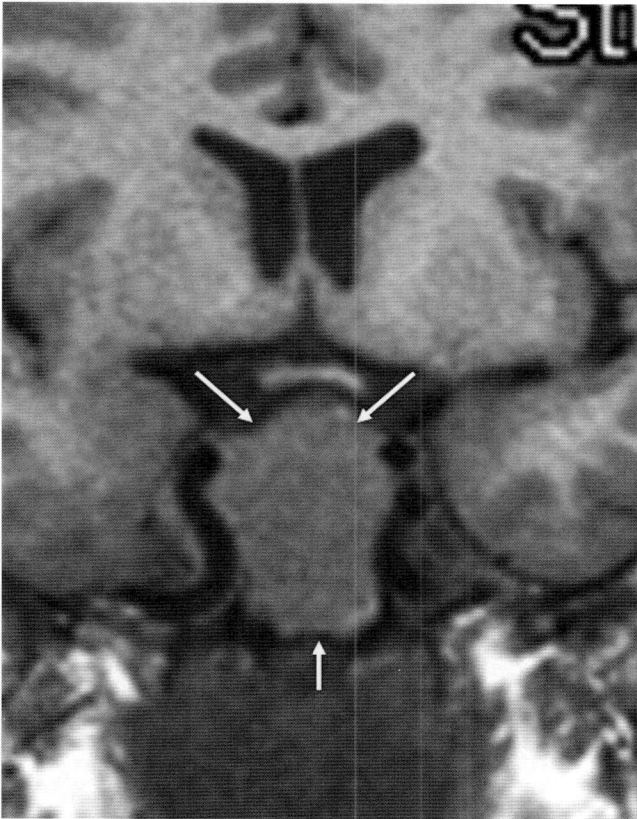

(A)

Fig. 4. Three consecutive precontrast T1-weighted coronal images of the pituitary gland in a 46-year-old patient with TSH-oma. (A) There is a large pituitary mass (arrows) that has destroyed the floor of sella turcica and has occupied the sphenoidal sinus. (B) Evidence of invasion of the right cavernous sinus with encasement of the right carotid artery (arrows). (C) Evidence of abutment of the right carotid artery and invasion of the right cavernous sinus (arrows). The adenoma has extended into the suprasellar cistern, but there is no compression of the optic chiasm.

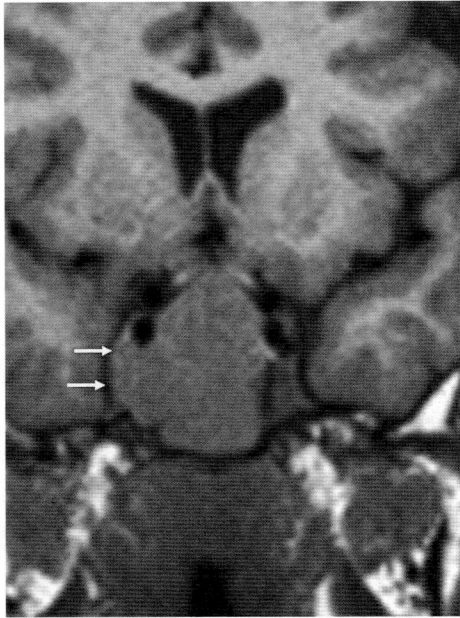

(B)

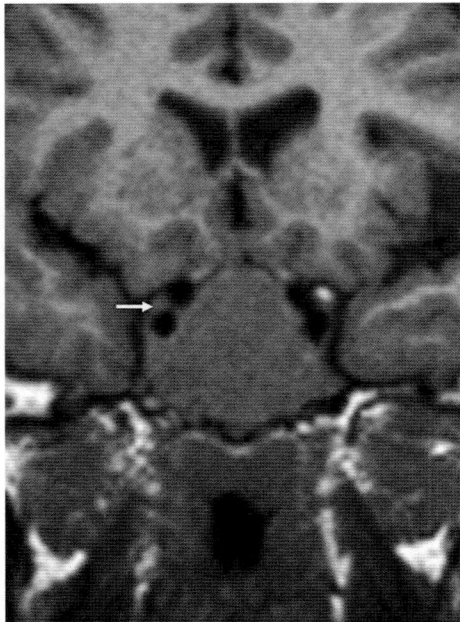

(C)

Fig. 4. (Continued)

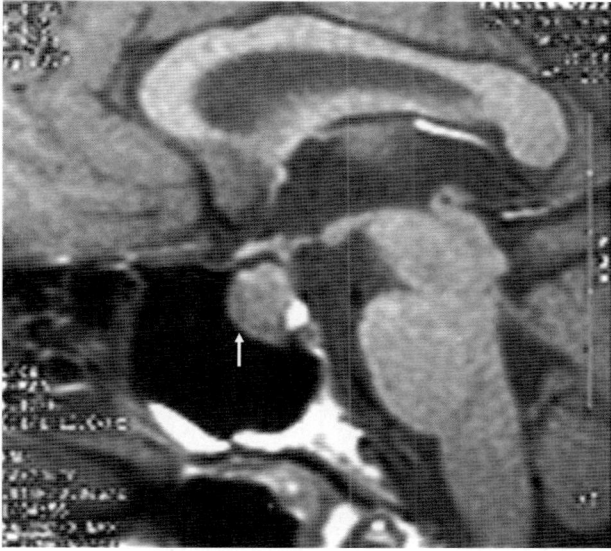
(A)

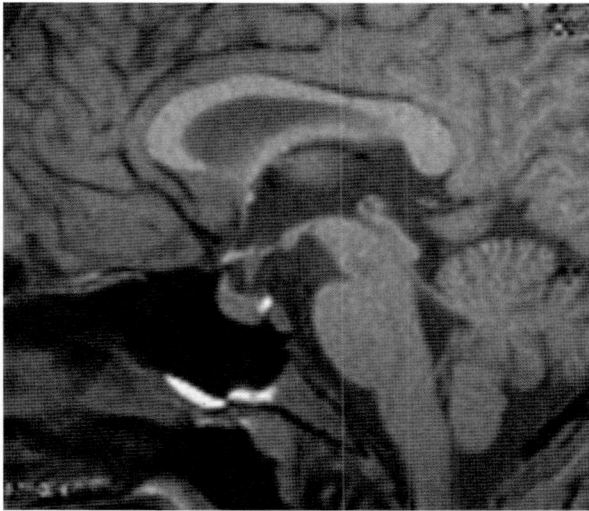
(B)

Fig. 5. Sagittal T1-weighted MRI scans of the pituitary in a 26-year-old woman with history of hypothyroidism. (A) The examination was performed prior to initiation of thyroid hormone therapy. There is enlargement of the pituitary gland extending above the diaphragm sella due to hyperplasia (arrow). (B) Image of the same patient on day 31 following initiation of thyroid hormone therapy. There is significant reduction in the size of the pituitary, which is now within the normal range for size.

which have superior ability to demonstrate tumor invasion into the cavernous sinus, optochiasmatic system, or parasellar areas *(104)*.

6.1. Somatostatin Analog Scintigraphy

Pituitary scintigram using radiolabeled octreotide has been used to image pituitary tumors expressing somatostatin receptors, especially GH-secreting tumors which are the most rich in somatostatin receptors; other pituitary tumors also express the receptors to a varying degree. TSH-omas have been successfully imaged using of [111]indium pentreotide single-photon emission tomography, thus confirming the presence of somatostatin receptors in these tumors *(105)*. Other labeled ligands, such I^{123}-Tyr^3- substituted octreotide, have also been used successfully *(106,107)*.

The role of scintigraphy is limited since its specificity is low and it cannot differentiate the type or functionality of the pituitary tumor. It cannot be used to guide therapy as the presence or absence of uptake does not predict the response to somatostatin analog. In the report of Socin et al. *(8)*, three out of seven patients undergoing octreotide scintigraphy had positive scans although all seven patients had a clinical response to analog with suppression of TSH on therapy. This imaging modality may play a role in the identification of ectopic tumors *(99)* or in the detection of metastasis in the rare cases of pituitary carcinoma.

6.2. Petrosal Sinus Sampling

Petrosal sinus sampling, an important tool in the differential diagnosis of hypercortisolism, has been used rarely to confirm the diagnosis of a TSH-secreting microadenoma. Blood is usually drawn simultaneously from the bilateral inferior petrosal sinus and from the peripheral vein before and after TRH stimulation *(108,109)*. In two patients, central to peripheral gradients of TSH confirmed the presence of TSH-oma and TSH levels differed between the right and left inferior petrosal sinuses, correctly localizing the side of the tumor *(108)*. In another case the absence of a central gradient in TSH concentrations confirmed thyroid hormone resistance and allowed the patient to avoid surgery *(109)*. These clinical experiences should be interpreted cautiously and this technique should not be relied upon to differentiate RTH from TSH-oma.

7. TREATMENT

7.1. Surgery

Surgical removal is the single best therapy for TSH-oma. Preoperative imaging is used to determine the surgical strategy; the transsphenoidal approach is preferred, although large tumors may rarely require a craniotomy *(9,110)*.

In the literature, about one-third of the patients are cured surgically, another third improve clinically, and the remainder are unchanged *(110,111)*. These dismal outcomes reflect the advanced stage at diagnosis and are similar to experiences with large GH adenomas with cavernous sinus invasion *(112)*. As in all pituitary tumors, the persistence of microscopic lateral dural invasion after surgery is a common cause of treatment failure *(113)*. The extensive fibrous nature of these tumors presents an additional challenge for the achievement of complete surgical removal of the tumor *(1,41)*.

The preoperative management includes restoring a euthyroid state in patients with moderate and severe hyperthyroidism to avoid intraoperative and postoperative complications *(114–116)*. Patients with mild hyperthyroidism can safely proceed with elective surgery or can be treated with beta-blockers only *(116)*. Somatostatin analogs, antithyroid medications, beta-blockers, or combinations of these drugs are conventionally used to diminish clinical signs and symptoms. Antithyroid medications such as propylthiouracil or methimazole usually reduce thyroid hormone production temporarily, but may require 6–8 weeks to achieve results *(114)*. Beta-blockers, particularly propranolol, are effective in the acute preoperative period and quickly ameliorate the symptoms of thyrotoxicosis *(117)*. Somatostatin analogs such as octreotide suppress TSH production within days and may reduce tumor size *(118)*. Recently, successful treatment of severe tumor-induced thyrotoxicosis with iopanoic acid has been described in two patients *(114)*.

With proper medical management, the surgical complications associated with TSH-oma are not different from those occurring after other pituitary tumors and are related to the size of the tumor and the experience of the surgeon. Serious complications such as CSF leak, meningitis, stroke, intracranial hemorrhage, and visual loss may occur in the immediate postoperative period in 3.4% of pituitary tumors *(119)*. A much more common postoperative problem is water balance instability. Transient diabetes insipidus occurs in up to half of all patients *(120)*. In a series of 92 surgical patients, isolated hyponatremia was detected in 25% of the cases on average 7 days postoperatively. Posterior pituitary damage and unregulated AVP release occurs with equal frequency in patients with TSH and ACTH-secreting or nonsecreting tumors *(121)*.

Another potential complication of the pituitary surgery is hypopituitarism. The loss of one or more anterior pituitary functional axes can occur in 3% of microadenomas and in 5% of macroadenomas *(119)*. Transient central hypothyroidism, secondary to normal thyrotroph suppression, is a desired outcome of surgery and may take 3–12 months to recover *(9)*, but thyroid hormone replacement is rarely needed.

7.2. External Radiation

Radiotherapy is recommended when surgery is not curative, contraindicated, or declined. Pituitary radiation results in tumor shrinkage and prevents regrowth in most patients *(122)*. Radiation should be performed when surgery is known to be incomplete, even if the patient is euthyroidic, as relapse is inevitable and the full effect of radiation is usually delayed for several months or even years. Common modalities employed for treatment of pituitary tumors are external photon-beam irradiation by use of conventional fractionation regimens *(123,124)* or stereotactic techniques including proton-beam irradiation *(125)* and gamma-knife radiosurgery *(126)*. Fractionated or conventional radiotherapy refers to the repeat administration of small doses of radiation in a relatively large target. Conventional dose fractionation schemes for pituitary tumors typically consist of 1.8–2.0 Gy in daily sessions with cumulative doses of no less than 45 Gy. Unfortunately, in the largest, most invasive tumors (2–3 cm), surgery and radiation therapy combined are not sufficient for control of the tumor *(9,110)*. There are potential long-term complications of external radiation, such as hypopituitarism, optic nerve neuropathy, impaired cognitive function, and increased risk of development of malignant brain tumors *(122)*. Another disadvantage of conventional fractionated radiotherapy is that the mean time to attain endocrine normalization is more than 5 years of therapy *(127)*.

Stereotactic radiotherapy has an advantage of targeted delivery of high-dose radiation to small intracranial tumors such as pituitary microadenoma with relatively few grouped beams and with almost no irradiation beyond the intended tissue *(125,128)*. The complications reported with this technique include hypopituitarism, focal temporal lobe injury, and injury to cranial nerves *(129)*. Doses and techniques range from single-fraction proton radiosurgery *(130)* to fractionated conformal proton-beam irradiation to doses of 50–54 Gy in 1.8-Gy to 2-Gy fractions *(125)*. Proton-beam stereotactic radiotherapy has been successfully employed in treatment of pituitary tumors, particularly GH-secreting and ACTH-secreting adenomas *(125,131)* with only limited experience in patients with TSH-oma *(125)*.

Radiosurgery with gamma knife has recently emerged as a treatment option for patients with residual or recurrent pituitary adenomas after surgical removal. The time required to achieve endocrine normalization is shorter than after conventional fractionated radiation therapy *(132)*. The limiting factor for the use of this technique in pituitary adenomas is proximity of the tumor to the optic chiasm and nerve that is the most radiosensitive tissue among neighboring structures *(132)*. The radiation dose required for tumor growth control is thought to be a minimum of 10–20 Gy *(133,134)*, and a higher dose is required for the endocrine control of pituitary tumors *(135)*. The possible complications are visual disturbance, hypopituitarism, injury to cranial nerves in the cavernous sinus, and radiation necrosis of the adjacent brain tissue *(136)*, but the risk may be less than with conventional fractionated radiotherapy *(132)*. There are few data published in the literature about use of this technique in patients with TSH-omas. Nevertheless, there are reports about the effective use of stereotactic surgery for the treatment of persistent or recurrent TSH-secreting adenomas, especially when the residual tissue invades the cavernous sinus *(9,126,137)*

7.3. Medical Therapy Targeted to the Tumor

Medical therapy is proposed for patients who remain hyperthyroid in spite of surgery, as an adjuvant to radiation therapy or in rare cases, as sole therapy.

7.3.1. SOMATOSTATIN ANALOGS

The analogs of somatostatin, octreotide, and lanreotide are the most effective therapy for the treatment of TSH-oma *(9,138–140)*. The abundant expression of somatostatin receptor subtypes two and five by most TSH-oma results in excellent responsivity to these agents *(141–143)*. In addition to decreasing TSH secretion, there is some evidence that somatostatin alters the bioactivity of TSH *(144)*. Taken together, the biological effects of somatostatin result in normalization of TSH in up to 79% of TSH-oma patients *(111)*. In some cases the marked suppression of TSH secretion results in hypothyroidism, requiring levothyroxine replacement *(28)*. Somatostatin therapy is the drug of choice when surgery cannot be performed as primary therapy *(145)*.

Somatostatin analogs are recognized to be tumoristatic in GH-secreting adenomas *(146,147)* and less so in nonsecreting pituitary adenomas. TSH-oma responds to somatostatin therapy with a size reduction observed in about 40% and resultant visual field improvement in 75% of patients *(111,140,148)*. Interestingly, the improvement in visual field defects has been reported to occur as soon as 3 h after initiation of treatment, while the tumor shrinkage is apparent after 3 months *(149,150)*.

The initial dose of the short-acting analog is usually 50 mcg subcutaneously twice daily. The dose is advanced to 100–200 mcg three times daily in 50 mcg increments at 2-week to 3-week intervals as tolerated. The goal of therapy is the titration of serum TSH and T4 concentrations to the normal range. The longer-acting compounds (SMS-LAR and lanreotide-SR) can be administered once every several weeks intramuscularly (monthly for SMS-LAR and 2–3 times per month for lanreotide-SR) *(151–153)*. These convenient preparations are effective in decreasing TSH secretion although their impact on tumor size is unknown *(19,38,154)*.

The side effects of octreotide include nausea, abdominal discomfort, diarrhea, glucose intolerance, and cholelithiasis. There is limited experience in pregnant women; somatostatin analog effectively restored euthyroidism in a mother and resulted in no serious adverse effects in the developing fetus, but its use is not approved during pregnancy (155,156).

Tachyphylaxis has been reported in 22% of patients requiring an increased dose (63). Escape from the inhibitory effects was recorded in 12% of patients and true resistance has been documented only in 5% of cases (63,148,157). The absence of effect of octreotide in some patients may be explained by the lack of sufficient somatostatin receptors or the presence of less effective subtypes of receptors on the tumor.

In conclusion, somatostatin analogs are highly effective in most patients with TSH-oma and can be used to reduced TSH secretion and potentially decrease tumor size. It is recommended primarily in the postoperative patient as an adjuvant to radiation therapy. It may be used as long as medical therapy is needed or until radiation therapy has its full effect.

7.3.2. DOPAMINE RECEPTOR AGONISTS

Prior to the availability of somatostatin analogs, dopamine receptor agonists such as bromocriptine were used with marginal effect at high doses (158). The newer, long-acting agonist cabergoline was demonstrated to have a good effect in a patient with mixed prolactin/TSH secretion with normalization of the pituitary hormone levels but without changes in tumor size (159,160). It has recently been reported that cabergoline and other ergot dopamine agonists are associated with increased risk of valvular heart disease in patients with Parkinson's disease (161,162). Although the doses of dopamine agonists used for endocrine disorders are lower than those used in Parkinson's disease, it is not known yet if long-term treatment with lower doses may lead to similar cardiac abnormalities.

7.3.3. THYROID HORMONE ANALOG

The sodium salt of 3,5,3'-triiodothyroacetic acid (TRIAC), a thyroid hormone analog that is not widely available, has been successfully used in several patients with TSH-omas (163,164). This compound is a natural metabolite of T3 and has altered peripheral metabolic activity, but retains inhibitory action at the pituitary. TRIAC effectively decreased TSH levels and circulating thyroid hormone levels with full clinical remission in five patients with TSH-producing tumors (164). No studies of the long-term effects of this thyroid hormone derivative on TSH-oma are available.

7.3.4. NUCLEAR RECEPTOR LIGANDS

TSH synthesis and secretion is regulated by the action of the thyroid receptor, a nuclear protein belonging to a family of nuclear receptors that includes the retinoids, vitamin D, and peroxisome proliferator-activated receptor (PPAR). There is emerging evidence that other agents may be used to decrease TSH secretion in the setting of TSH-oma.

The effects of retinol (vitamin A) on thyroid hormone production have been known since the 1940s, when Simkins et al. *(165)* demonstrated that patients with hyperthyroidism were successfully treated with massive doses of vitamin A *(166)*. Retinol and its metabolites are involved in the control of different biological processes *(167)* through two receptor types: retinoic acid receptors (RAR), which bind both all-*trans* retinoids and 9-*cis* retinoic acid, and retinoid receptors (RXR), which selectively bind 9-*cis* retinoic acid *(168)*. Retinoids are used in the treatment of dermatologic, hematopoietic, and oncologic diseases *(169,170)*. Central hypothyroidism has been described among the adverse effects of RXR-selective retinoids (rexinoids) including bexarotene *(171,172)*. Patients with cutaneous T-cell lymphoma treated with bexarotene had a 40-fold decrease in serum TSH and a 2-fold decrease in free thyroxine levels *(171)*. In normal volunteers, a single dose of bexarotene suppressed serum TSH by 78% within 8–12 h of administration *(173)*. Most cellular effects of these agents are mediated by RXR-alpha, RXR-beta, and RXR-gamma of which gamma is most abundantly expressed in the thyrotroph cells of the pituitary gland *(172)*. The RXR ligand, 9-*cis*-RA, causes central hypothyroidism by suppressing TSH beta gene expression in animals *(172)*. In summary, rexinoids can decrease TSH synthesis and deserve additional study in the treatment of states of inappropriate TSH secretion, including TSH-oma.

Recently, the presence of PPAR gamma has been described and confirmed immunohistochemically in cells from resected TSH-oma *(61,174)*. Moreover, Heaney et al. *(174)* demonstrated the suppression of tumor growth and GH, prolactin, and LH secretion with PPAR-gamma-activating thiazolidinediones (TZDs) in vivo and in vitro and proposed this agent as a novel treatment for control of pituitary tumors. The role of TZDs is as yet unexplored in patients with TSH-oma and may be a novel alternative or adjunct to current effective therapy.

7.4. Treatment Targeted to the Thyroid

Surgical or medical therapy directed at the thyroid gland was previously used in a large number of patients either because they were wrongly diagnosed with primary hyperthyroidism or in an attempt to control hyperthyroid symptoms. The success rate of these treatment modalities is low. Reduction in thyroid hormone secretion with thyroid-directed therapy does not suppress pituitary tumor activity and can in fact increase TSH secretion and stimulate tumor growth.

Moreover, the diagnosis in patients previously treated with antithyroid medications, surgery, or ablation is significantly delayed, increasing the invasiveness and aggressiveness of the tumor. In general, treatment with thyrostatic drugs, radioactive iodine, or thyroid surgery is not indicated in these patients and should be avoided. Occasionally, antithyroid medications can be used for short-term symptomatic relief of hyperthyroid symptoms in preparation for pituitary surgery. Many times due to mild symptoms, beta-adrenergic blockers such as propranolol are all that is needed to control thyrotoxicosis.

8. CRITERIA FOR CURE

There are no consensus criteria for cure of TSH-omas in the literature because of the rarity of the disease. Disappearance of neurological signs and symptoms and visual improvement is a good prognostic event but lacks sensitivity and specificity, because even debulking of the tumor may improve the above symptoms *(3)*. Cure has been defined as restoration of the euthyroidism and the absence of residual tumor on MRI *(9)*. Negative postoperative pituitary imaging is not sufficient alone to define cure as patients may have persistent TSH secretion and relapse due to microscopic dura invasion *(55)*.

Undetectable TSH levels after surgery are highly predictive of complete tumor removal in those patients who were hyperthyroid prior to surgery due to persistent suppression of normal thyrotropes *(55)*. Normalization of α-subunit or α-subunit/TSH molar ratio in patients with elevations in those parameters before surgery indicates complete resection of the tumor. In the late postoperative period, more comprehensive criteria of cure should be used, such as normalization dynamic testing of TSH secretion and imaging studies *(111)*. Some have suggested that normalization of T3 suppression test (decline of TSH to less than 10% of the baseline) may be the most predictive and most sensitive index of cure *(9,55)*. Resumption of a normal TSH response to TRH is suggestive of cure; however, a persistently abnormal TRH test is observed in cured patients with central postsurgical hypothyroidism.

It is recommended that pituitary imaging be performed every 2–3 years, but it should be done immediately if TSH levels are increased or if clinical symptoms reoccur. Because it may be hard to identify subtle changes in the postoperative sella on MRI, careful attention to TSH and α-subunit is recommended. In the case of persistent pituitary mass, close surveillance of visual fields is required.

9. CLINICAL OUTCOMES

Overall, with modern neurosurgical techniques and advances in external radiation therapy and medical therapy, patients with TSH-oma are expected to have excellent outcomes with control of tumor mass and thyrotoxicosis with limited morbidity. Early detection is necessary to achieve cure and requires widespread awareness of this disease entity and liberal thyroid hormone screening.

The historical surgical cure rate of 35% is too low *(6,9)*. With both surgery and radiotherapy, two-thirds of patients are clinically controlled, with less than 40% of patients cured (euthyroid state and eradication of the tumor) and an additional 30% of patients improved (biochemical control with residual tumor) *(63,126,175)*. Data on the recurrence rate or progression of TSH-oma after surgery and/or radiotherapy are still lacking and will be difficult to assess due to the rarity of the tumor. Postsurgical deaths are rare and have been reported in six cases *(9,29,78,176–178)*. The overall effect of therapies on survival is unknown.

10. CONCLUSION

The history of the diagnosis and medical therapy of thyrotropin-secreting pituitary adenomas is changing. Advances in early detection of TSH-oma will increase surgical cure rates. Thyrotoxicosis is effectively controlled with somatostatin analogs, thus decreasing morbidity without enhancing tumor growth as was seen with thyroid-specific therapy. Additional studies are required to assess the effect of newer methods to deliver radiation on the time to cure as well as novel pharmacologic therapies that are more cost-effective.

ACKNOWLEDGMENTS

We are indebted to Dr. Nicholas Patronas, Department of Radiology, Clinical Center, National Institutes of Health, for his thorough review of imaging studies and constructive comments and suggestions.

REFERENCES

1. McDermott MT, Ridgway EC. Central hyperthyroidism. Endocrinol Metab Clin North Am 1998;27:187–203.
2. Jailer JW, Holub DA. Remission of Graves' disease following radiotherapy of a pituitary neoplasm. Am J Med 1960;28:497–500.
3. Beck-Peccoz P, Persani L. Thyrotropin-Secreting Pituitary Adenomas: www. thyroid-manager.org, 2004.
4. Beck-Peccoz P, Persani L, Asteria C, et al. Thyrotropin-secreting pituitary tumors in hyper- and hypothyroidism. Acta Med Austriaca 1996;23:41–6.
5. Samuels MH, Ridgway EC. Glycoprotein-secreting pituitary adenomas. Baillieres Clin Endocrinol Metab 1995;9:337–58.
6. Mindermann T, Wilson CB. Thyrotropin-producing pituitary adenomas. J Neurosurg 1993;79:521–7.
7. Kourides IA. Inappropriate secretion of thyroid-stimulating hormone. Curr Ther Endocrinol Metab 1997;6:52–6.

8. Socin HV, Chanson P, Delemer B, et al. The changing spectrum of TSH-secreting pituitary adenomas: diagnosis and management in 43 patients. Eur J Endocrinol 2003;148:433–42.

9. Brucker-Davis F, Oldfield EH, Skarulis MC, Doppman JL, Weintraub BD. Thyrotropin-secreting pituitary tumors: diagnostic criteria, thyroid hormone sensitivity, and treatment outcome in 25 patients followed at the National Institutes of Health. J Clin Endocrinol Metab 1999;84:476–86.

10. Mantovani S, Beck-Peccoz P, Saccomanno K, et al. TSH-secreting pituitary adenomas are monoclonal in origin. 77th Annual Meeting of the Endocrine Society, Washington, DC, 1995.

11. Arafah BM, Nasrallah MP. Pituitary tumors: pathophysiology, clinical manifestations and management. Endocr Relat Cancer 2001;8:287–305.

12. Alexander JM, Biller BM, Bikkal H, Zervas NT, Arnold A, Klibanski A. Clinically nonfunctioning pituitary tumors are monoclonal in origin. J Clin Invest 1990;86:336–40.

13. Farfel Z, Bourne HR, Iiri T. The expanding spectrum of G protein diseases. N Engl J Med 1999;340:1012–20.

14. Chandrasekharappa SC, Guru SC, Manickam P, et al. Positional cloning of the gene for multiple endocrine neoplasia-type 1. Science 1997;276:404–7.

15. Zhuang Z, Ezzat SZ, Vortmeyer AO, et al. Mutations of the MEN1 tumor suppressor gene in pituitary tumors. Cancer Res 1997;57:5446–51.

16. Asteria C, Anagni M, Persani L, Beck-Peccoz P. Loss of heterozygosity of the MEN1 gene in a large series of TSH-secreting pituitary adenomas. J Endocrinol Invest 2001;24:796–801.

17. Poncin J, Stevenaert A, Beckers A. Somatic MEN1 gene mutation does not contribute significantly to sporadic pituitary tumorigenesis. Eur J Endocrinol 1999;140:573–6.

18. Burgess JR, Shepherd JJ, Greenaway TM. Thyrotropinomas in multiple endocrine neoplasia type 1 (MEN-1). Aust N Z J Med 1994;24:740–1.

19. Taylor TJ, Donlon SS, Bale AE, et al. Treatment of a thyrotropinoma with octreotide-LAR in a patient with multiple endocrine neoplasia-1. Thyroid 2000;10:1001–7.

20. Wynne AG, Gharib H, Scheithauer BW, Davis DH, Freeman SL, Horvath E. Hyperthyroidism due to inappropriate secretion of thyrotropin in 10 patients. Am J Med 1992;92:15–24.

21. Sanno N, Teramoto A, Matsuno A, Inada K, Itoh J, Osamura RY. Clinical and immunohistochemical studies on TSH-secreting pituitary adenoma: its multihormonality and expression of Pit-1. Mod Pathol 1994;7:893–9.

22. Pellegrini-Bouiller I, Morange-Ramos I, Barlier A, Gunz G, Enjalbert A, Jaquet P. Pit-1 gene expression in human pituitary adenomas. Horm Res 1997;47:251–8.

23. Umeoka K, Sanno N, Osamura RY, Teramoto A. Expression of GATA-2 in human pituitary adenomas. Mod Pathol 2002;15:11–7.

24. Ando S, Sarlis NJ, Krishnan J, et al. Aberrant alternative splicing of thyroid hormone receptor in a TSH-secreting pituitary tumor is a mechanism for hormone resistance. Mol Endocrinol 2001;15:1529–38.

25. Ando S, Sarlis NJ, Oldfield EH, Yen PM. Somatic mutation of TRbeta can cause a defect in negative regulation of TSH in a TSH-secreting pituitary tumor. J Clin Endocrinol Metab 2001;86:5572–6.

26. Gittoes NJ, McCabe CJ, Verhaeg J, Sheppard MC, Franklyn JA. An abnormality of thyroid hormone receptor expression may explain abnormal thyrotropin production in thyrotropin-secreting pituitary tumors. Thyroid 1998;8:9–14.

27. Dong Q, Brucker-Davis F, Weintraub BD, et al. Screening of candidate oncogenes in human thyrotroph tumors: absence of activating mutations of the G alpha q, G alpha

11, G alpha s, or thyrotropin-releasing hormone receptor genes. J Clin Endocrinol Metab 1996;81:1134–40.

28. Beck-Peccoz P, Persani L, Mantovani S, Cortelazzi D, Asteria C. Thyrotropin-secreting pituitary adenomas. Metabolism 1996;45:75–9.

29. Weintraub BD, Petrick PA, Gesundheit G, et al. TSH-secreting pituitary tumors. In: Medeiros-Neto G, Gaitan S, editors. Frontiers in Thyroidology. New York: Plenum; 1986. pp. 71–7.

30. Chanson P, Li JY, Le Dafniet M, et al. Absence of receptors for thyrotropin (TSH)-releasing hormone in human TSH-secreting pituitary adenomas associated with hyperthyroidism. J Clin Endocrinol Metab 1988;66:447–50.

31. Jaquet P, Hassoun J, Delori P, Gunz G, Grisoli F, Weintraub BD. A human pituitary adenoma secreting thyrotropin and prolactin: immunohistochemical, biochemical, and cell culture studies. J Clin Endocrinol Metab 1984;59:817–24.

32. Felix I, Asa SL, Kovacs K, Horvath E, Smyth HS. Recurrent plurihormonal bimorphous pituitary adenoma producing growth hormone, thyrotropin, and prolactin. Arch Pathol Lab Med 1994;118:66–70.

33. Dufy B, Mollard P, Dufy-Barbe L, Manciet G, Guerin J, Roger P. The electrophysiological effects of thyrotropin-releasing hormone are similar in human TSH- and prolactin-secreting pituitary cells. J Clin Endocrinol Metab 1988;67:1178–85.

34. Filetti S, Rapoport B, Aron DC, Greenspan FC, Wilson CB, Fraser W. TSH and TSH-subunit production by human thyrotrophic tumour cells in monolayer culture. Acta Endocrinol (Copenh) 1982;99:224–31.

35. Le Dafniet M, Brandi AM, Kujas M, Chanson P, Peillon F. Thyrotropin-releasing hormone (TRH) binding sites and thyrotropin response to TRH are regulated by thyroid hormones in human thyrotropic adenomas. Eur J Endocrinol 1994;130:559–64.

36. Spada A, Bassetti M, Martino E, et al. In vitro studies on TSH secretion and adenylate cyclase activity in a human TSH-secreting pituitary adenoma. Effects of somatostatin and dopamine. J Endocrinol Invest 1985;8:193–8.

37. Bertherat J, Brue T, Enjalbert A, et al. Somatostatin receptors on thyrotropin-secreting pituitary adenomas: comparison with the inhibitory effects of octreotide upon in vivo and in vitro hormonal secretions. J Clin Endocrinol Metab 1992;75:540–6.

38. Gancel A, Vuillermet P, Legrand A, Catus F, Thomas F, Kuhn JM. Effects of a slow-release formulation of the new somatostatin analogue lanreotide in TSH-secreting pituitary adenomas. Clin Endocrinol (Oxf) 1994;40:421–8.

39. Takano K, Ajima M, Teramoto A, Hata K, Yamashita N. Mechanisms of action of somatostatin on human TSH-secreting adenoma cells. Am J Physiol 1995;268: E558–64.

40. Webster J, Peters JR, John R, et al. Pituitary stone: two cases of densely calcified thyrotrophin-secreting pituitary adenomas. Clin Endocrinol (Oxf) 1994;40:137–43.

41. Sarlis NJ, Gourgiotis L, Koch CA, et al. MR imaging features of thyrotropin-secreting pituitary adenomas at initial presentation. AJR Am J Roentgenol 2003;181:577–82.

42. Ezzat S, Horvath E, Kovacs K, Smyth HS, Singer W, Asa SL. Basic fibroblast growth factor expression by two prolactin and thyrotropin-producing pituitary adenomas. Endocr Pathol 1995;6:125–134.

43. Mixson AJ, Friedman TC, Katz DA, et al. Thyrotropin-secreting pituitary carcinoma. J Clin Endocrinol Metab 1993;76:529–33.

44. Brown RL, Muzzafar T, Wollman R, Weiss RE. A pituitary carcinoma secreting TSH and prolactin: a non-secreting adenoma gone awry. Eur J Endocrinol 2006;154:639–43.

45. Terzolo M, Orlandi F, Bassetti M, et al. Hyperthyroidism due to a pituitary adenoma composed of two different cell types, one secreting alpha-subunit alone and another cosecreting alpha-subunit and thyrotropin. J Clin Endocrinol Metab 1991;72:415–21.

46. Beck-Peccoz P, Piscitelli G, Amr S, et al. Endocrine, biochemical, and morphological studies of a pituitary adenoma secreting growth hormone, thyrotropin (TSH), and alpha-subunit: evidence for secretion of TSH with increased bioactivity. J Clin Endocrinol Metab 1986;62:704–11.

47. Zemskova MS SM. Clinical features of thyrotropin-secreting pituitary adenomas. In press.

48. Kiso Y, Yoshida K, Kaise K, et al. A case of thyrotropin (TSH)-secreting tumor complicated by periodic paralysis. Jpn J Med 1990;29:399–404.

49. Alings AM, Fliers E, de Herder WW, et al. A thyrotropin-secreting pituitary adenoma as a cause of thyrotoxic periodic paralysis. J Endocrinol Invest 1998;21:703–6.

50. Hsu FS, Tsai WS, Chau T, Chen HH, Chen YC, Lin SH. Thyrotropin-secreting pituitary adenoma presenting as hypokalemic periodic paralysis. Am J Med Sci 2003;325:48–50.

51. Banerjee AK, Sharma BS, Kak VK. Clinically and biochemically silent thyrotroph adenoma with oncocytic change. Neurol India 2000;48:374–7.

52. Langlois MF, Lamarche JB, Bellabarba D. Long-standing goiter and hypothyroidism: an unusual presentation of a TSH-secreting adenoma. Thyroid 1996;6:329–35.

53. Ghannam NN, Hammami MM, Muttair Z, Bakheet SM. Primary hypothyroidism-associated TSH-secreting pituitary adenoma/hyperplasia presenting as a bleeding nasal mass and extremely elevated TSH level. J Endocrinol Invest 1999;22:419–23.

54. Losa M, Mortini P, Minelli R, Giovanelli M. Coexistence of TSH-secreting pituitary adenoma and autoimmune hypothyroidism. J Endocrinol Invest 2006;29:555–9.

55. Losa M, Giovanelli M, Persani L, Mortini P, Faglia G, Beck-Peccoz P. Criteria of cure and follow-up of central hyperthyroidism due to thyrotropin-secreting pituitary adenomas. J Clin Endocrinol Metab 1996;81:3084–90.

56. Beck-Peccoz P, Persani L. TSH adenomas: Clinical findings, endocrionology and treatment. In: Landolt A, Vance ML, Reily PL, editors. Pituitary Adenomas: Biology, Diagnosis and Treatment. London: Churchill Livingstone; 1996. pp. 139–55.

57. Sandler R. Recurrent hyperthyroidism in an acromegalic patient previously treated with proton beam irradiation: Graves' disease as probable etiology based on follow-up observations. J Clin Endocrinol Metab 1976;42:163–8.

58. O'donnell J, Hadden DR Weaver JA, Montgomery DAD. Thyrotoxicosis recurring after surgical removal of a thyrotrophin-secreting pituitary tumor. Proceedings of the Royal Society of Medicine, vol. 66, 1973.

59. Azukizawa M, Morimoto S, Miyai K, et al. TSH-producing pituitary adenoma associated with Graves' disease. In: Nagataki JSS, editor. Thyroid Research, vol. VII, Canberra: Australian Academy of Science; 1980. pp. 645–8.

60. Kamoi K, Mitsuma T, Sato H, et al. Hyperthyroidism caused by a pituitary thyrotrophin-secreting tumour with excessive secretion of thyrotrophin-releasing hormone and subsequently followed by Graves' disease in a middle-aged woman. Acta Endocrinol (Copenh) 1985;110:373–82.

61. Koriyama N, Nakazaki M, Hashiguchi H, et al. Thyrotropin-producing pituitary adenoma associated with Graves' disease. Eur J Endocrinol 2004;151:587–94.

62. Yovos JG, Falko JM, O'Dorisio TM, Malarkey WB, Cataland S, Capen CC. Thyrotoxicosis and a thyrotropin-secreting pituitary tumor causing unilateral exophthalmos. J Clin Endocrinol Metab 1981;53:338–43.

63. Beck-Peccoz P, Persani L. TSH-Producing adenomas. In: DeGroot L, Jameson JL, editors. Endocrinology, vol. 1, Philadelphia: Elsevier Saunders; 2006. pp. 475–84.

64. Borst GC, Eil C, Burman KD. Euthyroid hyperthyroxinemia. Ann Intern Med 1983; 98:366–78.
65. Refetoff S, DeWind LT, DeGroot LJ. Familial syndrome combining deaf-mutism, stuppled epiphyses, goiter and abnormally high PBI: possible target organ refractoriness to thyroid hormone. J Clin Endocrinol Metab 1967;27:279–94.
66. Beck-Peccoz P, Chatterjee VK. The variable clinical phenotype in thyroid hormone resistance syndrome. Thyroid 1994;4:225–32.
67. Watanabe K, Kameya T, Yamauchi A, et al. Thyrotropin-producing microadenoma associated with pituitary resistance to thyroid hormone. J Clin Endocrinol Metab 1993;76:1025–30.
68. Safer JD, Colan SD, Fraser LM, Wondisford FE. A pituitary tumor in a patient with thyroid hormone resistance: a diagnostic dilemma. Thyroid 2001;11:281–91.
69. Akiyoshi F, Okamura K, Fujikawa M, et al. Difficulty in differentiating thyrotropin secreting pituitary microadenoma from pituitary-selective thyroid hormone resistance accompanied by pituitary incidentaloma. Thyroid 1996;6:619–25.
70. Weintraub BD, Stannard BS, Magner JA, et al. Glycosylation and posttranslational processing of thyroid-stimulating hormone: clinical implications. Recent Prog Horm Res 1985;41:577–606.
71. Pierce JG, Parsons TF. Glycoprotein hormones: structure and function. Annu Rev Biochem 1981;50:465–95.
72. Magner JA. Thyroid-stimulating hormone: biosynthesis, cell biology, and bioactivity. Endocr Rev 1990;11:354–85.
73. Sergi I, Papandreou MJ, Medri G, Canonne C, Verrier B, Ronin C. Immunoreactive and bioactive isoforms of human thyrotropin. Endocrinology 1991;128:3259–68.
74. Ryan RJ, Charlesworth MC, McCormick DJ, Milius RP, Keutmann HT. The glyco-protein hormones: recent studies of structure-function relationships. Faseb J 1988;2: 2661–9.
75. Beck-Peccoz P, Persani L. Variable biological activity of thyroid-stimulating hormone. Eur J Endocrinol 1994;131:331–40.
76. Papandreou MJ, Persani L, Asteria C, Ronin C, Beck-Peccoz P. Variable carbohydrate structures of circulating thyrotropin as studied by lectin affinity chromatography in different clinical conditions. J Clin Endocrinol Metab 1993;77:393–8.
77. Magner J, Klibanski A, Fein H, et al. Ricin and lentil lectin-affinity chromatography reveals oligosaccharide heterogeneity of thyrotropin secreted by 12 human pituitary tumors. Metabolism 1992;41:1009–15.
78. Gesundheit N, Petrick PA, Nissim M, et al. Thyrotropin-secreting pituitary adenomas: clinical and biochemical heterogeneity. Case reports and follow-up of nine patients. Ann Intern Med 1989;111:827–35.
79. Patel YC, Alford FP, Burger HG. The 24-hour plasma thyrotrophin profile. Clin Sci 1972;43:71–7.
80. Weeke J. Circadian variation of the serum thyrotropin level in normal subjects. Scand J Clin Lab Invest 1973;31:337–42.
81. Caron PJ, Nieman LK, Rose SR, Nisula BC. Deficient nocturnal surge of thyrotropin in central hypothyroidism. J Clin Endocrinol Metab 1986;62:960–4.
82. Beckers A, Abs R, Mahler C, et al. Thyrotropin-secreting pituitary adenomas: report of seven cases. J Clin Endocrinol Metab 1991;72:477–83.
83. Weintraub BD, Gershengorn MC, Kourides IA, Fein H. Inappropriate secretion of thyroid-stimulating hormone. Ann Intern Med 1981;95:339–51.

84. Grisoli F, Leclercq T, Winteler JP, et al. Thyroid-stimulating hormone pituitary adenomas and hyperthyroidism. Surg Neurol 1986;25:361–8.
85. Tolis G, Bird C, Bertrand G, McKenzie JM, Ezrin C. Pituitary hyperthyroidism. Case report and review of the literature. Am J Med 1978;64:177–81.
86. Smallridge RC, Wartofsky L, Dimond RC. Inappropriate secretion of thyrotropin: discordance between the suppressive effects of corticosteroids and thyroid hormone. J Clin Endocrinol Metab 1979;48:700–5.
87. Turner HE, Vadivale A, Keenan J, Wass JA. A comparison of lanreotide and octreotide LAR for treatment of acromegaly. Clin Endocrinol (Oxf) 1999;51:275–80.
88. Mccutcheon IE, Olfield EH. Thyroid-Stimulating Hormone-Secreting Pituitary Tumors. In: Krisht AF, Tindall GT, editors. Pituitary Disorders: Comprehensive Management. Baltimore, MD: Lippincott Williams & Wikins; 1999. pp. 267–80.
89. Kourides IA, Ridgway EC, Weintraub BD, Bigos ST, Gershengorn MC, Maloof F. Thyrotropin-induced hyperthyroidism: use of alpha and beta subunit levels to identify patients with pituitary tumors. J Clin Endocrinol Metab 1977;45:534–43.
90. Beck-Peccoz P, Persani L, Faglia G. Glycoprotein hormone α-subunit in pituitary adenomas. Trends Endocrinol Metab 1992;3:41–45.
91. Beck-Peccoz P, Roncoroni R, Mariotti S, et al. Sex hormone-binding globulin measurement in patients with inappropriate secretion of thyrotropin (IST): evidence against selective pituitary thyroid hormone resistance in nonneoplastic IST. J Clin Endocrinol Metab 1990;71:19–25.
92. Persani L, Giammona E, Cortelazzi D, Beck-Peccoz P. Carboxyterminal cross-linked telopeptide of type I collagen (ICTP) as an index of thyroid hormone effects on the bone. 77th Annual Meeting of the Endocrine Society, 1995.
93. Refetoff S, Weiss RE, Usala SJ. The syndromes of resistance to thyroid hormone. Endocr Rev 1993;14:348–99.
94. Saad B, Liu A, Brucker-Davis F, Spencer C, LoPresti J, Nicoloff J. Simplified screening test for resistance to thyroid hormone (RTH)-the T3 challenge test (T3CT). 77th Annual Meet of The Endocrine Society, 1995.
95. Sarlis NJ, Brucker-Davis F, Doppman JL, Skarulis MC. MRI-demonstrable regression of a pituitary mass in a case of primary hypothyroidism after a week of acute thyroid hormone therapy. J Clin Endocrinol Metab 1997;82:808–11.
96. Beck-Peccoz P, Mariotti S, Guillausseau PJ, et al. Treatment of hyperthyroidism due to inappropriate secretion of thyrotropin with the somatostatin analog SMS 201–995. J Clin Endocrinol Metab 1989;68:208–14.
97. Hall WA, Luciano MG, Doppman JL, Patronas NJ, Oldfield EH. Pituitary magnetic resonance imaging in normal human volunteers: occult adenomas in the general population. Ann Intern Med 1994;120:817–20.
98. Molitch ME, Russell EJ. The pituitary "incidentaloma". Ann Intern Med 1990;112:925–31.
99. Cooper DS, Wenig BM. Hyperthyroidism caused by an ectopic TSH-secreting pituitary tumor. Thyroid 1996;6:337–43.
100. Collie RB, Collie MJ. Extracranial thyroid-stimulating hormone-secreting ectopic pituitary adenoma of the nasopharynx. Otolaryngol Head Neck Surg 2005;133:453–4.
101. Pasquini E, Faustini-Fustini M, Sciarretta V, et al. Ectopic TSH-secreting pituitary adenoma of the vomerosphenoidal junction. Eur J Endocrinol 2003;148:253–7.
102. Lamberts SW. Somatostatin analogs: their role in the treatment of growth hormone hypersecretion and excessive body growth. Growth Regul 1991;1:3–10.

103. Yamada T, Tsukui T, Ikejiri K, Yukimura Y, Kotani M. Volume of sella turcica in normal subjects and in patients with primary hypothyroidism and hyperthyroidism. J Clin Endocrinol Metab 1976;42:817–22.

104. Wolfsberger S, Ba-Ssalamah A, Pinker K, et al. Application of three-tesla magnetic resonance imaging for diagnosis and surgery of sellar lesions. J Neurosurg 2004;100: 278–86.

105. Melmed S. Evaluation of pituitary masses. In: DeGroot L, editor. Endocrinology, vol. 1, Philadelphia: Elsevier Saunders; 2006. pp. 388.

106. Lamberts SW, Bakker WH, Reubi JC, Krenning EP. Somatostatin-receptor imaging in the localization of endocrine tumors. N Engl J Med 1990;323:1246–9.

107. Lamberts SW, Krenning EP, Reubi JC. The role of somatostatin and its analogs in the diagnosis and treatment of tumors. Endocr Rev 1991;12:450–82.

108. Frank SJ, Gesundheit N, Doppman JL, et al. Preoperative lateralization of pituitary microadenomas by petrosal sinus sampling: utility in two patients with non-ACTH-secreting tumors. Am J Med 1989;87:679–82.

109. Itagaki Y, Yoshida K, Sakurada T, et al. A case of Refetoff syndrome: selective venous sampling for TSH is useful in differentiating thyroid hormone resistance from TSH secreting tumor. Tohoku J Exp Med 1989;157:69–78.

110. McCutcheon IE, Weintraub BD, Oldfield EH. Surgical treatment of thyrotropin-secreting pituitary adenomas. J Neurosurg 1990;73:674–83.

111. Beck-Peccoz P, Brucker-Davis F, Persani L, Smallridge RC, Weintraub BD. Thyrotropin-secreting pituitary tumors. Endocr Rev 1996;17:610–38.

112. Yamada S, Takada K, Ozawa Y, et al. The results of transsphenoidal surgery for 44 consecutive acromegalic patients. Endocr J 1997;44:395–402.

113. Penar PL, Nathan DJ, Nathan MH, Salsali A. Pituitary tumor diagnosis and treatment. Curr Neurol Neurosci Rep 2002;2:236–45.

114. Dhillon KS, Cohan P, Kelly DF, Darwin CH, Iyer KV, Chopra IJ. Treatment of hyper-thyroidism associated with thyrotropin-secreting pituitary adenomas with iopanoic acid. J Clin Endocrinol Metab 2004;89:708–11.

115. Nemergut EC, Dumont AS, Barry UT, Laws ER. Perioperative management of patients undergoing transsphenoidal pituitary surgery. Anesth Analg 2005;101:1170–81.

116. Schiff RL, Welsh GA. Perioperative evaluation and management of the patient with endocrine dysfunction. Med Clin North Am 2003;87:175–92.

117. Farling PA. Thyroid disease. Br J Anaesth 2000;85:15–28.

118. Caron P, Arlot S, Bauters C, et al. Efficacy of the long-acting octreotide formu-lation (octreotide-LAR) in patients with thyrotropin-secreting pituitary adenomas. J Clin Endocrinol Metab 2001;86:2849–53.

119. Thapar K, Laws ER. Pituitary Tumors. In: Kaya A, Laws ER, editors. Brain Tumors. London: Churchill Livingstone; 2001. pp. 804–54.

120. Hensen J, Henig A, Fahlbusch R, Meyer M, Boehnert M, Buchfelder M. Prevalence, predictors and patterns of postoperative polyuria and hyponatraemia in the immediate course after transsphenoidal surgery for pituitary adenomas. Clin Endocrinol (Oxf) 1999;50:431–9.

121. Olson BR, Rubino D, Gumowski J, Oldfield EH. Isolated hyponatremia after transsphe-noidal pituitary surgery. J Clin Endocrinol Metab 1995;80:85–91.

122. Plowman PN. Radiotherapy for pituitary tumours. Baillieres Clin Endocrinol Metab 1995;9:407–20.

123. Zierhut D, Flentje M, Adolph J, Erdmann J, Raue F, Wannenmacher M. External radio-therapy of pituitary adenomas. Int J Radiat Oncol Biol Phys 1995;33:307–14.

124. Sasaki R, Murakami M, Okamoto Y, et al. The efficacy of conventional radiation therapy in the management of pituitary adenoma. Int J Radiat Oncol Biol Phys 2000;47: 1337–45.
125. Ronson BB, Schulte RW, Han KP, Loredo LN, Slater JM, Slater JD. Fractionated proton beam irradiation of pituitary adenomas. Int J Radiat Oncol Biol Phys 2006;64:425–34.
126. Losa M, Mortini P, Franzin A, Barzaghi R, Mandelli C, Giovanelli M. Surgical management of thyrotropin-secreting pituitary adenomas. Pituitary 1999;2:127–31.
127. Landolt AM, Haller D, Lomax N, et al. Stereotactic radiosurgery for recurrent surgically treated acromegaly: comparison with fractionated radiotherapy. J Neurosurg 1998;88:1002–8.
128. Miller DW. A review of proton beam radiation therapy. Med Phys 1995;22:1943–54.
129. Kliman B, Kjellberg RN, Swisher B. Proton beam therapy of acromegaly: A 20-year experience. In: Ridgeway E, editor. Secretory tumors of the pituitary gland. New York: Raven Press; 1984. pp. 191–211.
130. Kjellberg RN, Shintani A, Frantz AG, Kliman B. Proton-beam therapy in acromegaly. N Engl J Med 1968;278:689–95.
131. Levy RP, Fabrikant JI, Frankel KA, Phillips MH, Lyman JT. Charged-particle radiosurgery of the brain. Neurosurg Clin N Am 1990;1:955–90.
132. Akabane A, Yamada S, Jokura H. Gamma knife radiosurgery for pituitary adenomas. Endocrine 2005;28:87–92.
133. Ganz JC, Backlund EO, Thorsen FA. The effects of gamma knife surgery of pituitary adenomas on tumor growth and endocrinopathies. Stereotact Funct Neurosurg 1993;61(Suppl 1):30–7.
134. Ganz JC. Gamma knife treatment of pituitary adenomas. Stereotact Funct Neurosurg 1995;64(Suppl 1):3–10.
135. Pollock BE, Nippoldt TB, Stafford SL, Foote RL, Abboud CF. Results of stereotactic radiosurgery in patients with hormone-producing pituitary adenomas: factors associated with endocrine normalization. J Neurosurg 2002;97:525–30.
136. Landolt A, Lomax N, Scheib SG. Stereotactic radiosurgery for pituitary adenoma. In: Pollock BE, editor. Contemporary Stereotactic Radiosurgery: Technique and Evaluation. New York: Futura Publishing Company; 2002. pp. 213–41.
137. Ohki M, Sato K, Tuchiya D, et al. A case of TSH-secreting pituitary adenoma associated with an unruptured aneurysm: successful treatment by two-stage operation and gamma-knife. No To Shinkei 1999;51:895–9.
138. Katznelson L, Oppenheim DS, Coughlin JF, Kliman B, Schoenfeld DA, Klibanski A. Chronic somatostatin analog administration in patients with alpha-subunit-secreting pituitary tumors. J Clin Endocrinol Metab 1992;75:1318–25.
139. Comi RJ, Gesundheit N, Murray L, Gorden P, Weintraub BD. Response of thyrotropin-secreting pituitary adenomas to a long-acting somatostatin analogue. N Engl J Med 1987;317:12–7.
140. Gorden P, Comi RJ, Maton PN, Go VL. NIH conference. Somatostatin and somatostatin analogue (SMS 201–995) in treatment of hormone-secreting tumors of the pituitary and gastrointestinal tract and non-neoplastic diseases of the gut. Ann Intern Med 1989;110: 35–50.
141. Ridgway EC, Klibanski A, Martorana MA, Milbury P, Kieffer JD, Chin WW. The effect of somatostatin on the release of thyrotropin and its subunits from bovine anterior pituitary cells in vitro. Endocrinology 1983;112:1937–42.
142. Shimon I, Yan X, Taylor JE, Weiss MH, Culler MD, Melmed S. Somatostatin receptor (SSTR) subtype-selective analogues differentially suppress in vitro growth hormone and

prolactin in human pituitary adenomas. Novel potential therapy for functional pituitary tumors. J Clin Invest 1997;100:2386–92.

143. Shimon I, Taylor JE, Dong JZ, et al. Somatostatin receptor subtype specificity in human fetal pituitary cultures. Differential role of SSTR2 and SSTR5 for growth hormone, thyroid-stimulating hormone, and prolactin regulation. J Clin Invest 1997;99:789–98.

144. Francis TB, Smallridge RC, Kane J, Magner JA. Octreotide changes serum thyrotropin (TSH) glycoisomer distribution as assessed by lectin chromatography in a TSH macroadenoma patient. J Clin Endocrinol Metab 1993;77:183–7.

145. Iglesias P, Diez JJ. Long-term preoperative management of thyrotropin-secreting pituitary adenoma with octreotide. J Endocrinol Invest 1998;21:775–8.

146. Ilias I, Mastorakos G. Complete regression of a somatotropin-secreting adenoma with lanreotide monotherapy. Presse Med 2000;29:1818–9.

147. Lamberts SW, Reubi JC, Krenning EP. Somatostatin analogs in the treatment of acromegaly. Endocrinol Metab Clin North Am 1992;21:737–52.

148. Chanson P, Weintraub BD, Harris AG. Octreotide therapy for thyroid-stimulating hormone-secreting pituitary adenomas. A follow-up of 52 patients. Ann Intern Med 1993;119:236–40.

149. Warnet A, Lajeunie E, Gelbert F, et al. Shrinkage of a primary thyrotropin-secreting pituitary adenoma treated with the long-acting somatostatin analogue octreotide (SMS 201–995). Acta Endocrinol (Copenh) 1991;124:487–91.

150. Mihailovic V, Feller MS, Kourides IA, Utiger RD. Hyperthyroidism due to excess thyrotropin secretion: follow-up studies. J Clin Endocrinol Metab 1980;50:1135–8.

151. Gillis JC, Noble S, Goa KL. Octreotide long-acting release (LAR). A review of its pharmacological properties and therapeutic use in the management of acromegaly. Drugs 1997;53:681–99.

152. Anthony LB. Long-acting formulations of somatostatin analogues. Ital J Gastroenterol Hepatol 1999;31(Suppl 2):S216–8.

153. Lancranjan I, Bruns C, Grass P, et al. Sandostatin LAR: a promising therapeutic tool in the management of acromegalic patients. Metabolism 1996;45:67–71.

154. Kuhn JM, Arlot S, Lefebvre H, et al. Evaluation of the treatment of thyrotropin-secreting pituitary adenomas with a slow release formulation of the somatostatin analog lanreotide. J Clin Endocrinol Metab 2000;85:1487–91.

155. Blackhurst G, Strachan MW, Collie D, Gregor A, Statham PF, Seckl JE. The treatment of a thyrotropin-secreting pituitary macroadenoma with octreotide in twin pregnancy. Clin Endocrinol (Oxf) 2002;57:401–4.

156. Caron P, Gerbeau C, Pradayrol L, Simonetta C, Bayard F. Successful pregnancy in an infertile woman with a thyrotropin-secreting macroadenoma treated with somatostatin analog (octreotide). J Clin Endocrinol Metab 1996;81:1164–8.

157. Karlsson FA, Burman P, Kampe O, Westlin JE, Wide L. Large somatostatin-insensitive thyrotrophin-secreting pituitary tumour responsive to D-thyroxine and dopamine agonists. Acta Endocrinol (Copenh) 1993;129:291–5.

158. Sriwatanakul K, McCormick K, Woolf P. Thyrotropin (TSH)-induced hyperthyroidism: response of TSH to dopamine and its agonists. J Clin Endocrinol Metab 1984;58:255–61.

159. Kerstens MN, Kapelle JW, van der Berg G. Partial remission with cabergoline pf a thyrotropin producing pituitary tumor cosecreting prolactin, 84th Annual Meeting of the Endocrine Society, San Francisco, CA, 2002.

160. Mulinda JR, Hasinski S, Rose LI. Successful therapy for a mixed thyrotropin-and prolactin-secreting pituitary macroadenoma with cabergoline. Endocr Pract 1999;5:76–9.

161. Zanettini R, Antonini A, Gatto G, Gentile R, Tesei S, Pezzoli G. Valvular heart disease and the use of dopamine agonists for Parkinson's disease. N Engl J Med 2007;356:39–46.

162. Schade R, Andersohn F, Suissa S, Haverkamp W, Garbe E. Dopamine agonists and the risk of cardiac-valve regurgitation. N Engl J Med 2007;356:29–38.

163. Beck-Peccoz P, Piscitelli G, Cattaneo MG, Faglia G. Successful treatment of hyperthyroidism due to nonneoplastic pituitary TSH hypersecretion with 3,5,3'-triiodothyroacetic acid (TRIAC). J Endocrinol Invest 1983;6:217–23.

164. Faglia G, Beck-Peccoz P, Piscitelli G, Medri G. Inappropriate secretion of thyrotropin by the pituitary. Horm Res 1987;26:79–99.

165. Simkins S. Use of massive doses of vitamin A in the treatment of hyperthyroidism. J Clin Endocrinol Metab 1947;7:574–85.

166. Sharma V, Hays WR, Wood WM, et al. Effects of rexinoids on thyrotrope function and the hypothalamic-pituitary-thyroid axis. Endocrinology 2006;147:1438–51.

167. Gudas LJ, Sporn MB, Roberts AB. Cellular biology and biochemistry of retinoids. In: Sporn MB, Roberts AB, Goodman DS, editors. The Retinoids. New York: Raven Press; 1994. pp. 443–520.

168. Aranda A, Pascual A. Nuclear hormone receptors and gene expression. Physiol Rev 2001;81:1269–304.

169. Orfanos CE. Treatment of psoriasis with retinoids: present status. Cutis 1999;64:347–53.

170. Altucci L, Wilhelm E, Gronemeyer H. Leukemia: beneficial actions of retinoids and rexinoids. Int J Biochem Cell Biol 2004;36:178–82.

171. Sherman SI, Gopal J, Haugen BR, et al. Central hypothyroidism associated with retinoid X receptor-selective ligands. N Engl J Med 1999;340:1075–9.

172. Haugen BR, Brown NS, Wood WM, Gordon DF, Ridgway EC. The thyrotrope-restricted isoform of the retinoid-X receptor-gamma1 mediates 9-*cis*-retinoic acid suppression of thyrotropin-beta promoter activity. Mol Endocrinol 1997;11:481–9.

173. Janssen JS, Sharma V, Berenz AJ, Golden WM, Hernandez TL, Hayes WR, Haugen BR. RXR-Selective Retinoids (Rexinoids) Affect TSH "Setpoint" in Thyrotropes., The Endocrine Society's 88th Annual Meeting, Boston, MA, 2006.

174. Heaney AP, Fernando M, Melmed S. PPAR-gamma receptor ligands: novel therapy for pituitary adenomas. J Clin Invest 2003;111:1381–8.

175. Greenman Y, Melmed S, Thyrotropin-secreting pituitary tumors. In: Melmed S, editor. The pituitary. Malden, MA: Blackwell Science; 2002. pp. 561–74.

176. Coculescu M, Pop A, Constantinovici A, Oprescu M, Temeli E, Marinescu I. Mixed TSH- and HGH-secreting pituitary adenoma. Endocrinologie 1982;20:209–16.

177. Menon PS, Suhasini G, Chawla MH, Modha PG, Damani BJ, Abhyankar SC. Thyrotoxicosis secondary to TSH secreting pituitary tumour. J Assoc Physicians India 1988;36: 283–5.

178. Azarnivar A, Chopra IJ. Tension Pneumocephalus After Transsphenoidal Resection of a Thyrotropin (TSH) Secreting Pituitary Adenoma. The Endocrinologist 1995:308–11.

14 Non-functioning Adenomas: *Diagnosis and Treatment*

Carrie R. Muh, MD, MS, and Nelson M. Oyesiku, MD, PhD, FACS

CONTENTS

1. INTRODUCTION
2. CLINICAL PRESENTATION
3. DIAGNOSIS
4. TREATMENT OPTIONS
5. PATHOLOGY
6. FOLLOW-UP
7. CONCLUSION

Summary

Nonfunctioning pituitary adenomas are benign lesions that generally present secondary to mass effect on the pituitary gland or optic nerves, leading to hypopituitarism and visual field defects. Surgical removal via a transsphenoidal approach is a safe and effective treatment for the vast majority of patients with these lesions. Here we will discuss the diagnosis and treatment of nonfunctioning pituitary adenomas.

Key Words: Nonfunctioning pituitary adenoma, Transsphenoidal surgery, Pituitary tumor.

1. INTRODUCTION

Pituitary tumors are neoplasms composed of adenohypophysial cells that constitute approximately 10–15% of all primary intracranial tumors *(1,2)*. Among pituitary tumors, approximately 30% are classified as nonfunctioning adenomas *(3)*.

The term nonfunctioning reflects the fact that these tumors do not cause clinical hormone hypersecretion and so do not cause hypersecretory syndromes

From: *Contemporary Endocrinology: Diagnosis and Management of Pituitary Disorders*
Edited by: B. Swearingen and B. M. K. Biller © Humana Press, Totowa, NJ

such as Cushing's disease, hyperprolactinemia, or acromegaly *(3)*. These tumors are uniquely heterogeneous, consisting of multiple histopathologic cell types *(4)*. Though they do not lead to clinical hormone hypersecretion, histopathologic evidence of hormone expression is evident in more than 40% *(5)*. These tumors are typically large upon presentation and manifest themselves via symptoms of mass effect, including headaches, visual field deficits, and hypopituitarism.

Enlargement of a nonfunctioning adenoma causes progressive bitemporal visual field loss and hypopituitarism, and puts the patient at risk for pituitary apoplexy. However, unlike the functional pituitary tumors that can be treated with bromocriptine or other chemical agents, there is no available effective medical therapy for nonfunctioning pituitary tumors. Surgical resection, generally via a transsphenoidal approach, is a safe and effective treatment for the vast majority of patients with these lesions. Throughout this chapter, we will discuss the diagnosis and treatment of these nonfunctioning pituitary adenomas.

1.1. Epidemiology

Pituitary adenomas have an annual incidence rate of 25 per one million people and comprise nearly 10% of all surgically resected brain tumors, with nonfunctioning adenomas and prolactinomas being the most common pituitary tumors *(6,7)*. Many of these lesions are subclinical and may never present during a patient's lifetime; autopsy studies have shown an 11–27% incidence of occult microadenomas *(1,2,8,9)*. Pituitary tumors are the third most common primary intracranial neoplasm after glioma and meningioma *(10)*, and are more common among African Americans where they account for more than 20% of central nervous system neoplasms *(11)*.

Microadenomas are most often found in women of childbearing age. Though studies in the 1970s seemed to reflect a higher incidence of adenomas among women than among men, it is unclear if there is actually a higher prevalence among women or if the effect of an adenoma on pituitary function and, therefore, reproduction leads to a higher rate of detection. Autopsy studies have shown no sex predominance *(7)*. Men with pituitary tumors more often present with macroadenomas in their fifth and sixth decades of life *(1)*.

1.2. Classification

The major classifications of pituitary tumors are based on their size, secretory abilities, and histology. Tumors measuring less than 10 mm in diameter are deemed to be microadenomas, while those measuring greater than 10 mm are macroadenomas. Those lesions that reach beyond the boundaries of the sella are considered to be giant adenomas.

Other chapters of this text discuss hormone-secreting lesions; however, even among nonfunctional tumors, multiple different tumor types are found. These include null cell tumors, oncocytoma, silent gonadotropin or glycopeptide-secreting tumors, silent corticotropin-secreting tumors, and silent somatotropin-secreting tumors *(4,12)*. Pathologic specimens of null cell adenomas do not express hormones and are present in oncocytic and nononcocytic varieties. Oncocytomas contain large amounts of mitochondria, produce hormones in vitro, and may show focal immunostaining for anterior pituitary hormones. Silent gonadotropes morphologically resemble glycopeptide-secreting tumors and stain positive for follicle-stimulating hormone (FSH), luteinizing hormone (LH), or their common alpha-subunit. Silent somatotropes stain positive for growth hormone (GH), while silent corticotrophs stain positive for adreno-corticotropic hormone (ACTH) on pathologic specimen but do not cause the clinical manifestations of acromegaly or hypercortisolemia.

According to the World Health Organization, tumors with benign histologic features are classified as typical pituitary adenomas while rare tumors that show invasive growth, an increased rate of mitosis, and extensive p53 nuclear reactivity are deemed atypical adenomas. The diagnosis of pituitary carcinoma is very rare, constituting less than 0.2% of pituitary tumors, and is made only when distant metastases are found *(13,14)*.

2. CLINICAL PRESENTATION

2.1. Mass Effect

The majority of nonfunctioning pituitary adenomas present with symptoms of mass effect *(15)*. Pressure on the pituitary gland can lead to hypopitu-itarism, resulting in decreased levels of anterior pituitary hormones. Generally, gonadotropins are the first hormones affected, then GH followed by TSH and ACTH. This hormone dysfunction may then lead to amenorrhea or hypogo-nadism and decreased libido due to low levels of LH or FSH; GH deficiency; or hypothyroidism with its associated weight gain, depression, fatigue, and mental slowing. These changes generally develop insidiously as the tumor grows over time, so the patient may not notice any change until the lesion is quite large. Adenomas may also lead to modest hyperprolactinemia as a result of mass effect on the pituitary stalk and subsequent disinhibition of hypothalamic dopamine on its target cells.

Any structure near the sella is at risk of compression. When these lesions enlarge superiorly, they put pressure on the optic chiasm, causing visual loss. Compression on the inferonasal fibers that are decussating at the anterior and inferior aspect of the chiasm leads to superior temporal quadrantanopia and then bitemporal hemianopia. An adenoma may grow laterally into the cavernous sinus, and though this rarely leads to extraocular muscle palsies, it may cause enough compression to cause deficits to sympathetic nerves and cranial nerves III, IV, or VI, leading to mydriasis, ptosis, facial pain, or, infrequently, diplopia. Headache due to pressure on the dura may occur as well.

Once a large tumor has extended out of the sella, it can cause pressure on the temporal or frontal lobes and even lead to hydrocephalus via obstruction of usual CSF pathways. Pituitary lesions may also be discovered incidentally during evaluations for other conditions or after trauma, often before the patient has noticed subtle hormone dysfunction or visual field abnormalities.

2.2. Apoplexy

Occasionally, pituitary adenomas become suddenly apparent due to apoplexy *(16,17)*. Pituitary apoplexy is a life-threatening situation in which the tumor undergoes sudden hemorrhage or infarction, causing significant expansion of the lesion with resulting compression of the pituitary gland, optic chiasm, optic nerves, and cavernous sinus. Nonfunctioning adenomas are the most common variety of pituitary lesion found in patients with apoplexy, that is in about 50% of such patients *(18)*. Presenting symptoms include sudden headache, visual loss, ophthalmoplegia, vomiting, impaired consciousness, and acute hormonal insufficiency *(4,16,19)*.

Hemorrhage or infarct can cause acute hypopituitarism, which may lead to cortisol deficiency and cardiovascular collapse. The apoplectic patient requires immediate corticosteroid supplementation as well as careful fluid and electrolyte monitoring and replacement. Long-term steroid or hormonal replacement may be necessary and visual field defects may be permanent after apoplexy. However, patients who undergo surgery quickly, within a few days of the apoplectic event, have a significantly better chance of recovering visual loss than do those in whom surgery is delayed by a week or more *(16,18)*. Patients with rapidly progressing visual or neurologic symptoms may have a lesion that is continuing to expand, and they therefore need to undergo urgent surgical evacuation of the lesion. Apoplexy should be considered in any patient with abrupt neuro-ophthalmologic deterioration and headache *(16)*.

Fortunately, this condition is quite rare. While clinically asymptomatic infarct or hemorrhage have been documented in up to 25% of pituitary adenomas *(17,20)*, significant infarct or hemorrhage leading to apoplexy is much less common. Though radiation treatment, endocrine changes, anticoagulation, and severe systemic illness may increase the risk of an apoplectic event, most cases appear to have no identifiable precipitating cause *(9,16)*.

2.3. Pediatric

Pituitary adenomas are rare in the pediatric population, comprising less than 3% of supratentorial pediatric tumors, and occurring at an incidence of 0.1 per one million children *(21)*. However, due to the location of these lesions and the importance of the anterior pituitary hormones on puberty, they can cause significant morbidity including delay in puberty, oligomenorrhea, and galactorrhea. The vast majority of pituitary lesions found in pediatric patients are macroadenomas; approximately 30% are nonfunctioning *(22)*. As tumor size is often proportional to endocrine and neurologic dysfunction, earlier detection of lesions may lead to better outcome; therefore adolescent patients with growth or pubertal abnormalities deserve an evaluation for a possible pituitary lesion *(23)*.

When a nonfunctional pituitary adenoma is discovered in a pediatric patient, the treatment is much the same as for an adult patient, generally consisting of surgical resection *(24,25)*.

3. DIAGNOSIS

Any patient presenting to a neurosurgeon with a pituitary lesion should undergo a complete neurologic and endocrinologic evaluation including a detailed history and examination to assess for signs or symptoms of Cushing's disease, hyperprolactinemia, or acromegaly.

Endocrinologic testing is needed to determine if there is a change in hormonal function. Important laboratory studies include prolactin, FSH, LH, GH, insulin-like growth factor 1 (IGF-1), ACTH, cortisol, thyroid-stimulating hormone (TSH), thyroxine, estradiol, and testosterone.

If patients have history, examination, or laboratory findings suggestive of a functional pituitary tumor, they may then need to undergo further studies such as an oral glucose tolerance test (OGTT), 24-h urine free cortisol (UFC), high-dose and low-dose dexamethasone suppression tests, or petrosal vein sampling. Hypersecretory syndromes have to be ruled out before the diagnosis of a nonfunctioning adenoma can be made. Glycoprotein-secreting nonfunctioning adenomas rarely secrete enough FSH or LH to cause a systemic elevation in the level of these hormones. A mildly elevated prolactin does not exclude a nonfunctioning tumor as the mass effect of a lesion distorting the pituitary stalk can lead to elevated prolactin levels up to 150 µg/ml via a phenomenon known as the "stalk effect."

Neuro-ophthalmologic examinations, including visual field testing and visual acuity, are necessary both preoperatively and postoperatively to document deficits and monitor changes.

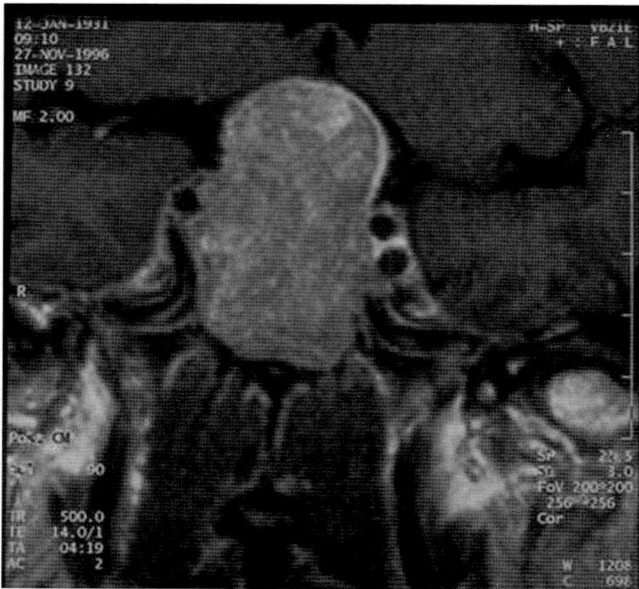

(A)

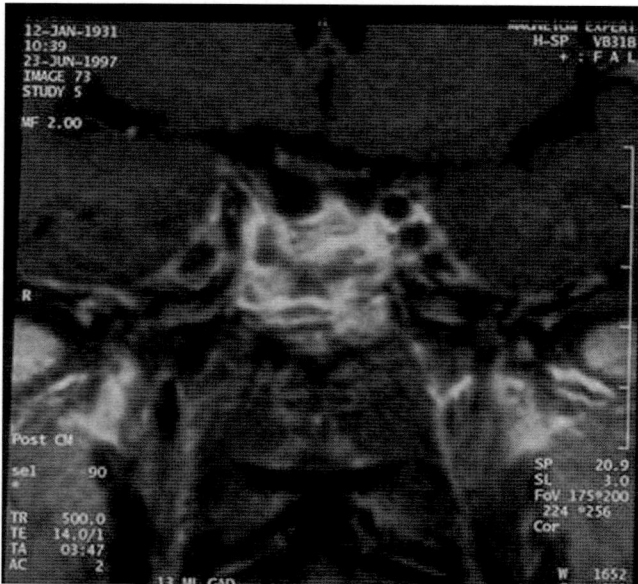

(B)

Fig. 1. (A) Coronal MRI with contrast. clinically nonfunctional pituitary macroadenoma (preoperative). (B) Coronal MRI with contrast. Clinically nonfunctional pituitary macroadenoma (postoperative).

On plain radiographs, an enlarged, rounded sella may be visible, and the sellar floor may appear doubled due to a thinned, asymmetrically worn lamina dura. Good-quality MRI and CT scans are needed to display the specific anatomical configuration of the adenoma *(26,27)*. High-resolution MRI with sagittal and coronal cuts through the sellar region is essential for surgical planning as it will show the exact size and location of the lesion as well as its relationship with the chiasm, cavernous sinus, and other surrounding structures (Fig. 1A,B) while CT will likely provide a better view of the anatomy of the sphenoid sinus.

Multiple other lesions must be considered in the differential diagnosis of a nonfunctioning pituitary adenoma, including multiple varieties of functioning pituitary tumors that should be able to be differentiated via laboratory results. A tuberculum sellae meningioma may grow to compress the chiasm; however, it will generally not show enlargement of the sella on imaging. A craniopharyngioma may be located in the sella turcica, though these are more often suprasellar lesions. A metastatic lesion to the sella would be likely to cause diabetes insipidus or extraocular muscle palsies, whereas these symptoms are rare among patients with pituitary adenomas. A Rathke's cleft cyst may appear similar to a cystic pituitary adenoma. An internal carotid artery aneurysm may fill the sella; however, this will appear as a flow void on MRI. Other lesions including a sarcoid granuloma or a tuberculoma are quite rare.

4. TREATMENT OPTIONS

4.1. Surgery

The standard treatment of a nonfunctioning pituitary adenoma is transsphenoidal resection of the tumor *(5,15,28,29)*. This is usually an elective procedure and is the first line of treatment for nearly all patients as it provides immediate relief from the mass effect and has a low rate of complications. An extended transsphenoidal approach may be needed when the tumor has reached beyond the sella *(30,31)* and a transcranial approach or combination transsphenoidal and transcranial approach should be considered if there is significant supratentorial tumor extension *(32,33)*. The goals of surgical resection are multifold; to eliminate mass effect from the pituitary and surrounding structure, to preserve or restore pituitary function, to preserve or restore visual and neurologic function, to resect enough lesion to prevent recurrence, and to obtain tissue for histologic and immunohistochemical study *(34)*.

4.1.1. Transsphenoidal Approach

Since Hermann Schloffer performed the first transsphenoidal resection of a pituitary tumor in 1907 *(35,36)* and Harvey Cushing popularized it in the decade that followed *(35,37)*, neurosurgeons have been trying to perfect the transsphenoidal approach. The standard methods in use today involve approaching the sella using either an endonasal or a sublabial approach.

Endonasal Transsphenoidal Approach. In the endonasal transsphenoidal approach, the patient's head is placed in the Mayfield head-holder; the body lies supine with the neck slightly extended and the head turned faintly toward the surgeon who is standing to the patient's right. This allows the surgeon a good view through the nares. Infusion of saline through a lumbar catheter may be helpful in permitting resection of the tumor.

A direct endonasal approach is an option in which one enters directly into the sphenoid sinus though the ostium. In the unilateral transseptal approach, a small incision is made in the right nostril and a submucosal plane is developed along the septum until the anterior wall of the sphenoid sinus is identified. A speculum is inserted and the septum is broken and deviated from left to right.

The operating microscope is brought into the field and the sphenoid sinus is opened with an osteotome and rongeurs. The opening is broadened to allow visualization of the lateral aspects of the sella and the speculum is advanced. At this point some surgeons choose to obtain fluoroscopic or image-guided confirmation of the sella position; however, direct visualization generally gives all the confirmation that one needs (Fig. 2A,B).

The sellar floor is then opened with an osteotome and an upbiting Kerrison rongeur. Once the dura is revealed, a midline vertical incision is made with a number 11 blade and upbiting scissors are used to open the dura and expose the tumor. The tumor is extracted in fragments using pituitary rongeurs, ring curettes, gentle suction, and irrigation (Fig. 3). There may be significant bleeding associated with adenoma removal, making adequate suction imperative, as bleeding generally only ceases once the tumor has been removed.

After resection of the lesion, a piece of fat harvested from the patient's abdomen is packed within the sphenoid sinus. The speculum is removed, the septum returned to midline, and the mucosa sutured shut at the inside edge of the nare with absorbable sutures. As the patient will have copious mucosal secretions in the immediate postoperative period, a nasal trumpet is placed in the nares to improve nasal respirations, and is removed the following day.

For patients with giant macroadenomas that cannot be completely resected using only a transsphenoidal approach, this surgery may be combined with a simultaneous pterional craniotomy. This provides significantly more exposure but also brings more risk and is needed for only a small subset of patients *(32)*.

Sublabial Transsphenoidal Approach. Pediatric patients with small nares and patients with large sellar tumors are often better served by a sublabial operation *(10)*. In this approach, the patient's upper lip is retracted and a horizontal incision is made in the upper gingival mucosa. The incision is

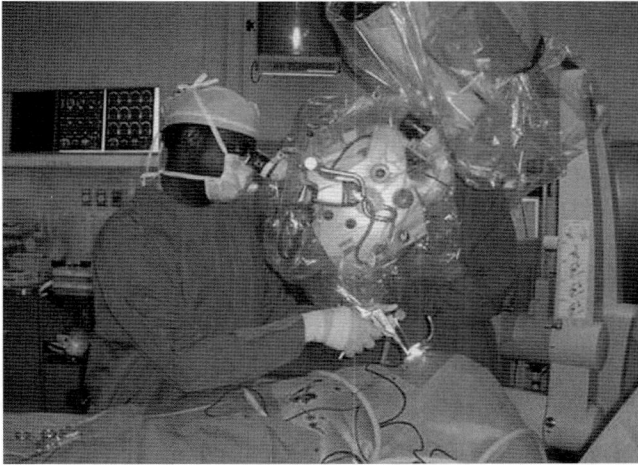

(A)

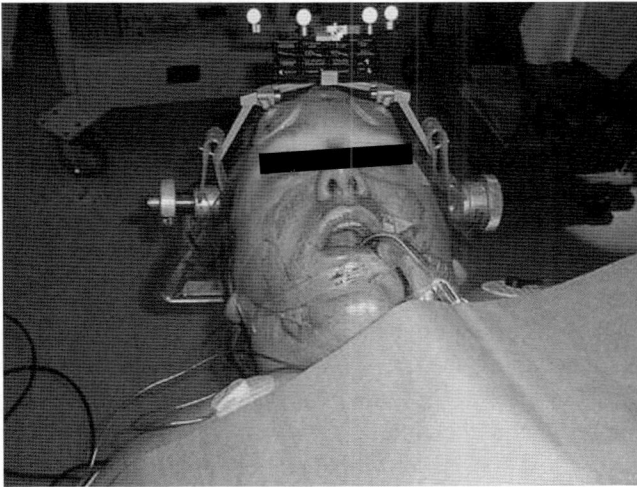

(B)

Fig. 2. Intraoperative setup. Transsphenoidal microsurgery.

followed down to the maxilla and floor of the nasal cavity. A vertical incision then separates the nasal mucosa from the septum. The anterior septum is broken and the speculum is inserted. The operating microscope is brought into the field and the operation continues in a similar fashion to the endonasal approach just described.

Neuronavigation or Endoscopy. The transsphenoidal operation may be performed with various assisting devices including frameless stereotactic

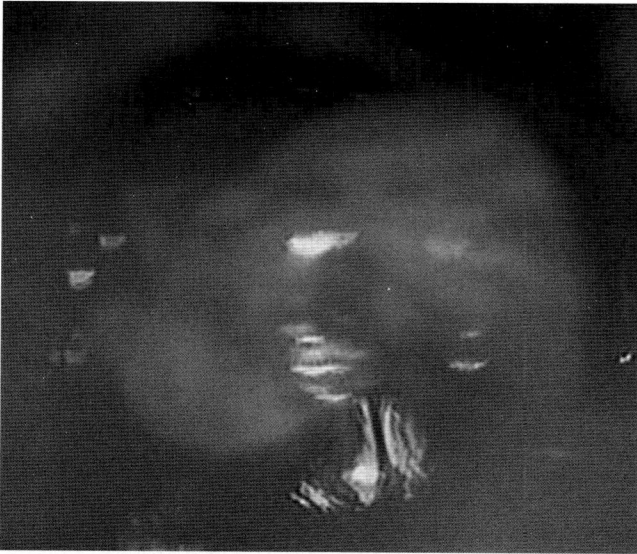

Fig. 3. Gross intraoperative appearance of pituitary adenoma.

neuronavigation or an endoscope. The benefit of neuronavigation is most significant with large or recurrent lesions where a prior operation has altered the normal anatomy *(38,39)*. The case is performed as described above; however, the surgeon is able to check his or her position at any point throughout the procedure to assess the proximity of surrounding structures or determine when he or she is approaching the outermost limits of the lesion.

When using the endoscope, the patient is positioned in a manner similar to that used for the standard endonasal approach. Once the posterior septum is reflected laterally and the anterior wall of the sphenoid is opened, a 4-mm or 2.7-mm endoscope is brought into the field in place of the operative microscope. The tumor is removed in the same manner as it is with the standard approach. The endoscope provides a wide field of view and angled scopes permit enhanced inspection of the walls of the sella and cavernous sinus to search for residual tumor. A fat graft is again used to pack the sphenoid sinus and tumor cavity, though the speculum is not needed with this approach *(36,40,41)*.

4.1.2. Outcomes

Mortality for patients undergoing transsphenoidal surgery is very low, approximately 0.5% *(42)*. Among giant macroadenomas, the mortality is slightly higher at approximately 1%. At 10-year follow-up, more than 80% of patients who underwent transsphenoidal resection of a nonfunctioning pituitary adenoma were alive and disease free *(11)*.

Complications from transsphenoidal surgery range from gravely serious, including intracranial hemorrhage, carotid artery injury, ischemic stroke, visual impairment, cerebrospinal fluid leak, and death, to more benign, including nasal septal perforation, fat graft hematoma, and epistaxis. The risk of stroke, death, or visual loss is less than 1%, while the risk of CSF rhinorrhea is 5% *(4)*.

After transsphenoidal removal of a pituitary adenoma, hormone levels must be closely followed as the patient is at risk for hypopituitarism. Patients are administered hydrocortisone postoperatively for 24 h and morning cortisol levels are checked for several days postoperatively. Patients with hypocortisolemia, less than 5–8 µg/dl, are treated with steroid replacement as needed.

Endocrine function is generally unchanged postoperatively, although tumor resection will frequently halt progressive loss of hormonal function. Unfortunately, approximately one-third of patients with nonfunctioning adenomas have some degree of hypopituitarism prior to their surgical treatment *(43)*. In one quarter of these patients, preoperative pituitary deficiencies will improve after surgery, although 10% of patients have some postoperative worsening of hormone function *(4,11)*. Fortunately, oral hormone replacement is generally sufficient for those patients whose pituitary deficiencies worsen or do not improve.

Diabetes insipidus and the syndrome of inappropriate antidiuretic hormone secretion (SIADH) are common, transient postoperative complications after transsphenoidal surgery. Up to 20% of patients will develop diabetes insipidus, though this rarely lasts permanently. It is therefore imperative to closely monitor postoperative fluid balance, serum sodium, and urine specific gravity.

In a small percentage of patients, hyponatremia can occur a week or more after the surgery. Temporary postoperative polyuria occurs in up to 30% of patients; however, this persists more than 1 week in less than 10% *(10)*.

Following operative decompression of a nonfunctioning adenoma, visual field defects will improve in 70–89% of patients *(44–46)*, approximately 7% will have no significant change, and visual fields will worsen in less than 4% of patients *(46,47)*.

Following resection of a giant macroadenoma, when it is likely that some residual tumor may remain, a rare but potentially fatal complication is postoperative apoplexy. In one study of 134 surgically resected giant adenomas, four patients suffered fatal postoperative pituitary apoplexy *(19)*. This must be closely monitored in these patients.

4.2. Medical Therapy

Medical therapy is frequently available for hypersecretory tumors; however, there are no available effective drug regimens for nonfunctioning pituitary lesions. Among tumors that were unable to be resected completely, medical and radiation therapy may be considered.

Multiple medical therapies have been tested. Dopamine agonists have been shown to lead to a small reduction in tumor size in less than 10% of patients, and visual deficits have improved among some patients with macroadenomas who were treated with octreotide *(44,45)*; however, most patients with nonfunctioning pituitary tumors have gained no clinical or biochemical benefit from medical agents.

4.3. Radiation Therapy

If the patient is elderly or medically unstable, radiation therapy may be the only viable treatment for a pituitary lesion. More often, however, radiation therapy is used in patients who have significant residual tumor or tumor recurrence after surgical resection *(48)*.

Radiation therapy controls tumor growth in 80–98% of patients with nonfunctioning tumors *(48)*. Stereotactic radiosurgery is preferable to conventional external-beam radiotherapy when there is a favorable configuration of tumor relative to the chiasm and optic nerves (Fig. 4A,B).

Conventional radiotherapy calls for fractionated doses of 1.6 to 2 Gy four or five times per week for 5 or 6 weeks, until a maximum dose of 45 to 50 Gy is achieved *(12)*. Pituitary adenomas respond rather slowly, with benefits delayed up to 1 year or more. Delayed hypopituitarism, radiation necrosis, optic neuropathy, neuropsychiatric changes, and development of a radiation-induced second neoplasm are among the risks of this therapy.

Because of these complications, stereotactic gamma knife, linear accelerator (LINAC), or fractionated stereotactic radiotherapy are now used more often than conventional radiotherapy. Stereotactic radiosurgery uses only a single session to deliver focused radiation to the lesion with significantly less radiation to surrounding structures. It is not risk free, however. The optic nerves and the optic chiasm are very radiation sensitive, and the radiation dose to the chiasm must be kept under 10 Gy *(49)*. Patients with adenomas closer than approximately 3 mm from the optic chiasm are therefore not candidates for stereotactic radiosurgery, though they may undergo conventional radiotherapy.

The risks of radiation-induced second neoplasm and neuropsychiatric changes are decreased with stereotactic radiosurgery versus with conventional radiotherapy. Hypopituitarism is the most common side effect of pituitary irradiation with an incidence of 13–56% *(50,51)*. Long-term overall risk for brain necrosis is estimated at 0.2%. Other side effects are rare; they include optic neuropathy in 1.7%, vascular changes in 6.3%, neuropsychological

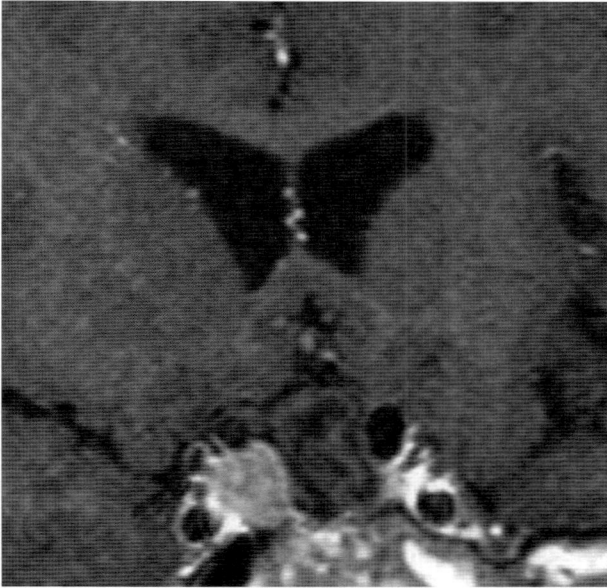

(A)

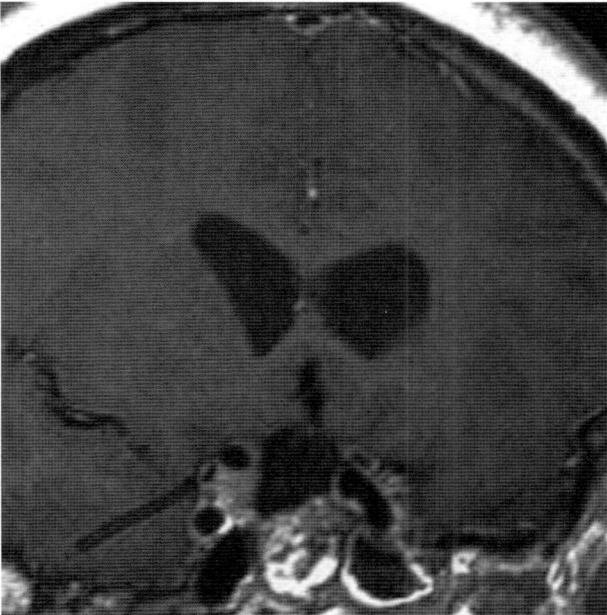

(B)

Fig. 4. (A) Residual pituitary adenoma following transsphenoidal surgery. Treated by stereotactic radiosurgery. (B) Residual pituitary adenoma following transsphenoidal surgery, 3 years after stereotactic radiosurgery.

problems in 0.7%, and secondary malignancies in 0.8% *(50)*. Both forms of radiation therapy have delayed benefits, though stereotactic radiosurgery induces remission more rapidly than does fractionated radiotherapy *(52,53)*. Patients may require hormonal supplementation or other medical therapy while awaiting the benefits of radiation.

4.4. Recurrent Lesions

Unfortunately, even after successful surgical resection, 10–20% of pituitary tumors recur within 5 to 6 years *(44,45)*. Some centers have therefore routinely treated pituitary adenoma patients with radiation after successful transsphenoidal resection. Even among these postoperatively radiated patients, however, 2–36% still develop tumor recurrence *(54)*. The risks associated with radiation therapy are low, but are not negligible, so this practice is becoming less common and is only rarely recommended in specific cases.

Recurrent tumors can be treated with repeated transsphenoidal resection, radiation therapy, or sometimes with medical therapy. For patients with recurrent adenomas that are not causing visual or significant endocrine abnormalities, observation of the lesion may often be the best next step.

5. PATHOLOGY

The touch preparation performed by pathologists at the time of surgery shows a monolayer of adenomatous cells. Staining of a pituitary adenoma with hematoxylin and eosin stain generally shows the cells arranged in a papillary fashion. Immunohistochemical staining may be negative or may show production of anterior pituitary hormones including FH, LSH, GH, or ACTH (Table 1).

cDNA microarray analysis has revealed that the folate receptor, FR-α, is overexpressed in nonfunctioning adenomas *(55)*. FR-α acts as a high-affinity

Table 1
Histopathologic Classification of Nonfunctioning Adenomas

Cell Type	Hormone Expression	Percentage (%) of NF Tumors
Silent gonadotrope	LH, FSH, or the alpha-subunit	40–79
Null cell	None	17
Silent corticotrope	ACTH	8
Oncocytoma	None	6
Silent somatotrope	GH	3

folate transporter that has been found to be overexpressed in other tumor types and may provide cells with a growth advantage. Studies using ^{3}H-labeled folate have shown that FR-α is capable of binding folate, so the overexpressed receptor may mediate vitamin uptake in the tumor cells. Comparison between varieties of nonfunctioning adenomas revealed that immunohistochemically negative tumors produce more FR-α than do those tumors that express hormones. Understanding the factors that enhance tumor growth may provide researchers with targets for future medical treatments.

6. FOLLOW-UP

Postoperative evaluation with MRI and CT is best delayed for at least 4 to 6 weeks postsurgery because of the difficulty in analyzing the tumor area in the midst of postoperative changes. Mass effect seen in the early postoperative period will generally resolve and can be documented with serial MRIs *(56)*. If the patient's vision is stable or improved following transsphenoidal resection, it may be best to simply follow up, even if there is persistent mass effect on the imaging studies.

Most patients with nonfunctioning pituitary adenomas should have annual MRI or CT scans, as well as visual and endocrine evaluations, whether or not they have had surgical or radiation treatment. If these tumors are not treated, they tend to grow slowly over months or years.

Because of the significant recurrence rate following transsphenoidal surgery and the considerable number of patients who develop hypopituitarism after radiation therapy, even successfully treated patients need to be followed closely by their medical team. They should also follow up with general practitioners who can closely monitor their general health as studies have demonstrated that patients who have a nonfunctioning pituitary adenoma, even those patients who do not undergo radiation, are at an increased risk of developing a second neoplasm elsewhere *(6,57)*.

7. CONCLUSION

Nonfunctioning pituitary adenomas most frequently present with visual field deficits secondary to mass effect; however, endocrine function must be fully evaluated in all patients. Transsphenoidal resection of nonfunctioning pituitary tumors has a low morbidity and mortality and very effectively relives the mass effect on the normal gland and visual apparatus. Radiation therapies and medical regimens are more appropriate for patients who cannot undergo surgical resection or who suffer from recurrent lesions.

Because of the need for close endocrine, visual, and neurologic monitoring of patients with pituitary tumors, it is important to have close collaboration among the multiple physicians treating each patient. We rely on our colleagues in endocrinology, neuro-ophthalmology, neuropathology, neuroradiology, and radiosurgery to assist in our care of each patient.

REFERENCES

1. Monson JP. The epidemiology of endocrine tumours. Endocr Relat Cancer 2000;7:29–36.
2. Clayton RN, Stewart PM, Shalet SM, Wass JA. Pituitary surgery for acromegaly. Should be done by specialists. BMJ 1999;319:588–9.
3. Asa SL, Kovacs K. Clinically non-functioning human pituitary adenomas. Can J Neuro Sci 1992;19:228–35.
4. Oyesiku NM. Nonfunctioning Pituitary Adenomas. In: Rengachary SS, Ellenbogen RG, editors. Principles of Neurosurgery, 2nd ed. New York: Elsevier Mosby; 2005. pp. 593–602.
5. Katznelson L, Alexander JM, Klibanski A. Clinically nonfunctioning pituitary adenomas. J Clin Endocrinol Metab 1993;76:1089–94.
6. Clayton RN. Sporadic pituitary tumours: from epidemiology to use of databases. Baillieres Best Pract Res Clin Endocrinol Metab 1999;13:451–60.
7. Buurman H, Saeger W. Subclinical adenomas in postmortem pituitaries: classification and correlations to clinical data. Euro J Endocrinol 2006;154:753–8.
8. Burrow GN, Wortzman G, Rewcastle MB, Holgate RC, Kovaks K. Microadenomas of the pituitary and abnormal sellar tomograms in an unselected autopsy series. N Engl J Med 1981;304:156–8.
9. Arita K, Tominaga A, Sugiyama K, et al. Natural course of incidentally found nonfunctioning pituitary adenoma, with special reference to pituitary apoplexy during follow-up examination. J Neurosurg 2006;104:884–91.
10. Jane JA, Jr., Laws ER, Jr. The management of non-functioning pituitary adenomas. Neurology India 2003;51:461–5.
11. Jane JA, Jr., Laws ER, Jr. Chapter 13: Surgical management of pituitary adenomas. In: Endotext.com; 2004.
12. Colin P, Jovenin N, Delemer B, et al. Treatment of pituitary adenomas by fractionated stereotactic radiotherapy: A prospective study of 110 patients Int J Radiat Oncol Biol Phys 2005;62:333–41.
13. Al-Shraim M, Asa SL. The 2004 World Health Organization classification of pituitary tumors: What is new? Acta Neuropathol 2006;111:1–7.
14. Ragel BT, Couldwell WT. Pituitary carcinoma: a review of the literature. Neurosurg Focus 2004;16:1–9.
15. Greenman Y, Melmed S. Diagnosis and management of nonfunctioning pituitary tumors. Annu Rev Med 1996;47:95–106.
16. Biousse V, Newman NJ, Oyesiku NM. Precipitating factors in pituitary apoplexy. J Neurol Neurosurg Psychiatr 2001;71:542–5.
17. Sibal L, Ball SG, Connolly V, et al. Pituitary apoplexy: a review of clinical presentation, management and outcome in 45 cases. Pituitary 2004;7:157–63.
18. Bills DC, Meyer FB, Laws ER, Jr., et al. A retrospective analysis of pituitary apoplexy. Neurosurgery 1993;33:602–9.
19. Ahmad FU, Pandey P, Mahapatra AK. Post operative 'pituitary apoplexy' in giant pituitary adenomas: a series of cases. Neurology India 2005;53:326–8.
20. Semple P, Laws E. Complications in a contemporary series of patients who underwent transsphenoidal surgery for Cushing's disease. J Neurosurg 1999;91:175–9.

21. Singh SK, Aggarwal R. Pituitary adenomas in childhood. Indian J Ped 2005;72:583–91.
22. De Menis E, Visentin A, Billeci D, et al. Pituitary adenomas in childhood and adolescence. Clinical analysis of 10 cases. J Endocrinol Invest 2001;24:92–7.
23. Artese R, D'Osvaldo DH, Molocznik I, et al. Pituitary tumors in adolescent patients. Neurol Res 1998;20:415–7.
24. Maira G, Anile C. Pituitary adenomas in childhood and adolescence. Can J Neurol Sci 1990;17:83–7.
25. Jagannathan J, Dumont AS, Jane JA, Jr. . Diagnosis and management of pediatric sellar lesions. Front Horm Res 2006;34:83–104.
26. Dolinskas C, Simeone F. Transsphenoidal hypophysectomy: postsurgical CT findings. Am J Neuroradiol 1985;6:45–50.
27. Mikhael MA, Ciric IS. MR imaging of pituitary tumors before and after surgical and/or medical treatment. J Computer Assisted Tomogr 1988;12:441–5.
28. Ebersold MJ, Quast LM, Laws ER, Scheithauer B, Randall RV. Long-term results in transsphenoidal removal of nonfunctioning pituitary adenomas. J Neurosurg 1986;64: 713–9.
29. Mortini P, Losa M, Barzaghi R, Boari N, Giovanello M. Results of transsphenoidal surgery in a large series of patients with pituitary adenoma. Neurosurgery 2005;56:1222–33.
30. Kaptain GJ, Vincent DA, Sheehan JP, Laws ER, Jr. Transsphenoidal approaches for the extracapsular resection of midline suprasellar and anterior cranial base lesions. Neurosurgery 2001:94–100.
31. Kouri JG, Chen MY, Watson JC, Oldfield EH. Resection of suprasellar tumors by using a modified transsphenoidal approach. Report of four cases. J Neurosurg 2000;92:1028–35.
32. Alleyne CHJ, Barrow DL, Oyesiku NM. Combined transsphenoidal and pterional craniotomy approach to giant pituitary tumors. Surg Neurol 2002;57:380–90.
33. Liu JK, Weiss MH, Couldwell WT. Surgical approaches to pituitary tumors. Neurosurg Clin N Am 2003;14:93–107.
34. De Divitiis E, Esposito F, Cavallo LM, Cappabianca P. Chapter 14A: Pituitary Adenomas and Craniopharyngiomas. Philadelphia: Lippincott, Williams and Wilkins; 2004.
35. Kante AS, Dumont AS, Asthagiri AR, Oskouian RJ, Jane JA, Jr., Laws ER, Jr. The transsphenoidal approach: a historical perspective. Neurosurg Focus 2005;18.
36. Kabil MS, Eby JB, Shahinian HK. Fully endoscopic endonasal vs. transseptal transsphenoidal pituitary surgery. Minim Invas Neurosurg 2005;48:348–54.
37. Cohen-Gadol AA, Liu JK, Laws ER, Jr. Cushing's first case of transsphenoidal surgery: the launch of the pituitary surgery era. J Neurosurg 2005;103:570–4.
38. Jane JA, Jr., Thapar K, Alden TD, Laws ER, Jr. Fluoroscopic frameless stereotaxy for transsphenoidal surgery. Neurosurgery 2001; 48:1302–8.
39. Elias WJ, Chadduck JB, Alden TD, Laws ER, Jr. Frameless stereotaxy for transsphenoidal surgery Neurosurgery 1999;45:271–5; discussion 5–7.
40. Jho HD, Alfieri A. Endoscopic endonasal pituitary surgery: evolution of surgical technique and equipment in 150 operations. Minim Invasive Neurosurg 2001;44:1–12.
41. Jho HD, Carrau RL. Endoscopic endonasal transsphenoidal surgery: experience with 50 patients. J Neurosurg 1997;87:44–51.
42. Trautmann JC, Laws ER, Jr. Visual status after transsphenoidal surgery at the Mayo Clinic, 1971–1982. Am J Ophthalmol 1983;96:200–8.
43. Flickinger JC, Nelson PB, Martinez AJ, Deutsch M, Taylor F. Radiotherapy of nonfunctional adenomas of the pituitary gland. Results with long-term follow-up. Cancer 1989;63:2409–14.

44. Shimon I, Melmed S. Management of pituitary tumors. Ann Intern Med 1998;129:472–83.
45. Orrego JJ, Barkan AL. Pituitary disorders. Drug treatment options. Drugs 2000;59:93–106.
46. Peter M, Tribolet N. Visual outcome after transsphenoidal surgery for pituitary adenomas. Br J Neurosurg 1995;9:151–7.
47. Powell M. Recovery of vision following transsphenoidal surgery for pituitary adenomas. Br J Neurosurg 1995;9:367–73.
48. Milker-Zabel S, Debus J, Thilmann C, Schlegel W, Wannenmacher M. Fractionated stereotactically guided radiotherapy and radiosurgery in the treatment of functional and nonfunctional adenomas of the pituitary gland. Int J Radiat Oncol Biol Phys 2001;50:1279–86.
49. Jackson IM, Noren G. Gamma knife radiosurgery for pituitary tumours. Baillieres Best Pract Res Clin Endocrinol Metab 1999;13:461–9.
50. Becker G, Kocher M, Kortmann RD, et al. Radiation therapy in the multimodal treatment approach of pituitary adenoma. Strahlenther Onkol 2002;178:173–86.
51. Benveniste RJ, King WA, Walsh J, Lee JS, Delman BN, Post KD. Repeated transsphenoidal surgery to treat recurrent or residual pituitary adenoma. J Neurosurg 2005;102:1004–12.
52. Powell JS, Wardlaw SL, Post KD, Freda PU. Outcome of radiotherapy for acromegaly using normalization of insulin-like growth factor I to define cure. J Clin Endocrinol Metab 2000;85:2068–71.
53. Zhang N, Pan L, Wang EM, Dai JZ, Wang BJ, Cai PW. Radiosurgery for growth hormone-producing pituitary adenomas. J Neurosurg 2000;93:6–9.
54. Dekkers OM, Pereira AM, Roelfsema F, et al. Observation alone after transsphenoidal surgery for nonfunctioning pituitary macroadenoma. J Clin Endocrinol Metab 2006;91:1796–801.
55. Evans CO, Young AN, Brown MR, et al. Novel patterns of gene expression in pituitary adenomas identified by complementary deoxyribonucleic acid microarrays and quantitative reverse transcription-polymerase chain reaction. J Clin Endocrinol Metab 2001;86:3097–107.
56. Rajaraman V, Schulder M. Postoperative MRI appearance after transsphenoidal pituitary tumor resection. Surg Neurol 1999;52:592–8.
57. Popovic V, Damjanovic S, Micic D, et al. Increased incidence of neoplasia in patients with pituitary adenomas. Clin Endocrinol 1998;49:441–5.

15 Pituitary Surgery: *Techniques*

William F. Chandler, MD, *and Ariel L. Barkan,* MD

CONTENTS

1. INTRODUCTION
2. TRANSSPHENOIDAL APPROACHES
3. TRANSCRANIAL APPROACHES
4. INDICATIONS FOR SURGERY
5. CHOICE OF APPROACH
6. REOPERATION

Summary

This chapter discusses the surgical techniques used in the management of pituitary tumors and other forms of sellar disease, with an emphasis on the transsphenoidal approach. Potential complications are described. Alternative techniques and their relative merits are presented.

Key Words: Transsphenoidal surgery.

1. INTRODUCTION

Although most tumors in the region of the sella can be approached via the sphenoid sinus, selected tumors require a different trajectory to maximize tumor removal and minimize the risk of the surgical procedure (Fig. 1). The development of these various approaches is based both on the historical progression of experience and on the development of new technology, but the major reason for the wide range of surgical choices is the unique location of the sella and the considerable variety of lesions occurring in and around the sella. We will describe both the transsphenoidal and transcranial approaches.

From: *Contemporary Endocrinology: Diagnosis and Management of Pituitary Disorders*
Edited by: B. Swearingen and B. M. K. Biller © Humana Press, Totowa, NJ

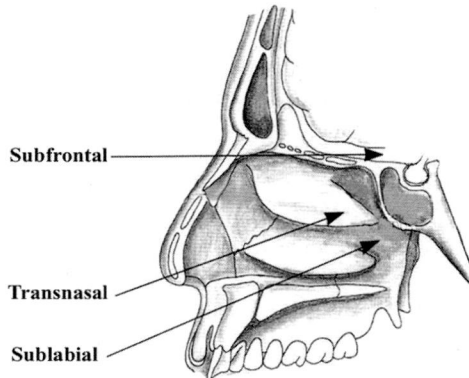

Fig. 1. Approaches to the sella. This midline sagittal view of the anterior skull base diagrams the three common approaches to the sella.

2. TRANSSPHENOIDAL APPROACHES

From 1979 to 1999 we used the "classic" sublabial transseptal approach to the sphenoid sinus, utilizing the operating microscope. Although this worked very well, with excellent tumor visualization and a minimal complication rate, it was uncomfortable for the patient and often resulted in numbness of the front teeth and sublabial area. Since 1999 we have used the direct transnasal approach to the sella with an overnight stay in the hospital. We still prefer the microscope with three-dimensional visualization to the endoscope, but use the endoscope available for selected situations. The various transsphenoidal approaches will be presented.

2.1. Transnasal Approach

2.1.1. TRANSNASAL—DIRECT TRANSSPHENOIDAL MICROSCOPE APPROACH

Griffith and Veerapen *(1)* in 1987 and Cooke and Jones *(2)* in 1994 described a transnasal approach involving placing a long narrow speculum directly into the nostril all the way back to the sphenoid ostia on one side. Until this time, most transnasal approaches involved an incision just inside the nose, with submucosal dissection all the way up along the septum. By making the mucosal incision at the very back of the nasal airway passage, there is no disruption of the midline septum of the nose and therefore less discomfort and minimal chance of a postoperative anterior septal perforation. The visualization of the sphenoid sinus and sella is excellent and is as good as the sublabial approach.

We have adopted this approach and our current technique involves the following steps:

1. Induction of general anesthesia, placement of Foley catheter.
2. Placement of the head in three-point fixation.
3. Lateral fluoroscopic imaging of sella, which provides localization of instruments in the up-down and front-back directions.
4. Registration of the patient using a frameless stereotactic system if the patient has a small sella and a microadenoma, which provides localization of instruments in the side-to-side direction.
5. Preparation of abdomen for fat graft.
6. Draping of all surgical areas and the operating microscope.
7. Placement of long self-retaining speculum (Kilian) in the right nostril and visualization using the operating microscope.
8. Identification of inferior and middle turbinates (laterally).
9. Placement of speculum just medial to middle turbinate.
10. Lateral fluoroscopic imaging to identify relationship to sphenoid sinus.
11. Removal of mucosa overlying rostrum of sphenoid sinus on the right and along the posterior midline by using a long Bovie tip.
12. Entering sphenoid sinus on the right by using small osteotome.
13. Undercutting the posterior midline nasal septum and gently pushing the septum toward the opposite side.
14. Moving the speculum deeper to the anterior border of the sphenoid sinus and fixing in the holding device.
15. Entering the sphenoid sinus and removing all septae.
16. Visualizing the sella with the microscope and confirming with fluoroscopy.
17. Identifying the midline in patients with a small sella by using a frameless stereotactic system.
18. Using a high-speed drill to open the sella and removing the bone with small Kerrison punches.
19. Opening the dura with a microblade avoiding the superior one-third to reduce CSF leakage.
20. Curetting out the macroadenoma (tumor) with various ring curettes.
21. Making an incision in the pituitary and exploring for the presence of a microadenoma.
22. After tumor is removed, placing the fat in the tumor cavity, reconstructing the sellar opening with an allograft, and filling the sphenoid sinus with fat and tissue glue.
23. Placing a small telfa pack over the sphenoid sinus opening and removing the speculum. The patient can breathe easily with the pack in place and it is removed at the bedside the next morning before discharge.
24. Discharging all patients on Cortef, 10 mg q am and 5 mg at noon. Other pituitary hormones are replaced as needed. Patients generally return in 4 weeks for their postoperative follow-up.

Intraoperative complications are fortunately rare, but include injury to the carotid artery, injury to the optic pathways, injury to the contents of the cavernous sinuses (cranial nerves III, IV, V, and VI), intracranial bleeding, and CSF leakage. It is not uncommon to encounter a small amount of CSF leakage during surgery. This minor "weeping" of CSF is usually treated by placing a small amount of fat harvested from the abdomen within the tumor cavity (intrasellar) and then fitting a piece of bone into the sellar opening. This bone may be from a sphenoid septum or from a banked iliac crest bone. We put tissue glue over the bone graft and then fill the entire sphenoid sinus with fat. Tissue glue is put over the opening to the sphenoid sinus to keep the fat in place. If there is a major amount of CSF leakage during surgery, it is carefully closed with the technique described above, plus a lumbar drain is placed at the termination of the procedure before the patient awakens from anesthesia. CSF is then drained for 2–3 days with a controlled drainage system at 10–12 cc per hour.

Injury to the carotid artery is fortunately very rare, but must be recognized and treated. If this is suspected the sphenoid sinus is vigorously packed to stop the bleeding and the patient is taken directly to angiography for assessment of the injured carotid artery. With current endovascular techniques it is often possible to reconstruct the area of injury with a stent, but in some cases involving a pseudoaneurysm it may be necessary to sacrifice the carotid artery after test occlusion.

Early postoperative complications are also uncommon, and include hematoma formation in the tumor cavity (with compression of cranial nerves II, III, or IV), CSF rhinorrhea, and epistaxis. It is critical to methodically check patients during the first night after surgery for any change in vision. This includes visual acuity and visual fields as well as extraocular eye movements. On several occasions over the years we have discovered patients to have either a cranial nerve III or cranial nerve VI palsy or diminished vision in one or both eyes within the first 12 h of surgery. Such patients should undergo emergent CT scanning to look for a hematoma within the tumor bed and then be returned immediately to the operating room for exploration of the operative site. We have seen this in five patients in nearly 2,000 operations and in every case the vision returned to the preoperative status or better. This complication is uncommon, but must be recognized and treated.

Delayed CSF leak (rhinorrhea) should be treated with a lumbar drain if adequate closure is accomplished at the initial procedure, but will occasionally require reoperation with further packing of the sellar opening plus a lumbar drain.

Epistaxis is very uncommon, but can occur a week or so after surgery. This requires a visit to the emergency room and usually just nasal packing to stop the bleeding. Careful visualization of nasal passages by either the original surgeon or a local ENT surgeon may be needed. In very rare cases embolization of the small sphenopalatine arteries in the sphenoid sinus may be necessary.

Postoperative endocrine issues will be covered in another chapter and include diabetes insipidus, hypocortisolemia, and electrolyte imbalance.

Although we do this approach without the assistance of an ENT surgeon, many neurosurgeons who do fewer transsphenoidal procedures will utilize the skills of a trained ENT nasal surgeon to assist with the approach to the sella. This approach generally allows gross total removal of macroadenomas and complete removal of microadenomas. Many pituitary adenomas are larger than 1 cm and somewhat invasive of the surrounding dura. We typically follow these tumors with yearly MRI for 5 years and biennially after that.

2.1.2. TRANSNASAL —DIRECT TRANSSPHENOIDAL ENDOSCOPIC APPROACH

It has been shown recently by Jho *(3)* that the entire procedure described above using the operating microscope can be duplicated using only the endoscope. This has the potential advantage of using smaller instruments, but has the significant disadvantage that only two-dimensional visualization is possible. The operator looks at a flat screen monitor while manipulating instruments in the surgical field. It is quite easy to pass the endoscope up the nasal passage to the sphenoid sinus and relatively easy to provide an opening into the sinus. The endoscope is then fixed in position by a holding device and standard instruments are used either along this same pathway or up the other nasal passage. The amount of retraction and bony opening is identical to that required by the direct microscopic approach. Whereas it is true that a 30–45°-angled endoscope will see further laterally in the sphenoid sinus, it unfortunately does not provide three-dimensional imaging of the sella and the pituitary tumor.

We believe the usefulness of an endoscope is in examining the skull base anatomy lateral and superior to the sella and occasionally in looking within a tumor for residual. We keep an endoscope available, but rarely use it during routine transsphenoidal procedures. With small microadenomas, such as in Cushing's disease, we would question whether the view afforded by the endoscope is adequate to perform careful dissection within the pituitary gland

2.1.3. TRANSNASAL—TRANSSEPTAL APPROACH

Hirsch *(4)* in 1910 described a transseptal approach to the sella that began with a small curved incision through the right septal mucosa via the right nostril. Once the submucosal plane is established, dissection is carried along the septum as deep as possible toward the sphenoid sinus. At this point the cartilage is divided and the opposite submucosal plane is developed. A long thin Kilian speculum is inserted on either side of the bony septum and the rostrum of the sphenoid sinus is identified. The posterior midline nasal septum is removed and the sphenoid sinus is entered. At this point the procedure is identical to the procedure described above, beginning at step 15. When the speculum is withdrawn the nasal mucosa is closed using absorbable chromic suture. If this approach is used, the nasal airways need to be packed bilaterally to compress the midline of the nose to prevent a septal hematoma.

The disadvantage of this approach is that there is a mandatory opening in the anterior nasal mucosa, which is not the case in the direct transnasal approach or the sublabial approach. This also requires uncomfortable postoperative nasal packing and allows the possibility of a postoperative septal perforation.

2.2. Sublabial Approach

The sublabial transseptal approach to the sphenoid sinus and sella has been used since the time of Harvey Cushing and allows the most midline trajectory to this region and the placement of a slightly larger speculum. We have described this approach previously *(5)*. It is also done exclusively with the operating microscope and involves making a 3-cm incision just above the incisors and then entering the nasal cavity submucosally. Dissection is carried submucosally along the midline and the cartilaginous portion of the septum is gently moved to the opposite side. Sizable portions of the vomer and perpendicular plate of the ethmoid are removed and eventually the midline rostrum of the sphenoid sinus is reached. A somewhat larger speculum than we use transnasally is placed and the anterior wall of the sphenoid sinus is removed as in step 15 above.

Unlike the transnasal transeptal approach described above, it is necessary to pack both sides of the nose extensively postoperatively to reoppose the mucosal walls of the midline septum. The most common unpleasant sequelae from this approach is numbness of the upper incisors and the gum area surrounding the sublabial incision. Although often transient, this is not uncommonly permanent.

2.3. Extended Transsphenoidal Approach

Any of these transsphenoidal approaches can be extended into the parasellar areas for more extensive tumor resection. Jho *(6)* and Kelly *(7)* have used the transnasal route for resection of meningiomas of the planum sphenoidale region. Oldfield *(8)* and Laws *(9)* have described a more extensive procedure in which the bone of the planum sphenoidale is removed and the underlying dura as well as the diaphragma sella are opened widely to expose the entire infundibulum and the optic chiasm. This is used for cases in which there is a relatively small, but hormonally active portion of the tumor attached to the pituitary stalk.

3. TRANSCRANIAL APPROACHES

It is interesting that all of the basic intracranial approaches used today were described in some form by 1914. Horsley *(10)* was the first surgeon to operate on a pituitary tumor in 1889 and described the subtemporal approach in 1906. Krause *(11)* described the subfrontal approach in 1914 and McArthur *(12)* and Frazier *(13)* described the extradural approach in 1912 and 1913. Heuer *(14)* devised the frontotemoral (pterional) approach in 1913, but was unable to report it until 1920.

3.1. Unilateral Subfrontal Approach

The right-sided unilateral subfrontal approach to the sella is the method that is most commonly used for a midline or eccentric right suprasellar lesion (Fig. 2). If the lesion is clearly eccentric to the left then a left subfrontal approach may be appropriate. If the lesion has a distinct middle fossa component, then a frontotemporal exposure is necessary. The classic subfrontal approach has been described in a step-by-step fashion by Symon *(15)*. This approach involves a transcoronal scalp incision to avoid a visible forehead scar and the elevation of a right frontal bone flap. The bone flap should extend from the midline to the frontozygomatic recess. Since the inferior aspect of the bone flap should be as low as possible, the frontal sinus is routinely entered.

The frontal lobe is gently elevated and the right optic nerve identified. A self-retaining retractor is placed beneath the frontal lobe and the microscope brought into position. Microdissection around the optic nerve is carried out and the tumor is usually evident beneath and medial to the optic nerve. Further

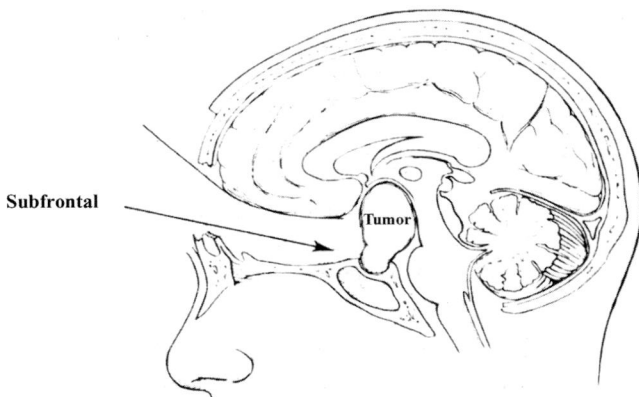

Fig. 2. Subfrontal approach. This midline sagittal view demonstrates the subfrontal approach to a sellar tumor.

elevation of the medial frontal lobe reveals the optic chiasm and the opposite optic nerve. Tumor removal is carried out using various instruments including the ring currettes used during transsphenoidal surgery. Intrasellar lesions may be approached in the window between the optic nerves and also in the window between the optic nerve and the ipsilateral carotid artery. The tumor can also be removed via the lamina terminalis if the tumor has grown into the third ventricle or if the chiasm is prefixed. Care must be taken to avoid injury to the pituitary stalk and to the undersurface of the optic chiasm.

After decompression of the optic pathways and maximum tumor removal, the retractors are removed and the craniotomy closed in the standard fashion. If the frontal sinus had been entered during the elevation of the bone flap then the sinus mucosa is obliterated and muscle or fat is packed into the frontal sinus. The pericranium can be separated from the scalp flap and folded down over the sinus opening, then held in place by the replacement of the bone flap.

In rare circumstances the contents of the sella cannot be adequately reached via this subfrontal approach and the "subfrontal transsphenoidal" approach is utilized. This technique involves drilling through the planum sphenoidale area down into the sphenoid sinus and then drilling or dissecting through the anterior wall of the sella to reach the tumor. With modern MRI most situations requiring this approach would be recognized preoperatively and likely be approached via the standard transsphenoidal route.

3.2. Pterional Approach

The pterional approach involves adding a temporal exposure to the frontal approach described above. This is not usually used for standard adenomas, but can be particularly useful for the resection of complex craniopharyngiomas. A curvilinear frontotemporal incision is made just to the hairline and a frontotemporal bone flap is elevated. The Sylvian fissure is gently opened and both the frontal and the anterior temporal lobes are elevated. This allows exposure of the optic chiasm as described above, but also allows a more lateral exposure of the space between the ipsilateral optic nerve and the carotid artery and also the space lateral to the carotid artery. Some parasellar tumors extend lateral and posterior enough to warrant this somewhat more extensive approach. This allows a view all the way back to the basilar artery if needed. This approach is useful for choristomas, which tend to arise more posteriorly and extend back to the brainstem.

4. INDICATIONS FOR SURGERY

The decision to proceed with surgery is based on a number of important factors. Ideally, every individual considered for surgery should be evaluated by both an endocrinologist and a neurosurgeon trained in pituitary surgery.

Although there are always a few patients who fall in the "gray areas" and can either be followed carefully or undergo tumor resection, most patients provide clear indications to their physicians as to whether they need surgery.

4.1. Nonfunctional Macroadenomas

Patients who have nonfunctional tumors that are large enough to cause loss of vision due to optic pathway compression clearly need surgery. Patients who have macroadenomas that cause loss of pituitary function need hormone replacement followed by tumor surgery. Some patients will enjoy at least a partial postoperative improvement in pituitary function and the remainder will be spared further loss of function. Patients who have debilitating headaches and only moderate size tumors will often experience relief with tumor resection. Sometimes surgery is necessary to reach a diagnosis. We have seen situations in which metastatic tumors, craniopharyngiomas, meningiomas, and abscesses have mimicked pituitary adenomas.

Incidentally found tumors often pose a treatment dilemma. The decision to operate on a tumor found incidentally depends on the size of the tumor, the function of the pituitary, and the age of the patient. We are more likely to operate on a patient who is younger since they have more years at risk.

4.2. Cushing's Disease

Virtually all patients with proven or suspected pituitary-dependent hypercortisolism need to have exploration of their pituitary. Fortunately, most of these patients have microadenomas. If a small tumor is identified on MRI, that becomes the target for the surgeon. If the imaging is negative, it is imperative to do inferior petrosal sinus sampling for ACTH levels. If that test shows a steep gradient in comparison with peripheral blood, then careful exploration within the pituitary is necessary. The petrosal sampling may be positive unilaterally, but that correlates only 70% of the time with the side of the tumor *(16)*. We use frameless stereotactic guidance system in all Cushing's cases with a normal size sella. We have been able to provide endocrine remission in 94% of over 200 patients with the microsurgical approach.

4.3. Acromegaly

The great majority of acromegalic patients have macroadenomas and all of these patients benefit from surgical debulking of their tumor. Although surgery only results in complete endocrine remission in about 30% of patients, it provides a very significant fall in GH and IGF-1 levels in most patients. This fall in hormone levels correlates very well with improvement in clinical symptoms. The majority of acromegalic patients need adjunctive therapy with either medication or radiation therapy. Currently we are using either long-acting somatostatin analogs (Sandostatin LAR) or pegvisomant (Somavert) before resorting to radiation therapy.

4.4. Prolactinoma

Most patients with prolactin-secreting tumors should be treated medically with dopamine agonists. This is clearly indicated in macroadenomas and, we believe, is also preferable as initial treatment for microadenomas. Only a few patients who cannot tolerate dopamine agonists or have prolactinomas that are resistant to medical therapy or harbor cystic or hemorrhagic components may require surgery. Although very high doses of cabergoline, such as used in patients with Parkinson's disease, have been associated with valvular heart disease, this has not been reported in the lower doses used to treat prolactinomas. Nervertheless, patients should be made aware of this potential complication and periodic echocardiograms are advised in patients on long term dopamine agonists.

4.5. Pituitary Apoplexy

Patients with suspected or proven acute hemorrhage and/or necrosis within a pituitary tumor that is accompanied by severe neurological signs (ophthamoplegia or loss of vision) often require emergent surgery. Whereas in the past we thought that all such patients required urgent surgery, it is now clear with modern imaging that patients with milder symptoms can be safely followed with MRI and may not require surgery. In some cases the tumor involutes after an event of apoplexy and simply stops growing. The management of pituitary apoplexy is described in Chapter 19.

4.6. Cysts

We see a number of patients that appear to have purely cystic lesions within the sella. If these are small and the pituitary function is normal they should be followed with MRI. If they enlarge or cause symptoms, then transsphenoidal surgery is indicated. If a craniopharyngioma or abscess is suspected then surgery should be carried out. The management of cystic lesions of the sella is described in Chapter 23.

4.7. Stalk and Hypothalmic Lesions

These lesions can be approached only through an intracranial approach, with panhypopituitarism being an almost inevitable consequence. Thus, a decision to operate on such lesions should never be taken lightly. Only tumors that are strongly suspected to be malignant or are severely affecting vision should be considered for surgical intervention. Small stalk lesions are often found incidentally and rarely progress. Close follow-up with MRI is mandatory.

5. CHOICE OF APPROACH

Well over 90% of sellar and parasellar tumors can be approached transsphenoidally. The only reason to utilize the transcranial approaches described above is for lesions that extend well into the middle fossa or have a large complex suprasellar component. If a tumor is clearly based above the pituitary, such as a craniopharyngioma or meningioma, then we prefer the subfrontal or pterional approach. If the tumor is based in the cavernous sinus or parasellar region, such as a schwannoma, then the intracranial approach is preferred.

How aggressive the surgeon should be is always a matter of judgment, based on both the anatomy and the biology of the tumor. Since all macroadenomas are invasive of the surrounding dura, it is rarely, if ever, possible to obtain 100% tumor removal. The goal is maximum safe removal—usually well over 95% of the tumor. Attempts to remove the intracavernous portions of the tumor or to strip the tumor fragments from the optic nerves are likely to result in neurological morbidity.

A few institutions have an MR scanner available in the operating room. Unfortunately, it is technically impossible for the MRI to clearly demarcate the residual tumor from the background of operative changes, thus making intraoperative MRI quite limited. This intraoperative imaging technique may result in slightly greater tumor removal in a few patients, but it is not clear that this changes short-term or long-term results. (Dr Fahlbusch would disagree.)

The goal with microadenomas, especially in Cushing's disease, is to remove the entire tumor. In Cushing's disease a bit of the surrounding normal pituitary is routinely taken in an attempt to obtain endocrine remission. If a tumor is found, but remission not accomplished, it is appropriate to go back and remove the entire gland.

The decision to utilize an endoscope during tumor removal is entirely up to the judgment and bias of the surgeon. We prefer to rely primarily on the three-dimensional view of the operating microscope, but others are satisfied with the wider, although two-dimensional view, with the endoscope. The rigid endoscope can provide a view somewhat lateral in the sphenoid sinus and is a handy adjunct to the microscope during surgery. We keep it available during surgery, but do not use it routinely.

The decision to use frameless stereotactic guidance during surgery is also up to the comfort and experience of the surgeon in combination with the size and location of the tumor. An experienced pituitary surgeon will need this less often, but it is a tremendous help when the sella is small and the anatomy of the sphenoid sinus is complex. It may be most beneficial for use by surgeons who do this operation only occasionally.

6. REOPERATION

The decision to reoperate on a pituitary tumor requires careful integration of all of the available information. It is easy to reach a decision if the first surgery was performed by an inexperienced surgeon and most of the tumor mass was left in place. However, if an experienced surgeon did not accomplish complete tumor removal because of invasiveness of the tumor, fibrotic consistency, or excessive vascularity, it is unlikely that further surgery will be successful and may result in significant morbidity. The goals of repeat surgery need to be clearly defined. It may be justified if vision is severely compromised, but should not be done just to improve the appearance on the MRI. The availability of alternative methods to deal with mass effect or hormonal hypersecretion should always be a factor in reaching a prudent decision.

We generally prefer giving radiation therapy if we see recurrence of a macroadenoma in the years following initial surgery (17). If a patient has been lost to follow-up and has a large recurrence, especially with visual impairment, we recommend repeat tumor debulking prior to radiation therapy. Patients with failed surgery for Cushing's disease or recurrence of the disease are often excellent candidates for repeat surgery. We rarely reoperate for treatment of continued biochemical evidence of acromegaly. Likewise, most patients with persistent prolactinomas may benefit from adjustment of medical therapy or occasionally from radiation. The radiotherapy of these tumors is described in Chapter 17.

REFERENCES

1. Griffith HB, Veerapen R. A direct transnasal approach to the sphenoid sinus. Technical note. J Neurosurg 1987;66:140–2
2. Cooke RS, Jones RA. Experience with the direct transnasal transsphenoidal approach to the pituitary fossa. Br J Neurosurg 1994;8:193–6
3. Jho HS, Carrau RL. Endoscopy assisted transsphenoidal surgery for pituitary adenoma. Acta Neurochir (Weien) 1996;138:1416–25
4. Hirsch O. Endonasal method of removal of hypophyseal tumors. JAMA 1910;55:772–4
5. Chandler WF. Transsphenoidal surgical treatment of Cushing's disease. In: Rengachary SS, Wilkins RH, editors., Neurosurgical Operative Atlas, vol. 4, , Park Ridge: American Association of Neurological Surgeons; 1995. p. 165–72
6. Jho, H. Endoscopic endonasal approach to the optic nerve: a technical note. Minim Invasive Neurosurg 2001;44(4):190–3
7. Dusick JR, Esposito. F., Kelly DF, et al. The extended direct endonasal transsphenoidal approach for nonadenomatous suprasellar tumors. J Neurosurg 2005;102(5):825–7.

8. Mason RB, Nieman LK, Doppman JL, Oldfield EH. Selective excision of adenomas originating in or extending into the pituitary stalk with preservation of pituitary function. J Neurosurg 1997;87:343–51.
9. Dumont AS, Kanter. AS., Jane JA Jr, Laws ER Jr. Extended transsphenoidal approach. Front Horm Res. 2006;34:29–45.
10. Horsley V. On the technique of operations on the central nervous system. Br Med J 1906;2:411–23
11. Krause F. Freilegung der hypophyse. In: Krause F, editor. Die Allgemeine Chirurgie der Gehirnkrankheiten, Part II, Stuttgart: Ferdinand Enke, 1914. p. 465–70
12. McArthur LL. An aseptic surgical approach to the pituitary body and its neighborhood. JAMA 1912;58:2009–11
13. Frazier CH. Lesions of the hypophysis from the viewpoint of the surgeon. SurgGynObst 1913;17:724–36
14. Heuer GJ. Surgical experiences with an intracranial approach to chiasmal lesions. Arch Surg 1920;1:368–381
15. Symon, L. Surgical technique: transcranial approach. In: Landolt AM, Vance ML, Reilly PL, editors. Pituitary Adenomas. New York: Churchill Livingstone; 1996. p. 295–306.
16. Oldfield EH, Chrousos GP, Schulte HM, et al. Preoperative lateralization of ACTH-secreting pituitary microadenomas by bilateral and simultaneous inferior petrosal venous sinus sampling. N Eng J Med 1985;312:100–3.
17. Park P, Chandler WF, Barkan AL, et al. The role of radiation therapy after surgical resection of nonfunctional pituitary macroadenomas. Neurosurgery 2004;55(1):100–7.

16 Pituitary Surgery: *Peri-operative Management*

Ariel L. Barkan, MD,
Howard Blank, MD,
and William F. Chandler, MD

CONTENTS

1. INTRODUCTION
2. PRE-OPERATIVE AND POST-OPERATIVE ASSESSMENT AND MANAGEMENT
3. DISORDERS OF WATER AND SALT METABOLISM IN THE POSTOPERATIVE PERIOD

Summary

This chapter describes the perioperative management of the patient undergoing surgery for pituitary disease, including preoperative and postoperative endocrine evaluation. The management of metabolic and endocrine abnormalities resulting from the surgery is described.

Key Words: Transsphenoidal surgery, SIADH, DI.

1. INTRODUCTION

Proper evaluation and therapy of a patient with suspected or established pituitary pathology requires joint involvement of several subspecialists. A dedicated pituitary endocrinologist and a dedicated pituitary neurosurgeon constitute the backbone of such a team. Multidisciplinary pituitary clinics in which patients are seen at the same time by both specialists are becoming more widespread in large academic medical centers. The advantage of such collaboration is obvious: both the neurological and the hormonal status of

From: *Contemporary Endocrinology: Diagnosis and Management of Pituitary Disorders*
Edited by: B. Swearingen and B. M. K. Biller © Humana Press, Totowa, NJ

the patient are assessed simultaneously, all pertinent information is immediately integrated, and treatment options are identified and presented to the patient. The same applies to the postoperative evaluation of the patient, when questions regarding the need for hormone replacement, long-term medical therapy, radiation therapy, or repeat surgery can be addressed and a treatment plan established.

In this chapter, we discuss the issues arising during the perioperative period that starts at the time of the first visit of the patient to the clinic and lasts at least until the patient's care is ready to be transferred back to his or her referring physician.

2. PRE-OPERATIVE AND POST-OPERATIVE ASSESSMENT AND MANAGEMENT

When a patient presents with a sellar mass, several interrelated questions need to be answered:

1. What is the likely nature of the mass?
2. Is there any compression (mass) effect?
3. Which, if any, hormone is overproduced?
4. Which, if any, hormone is lacking?

The answers to these questions will permit the physician to chart a rational therapeutic plan.

2.1. Question 1: What Is the Likely Nature of the Mass?

The list of potential sellar lesions is long and includes neoplastic processes, infiltrative/inflammatory processes, infections, and developmental malformations, as well as many other rare lesions.

From the practical point of view, the great majority of sellar lesions are likely to fall into a much tighter group consisting of pituitary adenomas, craniopharyngiomas/cysts, and meningiomas.

Examination of both precontrast and postcontrast T1 images as well as T2 images of a high-quality MRI is needed to correctly identify the nature of the lesion.

2.1.1. T1 Before Contrast

Solid tumors are, as a rule, isointense on precontrast T1 images. Bright areas on T1 images are due to the presence of either fat or blood. This may indicate the presence of fat tissue per se (inserted surgically to prevent CSF leak), high-cholesterol fluid in craniopharyngiomas, or hemorrhage within the tumor itself. A "bright spot" in the posterior part of the pituitary is normal and represents a healthy posterior lobe. The same spot located very high and accompanied by the "empty sella" may indicate congenital hypoplasia of the anterior pituitary.

2.1.2. T1 AFTER CONTRAST

Pituitary adenomas do not, as a rule, enhance after contrast administration nearly as much as the pituitary stalk and the surviving anterior pituitary tissue. The latter is often seen as a small bright streak at the periphery of the tumor, often contiguous with the stalk. T1 images with contrast are especially useful in delineating tumor margins. (Fig. 1)

2.1.3. T2

T2 images reverse the T1 picture: on T2 images the CSF looks bright and the soft tissues (including the brain and the pituitary) look dark. A pituitary mass that is isointense on T1 but is bright on T2 most likely represents a cyst filled with fluid. (Fig. 2)

CT scans are used infrequently, but may be valuable to demonstrate bone margins, calcifications within a craniopharyngioma, or acute hemorrhage. (Fig. 3)

Pituitary adenomas usually present radiologically as isointense lesions on precontrast T1 images. They usually remain hypointense after contrast in comparison with the normally enhancing gland tissue. Microadenomas are less than 10 mm in diameter. Macroadenomas are more than 10 mm in diameter, and the term "giant adenoma" is usually reserved for tumors that are bigger than 4 cm. Up to 20% of normal people will have evidence for microadenoma on MRI. Special caution needs to be exercised not to overdiagnose "microadenomas" in the posterior part of the pituitary, where artifacts are very prevalent.

Craniopharyngiomas may occur at any age, but are mostly found in children or in 40–50-year-old adults. They are typically partly cystic, partly solid, and

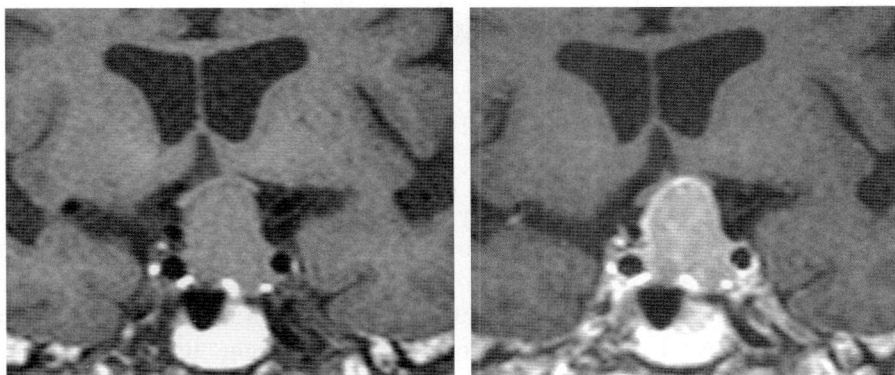

Fig. 1. Pituitary macroadenoma invading left cavernous sinus. *Left*: T1 without contrast shows diffusely isointense mass. *Right*: T1 with contrast shows bright rim of the residual normal pituitary, but the adenoma remains isointense.

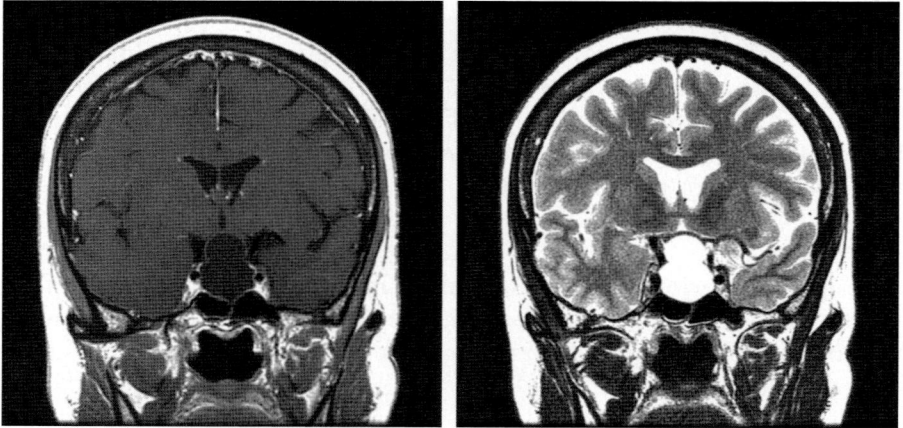

Fig. 2. Rathke's cleft cyst. *Left*: T1 with contrast. *Right*: T2 image. Note that cyst fluid is often isointense with CSF.

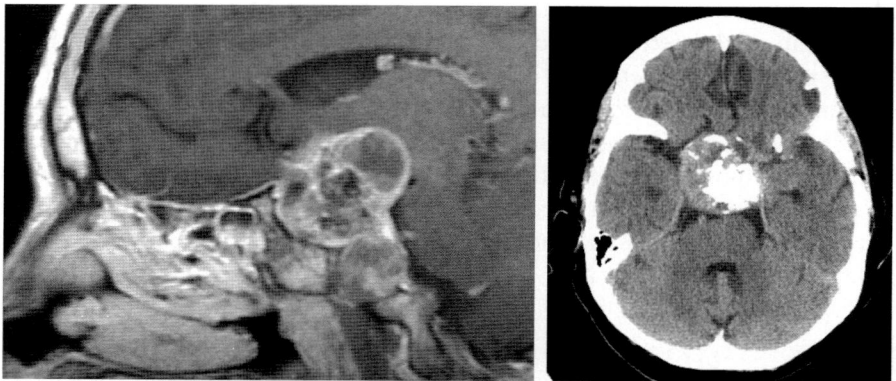

Fig. 3. Craniopharyngioma. *Left*: T1 with contrast shows partly cystic partly solid mass. *Right*: Noncontrast CT shows calcifications (bright areas) within the tumor.

often contain calcifications. They may arise from within the sella or from a suprasellar location. Very cystic craniopharyngiomas can be indistinguishable from a Rathke's cyst.

Meningioma involving sellar/parasellar space often arise from the planum sphenoidale. An MRI of a presellar mass with a straight, linear dural base can provide a clue. Meningiomas are as a rule isointense on T1 images and enhance after administration of gadolinium contrast (Fig. 4).

Less common lesions that need to be considered are as follows:

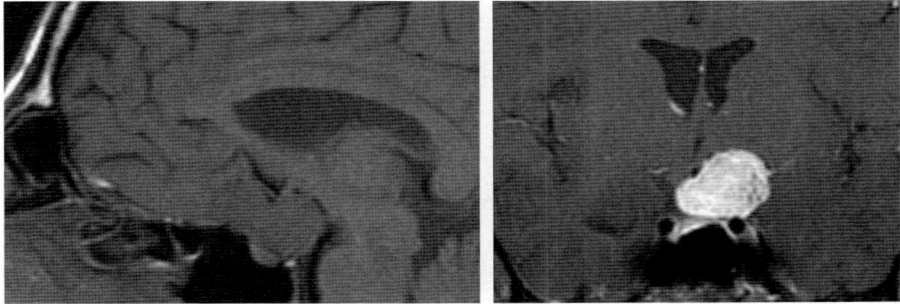

Fig. 4. meningioma. *Left*: Noncontrast T1 image shows large isointense mass with a linear dural base. *Right*: T1 after contrast administration shows major enhancement of the mass.

Pituitary hyperplasia presents with MRI of an enlarged pituitary that is usually very symmetric and enhances diffusely after contrast. This is occasionally seen in patients with severe primary hypothyroidism and is associated with a markedly elevated TSH. A mildly and diffusely enlarged gland is a frequent normal finding in pubertal children, especially in tall children. In addition, hyperplasia can be seen in those rare cases of ectopic tumors secreting releasing factors, such as adrenocorticotrophic-releasing hormone or growth hormone (GH)-releasing hormone. *Pituitary cysts* (Rathke's cysts or abscesses) are usually noninvasive, well-demarcated, and bright on T2 images like CSF.

Empty sella may be primary or secondary to such events as excision of a large pituitary mass or the spontaneous infarction of the tumor. Occasionally, it may be necessary to differentiate an empty sella from a large cyst. Examination of the postcontrast T1 images will usually provide an answer. In the case of empty sella, the bright streak of the stalk will go all the way to the bottom of the sella where the enhancing normal pituitary will be located in the inferior–posterior part of the sella. In the case of a large cyst, however, the stalk ends at a high position at the upper border of the mass with the pituitary tissue adjacent to it.

Many other disease processes may affect the hypothalamic–pituitary area and some have sufficient radiological features to allow a diagnosis preoperatively. Interpretation of pituitary MRI is best accomplished in consultation with a neuroradiologist or an experienced pituitary surgeon.

2.2. Question 2: Is There Any Mass Effect?

Small pituitary microadenomas are unlikely to produce mass effect and should not, as a rule, be blamed for headaches or hypopituitarism. Larger pituitary masses can expand upward and fill the suprasellar cistern laterally to invade the cavernous sinuses or downward to invade the sphenoid sinus. Occasionally, tumors may be large enough to compress or invade the temporal or frontal lobes, the hypothalamus, the ethmoid sinuses, or the orbits.

2.2.1. Suprasellar Expansion

Upward stretching of the diaphragma sella may produce headaches. If the tumor is large enough to compress the optic pathways, this usually causes a visual field defect. Examination with a small bright red object may disclose "red color desaturation" (sudden change in the intensity of the red color when the object is moved into the affected area) even in the patients who can still see the moving fingers in the same areas quite well. Bitemporal hemianopsia is the result of chiasmatic compression, but since the tumors are often irregular and the chiasm itself may be located anteriorly or posteriorly of the classic suprasellar position, many patients have other variations of visual field impairment. Consultation with a neuro-ophthalmologist and formal visual field testing is very useful.

2.2.2. Lateral Expansion

Invasion of a cavernous sinus puts the tumor in the vicinity of the third, fourth, sixth, and first two divisions of the fifth cranial nerves. As a rule, pituitary adenomas rarely cause impairment of these nerves' function. Usually, it is the result of a sudden expansion of volume within the cavernous sinus (pituitary apoplexy) that can be accompanied by sudden ophthalmoplegia and, often, severe headache and pituitary crisis (acute hypopituitarism). Subacute or chronic ophthalmoplegia with gradual onset is suggestive of a meningioma, pituitary metastasis (breast, prostate, and lung cancers), or aggressive granulomatous hypophysitis (tuberculosis, Tolosa–Hunt syndrome, etc.).

2.2.3. Downward Expansion

Invasion of the sphenoid sinus and, especially, penetration of the sphenoid sinus wall may be manifest by CSF rhinorrhea. Discharge of clear, watery fluid from the nose, especially on bending forward, is the typical presenting sign. This may also occur postoperatively, if the floor of the sella was not repaired well or, occasionally, after shrinkage of large and invasive prolactinomas by dopamine agonists. CSF rhinorrhea puts the patient in danger of developing meningitis and should not be left untreated.

Expansion of sellar masses in other directions occurs rarely, and may produce proptosis, blindness, or neurological syndromes (gelastic seizures, temporal epilepsy, etc.)

2.2.4. PITUITARY COMPRESSION

Any tumor large enough to compress the gland or to interfere with the hypothalamic–pituitary blood flow can produce anterior pituitary failure or the so-called stalk-section effect with resultant hyperprolactinemia. Thus, every patient with a large sellar mass should be deemed hypopituitary unless proven otherwise.

2.3. Question 3: Is There Any Evidence of Hormone Hypersecretion?

2.3.1. HYPERPROLACTINEMIA

Prolactinomas are the most frequent hormonally active pituitary tumors. Their preoperative diagnosis is crucial, since they are best treated medically (with dopamine agonist) instead of surgically. Recent data on the risk of cardiac valvular disease after use of cabergoline and pergolide may prompt a reexamination of this dictum in younger patients, especially those requiring high doses for tumor control. Nonetheless, prolactin must be measured in every patient with a sellar mass.

Functional hyperprolactinemia may also result from the effects of antidopaminergic drugs, estrogen excess (most often birth control pills or estrogen replacement), chest wall lesions, primary hypothyroidism, "stalk section" effect due to a non-prolactin-secreting tumor or from a hypothalamic damage most often due to an infiltrative process or previous radiation therapy. Thus, careful history and physical examination are indispensable. The hallmark of all these processes is a relatively modest elevation in prolactin levels, below 200 ng/ml. Only true prolactin-secreting tumors exhibit circulating prolactin levels in excess of 300 ng/ml and, usually over 200 ng/ml. Thus, a tumor of any size in the presence of prolactin above 200–300 ng/ml should be considered a prolactinoma. Since the degree of prolactin hypersecretion is roughly proportionate to tumor size, a sizable macroadenoma that is accompanied by only mildly elevated prolactin levels (<200 ng/ml) is unlikely to be a true prolactinoma. On the other hand, a microadenoma with modestly elevated prolactin level, below 200 ng/ml, may be a true prolactinoma. A therapeutic trial of dopamine agonist would be justified in such patients. Normalization of prolactin concentrations and shrinkage of the tumor will confirm the diagnosis.

Two laboratory pitfalls need to be remembered. The first one relates to the prolactin binding by circulating IgG that in effect acts as a binding protein. The bound prolactin (macroprolactin) circulates with extended half-life, and the apparent prolactin concentrations become modestly elevated. Most of these patients are asymptomatic and the finding of an apparently elevated prolactin in a patient with obviously normal gonadal axis should suggest the diagnosis of macroprolactinemia. However, since prolactin is usually measured in patients with symptoms of hypogonadism (abnormal menstrual cyclicity in women or sexual dysfunction in men), it is easy to make an incorrect diagnosis of hyperprolactinemia as a cause of the complaint. In case of doubt, repeat prolactin measurement after PEG precipitation of the IgG/prolactin complex will show normal prolactin levels and solve the diagnostic puzzle.

Another laboratory phenomenon is very rare but much more important. The modern two-site assays may erroneously report grossly elevated prolactin concentrations as normal or only mildly elevated. This is due to the saturation of binding sites on both antibodies by the extremely high prolactin concentrations; this prevents the formation of the "sandwich" structure (immobilized antibody–prolactin-signal antibody complex). This so-called high-dose hook effect may be seen in giant prolactinomas (>4 cm in diameter, as a rule) producing prolactin levels that exceed the performance parameters of a particular assay. There is no absolute value of prolactin concentrations that leads to "hook effect": it varies from assay to assay. In any patient with a very large sellar mass, prolactin needs to be assayed in the undiluted serum as well as in a diluted (1:100 or 1:1,000) sample. Even though the likelihood of finding true hyperprolactinemia that was masked by the "hook effect" is exceedingly small, its correct recognition is of major importance since it obviates the need for surgery (1).

2.3.2. GH HYPERSECRETION

This results in acromegaly if the disease process started after epiphyseal closure or gigantism if before. All pituitary giants have acromegalic features at the time of diagnosis or develop them subsequently.

Elevated IGF-1 is the biochemical hallmark of the disease, reflecting chronically elevated GH levels. Pitfalls include malnutrition of any origin, liver disease, or oral estrogen therapy. All these may decrease plasma IGF-1 to the point of apparent "normalcy" even in the patients with active GH hypersecretion. Puberty and pregnancy are normally associated with high IGF-1 levels. Nonsuppressibility of GH below 0.2–0.3 μg/l 60 min after oral 75 g glucose load is another biochemical hallmark of active disease.

The diagnosis of GH hypersecretion needs to be considered in every patient with a pituitary adenoma, especially in cases of apparent prolactinoma. It may change treatment strategy and will serve as an important marker postoperatively. Surgery is the primary treatment, although in some cases somatostatin analogs may be employed from the outset.

2.3.3. ACTH HYPERSECRETION

Tumors producing ACTH frequently result in Cushing's syndrome. Mostly they are small and in approximately 20% cannot be detected even by a sensitive MRI scan. Detailed differential diagnosis of Cushing's syndrome is described elsewhere in this volume. Surgery is currently the only rational initial treatment in Cushing's disease.

2.3.4. TSH HYPERSECRETION

Most of these tumors are large and invasive by the time of diagnosis. The patients are thyrotoxic, with high free T4 and free T3 concentrations but measurable or frankly elevated TSH levels. Free plasma a-subunit is almost always elevated. Concomitant hypersecretion of prolactin and/or GH is also often observed. The differential diagnosis is with pituitary hyperplasia due to insensitivity to thyroid hormone. Bolus dose of TRH results in no TSH response in case of the TSH-secreting tumor, but in exaggerated response in case of thyroid hormone insensitivity and pituitary hyperplasia. Another useful maneuver is a "T3 suppression test": 50 µg T3 given twice daily for 7–10 days does not suppress TSH in patients with TSH-producing tumors, but lowers it in those with thyrotrope hyperplasia. Surgery is the primary treatment of TSH adenomas and is often followed by somatostatin analogs.

2.3.5. GONADOTROPIN-PRODUCING TUMORS

Immunochemically, many of the so-called nonfunctioning pituitary tumors have scattered staining for gonadotropin subunits. True gonadotropinomas usually present as bulky, invasive tumors that are hormonally inactive but are often accompanied by hypopituitarism. Very rarely, in men, LH hypersecretion may cause high testosterone levels and FSH hypersecretion may result in enlargement of the testicles. In women, ovarian hyperstimulation syndrome has been described. Surgery is the best initial treatment for these tumors. Postoperatively, remnants may be treated with focused radiation. Dopamine agonists may occasionally be effective.

Overall, correct identification of the nature of the pituitary lesion allows the medical team to select an appropriate treatment plan and to choose the best surgical approach if surgery is needed.

2.4. Question 4: Is There Evidence Of Pituitary Hypofunction?

Normal pituitary function can be suppressed functionally (e.g., gonadotropins in case of a prolactinoma) or physically. The latter may be at least partially reversible if due to simple compression by a removable tumor mass, but may be permanent in case of pituitary destruction, as is often seen in craniopharyngiomas, metastatic lesions, or apoplexy.

If surgery is planned, detailed assessment of pituitary integrity is unnecessary as the results may change after tumor removal. Any patient with a sizeable pituitary lesion who is scheduled for surgery might be hypoadrenal, and hydrocortisone, 15–20 mg daily, should be given. The obvious exception is in patients

with Cushing's disease. The need for thyroid replacement is more controversial as hypothyroidism does not seem to affect the safety of the surgical
procedure. However, it is prudent to start L-thyroxine in replacement doses if
free T4 levels are subnormal. We do not routinely give testosterone preoperatively. Instead, we use it as a marker of surgical success, since normalization
of testosterone levels is good evidence of restoration of pituitary function.
Some patients with large suprasellar masses present with a clear history of
polydipsia and polyuria. They report repeated bouts of nocturia during which
they produce large amounts of dilute urine and experience severe thirst. The
diagnosis of diabetes insipidus (DI) is usually easily confirmed by the finding
of high normal serum osmolality in the presence of hypo-osmolar urine, usually
<300–400 mosm/kg (2). If the patient is scheduled for imminent surgery,
the overnight prolonged dehydration test is not necessary. Administration of
DDAVP (0.1–0.2 mg/day by mouth or 0.01–0.02 mg/day intranasally) will
usually be sufficient to relieve symptoms. If surgery is not contemplated, the
physician may decide to confirm the diagnosis using the prolonged dehydration
test. This should always be performed under direct observation and physician
supervision. Of note, patients with severe cortisol and thyroxine deficiencies
may not manifest polydipsia/polyuria even if ADH is lacking. Replacement of
cortisol and thyroxine may unmask the preexisting DI.

2.4.1. PERIOPERATIVE AND POSTOPERATIVE GLUCOCORTICOID REPLACEMENT

Surgery represents a classical "stress test" and the replacement hydrocortisone doses given preoperatively become insufficient in this situation. Again,
with the exception of cases of Cushing's disease, every patient undergoing
pituitary surgery should be given stress doses of glucocorticoids, irrespective of
prior replacement therapy. The magnitude of "stress" replacement is uncertain.
Usually, cortisol secretion rates increase 2–4 times in healthy subjects undergoing surgical procedure. Thus, a total daily dose of hydrocortisone of 50–
100 mg is sufficient on the day of surgery. Cortisol's half-life is 60–90 min,
dictating the need for repeat dosages to cover not only surgery itself (2–4 h)
but the immediate postoperative period as well (3).

We usually give 50 mg hydrocortisone IV at the induction of anesthesia,
another 25 mg immediately post surgery, and another 25 mg 8–12 h later. Close
monitoring of vital parameters, especially blood pressure, in the postoperative
period is mandatory, and additional boluses may be given as needed. This is
usually not necessary after uncomplicated transsphenoidal surgery, but may be
required in patients after a significantly more stressful subfrontal surgery when
they routinely stay in the neurosurgical ICU for 1–2 days postoperatively.
During this time, they should continue receiving 50–100 mg hydrocortisone

daily in the divided doses. As soon as the patient is well enough to be transferred to a general neurosurgical ward, replacement hydrocortisone doses 25 mg/day are usually sufficient *(4)*. Upon discharge, 10 mg orally at breakfast and 5–10 mg at lunchtime are recommended.

The need for permanent hydrocortisone replacement requires assessment of the endogenous pituitary ACTH secretion postoperatively. Some centers measure morning plasma cortisol on the second postoperative day after omitting the hydrocortisone dose on the preceding evening. We usually ask our patients to choose a convenient time 2–3 weeks post surgery, omit hydrocortisone for 24 h, and have a sample drawn early in the morning (8–9 a.m.) in a local laboratory.

The definition of "normalcy" is based on the measurements of plasma cortisol in patients without pituitary diseases who happen to undergo major physical stress: acute febrile illness, trauma, or surgery. Plasma cortisol at those times is elevated above 18 µg/dl and this is viewed as a minimal level sufficient to ensure survival. Insulin-induced hypoglycemia is a controlled model of stress. Acute fall in plasma glucose below 40 mg/dl reliably results in maximally stimulated ACTH and, subsequently, cortisol release. Cortisol levels above 18 mcg/dl, 30 min, after clinical and biochemical hypoglycemia strongly correlate with the spontaneous "stress" cortisol levels. This test requires medical supervision, is unpleasant, and is contraindicated in patients with arrhythmia, coronary disease, or seizures.

Thus, as a first step, early morning cortisol should be measured. If it is above 18 mcg/dl, no further investigation is needed and hydrocortisone replacement can be safely stopped. If it is below 5 µg/dl, there is an almost 100% certainty that the patient is ACTH deficient and that cortisol replacement needs to be continued for life *(5)*. Intermediate levels are less informative and, for example, a level of 10 mcg/dl has only a 50% predictive value for the diagnosis of ACTH deficiency. At that time, the physician should exercise clinical judgment to decide whether a hypoglycemia test or several more early morning cortisol measurements are indicated.

Attempts have been made to utilize an ACTH stimulation test (1 mcg or 250 mcg IV) to replace the insulin tolerance test *(6)*. The thinking is based on the premise that chronic ACTH deficiency results in adrenal cortical atrophy, so that even with the maximal stimulation by ACTH the adrenals do not respond in a normal fashion. We do not recommend this test as it is uninformative in cases of short-term ACTH deficiency as is the case soon after pituitary surgery. Even in cases of chronic, long-standing ACTH deficiency as proven by the insulin tolerance test, Cortrosyn stimulation test may be false-negative in more than a third of cases *(7)*. The reason is that even minimal residual ACTH secretion will maintain sufficiently trophic state of the adrenal cortex. Thus, when the cortex is challenged with a large bolus of *exogenous* ACTH, it will respond normally. However, the damaged pituitary will be unable to increase the output of *endogenous* ACTH during severe stress, and adrenal crisis may ensue. However, if this test is performed and indicates adrenal insufficiency, the reliability is good, particularly if the conventional rather than the low-dose test is used.

Every patient with ACTH deficiency needs to wear an identification necklace or bracelet specifying the loss of glucocorticoid function.

2.4.2. THYROXINE REPLACEMENT

The half-life of T4 is about 7 days. Thus, at least several weeks need to pass without thyroxine replacement to assess the final thyroid status. If deficient, L-thyroxine at 1.6 mcg/kg BW is given and free T4 is remeasured 2–3 months later for the final adjustment. Measurement of plasma TSH has no place in the follow-up of a patient with secondary hypothyroidism. Clinical assessment of thyroid status and plasma free T_4 should be followed instead.

2.4.3. GONADOTROPINS

In men, gonadotropin deficiency is managed on a chronic basis by replacing testosterone. In every man older than 50 years of age, PSA needs to be measured to exclude prostate cancer.

There are many testosterone preparations available including intramuscular injections, topical patches, gels and creams, and a buccal capsule. Intramuscular injections of depot testosterone are usually given at 200-mg doses every 2 weeks. In patients with severe and long-standing hypogonadism, we usually start at 100 mg a month to allow for the gradual adjustment. Sudden increase in testosterone in such patients may precipitate priapism or aggressive sexual behavior. Some patients exhibit good restoration of libido and potency for the first week after each injection, with gradually waning effect thereafter. Changing the regimen to 100–150 mg every week usually corrects the problem. Alternatively, testosterone gel 1% is recommended and the sufficient dose varies between 2.5 and 10 g/day.

Hematocrit is measured at 6–12-month intervals and the dose of testosterone is adjusted to ameliorate polycythemia. This is less of a problem with topical or buccal preparations as the blood levels are more stable without the large peaks that occur with intramuscular injection. PSA is measured as necessary using guidelines for healthy middle-aged or elderly men.

Hypogonadal women develop osteoporosis, flushes, and vaginal atrophy. The former can be managed using bisphosphonates but the latter two are best controlled with estrogen. We usually recommend estradiol skin patches at the lowest dose to control the symptoms. This can be given chronically in women post hysterectomy, but if the uterus is still intact, periodic withdrawal bleedings using progestagen are necessary to prevent endometrial cancer.

2.4.4. GH DEFICIENCY

Over the past 15–20 years, many studies were done to ascertain the role of GH replacement in adults with hypopituitarism. Current recommendations support the use of GH in adults with acquired severe GH deficiency, i.e., stimulated GH <3 mcg/l or in those with three or four other pituitary hormone deficiencies and low IGF-1 concentrations *(8)*. GH therapy decreases the amount of body fat, increases lean body mass and bone density, and improves patients' quality of life. Whether this is translated into alleviation of the metabolic syndrome, improved physical performance, and decreased fracture rate is still uncertain. Similarly, the question whether the improvement in the quality of life found in open-label studies is a real outcome or a placebo effect is still unresolved *(9)*. The cost of GH replacement in adults is not trivial, between $3,000 and $10,000 per year and this therapy is associated with edema, carpal tunnel syndrome, glucose intolerance, and joint aches. Thus, the risks and benefits of GH replacement in each individual patient need to be carefully considered.

3. DISORDERS OF WATER AND SALT METABOLISM IN THE POSTOPERATIVE PERIOD

Disorders of water–salt balance represent a major problem that requires close attention and prompt therapeutic decisions. Once sodium imbalance is identified in the postoperative pituitary surgery patient, a proper history and physical examination need to be performed. Along with a review of the patient's surgical procedure, including fluids administered and the calculation of fluid balance, a list of current medications the patient is receiving should be examined to evaluate the cause of the imbalance. Evaluation of intravascular and extravascular volume status and laboratory determination of plasma and urine osmolality along with plasma and urine sodium should be performed.

3.1. Hypernatremia

Hypernatremia is plasma sodium concentration more than 145 mmol/l *(2)*. It is associated with a relative sodium excess compared to whole body water and results from either net water loss or sodium loading of the body. Essentially, hypernatremia develops in those patients in whom the thirst mechanism is impaired or access to free water is restricted, as is often seen in postsurgical patients. The symptoms depend on the rapidity of the development of hypernatremia and include primarily neurological manifestations such as weakness,

altered mental status, seizures, and coma. History, physical examination, and a
review of the operative procedure can aid diagnosis in the postsurgery pituitary
patient.

3.1.1. DIABETES INSIPIDUS

Hypernatremia from DI may develop due to disruption of the hypothalamic–
pituitary axis after pituitary surgery. Surgery may cause injury to the hypothalamus, the stalk, or the pituitary leading to absent or insufficient antidiuretic
hormone (ADH) secretion. ADH aids water reabsorption in the collecting
tubules of the kidney; its absence leads to high volumes of maximally dilute
urine and hypernatremia. If a postsurgical patient develops DI and has impaired
access to free water, serum sodium will rise. Hyperosmolality, weight loss,
and urine output > 250 cc/h for 2 or more consecutive hours are usually seen.
Importantly, if the access to fluids is not impaired, DI will be manifest as
polyuria/polydipsia only, without obvious electrolyte abnormalities.

Many patients exhibit a triphasic course. The immediate postoperative phase
is characterized by the appearance of DI followed by a transient phase of
hyponatremia 7–10 days after surgery. DI reappears thereafter, and it may be
transient or permanent. This course may not be complete or clearly discernible;
the duration of each phase can be variable and of such inapparent magnitude
that is could be easily overlooked. Thus, pituitary surgery patients need to be
followed attentively postoperatively and the administration of any fluid therapy
needs to anticipate spontaneous changes in the water–electrolyte balance.

Treatment of DI depends on the clinical state of the patient. As soon as
postoperative patients regain access to free water, they are able to balance
their own fluid intake properly. This will typically allow correction of hypernatremia. Acute postoperative DI is easily corrected with DDAVP 1–2 mcg
i.v., s.c., i.m., or 0.1 mg orally. Chronically, nasal or oral DDAVP preparations
are preferred. A rule of thumb is that 1 mcg DDAVP i.m. is equivalent to 10
mcg nasally or 100 mcg of the oral preparation. The smallest dose providing
acceptable quality of life (such as uninterrupted sleep) should be used to avoid
hyponatremia. For some patients skipping the daytime dose once a week may
be advisable to correct incipient water accumulation. A patient with DI and
absent thirst presents a major therapeutic challenge. Both the patient and the
family need to be educated about mandatory scheduled fluid intake.

If a patient has hypernatremia and volume depletion, calculation of free
water deficit needs to be performed (*see* below) and caution should be used in
replacing water. The serum sodium should not be lowered by greater than 0.5
mmol/l/h. It is best to use free water replacement via mouth or NG tube.

The formula for calculating free water deficit is [(plasma Na – 140)/140] ×
(total body water). Urinary losses need to be accounted for as well.

The formula for calculating the change in serum Na is (infusate Na – serum Na)/(total body water + 1) may be used if IV fluids are utilized, though this method of replacement is not preferred.

3.1.2. OTHER CAUSES OF HYPERNATREMIA

Gastrointestinal sources of fluid loss and sodium loss (more free water is lost than sodium) along with an insensible loss from sweating can also cause hypernatremia when replacement with free water does not occur. Correction of these complications will help to improve free fluid loss. Replacement of volume with IV saline will correct the volume loss and hypernatremia. Again, care should be undertaken to avoid correcting the sodium imbalance too rapidly.

3.2. Hyponatremia

Hyponatremia is plasma sodium concentration less than 135 mmol/l *(10)*. It usually represents negative sodium balance in relation to total body water balance, though some causes of hyponatremia are related to isotonic and hypertonic states. Determining the serum osmolality aids diagnosis. Symptoms include nausea and vomiting with poor energy and headache. If it develops rapidly, extreme hyponatremia (<120 mmol/l) may be associated with elevated intracranial pressure, brain edema, and herniation, with injury to the brainstem. This requires urgent intervention to rapidly increase the plasma osmolality *(11)*.

If the patient tolerates the acute fall in plasma sodium and osmolality and enters the stage of chronic hyponatremia, brain edema abates and the blood–brain osmolality gradient vanishes. Rapid increase in plasma osmolality at that time may result in acute shift of water from the brain tissue to the blood and precipitate disseminated or focal cerebral myelinolysis. It is therefore imperative to determine clearly whether hyponatremia is acute or chronic. Since the brain's adaptation to acute change in osmolality takes 24–48 h, any hyponatremia of proven or suspected chronic duration should be treated as chronic. In practice the diagnosis of acute hyponatremia can be made only in a hospital setting, when plasma sodium has been documented by laboratory tests to be normal within the previous 24 h. Any other patient with hyponatremia should be treated as a case of chronic hyponatremia, with slow and cautious correction of the hypoosmolar state.

In isotonic hyponatremia the serum osmolality is normal and it may be due to elevated serum lipid and serum protein concentrations (pseudo-hyponatremia). Hyponatremia in this situation requires no further treatment. Hypertonic hyponatremia is usually due to hyperglycemia, such as in the case of uncontrolled diabetes mellitus. The elevated osmolality of hyperglycemia forces osmotic shift of water from intracellular spaces into the intravascular spaces, leading to true hyponatremia. Treating the uncontrolled diabetes improves the measurement of serum sodium.

Most etiologies of hyponatremia are associated with hypotonic (dilutional) states, those in which there is a relative excess of water compared to salt. This will be the focus of the remainder of the discussion on hyponatremia.

3.2.1. SIADH AND CEREBRAL SALT WASTING

In the postoperative pituitary surgery patient the most common causes of hypotonic hyponatremia are due to the syndrome of inappropriate secretion of antidiuretic hormone (SIADH) and the syndrome of cerebral salt wasting (CSW) *(12)*. SIADH is a volume-replete state in which ADH is secreted from the posterior pituitary despite adequate volume and low serum osmolality status. Hypertonic urine and elevated urine sodium are present despite hyponatremia and hypotonic plasma in SIADH. Intravascular and extravascular volumes are normal to mildly expanded due to free water retention from impaired renal water excretion but normal renal sodium excretion. Symptoms of SIADH may be expected to occur about 1 week after surgery, though hyponatremia could be present a couple of days before symptoms.

CSW is initiated by renal sodium wasting that in turn leads to volume depletion, as water excretion follows. This sodium wasting may be due to hormonal involvement, possibly from atrial natriuretic peptide (ANP) or brain natriuretic peptide (BNP), along with impaired neural input to the kidney. The resulting volume-depleted state appropriately causes ADH secretion, increasing free water retention and hyponatremia. CSW usually starts within 10 days of the surgery.

Laboratory findings may be similar in SIADH and CSW, including hyponatremia, elevated ADH, urine sodium, and decreased urine volume. SIADH may be associated with low serum uric acid levels. Signs and symptoms of volume status are the principal determinant differentiating the conditions as SIADH occurs with euvolemia or even mild hypervolemia and CSW occurs with intravascular and total volume depletion. Occasionally, invasive measures such as Swan–Ganz catheterization should be performed to differentiate hypovolemia from euvolemia, aiding the diagnosis.

3.2.2. TREATMENT OF SIADH AND CSW

Correct diagnosis of the cause of hyponatremia is important because management differs based on the etiology. Essentially, SIADH treatment involves fluid restriction, while CSW is treated with fluid supplementation with saline to aid intravascular fluid volume repletion. Fluid restriction involves limiting fluid intake to 1,000 ml/day with close electrolyte monitoring. If this does not correct the sodium over a few days, more stringent restriction should be attempted to 600 cc limitation per day *(13)*.

Adding loop diuretics (furosemide or ethacrinic acid) may increase free water excretion and accelerate resolution of hyponatremia. The recent development of the nonpeptidic vasopressin receptor antagonists will soon change our approach to therapy of hyponatremia in patients with SIADH *(14)*.

If the symptoms of hyponatremia are acutely developed and sodium is less than 120 mmol/l, then hypertonic saline may be cautiously given; the osmolality of the fluid given must be higher than the osmolality of the urine in order to avoid further worsening of serum sodium concentration and symptoms. Volume replenishment for CSW can occur with administration of intravenous saline to the point of euvolemia. Serum sodium concentration should not be raised more quickly than 0.5 mmol/l/h in order to avoid central myelinolysis (*see* formula below). Oral salt tablets can then be taken for about a month until CSW resolves.

3.2.3. OTHER CAUSES OF HYPOTONIC HYPONATREMIA

Other causes of hyponatremia need to be considered in making the diagnosis of hyponatremia in the setting of a postoperative pituitary surgery patient. Nonrenal sodium loss can occur from GI sources such as nasogastric intubation to aid gastrointestinal decompression, diarrhea, and vomiting, causing loss of hypertonic fluid and replacement with free water and resulting in hyponatremia. Insensible loss from sweating may also occur. Correction of these complications will help to reduce sodium loss. Replacement of volume with IV saline will correct the hyponatremia.

Hypothyroidism decreases cardiac output and leads to ADH secretion despite lowered glomerular filtration rate (GFR) and free water retention. Adrenal insufficiency and hypocortisolism allow for volume depletion with subsequent ADH release as well.

Edema from fluid overload occurs in congestive heart failure, renal failure with or without the presence of the nephrotic syndrome, and cirrhosis. These states effectively decrease GFR with a resulting increase of ADH and thirst. Therefore a paradoxical intake of free water exacerbates the fluid overload state and leads to hyponatremia. Addressing these complicating factors, including fluid restriction, will improve the clinical state.

REFERENCES

1. Barkan AL, Chandler WF. Giant pituitary prolactinoma with falsely-low serum prolactin: the pitfall of the "high-dose hook effect": case report. Neurosurgery 1998;42:913–5.
2. Adrogue HJ, Madias NE. Hypernatremia. NEJM 2000;20:1493–9.
3. Oelkers W. Adrenal insufficiency. N Engl J Med 1999;335:1206–12.
4. Dumont AS, Nemergut EC, Jane JA, Laws ER. Postoperative care following pituitary surgery. Journal of Intensive Care Medicine 2005;20:128–40.

5. Erturk E, Jaffe CA, Barkan AL. Evaluation of the integrity of the HPA axis by insulin hypoglycemia test. J Clin Endocrinol Metab 1998;83:2350–4.
6. Mayerknecht J, Diederich S, Bahr V, Plockinger U, Oelkers W. Comparison of low and high dose corticotrophin stimulation tests in patients with pituitary disease. J Clin Endocrinol Metab 1998;83:1558–62.
7. Dorin RI, Qualls CR, Crapo LM. Diagnosis of adrenal insufficiency. Ann Int Med 2003;139:194–204.
8. Molitch ME, Clemmons DR, Malozowski S, Merriam GR, Shalet SM, Vance ML. Endocrine Society Clinical Guidelines Subcommittee. Evaluation and treatment of adult onset growth hormone deficiency: Practical Guidelines. J Clin Endocrinol Metab 2006;91:1621–34.
9. Barkan AL, Clemmons DR, Molitch ME, Stewart PM, Young WF, Jr. Growth hormone therapy for hypopituitary adults: time for re-appraisal. Trends Endocrinol Metab 2000;11:238–45.
10. Adrogue HJ, Madias NE. Hyponatremia. NEJM 2000;21:1581–9.
11. Cole CD, Gottfried ON, Liu JK, Couldwell WT. Hyponatremia in the neurosurgical patient: diagnosis and management. Neurosurg Focus 2004;16:1–10.
12. Palmer BF. Hyponatremia in patients with central nervous system disease: SIADH versus CSW. Trends Endocrinol Metab 2003;14:182–7.
13. Reynolds RM, Seckl JR. Hyponatremia for the clinical endocrinologist. Clin Endocrinol 2005;63:366–74.
14. Ghali JK, Koren MJ, Taylor JR, et al. Efficacy and safety of oral conivaptan: a V_{1A}/V_2 vasopressin receptor antagonist, assessed in a randomized, placebo-controlled trial in patients with euvolemic or hypervolemic hyponatremia. J Clin Endocrinol Metab 2006;91:2145–52.

17 Radiation Therapy for Pituitary Adenomas

Helen A. Shih, MD, and Jay S. Loeffler, MD

CONTENTS

1. INTRODUCTION
2. MODALITIES OF RADIATION THERAPY
3. NONFUNCTIONING TUMORS
4. HORMONE-SECRETING TUMORS
5. RADIATION-RELATED ADVERSE EFFECTS
6. CONCLUSION

Summary

Radiation therapy offers another means of therapy for pituitary adenomas when roles for medical therapy and surgery have been exhausted. Technological advancements in medical physics have revolutionized modern day radiotherapy for pituitary adenomas. A variety of treatment modalities now exist, all of which offer higher degree of accuracy and safety in radiation delivery. Very high tumor local control rates and reasonably high hormonal response rates to radiation therapy can now be achieved with fairly low rates of treatment-related adverse effects. The exception to this remains radiation-induced hypopituitarism which remains an inherent limitation of irradiating the pituitary.

Key Words: Pituitary adenoma, Radiation therapy, Radiosurgery, Proton beam, LINAC, Gamma knife.

1. INTRODUCTION

Radiation therapy is generally not a primary treatment modality for pituitary adenomas. However, in patients with pituitary adenomas refractory to medical and/or surgical interventions, radiation can offer durable tumor control and

From: *Contemporary Endocrinology: Diagnosis and Management of Pituitary Disorders*
Edited by: B. Swearingen and B. M. K. Biller © Humana Press, Totowa, NJ

often biochemical remission for secretory tumors. Indications for radiation therapy vary by tumor type, size, and extrasellar extension. Radiation can be delivered in a single sitting by stereotactic radiosurgery (SRS) or in fractionated form of smaller doses delivered over typically 5–6 weeks in 25–30 treatments. A brief overview of forms of radiation modalities is followed by a discussion on the role of radiation therapy and the rationale of delivery method by adenoma type.

2. MODALITIES OF RADIATION THERAPY

Radiosurgery is defined as radiation delivered at a high dose to a single target at a single sitting; conventional fractionated radiotherapy involves multiple smaller doses, usually to a larger target, at multiple sittings. In order to minimize the dose to surrounding tissue, radiosurgical techniques employ stereotactic localization, where the target is localized in a coordinate reference system, usually by means of a frame affixed to the skull. There are a number of different forms of radiosurgery in use, with radiation delivered as photons (gamma knife (GK), LINAC) or charged particles (proton beam). Hybrid forms (stereotactic radiotherapy—SRT) that employ stereotactic aiming techniques with fractionated therapy have been developed.

2.1. GK Radiation Therapy

GK (Elekta, Stockholm, Sweden) is a form of SRS, a method of delivering high-dose radiation with high precision in a single sitting. It was first devised in 1951 by Lars Leksell, MD, a Swedish neurosurgeon. Following years of planning, the first clinical treatment facility was initiated by Leksell in 1968. Although it was initially used to treat arteriovenous malformations by a nonsurgical method, its use has expanded to include treatment of other small intracranial targets such as brain metastases and pituitary adenomas. GK utilizes cobalt-60 (^{60}Co), a radioactive isotope, as its radiation source. In its most common design, a total of 201 sources of ^{60}Co are distributed in a hemisphere. A metal frame is placed on the patient's head to bridge between the radioactive sources and the patient's head. The bores in the metal frame vary in size and determine the width of the radiation beams. Cobalt-60 has a half-life of 5.5 years and emits photons of an average energy of 1.25 MV. Its low megavoltage energy is ideal for limited tissue penetration such as in the head. The dose gradient between high and low doses is very narrow such that small targets can be treated to high doses yet be juxtaposed to radiation-sensitive structures that will receive negligible dose. These high-dose spots permit delivery of highly conformal treatments by treating clusters of spots that create the shape of the target. The dose heterogeneity between the edge of the treatment margin and the center of each pinpointed target is typically a 50 % dose gradient and this can be either very useful or sometimes harmful depending upon the tissue being irradiated. GK is the most widely published radiosurgical methodology used to treat pituitary adenomas.

2.2. Linear Accelerator-Based SRS

The linear accelerator (LINAC) is the most common technological equipment used today to deliver therapeutic radiation. Energy is accelerated, shaped, and delivered in the form of photons or electrons. LINACs have been adapted to deliver stereotactic treatments using small beams of photon radiation delivered in arcs to a fixed target of limited size in the head (1). Its application in the treatment of pituitary adenomas has been reported with comparable efficacy to GK in the literature (2,3). When LINACs are adapted to deliver high doses of radiation in a single session similar to GK treatment, a stereotactic frame is surgically fixed to the patient's head and the treatment is termed SRS. The frame used for SRS is adapted from similar stereotactic frames used during neurosurgery and involves using stabilization pins that fix the halo-shaped frame to the cranium, typically using four pins above the level of the brow. Local anesthesia is administered prior to pin placement. Frame placement can be performed in the outpatient sitting with the patient sitting upright. Radiation planning is based upon a CT scan that is subsequently obtained with the frame now fixed to the patient's head. During simulation, the frame attaches to the CT scanner platform in the same manner as it will during the time of treatment in a LINAC machine. Sometimes MRIs are used to facilitate treatment planning by fusing these images to the CT data set although this is rarely necessary when targeting the pituitary. Radiation delivered by LINAC-based SRS is more homogeneous in dose as compared to GK; this is helpful in avoiding hotspots when irradiated targets include radiation-sensitive normal tissues. Because treatment is delivered as moving arcs of radiation beams around a central axis, the treatment volume is spherical or elliptoid and can have an inferior conformality when treating irregularly shaped targets as compared to GK.

2.3. Stereotactic Radiotherapy

When LINAC-based stereotactic treatment is modified to deliver fractionated doses, this is termed SRT. SRT utilizes the same planning system as SRS but with the primary difference in alternate form of immobilization. Instead of the SRS frame that involves pins fixed to the cranium, SRT most commonly uses a dental mold fixed to a stereotactic frame. This setup can be replicated daily with no discomfort to the patient. Various customized head molds can also be made in the case of edentulous patients. Fractionation schedules most commonly used to treat pituitary adenomas are 1.8–2.0 Gy

per treatment, similar to other fractionated radiation therapy though some
investigators have employed hypofractionated schemes (e.g., 5 Gy for seven
fractions).

2.4. Three-Dimensional Conformal Radiation Therapy

Standard LINAC-based treatment has long been used to treat pituitary
adenomas. Three-dimensional conformal radiation therapy (3D-CRT) is the
most widely available form of radiation treatment. It utilizes CT-based planning
methods similar to stereotactic forms of delivery but uses immobilization and
planning systems that have slightly less stringency in setup replication. A
custom face mask is made during the planning process that utilizes a thermo-
plastic mesh that molds to the patient's facial contour and attaches directly
to the treatment machine. As in the other forms of immobilization, the mask
serves to keep the head in the same position for each treatment and minimizes
head rotation and chin tilt variation. It provides an easy and replicable method
for patient positioning; this technique is widely used but does not yield the
same degree of accuracy as the immobilization techniques used in GK or
LINAC-based SRS or SRT. To account for the potentially larger variation
in positioning, the treatment field using 3D-CRT is significantly larger as
compared to stereotactic methods. A variety of treatment beam directions can
be used but two or three fields are most commonly employed. The volume
of neighboring tissue irradiated and the dose to these areas are higher as
compared to stereotactic methods. Delivery is always fractionated. Because
doses required to control pituitary adenomas are generally within the accepted
tolerances of the surrounding normal tissues, this is a very effective and
acceptable alternative therapy when more advanced technological alternatives
are not available.

2.5. Proton Radiation Therapy

Protons are the nuclei of hydrogen atoms and are isolated by stripping off
the orbital electron from hydrogen. In regard to therapeutic radiation therapy,
proton radiation has similar biological effects as the energy delivered by
photons, but has a distinct benefit in physical properties, because of which
the surrounding nontarget tissues are exposed to less radiation. Due to the
complexity and expense of building and maintaining such facilities, there are
limited clinical proton treatment facilities in the United States, although this
number grew to five centers in 2006 and is expected to increase in the future.
Proton radiation can be delivered in a single fraction as proton SRS or in
multiple fractions depending upon the clinical scenario. While the pattern of
dose distribution is inherently more conformal than photon-based systems,
scarce resources limit its widespread use. The greatest benefit of using protons
to treat pituitary adenomas is in cases with larger target volumes, such as when

the entire enlarged sella is to be targeted or when extrasellar components exist. Significantly less radiation is delivered to the surrounding normal tissues as compared to photon-based methods.

3. NONFUNCTIONING TUMORS

The primary goal of radiation therapy in nonfunctioning pituitary adenomas is to arrest tumor growth. Partial tumor shrinkage can often be achieved and may alleviate symptoms related to tumor compression, although this is typically achieved by surgical decompression prior to radiotherapy. Gross totally resected or near-gross totally resected nonfunctioning pituitary adenomas typically do not require adjuvant radiation therapy since risk for recurrence is generally low, in the range of 0–15 % at 5 years (4–7). Immediate postoperative radiation decreases risk for recurrence, but reserving radiation for recurrent adenomas spares the majority of patients from exposure to radiation and can delay potential adverse effects (e.g., neuroendocrine dysfunction) related to radiation to a later time (6,7). Depending upon the size and extension of the recurrence, repeat resection prior to radiation can reduce the risk of potential radiation-related adverse effects.

Patients with subtotally resected nonfunctioning macroadenomas with extrasellar extension into the cavernous sinus, abutting or above the chiasm, or involving other neighboring tissues may often have tumor-related symptoms that persist postoperatively. Even among those patients that are asymptomatic, the risk of new or recurrent symptoms is high if the residual disease is left untreated. For such patients, postoperative radiation is recommended. Both SRS and fractionated radiation modalities have been used in such sittings. For residual disease that involves or is in close proximity to the chiasm or for tumors that involve the cavernous sinus, fractionated radiation is often a safer mode of radiation delivery with lower risks of normal tissue complications (3). Radiosurgical methods are often used and carefully target only the residual disease and avoid the surrounding critical structures. It is the preferred treatment modality if adequate sparing of radiation to normal tissues can be achieved. Doses typically delivered are 12–20 Gy for radiosurgical treatments and 45–54 Gy by fractionated methods. In centers without the option of SRT for fractionated treatments, a three-field plan with lateral or lateral obliques combined with a superior anterior oblique field is reasonable. Larger treatment fields are inherently at higher risk for normal tissue injury but this is partially offset by fractionation, which permits normal tissue repair (8).

A review of 17 radiosurgical series including 452 cases of nonfunctional pituitary adenomas achieved local control rates of 92–100 % at mostly 2–4 years follow-up (8). The predominant treatment modality was GK, with average tumor margin doses ranging from 14 to 25 Gy. Iwai et al. (9)

report their nonfunctioning adenomas experience following GK treatment. With median 5-year data on 31 patients, they achieved an actuarial local control rate of 93 %. Median marginal dose was 14 Gy. Similarly, Pollock (10) report on 33 patients treated with GK and a median marginal dose of 16 Gy. Five-year actuarial control was 97 %. Losa et al. (11) report a 5-year recurrence-free rate of 88 % based on 52 cases of nonfunctioning pituitary adenomas and two subsequent failures. Both failures occurred in the sella outside of the irradiated volume, which was limited to only the residual disease. Although there is an increase in regional failures associated with small treatment fields, the benefit of minimizing radiation toxicities outweighs this concern because recurrence is infrequent and salvage therapy by surgery or additional radiation is often possible (8).

Picozzi et al. (12) have recently reported a comparison study of 119 patients with nonfunctioning pituitary adenomas who either underwent surgical resection alone or surgery followed by GK radiosurgery within 1 year postoperatively. GK was given as adjuvant treatment and not for recurrence of tumor. Recurrence-free status at 5 years was 51.1 % in the surgery alone arm versus 89.8 % in the surgery and radiosurgery arm. There was both a significant reduction in recurrence rate and a reduction in size of residual tumor from a baseline of 2.4 ± 0.2 cc to 1.6 ± 0.2 cc. The authors show that preoperative tumor sizes are comparable between the two arms but do not comment on postoperative residual disease between the two groups. Although this was a nonrandomized retrospective series, it does suggest a role for postoperative adjuvant radiation particularly in cases where further surgery would be challenging or not possible.

Fractionated radiotherapy experiences of nonfunctioning adenomas have also achieved excellent local control rates. Milker-Zabel et al. (13) treated 42 patients with a mean dose of 50.4 Gy by SRT and reported only one failure at median follow-up of 38.7 months. Among another 65 patients with nonfunctioning adenomas treated with fractionated radiation, the 10-year local control rate was 98 % (14). In addition, 72 % of these patients experienced improvement of tumor-related symptoms, most commonly of visual disturbances or headaches.

Longer-term data following radiation therapy are limited. Van den Bergh et al. (15) reported on 122 patients with nonfunctioning adenomas predominantly treated with doses of 45–50.4 Gy. The 10-year local control rates after subtotal resection with or without immediate postoperative radiation was 95 % versus 22 %, respectively. The University of Pittsburgh experience with fractionated radiation to a median of 46.7 Gy suggests that failures do increase with time with actuarial tumor control rates of 87.5 %, 77.6 %, and 64.7 % at 10, 20, and 30 years, respectively (16). However, these data are derived from a series of 120 patients with median follow-up of 9 years. In another series of 22 patients with nonfunctioning adenomas treated with surgery and fractionated radiation to 50 Gy, 100% control was still maintained at 10 years *(17)*. Additional long-term data are needed to better define patterns of late failures.

Data on the use of proton radiation to treat nonfunctional pituitary adenomas are provided by Loma Linda's proton experience *(18)*. The majority of patients were referred for proton radiation as adjuvant therapy to partial resection, local recurrence, or inadequate hormonal control. Only 8.5% were treated as a primary modality of therapy. With an even mix of functional and nonfunctional pituitary adenomas treated with fractionated protons to a median dose of 54 GyE, local control was achieved in all 20 patients with nonfunctional adenomas available for assessment at a median of 47 months of radiographic follow-up.

In summary, radiation therapy for nonfunctioning adenomas may be indicated when residual extrasellar disease remains, particularly when the risk of surgical treatment is high. If only intrasellar residual tumor exists postoperatively, close surveillance with imaging studies is an option because these adenomas can be typically reresected with minimal morbidity should they show future evidence of regrowth. Radiation therapy can also be delivered at that time. In patients with tumors that recur and undergo a second resection, postoperative radiation is often recommended since these tumors are at high propensity for second recurrence. Choice of radiation modality partially depends upon the adjacent normal structures that are involved. In tumors involving the cavernous sinus or abutting the optic chiasm, fractionated radiation offers a lower risk of late tissue complications. Radiosurgical methods can be used where these normal tissue tolerances are not a concern, and doses of 14–17 Gy are frequently used with local control rates of 95% or greater at 5 years. Similar tumor control is achieved with fractionated doses of 45–50.4 Gy.

4. HORMONE-SECRETING TUMORS

Radiation therapy can be an effective means of controlling functional pituitary adenomas that are refractory to surgery and pharmacological interventions. SRS appears to produce faster hormonal ablative response than fractionated radiation in functional tumors *(3,19)*. In those patients with no residual tumor within 3–5 mm of the optic chiasm, radiosurgery is usually the preferred option and is more convenient for patients. When the tumor is in closer proximity to the chiasm or other critical structures such as brain parenchyma or other cranial nerves, fractionated treatment may offer lower treatment-related late effects than radiosurgery *(3)*. Local control of tumor growth is excellent, approximately 95 % at 5 years, similar to nonfunctioning adenomas *(8,20)*. Hormonal response, either complete or partial but sufficient to enable control in conjunction with medical therapy, is achieved in approximately 60–80 % of patients overall but reported results vary widely from 0 % to 100 % *(8,20,21)*.

4.1. Acromegaly

Growth hormone-secreting tumors are amongst the most radiosensitive of the functional pituitary adenomas *(8,14)*. A recent review of the published radiosurgical literature that included 22 GK series and 3 LINAC SRS reports involved a total of 420 patients with acromegaly who received marginal tumor doses of 15–34 Gy *(8)*. Definitions of endocrinologic cure varied between studies and ranged between 0 % and 100 %. One of the largest reported series of 68 patients treated with mean margin dose of 31 Gy achieved normalization of growth hormone level of 96 % at 24 months *(22)*. This was more than double of their 12-month response rate of 40 %, indicating that endocrine response following radiation therapy takes years to achieve its full effect. Castinetti et al. *(23)* report on 82 acromegalic patients also treated with GK having tumor margin dose range of 12–40 Gy at mean follow-up of 49.5 months who obtained a 40 % hormonal response in which either complete remission was achieved or decreased GH secretion could be effectively controlled by medical therapy. A recent report of 42 patients with growth hormone-producing tumors treated with GK after surgery achieved a significant to complete hormonal response ($\geq$50 % decrease in growth hormone) of 62 % with a median follow-up of 63 months *(24)*. Mean marginal dose was 18.9 Gy. Hormonal response is variable whereas tumor growth local control was 100 % in this series and similar across others *(8)*.

Fractionated radiation also achieves variable hormonal control. Among 36 patients with acromegaly treated with fractionated therapy to 40 Gy, 69 % achieved normalization of GH at 10 years *(25)*. Milker-Zabel et al. *(26)* report on 20 acromegalics treated with SRT to a median dose of 52.2 Gy who obtained 80 % normalization. Local tumor control was 100 %. Another fractionated series that included 17 acromegalics treated to a median dose of 51 Gy and followed for a median of 8.2 years achieved 80 % symptomatic improvement *(14)*. An experience with conventional fractionated radiation to 45–50 Gy among 47 patients provides some long-term data and demonstrates the progressive response to radiation over time, with GH normalization of 29 % at 5 years, of 52 % at 10 years, and of 77 % at 15 years *(27)*. Local tumor control remained at 95 % at 15 years. While multiple reports suggest the efficacy of radiation therapy in the management of acromegaly, at least one report differs. In a study that evaluated random GH and IGF-1 levels among 38 acromegalic patients treated with radiation therapy, 65 % of patients achieved random GH levels below 5 mcg/l off medical therapy at 5 years but only two patients (5 %) achieved normalization of IGF-1 *(28)* IGF-1 levels could not be correlated with a decrease in GH levels, suggesting that normalized GH levels may be overestimating the effectiveness of radiation.

Predictive factors of response to radiation therapy are not well defined but some suggestions have been made based on existing data. Pretreatment GH and IGF-1 levels appear to predict for treatment response, with lower levels correlating with higher probability of successful response *(23,29,30)*. Another observation in some series is that concurrent medical therapy during the time of radiosurgery may decrease the probability of radiation response *(23,31,32)*. These investigators recommend withholding medical therapy at the time of radiation; however, these studies are not prospective randomized trials and thus are subject to multiple biases. Another predictor of response may be radiation dose. Higher dose has been correlated with quicker clinical response such as time to resolution of disease-related hyperglycemia or hypertension *(22)*.

Results from proton radiation therapy are limited due to the limited number of treatment facilities, but are expected to have superior dose delivery and normal tissue sparing based on the inherent physical properties of protons. The initial report of the Massachusetts General Hospital (MGH) proton experience in treating acromegaly established efficacy of proton radiosurgery *(33)*. Current updates have also been favorable. Of 22 patients with persistent acromegaly treated with single-fraction proton radiosurgery, median dose of 20 GyE, 95 % have achieved at least a partial response at 6 years and 50 % have had a complete response *(34)*. Median time to complete response in those who responded was 30.5 months. One-third of patients developed at least one new pituitary deficiency, corrected with supplementation Loma Linda has reported on fractionated proton therapy for 21 patients with functional adenomas treated to a median dose of 54 GyE and followed for a median of 47 months. Biochemical control was obtained in 86 % of patients *(18)*. Subjectively, 71 % of patients reported symptomatic improvement.

4.2. Cushing's Disease

ACTH-secreting tumors that are persistent after surgery are typically referred for radiation management. Radiosurgical treatment offers faster response than fractionated treatment. In a review of 22 series and 314 patients treated radiosurgically for Cushing's disease, hormonal control was attained in 10–100 % of patients, a similarly wide spread of results as with radiosurgery for acromegaly *(8)*. Tumor margin dose varied between 15 and 32 Gy. One of the largest series was a report by Sheehan et al. *(35)* of 43 patients treated with GK to a mean margin dose of 20 Gy. With a median follow-up of 44 months, the investigators reported a 63 % success rate of hormonal control. Fractionated treatments are not as widely reported but 45–50 Gy has achieved laboratory testing response rates of 93 % among 40 Cushing's disease patients at 10 years (36). This is consistent with a similar review of 30 Cushing's disease patients that achieved clinical or diagnostic response of 83 % with a median follow-up of 42 months (37). Similarly, a third single institutional review of patients with pituitary adenomas treated with fractionated radiotherapy of 50.4 Gy reported hormonal normalization of 100 % response among 10 Cushing's disease patients with a median follow-up of 80 months (21).

The MGH proton experience includes 38 patients with persistent Cushing's disease following surgery treated with a median dose of 20 GyE and followed for a median time of 38 months (38). A response was obtained in 79 % of patients and normalization of cortisol levels was achieved in 50 % of patients. Median time to hormonal response was 14 months. New pituitary deficiency occurred in 36 % of patients.

Predictive factors to response of GK in Cushing's disease have included smaller tumor volume and being off of medical therapy at the time of irradiation (39). A limitation of this study is the inherent biases of retrospective analyses.

4.3. Prolactinoma

The application of radiation therapy in the management of prolactinomas is relatively uncommon because these adenomas are well managed with pharmacotherapy. Even in prolactin-secreting tumors that are refractory to medical therapy, surgery is frequently able to resolve the hyperprolactinemia or provide sufficient partial response that dopamine agonists can provide adequate hormonal control. In the rare circumstances of failed medical and surgical intervention, radiation therapy can also be given. Success of radiation in treating prolactin-secreting functional adenomas is somewhat less than with other adenomas (8,40). In the recent comprehensive literature review of radiosurgical experiences in treating pituitary adenomas by Sheehan et al. (8), 393 patients with prolactinomas were identified among 22 studies. Mean dose delivered to target margins ranged from 13.3 to 33 Gy and hormonal response rates varied between 0 % and 84 %. Response was assessed by normalization of prolactin levels, typically falling less than 20–30 ng/ml. By far the largest single series is reported by Pan et al. (40) who evaluated 128 cases of prolactinomas over a mean follow-up of 33 months. All patients were treated with GK to a mean tumor margin dose of 31.2 Gy. Local control and clinical curative hormonal response were achieved in 98 % and 52 % of cases, respectively. These investigators also found that higher treatment dose corresponded with increased endocrine response. Most patients were treated upfront with radiation perhaps partially in an effort to investigate alternate definitive first-line therapy for patients with prolactinomas with the hope of avoiding long-term medical therapy. It is unknown whether all prolactinomas share similar radiation sensitivity or if perhaps there exists biological variations in which tumors refractory to medical and surgical intervention may also be less responsive to radiation therapy. The true responsiveness and long-term hormonal control of prolactinomas by radiation therapy largely remains to be defined. Efficacy of fractionated radiation in prolactinomas exists in small series and results are similar to those of radiosurgery *(41)*.

Similar to findings in retrospective reports of GH-secreting tumors treated with radiation, there is the suggestion of decreased radiation efficacy if the patient was receiving concurrent medical therapy at the time of treatment. In one GK series of 20 patients with prolactinomas, a 25 % complete response and 55 % partial response was achieved at a median follow-up of 28.6 months following mean marginal dose of 25.2 Gy *(42)*. Nine patients were treated with a dopamine agonist at the time of GK radiosurgery; 11 patients were not on hormonal therapy. Although numbers are small, no patients experiencing a complete response were on dopamine agonists at the time of radiosurgery, supporting the hypothesis that concurrent hormonal therapy may decrease tumor susceptibility to radiation. However, these conclusions are purely observational and based on limited patient numbers.

4.4. Other Functional Adenomas

Experiences using radiation therapy to treat other types of hormone-secreting adenomas are far less common and sparsely reported. In general, functional adenomas appear to have a wide spectrum of response to radiation, probably a result of few numbers, short follow-up, and variable definitions of hormonal response.

5. RADIATION-RELATED ADVERSE EFFECTS

Technological advancements in radiation therapy increasingly improve accurate and high-dose delivery of therapeutic radiation to targets with steep dose gradients at target edges, thereby reducing unnecessary irradiation of juxtaposed normal tissues. While increasing treatment conformality with reduced treatment field sizes will translate into decrease of radiation-related toxicity, radiation-related adverse effects are still common.

5.1. Hypopituitarism

The loss of one or more hormonal functions of the hypothalamic–pituitary axis is the most common adverse effect of radiation therapy for pituitary adenomas. Patients should be counseled on the importance of regular endocrinologic evaluation. The majority of patients will develop a new hormonal deficiency of one or more axes and this risk increases with time. Hypopituitarism is largely unavoidable because it is a direct consequence of pituitary irradiation. The approximate risk of hypopituitarism is 20–50 % at 5 years (3,10,14,18,20,25,27,34,38,43). Biermasz et al. (25) report results of 36 acromegalics treated with fractionated 40 Gy; they found rates of hypopituitarism requiring replacement of 29 % at 5 years, 54 % at 10 years, and 58 % at 15 years. Along a similar trend, Minniti et al. (27) report long-term results of 47 patients with GH-secreting tumors and otherwise normal pituitary function prior to irradiation. New hypopituitarism developed following standard fractionated 45–50 Gy at a rate of 57 % at 5 years, 78 % at 10 years, and 85 % at 15 years, distributed over gonadal, thyroid, and cortisol insufficiency. Similar rates of hypopituitarism develop with either radiosurgery or fractionated therapy (3).

In an attempt to characterize susceptibility to radiation-associated hypopituitarism, a comparison study of two groups of patients with pituitary adenomas treated with GK and followed for a median of 5 years was performed; this study found that increased dose correlated with increased risk of postradiation hypopituitarism (44). The investigators also found that dose to the pituitary stalk increased the risk of pituitary dysfunction. Patient numbers were insufficient to further define the dose–hormonal insufficiency relationship. Similar risks of hypopituitarism with irradiation of the pituitary stalk or hypothalamus have been reported by others (20,45). Feigl et al. (20) report that the dose difference of 7.7 ± 3.7 Gy versus 5.5 ± 3 Gy to the infundibulum among 92 patients treated with GK for pituitary adenomas was statistically significant and correlated to pituitary dysfunction at 5 years. Moderate dose of 50 Gy to the hypothalamus has also been shown to be predictive of pituitary insufficiency (45). The effects of hypothalamic and stalk irradiation should be considered and minimized during radiation planning. Nonetheless, since hormonal deficiency is largely unavoidable but is correctable with pharmacotherapy, the importance of lifelong close surveillance should be discussed with patients who receive pituitary irradiation.

5.2. Visual Pathway Injury

Although uncommon, radiation-induced vision injury or blindness has a devastating impact on the quality of life of patients. Following their review of 1,621 patients from 35 studies of patients with pituitary adenomas treated with radiosurgery, Sheehan et al. (8) found 16 cases of vision injury with dose to the optic pathways ranging between 0.7 and 12 Gy. Most retrospective analyses attempting to determine the threshold of single-fraction radiation tolerance to the optic system report 8–10 Gy as the maximal tolerance, with

8 Gy considered as a safe threshold and rare occurrences of optic neuropathy at 10 Gy *(46,47)*. Leber et al. *(47)* studied 50 patients who underwent GK for benign tumors, not limited to pituitary adenomas, and found no cases of visual impairment among 31 patients whose optic system received less than 10 Gy; 26.7% rate of injury was found among 22 patients treated between doses of 10 to less than 15 Gy and 77.8% risk at doses of ≥15 Gy among 13 patients. However, case reports of optic nerve or chiasm injury at lower doses support the importance of minimizing unnecessary dose and volume of tissue exposed to radiation. Fractionated radiation is associated with substantially lower risk of optic pathway injury with an estimate of 1.5% at 20 years in one large series of 411 patients and no visual complications are often reported in smaller series *(3,48)*. Although fractionation can improve the rate of radiation side effects, the historical use of substantially larger treatment volumes may account for the 2% treatment-related vision impairment reported in some series *(49,50)*.

5.3. Other Cranial Nerve Deficits

Injury to other cranial nerves as a result of radiation therapy for pituitary adenomas is much less likely. The same review of 35 series by Sheehan et al. *(8)* found 21 cases of other cranial nerve injury, of which approximately half were transient symptoms. Many other smaller series report few, if any, cases of cranial neuropathies with single-fraction doses as high as 30 Gy to segments of nerves traversing through the cavernous sinus indicating the increased resiliency of these nerves *(47)*. Tischler et al. *(46)* report eight cases of cranial neuropathies of which two occurred against the background of prior high-dose irradiation, all others occurring at doses > 18 Gy, and at least three cases with symptoms that were either temporary or intermittent. History of prior irradiation and comorbidities such as baseline cranial nerve injury, diabetes mellitus, and vascular disease likely define an inherently higher risk population for nerve injury. Fractionation is an important means of decreasing this risk when a high dose is delivered to nerves that are unavoidably in the treatment field.

5.4. Brain Necrosis

Temporal lobe necrosis, seen most commonly with large conventional radiation fields, has become progressively uncommon with the use of modern stereotactic techniques that greatly reduce radiation exposure to nontarget tissues *(14)*. Although less common, brain parenchyma injury is also seen with modern radiosurgery, with 13 cases reported among the 35 series reviewed by Sheehan et al. *(8)*. Cases may remain clinically asymptomatic, detectable by imaging alone and sometimes self-resolving *(3,51)*. Prior irradiation appears to be a strong risk factor for radiation-induced brain necrosis *(8,51,52)*.

5.5. Second Tumors

The risk of radiation-induced neoplasm is low, but can be devastating when it occurs. Tsang et al. *(53)* report on long-term follow-up of 305 patients with pituitary adenomas who were treated with radiation, and found a rate of radiation-induced gliomas of 1.7% at 10 years and 2.7% at 15 years. Similarly, Brada et al. *(48)* reported on long-term results in 411 patients with pituitary adenomas and had a 20-year rate of radiation-induced tumors of 1.9%. Radiation treatments in the first study were delivered between 1972 and 1986 and in the second study between 1962 and 1986, both using antiquated methods that treated substantially larger volumes of tissue than would be treated using modern-day techniques of imaging, localization, and radiation delivery. Because the risk assessment of radiation-induced tumors requires long-term follow-up of ideally 10 or more years, there are currently insufficient data to accurately describe the risk with modern radiotherapy. Most common types of radiation-induced tumors include gliomas, meningiomas, and sarcomas with poor prognosis expected with malignant histologies *(48,54)*. Radiation-induced malignancies are particularly concerning in the setting of treating benign tumors such as pituitary adenomas; however, patients can be advised that the risk is expectedly much lower than those quoted from historical reports.

5.6. Internal Carotid Artery Stenosis

Vascular stenosis is an uncommon event reported in few series *(51,55,56)*. In one long-term analysis of 331 patients treated with fractionated radiation for pituitary adenomas, the investigators reported 5-year, 10-year, and 20-year risks for cerebrovascular accident of 4%, 11%, and 21%, respectively *(55)*. This approximate 1%/year rate of stroke was equivalent to a relative risk of 4.1 as compared to the normal population. In a recent review including 211 acromegalic patients treated with fractionated radiation using a traditional three-field technique, there was a significant increase in the standardized mortality ratio (4.42) among this cohort as compared to the local population *(57)*. Specific increase cause of death was due to cerebrovascular accidents. Concerns regarding both of these studies are the lack of other substantial data to support these findings and the lack of detail of the study population, including no information on types of strokes, possible inherent risk factors of patients, details of radiation, or locations of strokes. Whereas there may be little evidence consistent with radiation-related carotid stenosis, this risk currently appears to be minimal at a clinically significant level. As with all other tissues not intended for irradiation, treatment-related risks are best avoided by minimizing any unnecessary irradiation of neighboring tissues when possible.

6. CONCLUSION

Radiation therapy is not typically employed as a first-line therapy for pituitary adenomas but can present a useful treatment modality for otherwise refractory tumors. Radiation therapy can be delivered by a variety of modalities and patients should be evaluated by a radiation oncologist for recommendation of appropriate options. Radiation therapy controls tumor growth in approximately 95 % of pituitary adenomas and can frequently achieve either a complete or a partial hormonal response in functioning tumors. Hormonal response following radiation therapy requires many months to years to attain its full effect, with most responders having clinically appreciable changes by 2 years. Supplementation with medical therapy is required until adequate hormonal response has been demonstrated. Hypopituitarism is a common effect of radiation therapy, occurring in about a third of patients by 5 years after radiation treatment and with continued gradual rise with time. Advances in the delivery of radiation therapy continue to be associated with progressively lower rates of adverse effects, but these risks should still be recognized and discussed with patients prior to proceeding with treatment.

REFERENCES

1. Kooy HM, Nedzi LA, Loeffler JS, et al. Treatment planning for stereotactic radiosurgery of intra-cranial lesions. Int J Radiat Oncol Biol Phys 1991;21(3):683–93.
2. Yoon SC, Suh TS, Jang HS, et al. Clinical results of 24 pituitary macroadenomas with linac-based stereotactic radiosurgery. Int J Radiat Oncol Biol Phys 1998;41(4): 849–53.
3. Mitsumori M, Shrieve DC, Alexander E, et al. Initial clinical results of linac-based stereotactic radiosurgery and stereotactic radiotherapy for pituitary adenomas. Int J Radiat Oncol Biol Phys 1998;42(3):573–80.
4. 4. Alameda C, Lucas T, Pineda E, et al. Experience in management of 51 non-functioning pituitary adenomas: indications for post-operative radiotherapy. J Endocrinol Invest 2005;28(1):18–22.
5. Dekkers OM, Pereira AM, Roelfsema F, et al. Observation alone after transsphenoidal surgery for nonfunctioning pituitary macroadenoma. J Endocrinol Metab 2006;91(5): 1796–801.
6. Park P, Chandler WF, Barkan AL, et al. The role of radiation therapy after surgical resection of nonfunctional pituitary macroadenomas. Neurosurgery 2004;55(1):100–6.
7. Lillehei KO, Kirschman D, Kleinschmidt-DeMasters BK, et al. Reassessment of the role of radiation therapy in the treatment of endocrine-inactive pituitary macroadenomas. Neurosurgery1998;43(3):432–8.
8. Sheehan JP, Niranjan A, Sheehan JM, et al. Stereotactic radiosurgery for pituitary adenomas: an intermediate review of its safety, efficacy, and role in the neurosurgical treatment armamentarium. J Neurosurg 2005;102:678–91.
9. Iwai Y, Yamanaka K, Yoshioka K. Radiosurgery for nonfunctioning pituitary adenomas. Neurosurgery 2005;56:699–705.

10. Pollock BE, Carpenter PC. Stereotactic radiosurgery as an alternative to fractionated radiotherapy for patients with recurrent or residual nonfunctioning pituitary adenomas. Neurosurgery 2003;53(5):1086–94.

11. Losa M, Valle M, Mortini P, et al. Gamma knife surgery for treatment of residual nonfunctioning pituitary adenomas after surgical debulking. J Neurosurg 2004;100:438–44.

12. Picozzi P, Losa M, Mortini P, et al. Radiosurgery and the prevention of regrowth of incompletely removed nonfunctioning pituitary adenomas. J Neursurg 2005;102(Suppl): 71–4.

13. Milker-Zabel S, Debus J, Thilmann C, et al. Fractionated stereotactically guided radiotherapy and radiosurgery in the treatment of functional and nonfunctional adenomas of the pituitary gland. Int J Radiat Oncol Biol Phys 2001;50(5):1279–86.

14. Sasaki R, Murakami M, Okamoto Y, et al. The efficacy of conventional radiation therapy in the management of pituitary adenoma. Int J Radiat Oncol Biol Phys 2000;47(5):1337–45.

15. van den Bergh ACM, van den Berg G, Schoorl MA, et al. Immediate postoperative radiotherapy in residual nonfunctioning pituitary adenoma: beneficial effect on local control without additional negative impact on pituitary function and life expectancy. Int J Radiat Oncol Biol Phys 2007;67(3):863–9.

16. Breen P, Flickinger JC, Kondziolka D, et al. Radiotherapy for nonfunctioning pituitary adenoma: an analysis of long-term tumor control. J Neurosurg 1998;89(6):933–8.

17. Kokubo M, Sasai K, Shibamoto Y, et al. Long-term results of radiation therapy for pituitary adenoma. J Neurooncol 2000;47(1):79–84.

18. Ronson BB, Schulte RW, Han KP, et al. Fractionated proton beam irradiation of pituitary adenomas. Int J Radiat Oncol Biol Phys 2005;64(2):425–34.

19. Landolt AM, Haller D, Lomax, N, et al. Stereotactic radiosurgery for recurrent surgically treated acromegaly: comparison with fractionated radiotherapy. J Neurosurg 1998;88: 1002–8.

20. Feigl GC, Bonelli CM, Berghold A, et al. Effects of gamma knife radiosurgery of pituitary adenomas on pituitary function. J Neurosurg 2002;97(Suppl 5):415–21.

21. Colin P, Jovenin N, Delemer B, et al. Treatment of pituitary adenomas by fractionated stereotactic radiotherapy: a prospective study of 110 patients. Int J Radiat Oncol Biol Phys 2005;62(2):333–41.

22. Zhang N, Pan L, Wang EM, et al. Radiosurgery for growth hormone-producing pituitary adenomas. J Neurosurg 2000;93(Suppl 3):6–9.

23. Castinetti F, Taieb D, Kuhn J-M, et al. Outcome of gamma knife radiosurgery in 82 patients with acromegaly: correlation with initial hypersecretion. J Clin Endocrinol Metab 2005;90:4483–8.

24. Kobayashi T, Mori Y, Uchiyama Y, et al. Long-term results of gamma knife surgery for growth hormone-producing pituitary adenoma: is the disease difficult to cure? J Neurosurg 2005;102(Suppl):119–23.

25. Biermasz NR, van Dulken H, Roelfsema F. Long-term follow-up results of postoperative radiotherapy in 36 patients with acromegaly J Clin Endocrinol Metab 2000;85:2476–82.

26. Milker-Zabel S, Zabel A, Huber P, et al. Stereotactic conformal radiotherapy in patients with growth hormone-secreting pituitary adenoma. Int J Radiat Oncol Biol Phys 2004;59(4):1088–96.

27. Minniti G, Jaffrain-Rea M-L, Osti M, et al. The long-term efficacy of conventional radiotherapy in patients with GH-secreting pituitary adenomas. Clin Endocrinol 2005;62:210–6.

28. Barkan AL, Halasz I, Dornfeld KJ, et al. Pituitary irradiation is ineffective in normalizing plasma insulin-like growth factor I in patients with acromegaly. J Clin Endocrinol Metab 1997;82:3187–91.

29. Attanasio R, Epaminonda P, Motti E, et al. Gamma-knife radiosurgery in acromegaly: a 4-year follow-up study. J Clin Endocrinol Metab 2003;88:3105–12.
30. Littley MD, Shalet SM, Swindell R, et al. Low-dose pituitary irradiation for acromegaly. Clin Endocrinol (Oxf) 1990;32:261–70.
31. Pollock BE, Jacob JT, Brown PD, et al. Radiosurgery of growth hormone-producing pituitary adenomas: factors associated with biochemical remission. J Neurosurg 2007; 106:833–8.
32. Landolt AM, Haller D, Lomax N, et al. Octreotide may act as a radioprotective agent in acromegaly. J Clin Endocrinol Metab 2000;85:1287–9.
33. Kjellberg RN, Shintani A, Fanzt AG, et al. Proton beam therapy in acromegaly. N Engl J Med 1968;278:669–95.
34. Petit JH, Biller BMK, Swearingen B, et al. Proton stereotactic radiosurgery is effective and safe in the management of persistent acromegaly. The Endocrine Society, 88th Annual Meeting, Boston, MA, June 24–27, 2006.
35. Sheehan JM, Vance ML, Sheehan JP, et al. Radiosurgery for Cushing's disease after failed transsphenoidal surgery. J Neurosurg 2000;93:738–42.
36. Minniti G, Osti M, Jaffrain-Rea ML, et al. Long-term follow-up results of postoperative radiation therapy for Cushing's disease. J Neurooncol 2007; 84(1):79–84.
37. Estrada J, Boronat M, Mielgo M, et al. The long-term outcome of pituitary radiation therapy after unsuccessful transsphenoidal surgery in Cushing's disease. N Engl J Med 1997;336:172–7.
38. Petit JH, Biller BMK, Swearingen B, et al. Proton stereotactic radiosurgery is effective and safe in the management of Cushing's disease. The Endocrine Society, 88th Annual Meeting, Boston, MA, June 24–27, 2006
39. Castinetti F, Nagai M, Dufour H, et al. Gamma knife radiosurgery is a successful adjunctive treatment in Cushing's disease. Eur J Endocrinol 2007;156(1):91–8.
40. Pan L, Zhang N, Wang EM, et al. Gamma knife radiosurgery as a primary treatment for prolactinomas. J Neurosurg 2000;93(Suppl 3):10–3.
41. Tsagarakis S, Grossman A, Plowman PN, et al. Megavoltage pituitary irradiation in the management of prolactinomas: long-term follow-up. Clin Endocrinol (Oxf) 1991;34: 399–406.
42. Landolt AM, Lomax N. Gamma knife radiosurgery for prolactinomas. J Neurosurg 2000;93(Suppl 3):14–8.
43. Zierhut D, Flentje M, Adolph J, et al. External radiotherapy of pituitary adenomas. Int J Radiat Oncol Biol Phys 1995;33(2):307–14.
44. Vladyka V, Liscak R, Novotny J, et al. Radiation tolerance of functioning pituitary tissue in gamma knife surgery for pituitary adenomas. Neurosurgery 2003;52(2):309–17.
45. Pai HH, Thornton A, Katznelson L, et al. Hypothalamic/pituitary function following high-dose conformal radiotherapy to the base of skull: demonstration of a dose-effect relationship using dose-volume histogram analysis. Int J Radiat Oncol Biol Phys 2001;49(4):1079–92.
46. Tischler RB, Loeffler JS, Lunsford LD, et al. Tolerance of cranial nerves of the cavernous sinus to radiosurgery. Int J Radiat Oncol Biol Phys 1993;27:215–21.
47. Leber KA, Berglöff J, Pendl G. Dose-response tolerance of the visual pathways and cranial nerves of the cavernous sinus to stereotactic radiosurgery. J Neurosurg 1998;88:43–50.
48. Brada M, Rajan B, Traish D, et al. The long-term efficacy of conservative surgery and radiotherapy in the control of pituitary adenomas. Clin Endocrinol (Oxf) 1993;38:571–8.
49. Parsons JT, Bova FJ, Fitzgerald CR, et al. Radiation optic neuropathy after megavoltage external-beam irradiation: analysis of time-dose factors. Int J Radiat Oncol Biol Phys 1994;30(4):755–63.

50. McCord MW, Buatti JM, Fennell EM, et al. Radiotherapy for pituitary adenoma: long-term outcome and sequelae. Int J Radiat Oncol Biol Phys 1997;39(2):437–44.
51. Pollock BE, Nippoldt TB, Stafford SL, et al. Results of stereotactic radiosurgery in patients with hormone-producing pituitary adenomas: factors associated with endocrine normalization. J Neurosurg 2002;97:525–30.
52. Izawa M, Hayashi M, Nakaya K, et al. Gamma knife radiosurgery for pituitary adenomas. J Neurosurg 2000;93(Suppl 3):19–22.
53. Tsang RW, Laperriere NJ, Simpson WJ, et al. Glioma arising after radiation therapy for pituitary adenoma. Cancer 1993;72:2227–33.
54. Bembo SA, Pasmantier R, Davis RP, et al. Osteogenic sarcoma of the sella after radiation treatment of a pituitary adenoma. Endocr Pract 2004;10(4):335–8.
55. Brada M, Burchell L, Ashley S, et al. The incidence of cerebrovascular accidents in patients with pituitary adenoma. Int J Radiat Oncol Biol Phys 1999;45(3):693–8.
56. Lim YJ, Leem W, Park JT, et al. Cerebral infarction with ICA occlusion after gamma knife radiosurgery for pituitary adenoma: a case report. Stereotact Funct Neurosurg 1999;72(Suppl 1):132–9.
57. Ayuk J, Clayton RN, Holder G, et al. Growth hormone and pituitary radiotherapy, but not serum insulin-like growth factor-I concentrations, predict excess mortality in patients with acromegaly. J Clin Endocrinol Metab 2004;89(4):1613–7.

18 Lymphocytic Hypophysitis and Inflammatory Disease of the Pituitary

Stephan Ulmer, MD, and Thomas N. Byrne, MD

CONTENTS

1. DIFFERENTIAL DIAGNOSIS OF INFLAMMATORY DISEASE OF THE PITUITARY
2. MANAGEMENT OF LH

Summary

The most common form of primary hypophysitis is lymphocytic hypophysitis (LH), which is a rare inflammatory disorder of the pituitary that may present both as a sellar mass extending into the suprasellar space and as hypopituitarism. It is often confused radiographically with pituitary tumors. It usually presents in the peripartum period and may be associated with autoimmune diseases. The clinical context is usually quite important in raising the clinical suspicion of this disorder. This chapter discusses the epidemiology, pathogenesis, clinical presentation, imaging, differential diagnosis, and management of LH.

Key Words: Lymphocytic hypophysitis, Autoimmune.

1. DIFFERENTIAL DIAGNOSIS OF INFLAMMATORY DISEASE OF THE PITUITARY

1.1. Lymphocytic Hypophysitis

Patients clinically presenting with hypopituitarism and a contrast-enhancing lesion on magnetic resonance imaging (MRI) in the sella and/or suprasellar space are generally considered to harbor a neoplasm (Fig. 1). However,

From: *Contemporary Endocrinology: Diagnosis and Management of Pituitary Disorders*
Edited by: B. Swearingen and B. M. K. Biller © Humana Press, Totowa, NJ

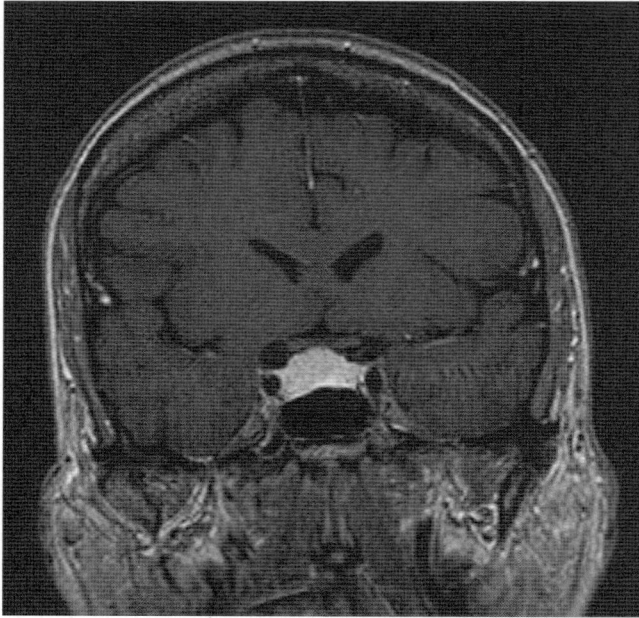

(A)

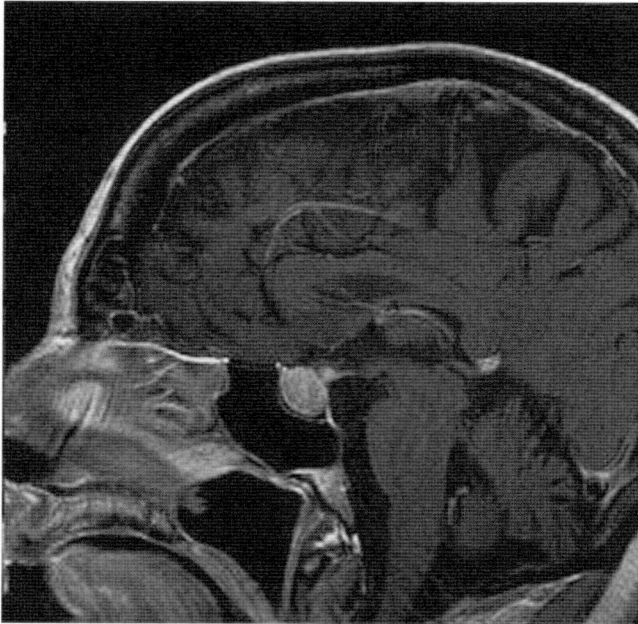

(B)

Fig. 1.

rarely, inflammatory disease may be the cause. While it has long been recognized that the pituitary may be damaged by systemic inflammatory disease such as sarcoidosis and tuberculosis affecting the basilar meninges, more recently there is increasing awareness of autoimmune inflammatory diseases affecting the pituitary alone or in association with other systemic autoimmune phenomena. When the pituitary is the primary target of such autoimmunity it is generally termed lymphocytic hypophysitis (LH) or autoimmune hypophysitis *(1,2)*. LH is a rare disorder; Caturegli et al. reported a prevalence of 8 cases in 905 surgical pituitary specimens (0.88%) from 1986 to 2004 at Johns Hopkins Hospital *(2)*. Even more uncommon are granulomatous and xanthomatous hypophysitis, which do not appear to be associated with other autoimmune diseases and have also been described histopathologically as a form of primary hypophysitis *(3)*. This chapter will principally discuss LH.

One possible reason for the increased awareness of LH may be the advances in modern imaging. Whereas previously these patients may have presented with idiopathic hypopituitarism or diabetes insipidus, current imaging in these patients may reveal abnormalities, which leads to the clinical suspicion of LH and subsequent biopsy and histological proof of the disorder *(4)*. Clinically, LH may affect the function of the anterior pituitary alone, the posterior pituitary alone, or both anterior and posterior in combination. When the anterior pituitary is the sole target, patients typically present with loss of anterior pituitary function and the disorder is termed lymphocytic adenohypophysitis (LAH). When the posterior pituitary or stalk is the sole locus of inflammation, patients often present with diabetes insipidus and the condition may be called lymphocytic infundibulohypophysitis (LINH). When both anterior and posterior segments of the pituitary are involved it may be called lymphocytic panhypophysitis (LPH). In this chapter, the classification and pathogenesis of these autoimmune inflammatory diseases as well as their clinical manifestations, imaging, and management approaches are discussed.

1.1.1. CLASSIFICATION, PATHOGENESIS, AND HISTOLOGY

An early description of LAH offers a glimpse at both a common clinical presentation and the pathogenesis of the disorder *(5)*. A young postpartum

Fig. 1. The spontaneous development of hypopituitarism in a 63-year-old woman; MRI demonstrated the homogeneous enlargement of the pituitary on coronal (1a) and sagittal (1b) views, without a clearly identified adenoma. Transsphenoidal biopsy with removal of minimal tissue demonstrated chronic and acute inflammation. Postoperative MRI without further treatment (beyond replacement glucocorticoids) showed partial resolution of pituitary enlargement, representing spontaneous resolution of the acute inflammation, although hormone function did not recover.

woman developed hypothyroidism, amenorrhea, and hypoadrenalism. About 1 year later she underwent an appendectomy and died. At autopsy, lymphocytic infiltration of the thyroid (Hashimoto's thyroiditis) and adrenal atrophy were found. The anterior pituitary was infiltrated with lymphocytes and showed atrophy but the neurohypophysis was normal. The authors recognized that this could represent an autoimmune disease related to her pregnancy. Since that report in the 1960s, LH has been increasingly recognized to occur more commonly in women, in the peripartum period, and in association with other autoimmune disorders; however, it has been described in men as well. LAH has been reported to occur in a female to male ratio of 6:1 (2). There is an association with autoimmune thyroid disease in up to 25%, most frequently Hashimoto's thyroiditis, although other associated autoimmune disorders have been reported (1,6).

Autoantibodies targeted against a 49-kDa cytosolic protein known as alpha-enolase have been found in the sera of patients with LH by Crock (7). However, presence of this antibody has also been found in pituitary neoplasms and other disorders (1,8). More recently, antibodies directed against gamma-enolase, more commonly known as neuron-specific enolase (NSE), have been reported in patients with LH (9). Since pituitary autoimmunity is strongly associated with pregnancy, the authors sought and identified NSE in placenta and autoantibodies in sera from patients with peripartum LH that also recognize NSE in the placenta. The authors concluded that the presence of NSE in the placenta and autoantibodies targeted against this antigen provides a theoretical basis for the predilection of LH to occur during pregnancy and the postpartum period. In Sheehan's syndrome with postpartum hemorrhage, pituitary necrosis, lactation failure, and hypopituitarism, antibodies against NSE have also been found, suggesting that patients with severe postpartum hemorrhage might also have evidence for pituitary autoimmunity (10). Autoantibodies directed against other pituitary constituents have been reported in cases of LH. Bensing et al. (2007) (11) reported a patient who presented with partial pituitary deficiency, an empty sella, and autoantibodies against secretogranin II, a protein frequently present in human gonadotrophs, thyrotrophs, and corticotrophs. They concluded that secretogranin II autoantibodies could serve as markers for LH. In contrast, Nishiki et al. (12) reported that serum antipituitary antibodies to human pituitary membrane antigens were found in a minority of patients with autoimmune LAH and LINH.

Lymphocytic infundibuloneurohypophysitis (LINH) causing diabetes insipidus has been reported to occur equally in men and women and is not associated with pregnancy (2). LINH has also been linked to autoantibodies targeted against arginine vasopressin (AVP). As discussed below, thickening of the pituitary stalk on MRI scan has been reported to be correlated pathologically with lymphocytic infiltration in LINH. De Bellis et al. *(13)* have reported a series of patients with idiopathic complete central diabetes insipidus (CDI) in which pituitary stalk thickening as demonstrated on MRI was present in patients with autoantibodies to AVP-secreting cells, but not in those without autoantibodies to AVP-secreting cells. This could indicate a strong relationship between the occurrence of these antibodies, markers of autoimmune hypothalamic involvement, and the lymphocytic infundibuloneurohypophysitis. More recently, Maghnie et al. *(14)* have reported circulating vasopressin-cell autoantibodies in 75% of 20 young patients with idiopathic CDI. However, these autoantibodies were also found in patients with CDI due to Langerhans cell histiocytosis (LCH) and germinoma, indicating that vasopressin-cell autoantibodies cannot be considered completely reliable markers of autoimmune CDI.

In summary, although there is circumstantial and indirect evidence that LH is an autoimmune disease, the absence of pituitary autoantibodies in some cases of LH, the presence of pituitary autoantibodies in conditions other than LH, as well as the lack of transmission of the disease from mother to newborn have raised questions as to their significance in making a diagnosis of LH. It remains unclear whether they have a pathogenetic role or, alternatively, they are epiphenomena *(1,2,12)*.

1.1.2. CLINICAL PRESENTATION

LH typically presents as a sellar mass, anterior pituitary dysfunction, diabetes insipidus, and/or hyperprolactinemia. Given the epidemiology of LH, it is typically suspected in a young pregnant or postpartum woman with symptoms and signs of a sellar mass and/or pituitary dysfunction, although Sheehan's syndrome and neoplastic lesions may also occur in this group *(15,16)*. In various series, it has been reported that approximately one-third to two-thirds of cases of LH occur during pregnancy or up to 6 months following delivery *(1–3,17)*. However, as more cases are reported, it is clear that males are affected and the age spectrum is expanding.

When the symptoms are those of sellar mass effect, the most common clinical presentation, patients have recent-onset headache, visual field loss if the chiasm is compressed, and may have isolated or multiple pituitary hormone deficiencies *(1)*. When present, the headache is typically bilateral frontal, retro-orbital, or temporal *(18)*. In other cases the clinical presentation may be insidious pituitary failure without symptoms or signs of mass effect. With or without headache, pituitary hormone deficiencies have been reported to occur in the majority of patients *(1,6,17)*. In a 1977 review of 124 cases by Hashimoto *(6)*, impairment of ACTH secretion was most frequent followed by TSH, gonadotrophin, growth hormone (GH), and prolactin deficiency. Hyperprolactinemia was found in one-third of cases. About 16% of patients had diabetes insipidus. However, isolated ACTH deficiency has been reported in LH *(19)*. In other cases the presentation may be a meningitic syndrome *(15,20,21)*.

Lymphocytic infundibuloneurohypophysitis (LINH) characteristically presents with diabetes insipidus. In a series of 17 patients with idiopathic diabetes insipidus of a few months to several years duration reported by Imura et al. *(4)*, 13 were women and the diabetes insipidus spontaneously improved in about half. Biopsy of two cases revealed infiltration primarily with lymphocytes and plasma cells. None of the patients in this series developed clinical symptoms or signs of hypopituitarism or hypothalamic dysfunction other than diabetes insipidus; however, several had impaired secretory responses of GH to insulin-induced hypoglycemia *(4)*. Patients with LINH may also have headache and mass-effect symptoms.

1.1.3. IMAGING

As for other intrasellar or suprasellar lesions, MRI is the imaging modality of choice. LH may be difficult to differentiate from pituitary adenomas or other mass lesions in the sella and suprasellar space. Although not diagnostic, imaging features that may suggest a preoperative diagnosis of LH include symmetric enlargement of the gland with diffuse contrast enhancement extending into the stalk and basal hypothalamus in a tongue-like fashion without erosion of the sella floor. In contrast, pituitary macroadenomas commonly are asymmetric masses that may erode the sella floor and displace the stalk *(2,15,16,20,22,23)*. However, no radiographic or MRI feature is pathognomonic, as other infiltrative disorders and some neoplasms may have a similar appearance.

LINH may show thickening of the stalk with enhancement and loss of the normal hyperintense signal of the neurohypophysis *(2,4)*. However, thickening of the pituitary stalk can also be seen in Langerhans cell histiocytosis (LCH), granulomatous diseases such as sarcoid and tuberculosis, and neoplasms such as craniopharyngioma, germinoma, lymphoma, and metastases *(24,25)*. De Bellis et al. *(13)* reported that, in patients with autoimmune CDI, the stalk thickening markedly improved over time in all patients during the follow-up; this may help make the diagnosis.

Imaging of LH can rarely reveal extension into the cavernous sinuses *(26)* and even clival involvement has been reported *(27)*. Additionally, LH may present as a cystic ring-enhancing lesion *(16,22)*. Because of the rarity of LH and the protean clinical and imaging manifestations, diagnosis of LH often requires biopsy.

1.1.4. SUMMARY OF THE DIAGNOSTIC CHALLENGE

The gold standard for diagnosis of LH is biopsy *(2,28)*. However, in their excellent review of autoimmune hypophysitis, Caturegli et al. *(2)* identified histological findings of LH in 14 reported cases due to the following lesions: five germinomas, four Rathke's cleft cysts, three craniopharyngiomas, and two adenomas. This underscores the fact that rarely even a biopsy may be misleading.

As discussed above, unfortunately, even organ-specific antibodies that may be good markers of many autoimmune endocrine diseases have been reported to be present against constituents of the pituitary in a variety of pituitary diseases and in postpartum women who have not developed hypophysitis. Accordingly, the pathogenetic and diagnostic role of antipituitary antibodies is controversial *(2,28)*.

Although there are no pathognomonic clinical, laboratory, or imaging signs there are features that can help in the differential diagnosis. Features that suggest LH include the onset in the peripartum period and hypopituitarism that is out of proportion to the relatively small pituitary mass seen on imaging. Endocrinological findings that suggest LH include prominent ACTH deficiency followed by TSH and gonadotrophic deficiency, but again these are not specific for LH and may not be always seen in LH *(2)*. Other systemic autoimmune diseases are common in LH as well *(1)*. The imaging features suggestive of LH are discussed above. Sheehan's syndrome (pituitary apoplexy) in the postpartum period thought to be due to hypotension from uterine hemorrhage may present as an acute disease or slowly evolving hypopituitarism. As mentioned above, however, pituitary autoantibodies may also be found in Sheehan's syndrome.

Caturegli et al. *(2)* culled the pituitary autoantibody results from several articles and found that using immunofluorescence, antibodies were positive in 14 of 39 (36%) patients with LAH; in none of 5 (0%) patients with LINH, and in 2 of 19 (10%) patients with LPH. Using an immunoblotting assay, positive antibodies were found in 11 of 16 (67%) patients with LAH, in 1 of 3 (33%) patients with LINH, and in 4 of 5 (80%) patients with LPH. The relatively low sensitivities and the few patients assayed lead to their questionable utility. The reviewers emphasize that the specificity of these antibodies is also dubious, in that autoantibodies are found in several other disease states such as pituitary adenomas, empty sella, Sheehan's syndrome, thyroid diseases, diabetes mellitus, and multiple sclerosis *(29–33)*.

2. MANAGEMENT OF LH

Management of LH may include replacement of hormone deficiencies, as well as surgical biopsy and/or debulking, glucocorticoids or other immunosuppressive agents such as azathoprine and methotrexate, and radiotherapy. Assessment of the efficacy of these treatments is complicated by the fact that the natural course is quite variable with some patients succumbing to the disease, others being left with permanent hypopituitarism and still others experiencing spontaneous recovery *(1,2,17)*.

Surgical resection was performed in 243 (64%) of 349 reported cases *(2)*. The benefits of surgery include histological confirmation of the diagnosis and decompression of normal tissues. However, surgery can lead to further endocrinological deficits. Thus the role of surgery in management is controversial, *(2,17)* but may be necessary if the diagnosis is unclear.

Glucocorticoids have been reported to be effective in diminishing the size of the region of enhancement *(6)*. Kristoff et al. *(20)* reported the results of a prospective high-dose methylprednisolone pulse therapy in nine patients, three of whom had a histological diagnosis of LH. The MRI improved in seven patients, anterior pituitary function improved in four of nine patients, and diabetes insipidus improved in all four in whom it occurred. The authors concluded that high-dose methylprednisolone therapy may improve clinical, endocrinological, and MRI findings. However, the benefit of high-dose steroids is difficult to assess from this uncontrolled trial as other articles have failed to confirm the benefits of high-dose steroids *(34–36)* and there have been cases of LH that resolve spontaneously *(17,21)*.

Accordingly, the management of LH remains controversial *(2,21,34,37)*. Despite this uncertainty, Caturegli et al. *(2)* concluded that it is reasonable to advocate the use of supraphysiological doses of glucocorticoids; a detailed discussion can be found in their review *(2)*. Alternatively, Matta et al. *(21)* have questioned the benefit of high-dose steroids citing cases that have responded to replacement doses of steroids. Because of the lack of large controlled trials showing the benefit of high-dose steroids, a number of centers confirm the diagnosis by biopsy, then follow the patient carefully with regular neurological, ophthalmological, endocrinological evaluations and serial MRI scans, and treat hormone deficiencies, reserving high-dose steroids for patients with symptomatic chiasm compression or other signs of mass effect. Other immunosuppressive agents such as azathioprine and methotrexate have also been used, but these are not routinely employed *(26,37,38)*. On long-term follow-up, the majority of patients require pituitary hormone replacement. However, spontaneous recovery without treatment as well as death from LH have been reported *(2)*.

2.1. Granulomatous and Xanthomatous Hypophysitis

Two other forms of primary hypophysitis, granulomatous and xanthomatous, are extremely rare. Because of the rare occurrence of these and their similar clinical and neuroradiological presentations, it remains unclear whether the subtypes are really distinct entities or represent the same disease with slightly different expression. A differentiation is made by histopathological examination. In a series of 31 patients with primary hypophysitis, Gutenberg et al. *(3)* reported 21 lymphocytic, 6 granulomatous, and 4 xanthomatous cases. While both the granulomatous and lymphocytic forms often caused both anterior and posterior pituitary dysfunction, the xanthomatous cases caused mild anterior pituitary failure and rarely posterior pituitary involvement in this series. Only LH was associated with pregnancy and other autoimmune diseases. The authors found that while glucocorticoid therapy appeared to be effective in reducing the pituitary size in 75% of lymphocytic cases, it was less effective in granulomatous and xanthomatous hypophysitis.

2.2. Secondary Hypophysitis

Secondary hypophysitis can occasionally be seen as a result of systemic inflammatory or infectious disease, which can rarely present as primary pituitary insufficiency (Fig. 2). Tuberculosis and syphilis are infectious causes; however, the most commonly encountered systemic diseases that may cause this are sarcoidosis, LCH *(39)*, and Wegener's granulomatosis *(40)*.

2.2.1. HYPOTHALAMIC–PITUITARY SARCOIDOSIS

Sarcoidosis, a disease of unknown etiology, is characterized pathologically by noncaseating granulomata. Neurosarcoidosis occurs in approximately 5% of systemic cases with the seventh cranial nerve as the most commonly affected *(41,42)*. When the hypothalamic–pituitary axis is involved, patients commonly present with polyuria and polydipsia. Abnormalities in pituitary endocrine function, obesity, personality change, somnolence, and variations in body temperature may also be seen *(42)*. The diagnosis of neurosarcoidosis typically requires evidence of systemic disease with pathological confirmation as well

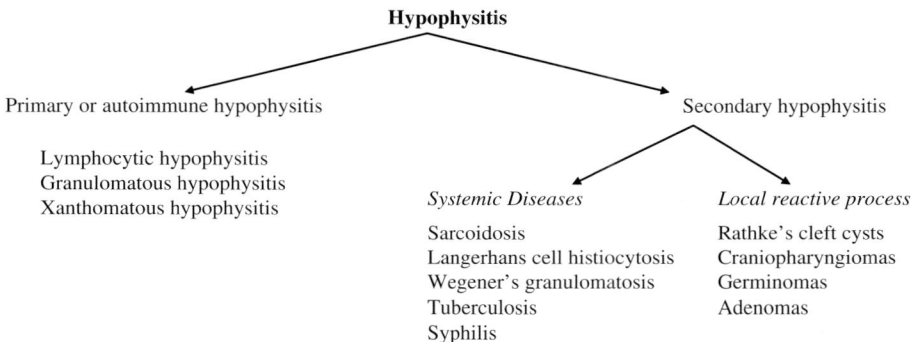

Fig. 2. Major forms of hypophysitis.

as compatible clinical and imaging findings. The cerebrospinal fluid shows nonspecific abnormalities such as mild pleocytosis and elevated protein in about half of cases. Serum and CSF angiotensin-converting enzyme elevations may be helpful but are often normal *(42)*. Glucocorticoids are the mainstay of therapy in an attempt to suppress pro-inflammatory cytokines and chemokines that are involved in the cell-mediated immune response and formation of nonnecrotizing granulomas. In patients who are unresponsive to corticosteroids or when steroid-sparing regimens are preferred, immunosuppressive agents such as azathioprine, methotrexate, or chloroquine have been used *(42–44)*. Recently, infliximab, a tumor necrosis factor inhibitor, has been reported to be effective in the case of sarcoid involving the pituitary that had been refractory to corticosteroids, methotrexate, and cyclophosphamide *(45)*.

2.2.2. LANGERHANS CELL HISTIOCYTOSIS

LCH is a systemic disease caused by monoclonal expansion of dendritic cells most commonly involving bones, skin, and lungs. The hypothalamus and pituitary are also common sites of involvement and LCH is a systemic disease that, when present, is a common cause of Central diabetes insipidus *(46)*.

Makras et al. *(47)* have reported the anterior and posterior pituitary gland function and morphology on MRI in 17 adults with multisystem LCH. Of the 17 patients, 14 (82%) had abnormal hypothalamic–pituitary imaging. Lack of the normal posterior pituitary lobe bright spot was found in all patients with diabetes insipidus; infundibular enlargement in 47%; pituitary infiltration in 35%; and hypothalamic infiltration in 18%. Diabetes insipidus was found in 94% and anterior pituitary dysfunction in 59%. The authors concluded that diabetes insipidus and anterior pituitary deficiency are common in patients with multisystem LCH.

The imaging of LCH can mimic that of germinoma and other diseases. Prosch et al. *(46)* report a case in which a thickened pituitary stalk suggested LCH that was later was found to be a germinoma.

In summary, inflammatory disorders of the pituitary gland may present with mass effect, anterior and posterior pituitary dysfunction, and may be mistaken radiographically for pituitary adenomas. The causes and optimal treatment remain controversial. Further investigation as to the etiology and treatment of this heterogeneous group of disorders will be important.

REFERENCES

1. Rivera JA. Lymphocytic hypophysitis: disease spectrum and approach to diagnosis and therapy. Pituitary 2006;9(1):35–45.
2. Caturegli P, Newschaffer C, Olivi A, Pomper MG, Burger PC, Rose NR. Autoimmune hypophysitis. Endocr Rev 2005;26(5):599–614.

3. Gutenberg A, Hans V, Puchner MJ, et al. Primary hypophysitis: clinical-pathological correlations. Eur J Endocrinol 2006;155(1):101–7.
4. Imura H, Nakao K, Shimatsu A, et al. Lymphocytic infundibuloneurohypophysitis as a cause of central diabetes insipidus. N Engl J Med 1993;329(10):683–9.
5. Goudie RB, Pinkerton PH. Anterior hypophysitis and Hashimoto's disease in a young woman. J Pathol Bacteriol 1962;83:584–5.
6. Hashimoto K, Takao T, Makino S. Lymphocytic adenohypophysitis and lymphocytic infundibuloneurohypophysitis. Endocr J 1997;44(1):1–10.
7. Crock PA. Cytosolic autoantigens in lymphocytic hypophysitis. J Clin Endocrinol Metab 1998;83(2):609–18.
8. Tanaka S, Tatsumi KI, Takano T, et al. Anti-alpha-enolase antibodies in pituitary disease. Endocr J 2003;50(6):697–702.
9. O'Dwyer DT, Clifton V, Hall A, Smith R, Robinson PJ, Crock PA. Pituitary autoantibodies in lymphocytic hypophysitis target both gamma- and alpha-Enolase – a link with pregnancy? Arch Physiol Biochem 2002;110(1–2):94–8.
10. Goswami R, Kochupillai N, Crock PA, Jaleel A, Gupta N. Pituitary autoimmunity in patients with Sheehan's syndrome. J Clin Endocrinol Metab 2002;87(9):4137–41.
11. Bensing S, Hulting AL, Hoog A, Ericson K, Kampe O. Lymphocytic hypophysitis: report of two biopsy-proven cases and one suspected case with pituitary autoantibodies. J Endocrinol Invest 2007;30(2):153–62.
12. Nishiki M, Murakami Y, Ozawa Y, Kato Y. Serum antibodies to human pituitary membrane antigens in patients with autoimmune lymphocytic hypophysitis and infundibuloneurohypophysitis. Clin Endocrinol (Oxf) 2001;54(3):327–33.
13. De Bellis A, Colao A, Bizzarro A, et al. Longitudinal study of vasopressin-cell antibodies and of hypothalamic-pituitary region on magnetic resonance imaging in patients with autoimmune and idiopathic complete central diabetes insipidus. J Clin Endocrinol Metab 2002;87(8):3825–9.
14. Maghnie M, Ghirardello S, De Bellis A, et al. Idiopathic central diabetes insipidus in children and young adults is commonly associated with vasopressin-cell antibodies and markers of autoimmunity. Clin Endocrinol (Oxf) 2006;65(4):470–8.
15. Bellastella A, Bizzarro A, Coronella C, Bellastella G, Sinisi AA, De Bellis A. Lymphocytic hypophysitis: a rare or underestimated disease? Eur J Endocrinol 2003;149(5):363–76.
16. Flanagan DE, Ibrahim AE, Ellison DW, Armitage M, Gawne-Cain M, Lees PD. Inflammatory hypophysitis – the spectrum of disease. Acta Neurochir (Wien) 2002;144(1):47–56.
17. Thodou E, Asa SL, Kontogeorgos G, Kovacs K, Horvath E, Ezzat S. Clinical case seminar: lymphocytic hypophysitis: clinicopathological findings. J Clin Endocrinol Metab 1995;80(8):2302–11.
18. Beressi N, Beressi JP, Cohen R, Modigliani E. Lymphocytic hypophysitis. A review of 145 cases. Ann Med Interne (Paris) 1999;150(4):327–41.
19. Jensen MD, Handwerger BS, Scheithauer BW, Carpenter PC, Mirakian R, Banks PM. Lymphocytic hypophysitis with isolated corticotropin deficiency. Ann Intern Med 1986;105(2):200–3.
20. Kristof RA, Van Roost D, Klingmuller D, Springer W, Schramm J. Lymphocytic hypophysitis: non-invasive diagnosis and treatment by high dose methylprednisolone pulse therapy? J Neurol Neurosurg Psychiatry 1999;67(3):398–402.
21. Matta MP, Kany M, Delisle MB, Lagarrigue J, Caron PH. A relapsing remitting lymphocytic hypophysitis. Pituitary 2002;5(1):37–44.
22. Perez-Nunez A, Miranda P, Arrese I, Gonzalez P, Ramos A, Lobato RD. Lymphocytic hypophysitis with cystic MRI appearance. Acta Neurochir (Wien) 2005;147(12):1297–300.

23. Tamiya A, Saeki N, Kubota M, Oheda T, Yamaura A. Unusual MRI findings in lymphocytic hypophysitis with central diabetes insipidus. Neuroradiology 1999;41(12):899–900.
24. Ozbey N, Sencer A, Tanyolac S, et al. An intrasellar germinoma with normal cerebrospinal fluid beta-HCG concentrations misdiagnosed as hypophysitis. Hormones (Athens) 2006;5(1):67–71.
25. Shin JH, Lee HK, Choi CG, et al. MR imaging of central diabetes insipidus: a pictorial essay. Korean J Radiol 2001;2(4):222–30.
26. Tubridy N, Saunders D, Thom M, et al. Infundibulohypophysitis in a man presenting with diabetes insipidus and cavernous sinus involvement. J Neurol Neurosurg Psychiatry 2001;71(6):798–801.
27. Kartal I, Yarman S, Tanakol R, Bilgic B. Lymphocytic panhypophysitis in a young man with involvement of the cavernous sinus and clivus. Pituitary 2007;10(1):75–80.
28. De Bellis A, Bizzarro A, Bellastella A. Pituitary antibodies and lymphocytic hypophysitis. Best Pract Res Clin Endocrinol Metab 2005;19(1):67–84.
29. Keda YM, Krjukova IV, Ilovaiskaia IA, et al. Antibodies to pituitary surface antigens during various pituitary disease states. J Endocrinol 2002;175(2):417–23.
30. Kobayashi T, Yabe S, Kikuchi T, Kanda T, Kobayashi I. Presence of anti-pituitary antibodies and GAD antibodies in NIDDM and IDDM. Diabetes Care 1997;20(5):864–6.
31. Komatsu M, Kondo T, Yamauchi K, et al. Antipituitary antibodies in patients with the primary empty sella syndrome. J Clin Endocrinol Metab 1988;67(4):633–8.
32. Mau M, Phillips TM, Ratner RE. Presence of anti-pituitary hormone antibodies in patients with empty sella syndrome and pituitary tumours. Clin Endocrinol (Oxf) 1993;38(5): 495–500.
33. Scherbaum WA, Schrell U, Gluck M, Fahlbusch R, Pfeiffer EF. Autoantibodies to pituitary corticotropin-producing cells: possible marker for unfavourable outcome after pituitary microsurgery for Cushing's disease. Lancet 1987;1(8547):1394–8.
34. Case records of the Massachusetts General Hospital. Weekly clinicopathological exercises. Case 25–1995. A 44-year-old woman with headache, blurred vision, and an intrasellar mass. N Engl J Med 1995;333(7):441–7.
35. Cemeroglu AP, Blaivas M, Muraszko KM, Robertson PL, Vazquez DM. Lymphocytic hypophysitis presenting with diabetes insipidus in a 14-year-old girl: case report and review of the literature. Eur J Pediatr 1997;156(9):684–8.
36. Selch MT, DeSalles AA, Kelly DF, et al. Stereotactic radiotherapy for the treatment of lymphocytic hypophysitis. Report of two cases. J Neurosurg 2003;99(3):591–6.
37. Leung GK, Lopes MB, Thorner MO, Vance ML, Laws ER, Jr. Primary hypophysitis: a single-center experience in 16 cases. J Neurosurg 2004;101(2):262–71.
38. Lecube A, Francisco G, Rodriguez D, et al. Lymphocytic hypophysitis successfully treated with azathioprine: first case report. J Neurol Neurosurg Psychiatry 2003;74(11):1581–3.
39. Donadieu J, Rolon MA, Thomas C, et al. Endocrine involvement in pediatric-onset Langerhans' cell histiocytosis: a population-based study. J Pediatr 2004;144(3):344–50.
40. Goyal M, Kucharczyk W, Keystone E. Granulomatous hypophysitis due to Wegener's granulomatosis. AJNR Am J Neuroradiol 2000;21(8):1466–9.
41. Newman LS, Rose CS, Maier LA. Sarcoidosis. N Engl J Med 1997;336(17):1224–34.
42. Porter N, Beynon HL, Randeva HS. Endocrine and reproductive manifestations of sarcoidosis. QJM 2003;96(8):553–61.
43. Lower EE, Broderick JP, Brott TG, Baughman RP. Diagnosis and management of neurological sarcoidosis. Arch Intern Med 1997;157(16):1864–8.
44. Sharma OP. Effectiveness of chloroquine and hydroxychloroquine in treating selected patients with sarcoidosis with neurological involvement. Arch Neurol 1998;55(9):1248–54.

45. Carter JD, Valeriano J, Vasey FB, Bognar B. Refractory neurosarcoidosis: a dramatic response to infliximab. Am J Med 2004;117(4):277–9.
46. Prosch H, Grois N, Prayer D, et al. Central diabetes insipidus as presenting symptom of Langerhans cell histiocytosis. Pediatr Blood Cancer 2004;43(5):594–9.
47. Makras P, Samara C, Antoniou M, et al. Evolving radiological features of hypothalamo-pituitary lesions in adult patients with Langerhans cell histiocytosis (LCH). Neuroradiology 2006;48(1):37–44.

19   Pituitary Apoplexy

Steven J. Russell, MD, PhD, and Karen Klahr Miller, MD

CONTENTS

Summary

Pituitary apoplexy (apoplexy—to disable by a stroke) is a clinical syndrome characterized by the abrupt onset of characteristic signs and symptoms, most commonly headache, nausea, visual disturbance, and ophthalmoplegia, in association with hemorrhage or infarction within the pituitary fossa. Because pituitary apoplexy is rare, and because most cases occur suddenly in the absence of prior suspicion for pituitary pathology, it has been a difficult condition to study. Regardless, if apoplexy is diagnosed in a timely fashion and managed appropriately, death should be rare and permanent neurologic complication of the acute event should be uncommon. This chapter will review what is known of the epidemiology of pituitary apoplexy as well as its clinical presentation, management, and prognosis.

Key Words: Pituitary apoplexy.

From: *Contemporary Endocrinology: Diagnosis and Management of Pituitary Disorders*
Edited by: B. Swearingen and B. M. K. Biller © Humana Press, Totowa, NJ

1. INTRODUCTION

Pituitary apoplexy (apoplexy —to disable by a stroke) is a clinical syndrome characterized by the abrupt onset of characteristic signs and symptoms, most commonly headache, nausea, visual disturbance, and ophthalmoplegia, in association with hemorrhage or infarction within the pituitary fossa. The first widely cited case of pituitary apoplexy was reported by Dr Pearce Bailey in 1898 as a case of "hemorrhage into the pituitary" *(1)*. The patient had suffered from "dimness of vision" for 5 months when he was "suddenly taken with severe headache, nausea, vomiting, and blindness." Physical examination was significant for "restlessness and stupor," weak pulses, varying degrees of ophthalmoplegia of both eyes, and ptosis of the right eyelid. His condition rapidly deteriorated, and he died within 24 h of presentation. Autopsy revealed that "Occupying the sella turcica and projecting about 3 cm above it was a mass …" that on microscopic examination was identified as "… the encapsulated pituitary, enlarged to three or four times its natural size, in which an extensive hemorrhage had recently taken place."

Several similar cases of hemorrhage within the pituitary gland found on autopsy were subsequently reported in the literature, but the syndrome was first described as "pituitary apoplexy" in a case series and review of the literature in 1950 *(2)*. The authors presented ten cases and described a clinically and pathologically defined syndrome in which patients "quite abruptly develop headache, amblyopia, diplopia, drowsiness, confusion, or coma," and autopsy reveals hemorrhage and necrosis of pituitary adenomas. All of the patients presented had died shortly after presentation. However, the authors cited two reports describing successful operative management of patients found to have hemorrhagic pituitary adenomas *(3,4)*. Interestingly, one of these surgical papers included as authors Pearce Bailey, credited with the first description of apoplexy, and Harvey Cushing.

Since that time, an extensive descriptive literature on pituitary apoplexy has emerged, mostly in the form of case reports and small series. Because pituitary apoplexy is rare, and because most cases occur suddenly in the absence of prior suspicion for pituitary pathology, it has been a difficult condition to study. Regardless, if apoplexy is diagnosed in a timely fashion and managed appropriately, death should be rare and permanent neurologic complication of the acute event should be uncommon. This chapter will review what is known of the epidemiology of pituitary apoplexy as well as its clinical presentation, management, and prognosis.

2. EPIDEMIOLOGY OF PITUITARY APOPLEXY

Most of what has been published about the frequency of pituitary apoplexy is derived from surgical series of patients treated operatively for pituitary tumors. In six published series (>20 patients each) of patients with surgically verified pituitary adenomas, 5% (248/5,197) presented with classical apoplexy *(5–10)*. Incidentally found radiologic evidence of pituitary hemorrhage or infarction, found in an additional 4.9% (109/1,146) of patients in surgical series *(9,10)*, does not meet the criteria for diagnosis of apoplexy. The term "pituitary apoplexy" should be reserved for cases in which hemorrhage is accompanied by the acute onset of symptoms. The vast majority of apoplexy cases arise in the setting of a preexisting pituitary tumor, but in 83% of cases the tumor was not previously known (40/229 patients) *(8,11–15)*

Surgical series of pituitary adenomas and apoplexy are biased to include patients with larger or more symptomatic tumors, as these are routinely referred for surgical consultation, whereas many prolactinomas and nonfunctioning microadenomas are not. It might therefore be expected that the rate of pituitary apoplexy would be lower in an unselected series of true incidentalomas. Surprisingly, this was not the case in a prospective study of patients with pituitary adenomas found incidentally by magnetic resonance imaging (MRI) *(16)*. Each patient underwent a complete endocrinologic evaluation and visual perimetry and was excluded from the analysis if there was evidence of endocrine hypersecretion, visual field defect, or panhypopituitarism. A total of 42 patients were included in the study, and their adenomas designated as "incidentally found," although 13 patients had the initial MRI performed due to chronic headache. During a mean follow-up period of 62 months, four patients (9.5%) developed classically symptomatic pituitary apoplexy with evidence of new hemorrhage within the tumor by MRI. The tumors in which apoplexy occurred ranged in size from 18 to 24 mm prior to the hemorrhagic event, and apoplexy occurred at a mean of 32 months (range 20–56 months) after diagnosis of the pituitary adenoma. Although small, this study is consistent with a fairly high rate of apoplexy in pituitary macroadenomas. Longer-term follow-up of this cohort would be helpful to determine whether the observed rate of apoplexy incidence will be sustained, and similar studies would be helpful in evaluating the reproducibility of this finding.

The higher rate of apoplexy observed in the prospective study of Arita et al. *(16)* as compared to surgical series may be related to the requirement that the tumors be nonfunctioning. In eight series (>20 patients) of patients with apoplexy for which immunohistochemical data were available, the majority of tumors were clinically nonfunctioning adenomas. Nonstaining tumors comprised 55%, whereas 7% stained for FSH, LH, alpha-subunit, or a combination of these. Tumors staining for prolactin accounted for 12%, growth hormone (GH) for 10%, corticotroph (ACTH) for 9%, and mixed staining for 1% of tumors (total n = 213) *(5,6,8,9,11,13–15)*. In support of this hypothesis, a surgical series that included only nonfunctioning pituitary adenomas found a much higher rate of pituitary apoplexy (21%) than in series including all surgically treated pituitary adenomas *(17)*. This tendency for apoplexy to occur in nonfunctioning tumors could be secondary to inherent differences in tumor biology, but could also be due to enhanced detection of secreting tumors prior to the development of apoplexy. Unfortunately, it is impossible to determine preapoplexy tumor size when the only imaging is performed after the event. Therefore, the available data do not allow testing of the hypothesis that greater size is an important contributor to the risk of hemorrhage or infarction in nonfunctioning tumors.

Pituitary apoplexy is slightly more common in males (60% of cases) than in females *(5–9,11–15)* possibly because amenorrhea prompts diagnosis of pituitary tumors earlier in women. The mean age of onset in surgical series is 50 years, but the ages at diagnosis ranged from 15 to 90 years of age, mandating consideration of pituitary apoplexy at any stage of life *(5–9,11–15)*.

No population-based reports of the incidence of pituitary apoplexy have been published. However, there are data available on the prevalence of pituitary tumors, the substrate for pituitary apoplexy. A systematic review found that the prevalence of pituitary tumors in unselected autopsy series was 14% and in radiologic studies was 22% *(18)*. A second meta-analysis including only autopsy series (including some overlap with the group of studies included in reference *(17)*) found a 11% incidence of pituitary tumors *(19)*. A very small percentage of lesions found in population-based studies are macroadenomas (>10 mm). In one study of 1,000 unselected autopsy specimens, no adenomas larger than 6 mm were found, although 3% of subjects had microadenomas *(20)*. An MRI study of 100 volunteers not suspected of having pituitary disease found a 10% incidence of presumed microadenomas (by imaging character- istics), but no lesions larger than 6 mm *(21)*. A meta-analysis of autopsy series including over 9,737 subjects found a macroadenoma rate of 0.03% *(19)*, whereas a population-based MRI study including 3,672 subjects found lesions consistent with macroadenomas in 0.16% *(22)*. If we extrapolate an incidence rate of apoplexy in nonsurgically treated macroadenomas of 1.8% per year from the data of Arita et al. *(16)* (9.5% incidence over 62 months) and assume a prevalence of macroadenomas of approximately 0.1%, the annual incidence of apoplexy is predicted to be approximately 18 per million. This is higher incidence than clinical experience would suggest is the case. A population- based study of apoplexy incidence would be necessary to resolve this apparent paradox. It seems likely that the rate of pituitary apoplexy will be lower in populations with better access to health care, and therefore fewer macroade- nomas left undetected and untreated.

3. THE CLINICAL SYNDROME OF PITUITARY APOPLEXY

Because of the unique anatomy of this region (Fig. 1), an expanding mass arising from within the sella turcica can impinge on the optic chiasm of cranial nerve II superiorly, or cranial nerves III. IV, V (ophthalmic and maxillary divisions), and VI as they pass through the cavernous sinus lateral to the sella. Also passing through the cavernous sinus is the internal carotid artery, which in rare cases may be obstructed by an expansile sellar mass *(23,24)*. These anatomic considerations account for characteristic neurologic signs associated with apoplexy.

The frequencies of the most common symptoms and signs in the following discussion have been determined by aggregating data from 11 independent surgical series, all including more than 20 patients ($n = 442$) from 1950 to 2005 *(5–15)* and are shown in Table 1. The most commons symptoms were sudden headache in 89% and nausea/vomiting in 57%. More than 50% of patients complained of visual disturbance, variously defined. Photophobia (40%) and facial pain or numbness (7%) were less common. The most common signs included decreased visual acuity in up to 56% and diminishment of visual fields in 28%, although the extent to which these were new deficits could not be determined. Visual defects included monocular or complete blindness in a very small number of patients, 5% and 10%, respectively, in two series *(5–15)*, but less than 2% of patients overall were specifically reported to suffer blindness in one or more eyes. Ophthalmoplegia was observed in at least 46% of patients *(5–15)*. Cranial nerve III (oculomotor nerve) was most commonly affected, with signs including ptosis, mydriasis, lack of pupillary light and/or accommodation reflex, and/or deviation of the affected eye downward and laterally reported

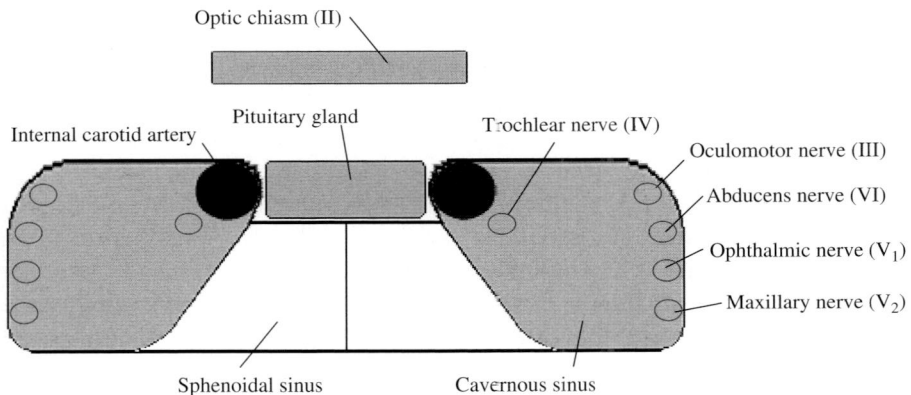

Optic chiasm (II)

Internal carotid artery

Pituitary gland

Trochlear nerve (IV)

Oculomotor nerve (III)

Abducens nerve (VI)

Ophthalmic nerve (V_1)

Maxillary nerve (V_2)

Sphenoidal sinus   Cavernous sinus

Fig. 1. Schematic of coronal section through pituitary and adjacent structures.

Table 1
Frequency of Symptoms and Signs of Pituitary Apoplexy

	Frequency (%)	*n*
Symptoms		
Headache	89	442
Nausea/vomiting	57	326
Visual disturbance	51	396
Photophobia	40	80
Facial pain/numbness	7	76
Signs		
Ophthalmoplegia	46	440
CN III	51	140
CN VI	29	140
CN IV	9	140
Decreased visual acuity	56	179
Subarachnoid hemorrhage	40	126
Visual field defect	28	388
Meningismus	25	8
Fever	16	155
Altered mental status or seizure	14	403

Data derived from references *(5–15)* ($n = 442$). Frequencies were calculated only for those studies explicitly reporting the data, and n represents the total number of patients for whom the presence or absence of a given finding is reported. Therefore, the frequency of certain signs or symptoms with $n<442$ may be overestimated. Most studies documented the presence or absence of ophthalmoplegia, but data on specific cranial nerve defects were reported in sufficient detail only in references *(6,8,13,14)* ($n = 140$).

in 51% of patients *(6,8,13,14)*. Cranial nerve VI (abducens) defects, including restriction of abduction and inward gaze, were found in 29%. Cranial nerve IV (trochlear) involvement, which is difficult to detect on examination, but can cause inward gaze of the affected eye or diplopia corrected by head tilt, was found in 9% *(6,8,13,14)*. Much less common was involvement of cranial nerve V_1 and V_2 (ophthalmic and maxillary divisions of the trigeminal) manifested as facial pain or numbness. Abnormalities of cranial nerves VI and IV may not be detected by superficial examination because patients can compensate for the resulting diplopia with head movement. Accordingly, a complete assessment of extraocular movements is required.

Hemorrhage may not be limited to the tumor within which it arises. Microscopic, or less commonly gross, subarachnoid hemorrhage has been reported in a substantial minority (up to 40%) of apoplexy cases *(6,25)*. Fever was specifically reported in four studies (16% of patients) *(8,9,11,14)* and meningismus in only one study (25% of patients) *(13,*. Altered mental status or seizures were reported in 14% of patients *(5–15)*, and may be related to meningeal irritation, hyponatremia, and adrenal insufficiency. Other signs rarely reported include epistaxis and CSF rhinorrhea. In rare cases, mass effect or spasm of the portion of the internal carotid artery passing through the cavernous sinus can result in seizures or hemiparesis *(26–28)* (Table 1).

Because the bony sella turcica limits expansion of any mass within it, infarction with attendant edema or hemorrhage within a pituitary tumor results in a dramatic increase in intrasellar pressure *(29)*. This, possibly combined with direct disruption of blood vessels supplying the pituitary, frequently results in necrosis of the sellar contents beyond the histologic bounds of hemorrhagic areas. Not surprisingly, deficiency of at least one pituitary hormone has been documented in up to 90% of patients after apoplexy *(11,13,14)*, although some series have found a lower proportion (40–50%) requiring long-term hormone therapy despite a classical presentation *(7,12)*. The degree to which the apoplexy event can be implicated in the acute development of hormone deficiencies is not clear. In retrospect, signs and symptoms consistent with hypopituitarism were often present prior to apoplexy *(6,8)*. Hypothyroidism was present in 55% of patients at the time of apoplexy in one series *(15)*. Given the half-life of levothyroxine, the hypothyroidism likely predated the apoplexy. Central adrenal insufficiency is common (61%) in the acute phase *(15)*, in some cases leading to hypotension or shock if glucocorticoid therapy is not instituted promptly. Transient disorders of sodium homeostasis are common due to the syndrome of inappropriate ADH and diabetes insipidus, but permanent diabetes insipidus occurs in less than 10% *(5,7,8)*.

4. PATHOPHYSIOLOGY OF PITUITARY APOPLEXY AND REPORTED PREDISPOSING FACTORS

Several theories have been elaborated to explain the onset of pituitary apoplexy. Some authors have postulated that large tumors outgrow their blood supply then suffer infarction followed in some cases by secondary hemorrhage *(2)*. Others have argued that larger tumors compress their own blood supply leading to infarction and secondary hemorrhage *(30)*. In fact, pituitary tumors usually grow very slowly, while apoplexy is an abrupt process, necessitating that one imagine a "tipping point" at which limitations in blood supply become critical or that some predisposing factor initiates the apoplectic event. A variant of the above theories is that an abrupt increase in the metabolic activity of the pituitary can precipitate apoplexy if blood flow cannot be increased to compensate *(12)*. Any process that causes edema within the confines of the sella is expected to increase intrasellar pressure and further restrict blood supply, potentially leading to infarction. In support of this proposal, increased intrasellar pressures (by an average of 10 mmHg) have been documented in patients undergoing surgery for apoplexy versus surgery for nonapoplectic macroadenomas *(29)*. Another theory is that the blood vessels within the tumor are abnormally fragile, and are therefore predisposed to hemorrhage *(31)*. Finally, a few case reports have ascribed apoplectic episodes due to embolic disease *(32)*.

Based on these theories of pathophysiology, a number of comorbid conditions, procedures, and drugs associated with the onset of pituitary apoplexy have been described as predisposing factors, though causality is difficult to establish. A list of such factors associated with pituitary apoplexy in the medical literature and accompanying references is found in Table 2. Among the most commonly cited factors are those that might reasonably compromise the integrity of tumor vessels, impair effective hemostasis, or cause rapid changes in intravascular pressure. These include hypertension, altered coagulation or platelet function, radiation therapy of known pituitary tumors, head trauma, and surgery. Another set of reported predisposing factors includes interventions, physiologic states, or drugs known or expected to change the endocrine activity of the pituitary gland or a pituitary tumor. Stimulation tests of anterior pituitary function deserve special mention because they are more commonly performed in patients with pituitary tumors and there are many reports of pituitary apoplexy apparently precipitated by stimulation tests. As shown in Table 2, pituitary apoplexy has been reported to occur shortly after multiple endocrine stimulation tests, including CRH *(57,58)*, TRH *(62,63)*, and metyrapone *(5,14)* stimulation as well as protocols for combined anterior pituitary function testing *(26,64–67)*. Interestingly, there have been no reports in the literature of pituitary apoplexy associated with cosyntropin testing of adrenal reserve, probably the most common provocative test performed on patients with untreated pituitary macroadenomas. The association of apoplexy with dopamine agonist treatment of prolactinomas or the withdrawal of such therapy is of particular importance. Dopamine agonists might reasonably precipitate apoplexy by disruption of the blood supply during rapid involution of dopamine-producing tumors, or during rapid regrowth after withdrawal of treatment. Both hemorrhage and infarction within the pituitary are well described during pregnancy and delivery. Because the pituitary is physiologically enlarged during pregnancy it is thought to be more vulnerable to a sudden decrease in perfusion associated with postpartum hemorrhage. Pituitary infarction in this setting is known as Sheehan's syndrome. Some reported "predisposing factors" for pituitary apoplexy stretch credulity, such as lower limb cellulitis *(12)* and upper respiratory infection *(46)*, emphasizing the point that association does not prove causality.

Even using very inclusive criteria to identify predisposing factors for apoplexy, no such factor can be identified in many cases. Predisposing factors

Table 2
Factors Reported to be Associated with Pituitary Apoplexy

Factors possibly affecting vascular integrity, hemostasis, or intravascular pressure:

Hypertension *(8,11,14,33,34)*
Anti-coagulation or anti-platelet pharmacotherapy *(6,8,11,12,14,30)*
Thrombolytic therapy *(12)*
Bleeding disorders *(11)*
Factor V Leiden mutation *(14)*
Idiopathic thrombocytopenic purpura *(35,36)*
Polycythemia *(14)*
Thrombocytopenia *(37)*
Chronic renal failure or hemodialysis *(33,38)*
Radiation therapy of known pituitary tumors *(3,5,33,34,39–41,105,106)*
Atherosclerosis *(32)*
Diabetes mellitus *(33,34,42,43)*
Head trauma *(6,39,41,44,45)*
Barotrauma *(44)*
Angiography *(5,46)*
Cardiac surgery with cardiopulmonary bypass *(12,39,47)*
Surgery *(6,11,12,14,33)*
Air encephalography *(48)*
Spinal anesthesia *(49)*
Gadolinium-contrast administration *(50)*
Isosorbide dinitrate administration *(51)*
Dental extraction *(44)*

Conditions affecting endocrine activity of the pituitary:

Nelson's syndrome *(11)*
Pregnancy or delivery *(5,12,14,25,41,52)*
Medications or provocative endocrine testing:
Oral contraceptive pills *(14,34,42)*
Withdrawal of corticosteroids *(5)*
Leuprolide *(53)*
Clomiphene *(54)*
Goserelin*(55,56)*
CRH *(57,58)*
GnRH *(59–61)*
TRH *(62,63)*
Combined anterior pituitary function testing *(26,64–67)*
Metyrapone testing *(5,14)*
Discontinuation of octreotide *(14)*
Dopamine agonist treatment or withdrawal of treatment *(5,11,12,33,34,40,41–44)*

have been cited in 4% *(39)* to 63% *(42)* of cases, with estimates varying with the size of the study, and presumably with the inclusiveness of the criteria *(5,6,11,12,14,33)*. While some of the reported predisposing factors seem more plausible than others, no causative relationships have been proven. Clearly, many of the predisposing factors, such as diabetes mellitus and hypertension, are very common and a causative relationship would be nearly impossible to establish given the rarity of apoplexy. The difficulty is compounded by the fact that apoplexy often represents the initial presentation of the pituitary tumor. Practically speaking, one should always consider apoplexy in a patient with components of the syndrome regardless of the setting, and the index of suspicion should perhaps be even higher in the setting of these reported predisposing factors.

5. DIAGNOSIS OF PITUITARY APOPLEXY

The primary challenge in making the diagnosis of pituitary apoplexy is considering the diagnosis, as only 17% of cases arise in a known pituitary tumor *(8,11–15)*, and delays in diagnosis have therefore been common. In relatively mild cases, consideration of the diagnosis along with more common etiologies for headache, nausea, and visual disturbance, such as migraine, is essential. The presence of visual symptoms or ophthalmoplegia associated with the rapid onset of severe headache should prompt consideration of pituitary apoplexy, although other "apoplectic" events such as subarachnoid hemorrhage should also be considered. In many cases, there is a history suggestive of pituitary hormone abnormality or tumor mass effect that may arouse suspicion for apoplexy if the proper questions are asked. The occurrence of apoplexy during surgery, or in patients who are otherwise unresponsive or uncooperative, can be especially challenging to diagnose.

Although pituitary apoplexy is primarily a clinical diagnosis, imaging studies have an important role in the diagnosis. Because the presentation of pituitary apoplexy may suggest the diagnosis of subarachnoid hemorrhage or other intracranial hemorrhage, or include mental status changes, a noncontrast head computed tomography (CT) is often the first radiological study performed. While CT does not reliably allow detection of hemorrhage or infarction in pituitary tumors *(6–8,13,14)*, the presence of a mass arising from the pituitary in the setting of symptoms consistent with apoplexy should prompt evaluation with MRI.

The ability of a pituitary protocol MRI scan to demonstrate the anatomy of the sellar region makes it the study of choice for diagnosis of this condition *(6–8,13,14)*. MRI has consistently been shown to be superior to CT in demonstrating apoplexy. Whereas CT is quite reliable in identifying pituitary tumors in patients with apoplexy, it has been able to demonstrate apoplexy in only in 21–82%, compared to 68–100% for MRI. Hemorrhage is most often seen as high signal intensity on noncontrast T1-weighted images, and infarction as peripheral or inhomogeneous enhancement after administration of gadolinium *(68)*. MRI with diffusion-weighted imaging may also demonstrate high signal intensity in cases of hemorrhage or infarction and necrosis without hemorrhage *(69)*.

The imaging findings vary with time after apoplexy, as the MRI characteristics of hemorrhage vary with time. Very early changes are related to hemorrhage or infarction, but disruption in the vascular network may also be manifested as thickening of the sphenoidal sinus mucosa on MRIs. Thickened mucosa was observed in 79% of 28 patients presenting with pituitary apoplexy between 1996 and 2005 who had MRI less than 7 days after presentation *(7)*. Interestingly, thickened sphenoidal sinus mucosa was associated with larger tumors, a higher rate of cranial nerve defects, and a higher rate of hypopituitarism than those without this finding. As necrosis leads to liquefaction, fluid levels may develop and ring enhancement becomes common *(33,70)*. In the long term, even patients not operatively managed may develop an empty or partially empty sella as necrotic tissue is remodeled and removed *(13,42,70)*. Subarachnoid hemorrhage may be associated with pituitary apoplexy, presumably because hemorrhage may breach the pituitary capsule. This may be demonstrated on noncontrast CT and/or by lumbar puncture. Lumbar puncture is not necessary to make the diagnosis of pituitary apoplexy, but may be performed in the setting of a presentation mimicking subarachnoid hemorrhage. The CSF in the setting of apoplexy may be grossly or microscopically bloody or xanthochromic, and most commonly has increased protein *(6,25)*.

Although most cases of apoplexy occur in pituitary adenomas, there are numerous case reports of a syndrome very similar to pituitary apoplexy caused by infarction or hemorrhage into nonadenomatous tissue within or near the sella turcica. These variant syndromes have been reported in the setting of lymphocytic hypophysitis *(71)*, Rathke's cleft cysts *(72–74)*, malignant tumors arising within the sella, or metastatic to the normal pituitary or a preexisting pituitary tumor *(75–78)*, intrasellar tuberculomas *(79)*, chondroid chordomas *(80)*, and pituitary abcesses *(81)*. Because hemorrhage into the sella puts normal pituitary tissue at risk regardless of the pathophysiology, hypopituitarism is common in these variant syndromes as well.

Mimics of apoplexy have included rupture of carotid intracavernous aneurysm *(82,83)*, internal carotid artery dissection *(84)*, intrasellar or suprasellar meningioma *(85)*, epidermoid cyst of the sphenoid sinus *(86)*, and granuloma *(87)*. Because only a subset of the possible signs and symptoms of apoplexy may be manifest in any given patient, and because apoplexy may be associated with subarachnoid or even intracerebral hemorrhage, other diagnoses entertained in cases of pituitary apoplexy have included expanding aneurysm or spontaneous subarachnoid hemorrhage *(44,88)*, ruptured anterior cerebral artery aneurysm *(89)*, meningitis *(90–92)*, meningo-encephalitis *(44,93)*, carotid artery dissection *(94)*, cavernous sinus thrombosis, midbrain infarction, acute optic neuritis *(95)*, and migraine headache *(44,96)*.

While dopamine agonist therapy of prolactin-producing tumors has been associated with pituitary apoplexy *(5,11,12,33,34,40–44)*, visual defects can occur in this setting even in the absence of apoplexy. Chiasmal herniation into the pituitary fossa associated with visual loss may be confused with apoplexy. This complication may occur when traction on the chiasm is caused by a rapidly shrinking tumor. MRI is the study of choice to document this condition. Chiasmal herniation in this setting can be successfully managed by discontinuing or reducing the dose of dopamine agonist *(84)*.

6. STABILIZATION AND MEDICAL EVALUATION OF PATIENTS WITH PITUITARY APOPLEXY

Even before the diagnosis is confirmed, any serious consideration of pituitary apoplexy should prompt the immediate, empiric, administration of high "stress-dose" glucocorticoid therapy. This is mandated by the high prevalence of adrenal insufficiency in patients with apoplexy and the dire consequences of failing to replace glucocorticoids in the setting of a severe physiologic stress. High-dose steroids may also improve the attendant neurologic deficits via their antiedema effects. Stress-dose glucocorticoids should be continued until the diagnosis of pituitary apoplexy can be ruled out. Detection and management of electrolyte abnormalities, primarily disorders of sodium regulation, is the next priority. Although hyponatremia may be caused by SIADH in this setting, it may also be secondary to adrenal insufficiency, providing another rationale for empiric glucocorticoid therapy.

Although treatment of possible adrenal insufficiency should be initiated empirically and normalization of electrolytes is important prior to surgery, treatment of any other endocrine abnormalities can usually be delayed until a new baseline is reached. Nonetheless, it is useful to document evidence for any other endocrine abnormalities at the time of presentation. Diagnosis of a hyper-secretion syndrome may influence choice of therapy and provides an important guide to long-term monitoring for recurrence after acute management. In the setting of acute illness, laboratory evaluation of cortisol hypersecretion is difficult because normal individuals dramatically increase cortisol secretion in such circumstances. However, measurements of prolactin, free thyroxine, and IGF-1 may be helpful if elevated. Documentation of hypersecretion prior to surgery may be the only information on tumor type available after apoplexy of a pituitary adenoma. Due to extensive tissue necrosis, immunohistochemical

diagnosis has been available for only 65% of patients in surgical series
(5,6,8,9,11,13,14,39).

Documenting hormone deficiencies is of limited utility in the acute and
subacute phase, as some degree of apparent hypogonadism, hypothyroidism
(nonthyroidal illness syndrome), and GH deficiency are to be expected in
the setting of acute illness. Documentation of a low free T4 dose implies
hypothyroidism predating the onset of apoplexy because of the long half-life
of levothyroxine. Decompression of normal pituitary tissue may lead to full
or partial recovery of pituitary function; however, rendering the preoperative
diagnosis of deficiency states moot in many cases.

7. ACUTE MANAGEMENT OF PITUITARY APOPLEXY

Rapid surgical decompression remains the therapy of choice for pituitary
apoplexy, but recent data suggest that a subset of patients might be managed
expectantly. The primary rationale for prompt surgical management has been
the recovery and preservation of neurologic function, with several authors
reporting better recovery of vision if surgery was performed soon after presentation *(6,8)* In one series, surgery led to compete resolution of visual acuity
deficits (defined as at least 20/25 vision or return to documented baseline) in
100% ($n = 7$), normalization of visual fields in 50% ($n = 10$), and resolution of
ocular paresis in 65% ($n = 12$) of patients when performed within 7 days *(6)*.
In another series, defects in visual acuity resolved in 100% ($n = 10$), visual
fields normalized in 75% ($n = 11$), and ocular paresis resolved in 73% ($n = 11$)
when surgery was performed within 8 days *(8)*.

In both studies, there was a significantly worse outcome in visual acuity
when surgery was performed more than 1 week after the apoplectic event. In the
first study, surgery more than 7 days after apoplexy led to complete resolution
of visual acuity in 45% ($n = 9$) , whereas 100% ($n = 7$) recovered when surgery
was performed within 7 days ($p = 0.03$) *(6)*. In the other study, 46% of those
with surgery more than 8 days after apoplexy ($n = 13$) versus 100% of those
with surgery within 8 days ($n = 10$) had complete resolution of visual acuity
($p = 0.007$) *(8)*. One study found a significant improvement in visual field
recovery with early surgery (75%, $n = 11$ versus 23%, $n = 13$, $p = 0.004$) *(8)*, but
a less dramatic trend was nonsignificant in the other *(6)*. Neither study found
any significant differences in the resolution of ophthalmoplegia with early
versus delayed surgery, primarily because ophthalmoplegia resolved regardless
of timing of surgery.

Two other surgical series reported visual outcomes, but did not document
the timing of surgery. In one, 80% ($n = 10$) of those patients with diminished
visual acuity on presentation showed improvement in at least one eye, although
only one patient had complete resolution. Of those with ophthalmoplegia, all

had dramatic improvement and 50% resolved completely *(48)*. In the other, 50% had complete resolution of visual acuity (*n* = 4), 60% had complete recovery of diminished visual fields (*n* = 5), and 71% had resolution of ophthalmoplegia *(98)*. Other surgical series either included very small numbers of patients or did not document visual improvement in sufficient detail, sometimes reporting the visual outcome in all patients rather than those with visual deficits at the time of presentation. It should be noted that in many cases detailed information on visual function prior to apoplexy was not known. Therefore, residual dysfunction after surgery could have been chronic but not previously appreciated.

In most surgical series, at least a small percentage of patients were reported to be medically or conservatively managed, or surgery was significantly delayed because either symptoms were not severe or coexisting conditions made the patient a poor surgical risk. In most of these cases, ophthalmoplegia *(6,15,98)* and visual function *(44,98)* improved without surgical decompression, although this was not always true, particularly when surgery was delayed due to severe intercurrent or underlying illness *(99)*. Whether recovery would have been more complete or more rapid with decompression is unclear. In some cases, recovery without surgery could be explained by shrinkage of prolactinomas by dopamine agonist treatment, but in others, no specific therapy other than glucocorticoids was administered. This observation raised the possibility that some patients might be managed conservatively with good outcome.

A small prospective, nonrandomized study of conservative management for pituitary apoplexy included 12 consecutive patients with classical apoplexy *(33)*. All patients presented with sudden onset of headache and either visual symptoms (ranging from blurred vision to bilateral blindness) or ophthalmoplegia of at least one eye, and three patients had impaired consciousness. Patients were treated with relatively high doses of dexamethasone (up to 16 mg per day) and underwent surgery if visual loss or impaired consciousness did not improve within the first week or if there was neurologic deterioration after discontinuation of dexamethasone. Seven patients did not require surgery by these criteria. All seven patients conservatively treated had presented with ophthalmoplegia, and six (86%) had complete recovery within 6 weeks. Two conservatively treated patients presented with blurred vision that resolved, but these patients also experienced severe hyperglycemia. Insulin treatment might have accounted for resolution of visual symptoms in these patients. All patients requiring surgery had at least unilateral blindness on presentation and all improved after surgery, although only one recovered completely.

More recently, three fairly large retrospective series that included a significant proportion of nonsurgically managed apoplexy patients have been published, all from referral hospitals in the United Kingdom *(13,14,100)*. All patients had sudden onset of signs and symptoms consistent with apoplexy in the setting of a pituitary mass, and most had CT, MRI, and/or histological evidence of hemorrhage or necrosis within the pituitary gland. Combining data from the three studies ($n = 108$), 97% of patients presented with headache, 80% with nausea/vomiting, 57% with ophthalmoplegia, 50% with visual field deficits, and 50% with abnormal visual fields. Thus, the clinical presentations of apoplexy in these series were similar to those reported in earlier surgical series. Almost all patients (96%) were treated with empiric glucocorticoid replacement therapy. A total of 47 patients underwent transsphenoidal surgery, 4 underwent craniotomy, and 56 (53%) were managed conservatively. Only three of the conservatively managed patients were thought to have prolactinomas on the basis of very high prolactin levels and were treated with dopamine agonists. In the series of Ayuk et al. *(13)*, the criteria for surgical management were worsening visual deficits or alterations in consciousness. Sibal et al. did not specifically state the criteria for surgical management, but patients with visual field deficits were significantly more likely to be managed surgically (64%) than conservatively (24%) *(14)*. The indications for surgery in the report by Gruber et al. were chiasmal compression in most cases (7/9) or tumor size (2/9) and patients with more severe visual deficits were more likely to undergo surgery *(100)*. The median times to surgery were 4, 6, and 8 days, respectively *(13,14,100)*. On average, patients managed conservatively had better neurologic outcomes than patients managed surgically. Visual field defects (excluding blindness) resolved in 45% (13/29) of surgically managed patients and 79% (11/14) of conservatively managed patients. Similarly, ophthalmoplegia resolved in 64% (16/25) of surgical patients and 87% (23/27) of conservatively managed patients. There was no significant difference in persistent hypopituitarism between the two groups. Notably, there was also no significant difference in neuro-ophthalmologic outcome in patients who had surgery within 7 days of presentation versus those managed surgically more than 7 days after presentation in one of the studies *(14)*, in contrast to the earlier referenced studies addressing this question *(6,8)*. Only one of the 108 patients included in the three studies died, a conservatively managed elderly patient with multiple comorbidities *(100)*. The superior neurologic outcomes of patients treated conservatively likely reflects the assignment of patients with more severe neurologic compromise to the surgical groups. Consequently, these data should not be interpreted to mean that medical management is superior to surgical management in an unselected population. However, these data do suggest that if patients are appropriately selected and closely monitored, neurologic outcomes can be favorable without surgery.

Based on all of the available evidence, rapid (within one week) surgical decompression is indicated for the majority of patients presenting with pituitary apoplexy. The best candidates for medical management of apoplexy would be those patients with only ocular palsy or mild and nonprogressive visual loss that is rapidly reversible with steroid treatment. Because none of the studies comparing surgical and conservative management strategies were randomized, it is not possible to determine whether even better outcomes might have been obtained in conservatively managed patients if surgery had been performed. Only data from a randomized trial will elucidate the optimal therapeutic strategy. One setting in which medical management is particularly attractive is that of apoplexy into a prolactinoma if there is a significant portion of the tumor that remains viable. In such a case, dopamine agonist treatment may cause rapid involution of noninfarcted areas of the tumor, leading to clinical improvement *(7,101)* In practice, the threshold of symptom and sign severity above which surgical management should be recommended is likely to depend in part on the availability of an experienced pituitary surgeon. Outcomes after transsphenoidal surgery are better for higher volume centers and surgeons *(102)*. For instance, mortality for all transsphenoidal surgeries was over twofold lower (0.4% vs. 0.9%) at hospitals with highest quartile versus lowest quartile volumes *(102)*. In cases where surgery is mandated by the severity of the presentation, transfer to a high-volume center may be beneficial if the patient is sufficiently stable and the transfer can occur quickly.

If appropriately managed, the risk of death after pituitary apoplexy is relatively low. In series including more than 20 patients, and therefore presumably from fairly high-volume centers, short-term mortality (within three months after presentation) for all patients presenting with apoplexy was 1.6% ($n = 353$). There were no deaths in the 64 patients in these series treated conservatively, so that mortality of patients managed surgically ($n = 378$) was 1.9% *(5,8–15)*. However, it should be emphasized that relatively few patients were managed conservatively, and clinical deterioration was an indication for surgery, ensuring that most of the mortality would occur in the surgical group.

8. INTERMEDIATE AND LONG-TERM MANAGEMENT AFTER PITUITARY APOPLEXY

Many patients are left with permanent endocrine deficits requiring long-term management after pituitary apoplexy. Up to 90% of patients require replacement of at least one anterior pituitary hormone, although other studies report lower rates *(5,12–14,17,33,43)*. In aggregate data from several series, the rate of hypoadrenalism was 74% ($n = 125$). Hypothyroidism was found in 70% ($n = 122$), and hypogonadism in 67% ($n = 121$) *(6,8,11,13)* (Table 3). Conversely, endocrine hypersecretion may persist if a secreting tumor in which apoplexy arose is not completely removed or entirely necrotic, or may recur after long remissions *(14,103)*. Disorders of sodium homeostasis, while

Table 3
Frequency of Pituitary Hormone Deficits after Apoplexy

Endocrine deficiency	Frequency (%)	n
Any deficiency	85	108
Adrenal insufficiency	74	125
Hypothyroidism	70	122
Hypogonadism	67	121
Diabetes insipidus	9	95

Data derived from references)6,8,11,13–15). Data for any deficiency from references (11,14,15). Data for hypoadrenalism, hypothyroidism, and hypogonadism from (6,8,11,13). Data for DI from (6,15). The total number of patients for which the presence or absence of a finding was reported is defined as n.

common, are usually transient. Diabetes insipidus may become permanent in approximately 10% of patients and require continuing management (6,15). Finally, tumors may exhibit regrowth after either medical or surgical management of apoplexy (5,13,14), and there are examples of second episodes of apoplexy occurring in residual or recurring tumors (33). These considerations mandate comprehensive postapoplexy endocrine evaluation followed by continued endocrine monitoring as well as periodic imaging.

In the short term, a complete evaluation of anterior pituitary hormone function should be performed approximately 6 weeks after presentation with apoplexy or surgery. Empiric glucocorticoid therapy should continue until adequate functioning of the hypothalamic–pituitary–adrenal axis is established. This can be demonstrated convincingly by measurement of a serum cortisol of greater than 18 mcg/dl, most commonly captured on an early morning sample. The cosyntropin test can also be used to demonstrate adequate adrenal reserve, but due to the nature of the test, must be performed at least 6–8 weeks after any acute event. Earlier testing may falsely reassure the clinician that cortisol secretory function is intact, when in fact there has not been sufficient time for adrenocortical atrophy in the absence of endogenous ACTH stimulation (92).

In the long term, patients who had evidence of pituitary hormone hypersecretion should be periodically monitored for recurrence. The type of monitoring should be informed by any evidence of hypersecretion documented at the time of presentation and by immunohistochemical staining of the tumor. A postoperative MRI performed after time for resolution of edema and healing (e.g., at least 2–3 months after surgery or, in the case of conservative management, after corticosteroids are reduced to replacement levels or discontinued) provides a new baseline to which future imaging studies can be compared, although continued involution of necrotic adenoma can occur for some months after presentation. Although no data are available on the optimal imaging schedule, a reasonable approach is to repeat imaging in 6 months, then annually unless there is evidence of residual tumor growth or patient develops new or recurrent neurologic symptoms. If several years pass without evidence of recurrence, the interval between imaging studies may be extended.

9. CONCLUSIONS

Pituitary apoplexy is a clinical syndrome caused by hemorrhage or infarct within a preexisting pituitary mass lesion. The resulting expansion of the mass leads to compression of adjacent structures, resulting in the characteristic pattern of signs and symptoms, which include headache, nausea, ophthalmoplegia, and visual disturbance. Prompt diagnosis is important because failure to treat the commonly associated adrenal insufficiency can prove fatal, and early treatment improves neurologic outcome. When properly managed, the outcomes are generally good, with low mortality and the majority of patients achieving complete resolution of neurologic deficits. Most patients require rapid surgical decompression. Although some patients may be treated nonsurgically, the criteria for selecting such patients are not well defined. Further research is needed to define optimal management strategies. Hypopituitarism is common even after successful treatment, requiring long-term endocrinologic follow-up. The possibility of tumor recurrence mandates both long-term endocrinologic and imaging surveillance for all patients recovering from pituitary apoplexy.

REFERENCES

1. Bailey P. Pathological report of a case of akromegaly, with especial reference to the lesions in the hypophysis cerebri and in the thyroid gland; and of a case of hemorrhage into the pituitary. Philadelphia Med J 1898;1(18):789–92.
2. Brougham M, Heusner AP, Adams RD. Acute degenerative changes in adenomas of the pituitary body – with special reference to pituitary apoplexy. J Neurosurg 1950;7(5): 421–39.
3. Sosman MC. The roentgen therapy of pituitary adenoma. J Am Med Assoc 1939;113:1282–5.
4. Dott NM, Bailey P, Cushinhg H. A consideration of the hypophyseal adenomata. Br J Surg 1925;13:814–66.
5. Bonicki W, Kasperlik-Zaluska A, Koszewski W, Zgliczynski W, Wislawski J. Pituitary apoplexy: endocrine, surgical and oncological emergency. Incidence, clinical course and treatment with reference to 799 cases of pituitary adenomas. Acta Neurochir (Wien) 1993;120(3–4):118–22.
6. Bills DC, Meyer FB, Laws ER, Jr, et al. A retrospective analysis of pituitary apoplexy. Neurosurgery 1993;33(4):602–8; discussion 8–9.

7. Liu JK, Couldwell WT. Pituitary apoplexy in the magnetic resonance imaging era: clinical significance of sphenoid sinus mucosal thickening. J Neurosurg 2006;104(6):892–8.

8. Randeva HS, Schoebel J, Byrne J, Esiri M, Adams CB, Wass JA. Classical pituitary apoplexy: clinical features, management and outcome. Clin Endocrinol (Oxf) 1999;51(2):181–8.

9. Wakai S, Fukushima T, Teramoto A, Sano K. Pituitary apoplexy: its incidence and clinical significance. J Neurosurg 1981;55(2):187–93.

10. Muller-Jensen A, Ludecke D. Clinical aspects of spontaneous necrosis of pituitary tumors (pituitary apoplexy). J Neurol 1981;224(4):267–71.

11. Dubuisson AS, Beckers A, Stevenaert A. Classical pituitary tumour apoplexy: Clinical features, management and outcomes in a series of 24 patients. Clin Neurol Neurosurg 2006;109(1):63–70.

12. Biousse V, Newman NJ, Oyesiku NM. Precipitating factors in pituitary apoplexy. J Neurol Neurosurg Psychiatry 2001;71(4):542–5.

13. Ayuk J, McGregor EJ, Mitchell RD, Gittoes NJ. Acute management of pituitary apoplexy – surgery or conservative management? Clin Endocrinol (Oxf) 2004;61(6):747–52.

14. Sibal L, Ball SG, Connolly V, et al. Pituitary apoplexy: a review of clinical presentation, management and outcome in 45 cases. Pituitary 2004;7(3):157–63.

15. Semple PL, Webb MK, de Villiers JC, Laws ER, Jr. Pituitary apoplexy. Neurosurgery 2005;56(1):65–72; discussion 3.

16. Arita K, Tominaga A, Sugiyama K, et al. Natural course of incidentally found nonfunctioning pituitary adenoma, with special reference to pituitary apoplexy during follow-up examination. J Neurosurg 2006;104(6):884–91.

17. Nielsen EH, Lindholm J, Bjerre P, et al. Frequent occurrence of pituitary apoplexy in patients with non-functioning pituitary adenoma. Clin Endocrinol (Oxf) 2006;64(3): 319–22.

18. Ezzat S, Asa SL, Couldwell WT, et al. The prevalence of pituitary adenomas. Cancer 2004;101:613–9.

19. Molitch ME, Russell EJ. The pituitary "incidentaloma." Ann Intern Med 1990; 112(12):925–31.

20. Teramoto A, Hirakawa K, Sanno N, Osamura Y. Incidental pituitary lesions in 1,000 unselected autopsy specimens. Radiology 1994;193(1):161–4.

21. Hall WA, Luciano MG, Doppman JL, Patronas NJ, Oldfield EH. Pituitary magnetic resonance imaging in normal human volunteers: occult adenomas in the general population. Ann Intern Med 1994;120(10):817–20.

22. Yue NC, Longstreth WT, Jr, Elster AD, Jungreis CA, O'Leary DH, Poirier VC. Clinically serious abnormalities found incidentally at MR imaging of the brain: data from the Cardiovascular Health Study. Radiology 1997;202(1):41–6.

23. Kurschel S, Leber KA, Scarpatetti M, Roll P. Rare fatal vascular complication of transsphenoidal surgery. Acta Neurochir (Wien) 2005;147(3):321–5; discussion 5.

24. Rodier G, Mootien Y, Battaglia F, Martinet O, Cohen E. Bilateral stroke secondary to pituitary apoplexy. J Neurol 2003;250(4):494–5.

25. Fraioli B, Esposito V, Palma L, Cantore G. Hemorrhagic pituitary adenomas: clinicopathological features and surgical treatment. Neurosurgery 1990;27(5):741–7; discussion 7–8.

26. Bernstein M, Hegele RA, Gentili F, et al. Pituitary apoplexy associated with a triple bolus test. Case report. J Neurosurg 1984;61(3):586–90.

27. Clark JD, Freer CE, Wheatley T. Pituitary apoplexy: an unusual cause of stroke. Clin Radiol 1987;38(1):75–7.

28. Rosenbaum TJ, Houser W, Laws ER. Pituitary apoplexy producing internal carotid artery occlusion: case report. J Neurosurgery 1977;47:599–604.
29. Zayour DH, Selman WR, Arafah BM. Extreme elevation of intrasellar pressure in patients with pituitary tumor apoplexy: relation to pituitary function. J Clin Endocrinol Metab 2004;89(11):5649–54.
30. Rovit RL, Fein JM. Pituitary apoplexy: a review and reappraisal. J Neurosurg 1972;37(3):280–8.
31. Mohanty S, Tandon PN, Banerji AK, Prakash B. Haemorrhage into pituitary adenomas. J Neurol Neurosurg Psychiatry 1977;40(10):987–91.
32. Sussman EB, Porro RS. Pituitary apoplexy: the role of atheromatous emboli. Stroke 1974;5(3):318–23.
33. Maccagnan P, Macedo CL, Kayath MJ, Nogueira RG, Abucham J. Conservative management of pituitary apoplexy: a prospective study. J Clin Endocrinol Metab 1995;80(7):2190–7.
34. da Motta LA, de Mello PA, de Lacerda CM, Neto AP, da Motta LD, Filho MF. Pituitary apoplexy. Clinical course, endocrine evaluations and treatment analysis. J Neurosurg Sci 1999;43(1):25–36.
35. Maiza JC, Bennet A, Thorn-Kany M, Lagarrigue J, Caron P. Pituitary apoplexy and idiopathic thrombocytopenic purpura: a new case and review of the literature. Pituitary 2004;7(3):189–92.
36. Lenthall R, Gonugunta V, Jaspan T. Pituitary apoplexy with optic tract oedema and haemorrhage in a patient with idiopathic thrombocytopenic purpura. Neuroradiology 2001;43(2):156–8.
37. Wongpraparut N, Pleanboonlers N, Suwattee P, et al. Pituitary apoplexy in a patient with acute myeloid leukemia and thrombocytopenia. Pituitary 2000;3(2):113–6.
38. De la Torre M, Alcazar R, Aguirre M, Ferreras I. The dialysis patient with headache and sudden hypotension: consider pituitary apoplexy. Nephrol Dial Transplant 1998;13(3): 787–8.
39. Semple PL, De Villiers JC, Bowen RM, Lopes MB, Laws ER, Jr. Pituitary apoplexy: do histological features influence the clinical presentation and outcome? J Neurosurg 2006;104(6):931–7.
40. Wakai S, Fukushima T, Furihata T, Sano K. Association of cerebral aneurysm with pituitary adenoma. Surg Neurol 1979;12(6):503–7.
41. Onesti ST, Wisniewski T, Post KD. Clinical versus subclinical pituitary apoplexy: presentation, surgical management, and outcome in 21 patients. Neurosurgery 1990;26(6):980–6.
42. Elsasser Imboden PN, De Tribolet N, Lobrinus A, et al. Apoplexy in pituitary macroadenoma: eight patients presenting in 12 months. Medicine (Baltimore) 2005;84(3):188–96.
43. Veldhuis JD, Hammond JM. Endocrine function after spontaneous infarction of the human pituitary: report, review, and reappraisal. Endocr Rev 1980;1(1):100–7.
44. McFadzean RM, Doyle D, Rampling R, Teasdale E, Teasdale G. Pituitary apoplexy and its effect on vision. Neurosurgery 1991;29(5):669–75.
45. Tsementzis SA, Loizou LA. Pituitary apoplexy. Neurochirurgia (Stuttg) 1986;29(3):90–2.
46. Dawson BH, Kothandaram P. Acute massive infarction of pituitary adenomas. J Neurosurg 1972;37:275–9.
47. Cooper DM, Bazaral MG, Furlan AJ, et al. Pituitary apoplexy: a complication of cardiac surgery. Ann Thorac Surg 1986;41(5):547–50.
48. Tsitsopoulos P, Andrew J, Harrison MJ. Pituitary apoplexy and haemorrhage into adenomas. Postgrad Med J 1986;62(729):623–6.

49. Lennon M, Seigne P, Cunningham AJ. Pituitary apoplexy after spinal anaesthesia. Br J Anaesth 1998;81(4):616–8.
50. Wichers M, Kristof RA, Springer W, Schramm J, Klingmuller D. Pituitary apoplexy with spontaneous cure of acromegaly and its possible relation to Gd-DTPA-administration. Acta Neurochir (Wien) 1997;139(10):992–4.
51. Bevan JS, Oza AM, Burke CW, Adams CB. Pituitary apoplexy following isosorbide administration. J Neurol Neurosurg Psychiatry 1987;50(5):636–7.
52. O'Donovan PA, O'Donovan PJ, Ritchie EH, Felly M, Jenkins DM. Apoplexy into a prolactin secreting macroadenoma during early pregnancy with successful outcome; case report. Br J Obstet Gynecol 1986;93:389–91.
53. Engel G, Huston M, Oshima S, et al. Pituitary apoplexy after leuprolide injection for ovum donation. J Adolesc Health 2003;32(1):89–93.
54. Walker AB, Eldridge PR, MacFarlane IA. Clomiphene-induced pituitary apoplexy in a patient with acromegaly. Postgrad Med J 1996;72(845):172–3.
55. Eaton HJ, Phillips PJ, Hanieh A, Cooper J, Bolt J, Torpy DJ. Rapid onset of pituitary apoplexy after goserelin implant for prostate cancer: need for heightened awareness. Intern Med J 2001;31(5):313–4.
56. Blaut K, Wisniewski P, Syrenicz A, Sworczak K. Apoplexy of clinically silent pituitary adenoma during prostate cancer treatment with LHRH analog. Neuro Endocrinol Lett 2006;27(5):569–72.
57. Levy A. Hazards of dynamic testing of pituitary function. Clin Endocrinol (Oxf) 2003;58(5):543–4.
58. Rotman-Pikielny P, Patronas N, Papanicolaou DA. Pituitary apoplexy induced by corticotrophin-releasing hormone in a patient with Cushing's disease. Clin Endocrinol (Oxf) 2003;58(5):545–9.
59. Masson EA, Atkin SL, Diver M, White MC. Pituitary apoplexy and sudden blindness following the administration of gonadotrophin releasing hormone. Clin Endocrinol (Oxf) 1993;38(1):109–10.
60. Reznik Y, Chapon F, Lahlou N, Deboucher N, Mahoudeau J. Pituitary apoplexy of a gonadotroph adenoma following gonadotrophin releasing hormone agonist therapy for prostatic cancer. J Endocrinol Invest 1997;20(9):566–8.
61. Arafah BM, Taylor HC, Salazar R, Saadi H, Selman WR. Apoplexy of a pituitary adenoma after dynamic testing with gonadotropin-releasing hormone. Am J Med 1989;87(1):103–5.
62. Masago A, Ueda Y, Kanai H, Nagai H, Umemura S. Pituitary apoplexy after pituitary function test: a report of two cases and review of the literature. Surg Neurol 1995;43(2):158–64; discussion 65.
63. Szabolcs I, Kesmarki N, Bor K, et al. Apoplexy of a pituitary macroadenoma as a severe complication of preoperative thyrotropin-releasing hormone (TRH) testing. Exp Clin Endocrinol Diabetes 1997;105(4):234–6.
64. Matsuura I, Saeki N, Kubota M, Murai H, Yamaura A. Infarction followed by hemorrhage in pituitary adenoma due to endocrine stimulation test. Endocr J 2001;48(4):493–8.
65. Chapman AJ, Williams G, Hockley AD, London DR. Pituitary apoplexy after combined test of anterior pituitary function. Br Med J (Clin Res Ed) 1985;291(6487):26.
66. Mikhailidis DP, Fonseca V, Dandona P. Pituitary apoplexy. Br Med J (Clin Res Ed) 1985;291(6493):488–9.
67. Otsuka F, Kageyama J, Ogura T, Makino H. Pituitary apoplexy induced by a combined anterior pituitary test: case report and literature review. Endocr J 1998;45(3):393–8.

68. Piotin M, Tampieri D, Rufenacht DA, et al. The various MRI patterns of pituitary apoplexy. Eur Radiol 1999;9(5):918–23.

69. Rogg JM, Tung GA, Anderson G, Cortez S. Pituitary apoplexy: early detection with diffusion-weighted MR imaging. AJNR Am J Neuroradiol 2002;23(7):1240–5.

70. Ahmed M, Rifai A, Al-Jurf M, Akhtar M, Woodhouse N. Classical pituitary apoplexy presentation and a follow-up of 13 patients. Horm Res 1989;31(3):125–32.

71. Lee MS, Pless M. Apoplectic lymphocytic hypophysitis. Case report. J Neurosurg 2003;98(1):183–5.

72. Rosales MY, Smith TW, Safran M. Hemorrhagic Rathke's cleft cyst presenting as diplopia. Endocr Pract 2004;10(2):129–34.

73. Pawar SJ, Sharma RR, Lad SD, Dev E, Devadas RV. Rathke's cleft cyst presenting as pituitary apoplexy. J Clin Neurosci 2002;9(1):76–9.

74. Nishioka H, Ito H, Miki T, Hashimoto T, Nojima H, Matsumura H. Rathke's cleft cyst with pituitary apoplexy: case report. Neuroradiology 1999;41(11):832–4.

75. Fernandez-Real JM, Villabona C, Acebes JJ, Gomez-Saez JM, Soler J. Pituitary apoplexy into nonadenomatous tissue: case report and review. Am J Med Sci 1995;310(2):68–70.

76. Furuta S, Hatakeyama T, Zenke K, Fukumoto S. Pituitary metastasis from carcinoma of the urinary bladder mimicking pituitary apoplexy – case report. Neurol Med Chir (Tokyo) 1999;39(2):165–8.

77. Hanna FW, Williams OM, Davies JS, Dawson T, Neal J, Scanlon MF. Pituitary apoplexy following metastasis of bronchogenic adenocarcinoma to a prolactinoma. Clin Endocrinol (Oxf) 1999;51(3):377–81.

78. Lieschke GJ, Tress B, Chambers D. Endometrial adenocarcinoma presenting as pituitary apoplexy. Aust N Z J Med 1990;20(1):81–4.

79. Arunkumar MJ, Rajshekhar V. Intrasellar tuberculoma presenting as pituitary apoplexy. Neurol India 2001;49(4):407–10.

80. Lee HJ, Kalnin AJ, Holodny AI, Schulder M, Grigorian A, Sharer LR. Hemorrhagic chondroid chordoma mimicking pituitary apoplexy. Neuroradiology 1998;40(11): 720–3.

81. Kingdon CC, Sidhu PS, Cohen J. Pituitary apoplexy secondary to an underlying abscess. J Infect 1996;33(1):53–5.

82. Suzuki H, Muramatsu M, Murao K, Kawaguchi K, Shimizu T. Pituitary apoplexy caused by ruptured internal carotid artery aneurysm. Stroke 2001;32(2):567–9.

83. Romano A, Chibbaro S, Marsella M, Ippolito S, Benericetti E. Carotid cavernous aneurysm presenting as pituitary apoplexy. J Clin Neurosci 2006;13(4):476–9.

84. Provenzale JM, Hacein-Bey L, Taveras JM. Internal carotid artery dissection associated with pituitary apoplexy: MR findings. J Comput Assist Tomogr 1995;19(1):150–2.

85. Orakdogeny M, Karadereler S, Berkman Z, Ersahin M, Ozdogan C, Aker F. Intra-suprasellar meningioma mimicking pituitary apoplexy. Acta Neurochir (Wien) 2004;146(5):511–5.

86. Sani S, Smith A, Leppla DC, Ilangovan S, Glick R. Epidermoid cyst of the sphenoid sinus with extension into the sella turcica presenting as pituitary apoplexy: case report. Surg Neurol 2005;63(4):394–7; discussion 7.

87. Matsumoto K, Kohmura E, Tsuruzono K, Mori K, Kawano K, Tsujimura T. Silicone plate-induced granuloma presenting pituitary apoplexy-like symptoms: case report. Surg Neurol 1995;43(2):166–9.

88. Oliver RM, Craft TM, Shaw KM. Bleeding intracranial aneurysm? Pituitary apoplexy! Br J Clin Pract 1991;45(2):150–1.

89. Chen ST, Chen SD, Ryu SJ, Hsu TF, Heimburger RF. Pituitary apoplexy with intracerebral hemorrhage simulating rupture of an anterior cerebral artery aneurysm. Surg Neurol 1988;29(4):322–5.
90. Winer JB, Plant G. Stuttering pituitary apoplexy resembling meningitis. J Neurol Neurosurg Psychiatry 1990;53(5):440.
91. Bjerre P, Lindholm J. Pituitary apoplexy with sterile meningitis. Acta Neurol Scand 1986;74(4):304–7.
92. Brouns R, Crols R, Engelborghs S, De Deyn PP. Pituitary apoplexy presenting as chemical meningitis. Lancet 2004;364(9433):502.
93. Jassal DS, McGinn G, Embil JM. Pituitary apoplexy masquerading as meningoencephalitis. Headache 2004;44(1):75–8.
94. Shin RK, Cucchiara BL, Liebeskind DS, Liu GT, Balcer LJ. Pituitary apoplexy causing optic neuropathy and Horner syndrome without ophthalmoplegia. J Neuroophthalmol 2003;23(3):208–10.
95. Jellinek EH. Empty sella syndrome and pituitary apoplexy. Lancet 1988;1(8593):1053.
96. Silvestrini M, Matteis M, Cupini LM, Troisi E, Bernardi G, Floris R. Ophthalmoplegic migraine-like syndrome due to pituitary apoplexy. Headache 1994;34(8):484–6.
97. Jones SE, James RA, Hall K, Kendall-Taylor P. Optic chiasmal herniation – an under recognized complication of dopamine agonist therapy for macroprolactinoma. Clin Endocrinol (Oxf) 2000;53(4):529–34.
98. Vidal E, Cevallos R, Vidal J, et al. Twelve cases of pituitary apoplexy. Arch Intern Med 1992;152(9):1893–9.
99. Chuang CC, Chang CN, Wei KC, et al. Surgical treatment for severe visual compromised patients after pituitary apoplexy. J Neurooncol 2006;80(1):39–47.
100. Gruber A, Clayton J, Kumar S, Robertson I, Howlett TA, Mansell P. Pituitary apoplexy: retrospective review of 30 patients – is surgical intervention always necessary? Br J Neurosurg 2006;20(6):379–85.
101. Brisman MH, Katz G, Post KD. Symptoms of pituitary apoplexy rapidly reversed with bromocriptine. Case report. J Neurosurg 1996;85(6):1153–5.
102. Barker FG, 2nd, Klibanski A, Swearingen B. Transsphenoidal surgery for pituitary tumors in the United States, 1996–2000: mortality, morbidity, and the effects of hospital and surgeon volume. J Clin Endocrinol Metab 2003;88(10):4709–19.
103. Kamiya Y, Jin-No YT, K., Suzuki T, et al. Recurrence of Cushing's disease after long-term remission due to pituitary apoplexy. Endocrine Journal 2000;47:793–7.
104. Cunningham SK, Moore A, McKenna TJ. Normal cortisol response to corticotropin in patients with secondary adrenal failure. Arch Intern Med 1983;143(12):2276–9.
105. Post MJ, David NJ, Glaser JS, Safran A. Pituitary apoplexy: diagnosis by computed tomography. Radiology 1980;134(3):665–70.
106. Weisberg LA. Pituitary apoplexy. Association of degenerative change in pituitary adenoma with radiotherapy and detection by cerebral computed tomography. Am J Med 1977;63(1):109–15.

20 Pituitary Tumors and Pregnancy

Mark E. Molitch, MD

CONTENTS

Summary

Pituitary adenomas may cause problems during pregnancy because of oversecretion of hormones and hypopituitarism. Hyperprolactinemia and Cushing's syndrome may need to be controlled to allow conception. Maternal morbidity and fetal mortality and morbidity may be affected by the hormone oversecretion in Cushing's disease, acromegaly, and TSH-secreting adenomas. Treatment of hyperprolactinemia and acromegaly during pregnancy is not necessary but resection of ACTH-secreting adenomas during pregnancy and medical treatment of hyperthyroidism are warranted. Reinstitution of dopamine agonists may be indicated in the 30% of macroprolactinomas that enlarge symptomatically during pregnancy. In hypopituitary patients, thyroid hormone levels should be increased empirically each trimester but no increase in steroid hormones is needed except during additional stress and labor. Lymphocytic hypophysitis may cause mass effects and hypopituitarism, both of which may need treatment. Sheehan's syndrome has both acute and chronic forms which need appropriate evaluation and treatment.

Key Words: Pregnancy, Pituitary adenoma, Acromegaly, Prolactinoma, Cushing's syndrome.

1. ANTERIOR PITUITARY GLAND AND PREGNANCY

Pituitary adenomas comprise 6% of intracranial (malignant and nonmalignant) neoplasms *(1)*. They may cause problems because of oversecretion of hormones by the tumor besides causing hypopituitarism, thereby affecting

From: *Contemporary Endocrinology: Diagnosis and Management of Pituitary Disorders*
Edited by: B. Swearingen and B. M. K. Biller © Humana Press, Totowa, NJ

fertility and pregnancy outcome if pregnancy does ensue. In addition, the pregnancy itself alters hormone secretion and pituitary function, complicating the evaluation of patients with pituitary neoplasms. The influence of various types of therapy on the developing fetus also affects therapeutic decision making.

During pregnancy, the normal pituitary gland enlarges considerably, due to estrogen-stimulated hyperplasia and hypertrophy of the prolactin (PRL)-producing lactotrophs (2,3). Concomitantly, PRL levels rise gradually throughout gestation (4). The elevated PRL levels found at term prepare the breast for lactation. Thus, the finding of amenorrhea associated with hyperprolactinemia could well be due to pregnancy and not due to pathologic hyperprolactinemia. This lactotroph hyperplasia results in an increase in overall pituitary size as seen on magnetic resonance imaging (MRI) scans, with the peak size occurring in the first few days postpartum when gland heights up to 12 mm may be seen (5–7). Following delivery there is a rapid involution of the gland, so that normal pituitary size is found by 6 months postpartum (6,7). This stimulatory effect of pregnancy on the pituitary has important implications for the patient with a prolactinoma who desires pregnancy.

Beginning in the second half of pregnancy, pituitary growth hormone (GH) secretion decreases and the circulating level of a GH variant made by the syncytiotrophoblastic epithelium of the placenta increases to as high as 10–20 ng/Ml (8,9). The decreased production of normal pituitary GH is likely due to negative feedback effects of insulin-like growth factor 1 (IGF-1), which is stimulated by the placentally produced GH variant (8,9). In patients with acromegaly who have autonomous GH secretion and become pregnant, both forms of GH persist in the blood throughout pregnancy (10).

Over the course of gestation, cortisol levels rise progressively, resulting in a twofold to threefold increase by term (11). Most of the elevation of cortisol levels is due to the estrogen-induced increase in cortisol binding globulin (CBG) levels (12). However, the bioactive "free" fraction is also elevated threefold and the cortisol production rate is increased, so that there is a twofold to threefold elevation in urinary free cortisol level (11,12). ACTH levels have been variously reported as being normal, suppressed, or elevated early in gestation (11,13). However, later in the pregnancy, there is a progressive rise, followed by a final surge of ACTH and cortisol levels during labor (11). ACTH does not cross the placenta but it is also manufactured by the placenta (13). The amount of ACTH in serum that is of placental as compared to pituitary origin at various stages of gestation is not known. Corticotropin-releasing hormone (CRH) is also produced by the placenta and is released into maternal plasma (14). The CRH is bioactive and may release ACTH both from the placenta, in a paracrine fashion, and from the maternal pituitary (14). The role of placental

CRH in regulating ACTH and cortisol secretion during pregnancy in humans is still unclear but it may be driving the marked increase in ACTH and cortisol in the third trimester *(15)*.

TSH levels fall in the first trimester, in response to the rise in thyroid hormone levels, which are stimulated by hCG, but return to the normal range by the third trimester *(16)*. In response to placental sex steroid production, both hypothalamic gonadotropin-releasing hormone (GnRH) and pituitary gonadotropin (FSH/LH) levels decline in the first trimester of pregnancy, with a blunted gonadotropin response to GnRH *(17)*.

2. PROLACTINOMA

Hyperprolactinemia is responsible for about one-third of all cases of female infertility *(18)*. Hyperprolactinemia impairs the hypothalamic–pituitary–ovarian axis at several levels, the primary site of inhibition being at the hypothalamus where it inhibits the pulsatile secretion of GnRH *(19)*. The differential diagnosis of hyperprolactinemia is extensive *(20)*, but this discussion will focus on the patient with a prolactinoma.

For patients with prolactinomas, the choice of therapy may have important consequences for decisions regarding pregnancy. Transsphenoidal surgery is curative in 50–60% of cases and rarely causes hypopituitarism when it is performed on women with microadenomas. For patients with macroadenomas, surgery cures a much smaller number with a considerably greater risk of causing hypopituitarism, and may therefore affect fertility *(19)*.

Dopamine agonists, including bromocriptine, pergolide (not approved in the United States), quinagolide (not approved in the United States), and cabergoline, have become the primary mode of therapy for virtually all patients with prolactinomas *(20)*. Bromocriptine, pergolide, and quinagolide can restore ovulatory menses in 70–80% of women and cabergoline can do so in over 90% *(19–21)*. Once ovulatory menses have been established, mechanical contraception is used until the first two or three cycles have occurred, so that an intermenstrual interval can be determined. Thus, a woman will know when she has missed a menstrual period; a pregnancy test can be performed quickly and the precise gestational age of the fetus will be known. In this way, these drugs will have been given for only about 3–4 weeks of gestation. However, because of its long half-life in the body, cabergoline cessation at that point will still result in a further fetal exposure for several additional weeks.

In addition to their efficacy in lowering PRL levels, the dopamine agonists often reduce tumor size of PRL-secreting macroadenomas, bromocriptine reducing the size by $\geq 50\%$ in 50–75% of patients, pergolide doing so in 80–90% of patients, and cabergoline achieving such reductions in over 90% of patients in some series *(19,22–24)*.

About 10–15% of patients are relatively resistant to the action of dopamine agonists and may require larger-than-usual doses to achieve normal or near-normal PRL levels *(25)*. Recently, the very large doses of pergolide and cabergoline used in patients with Parkinson's disease have been found to be associated with cardiac valvular lesions *(26,27)*. Because of this, such patients should be monitored with echocardiography; in the United States pergolide has been withdrawn from use because of this.

2.1. Effects of Pregnancy on Prolactinoma Growth

In women with prolactinomas, the stimulatory effect of the hormonal milieu of pregnancy may result in significant tumor enlargement during gestation (Fig. 1). This is then combined with the fact that the dopamine agonist that had caused the tumor to shrink has now been discontinued. Five reports

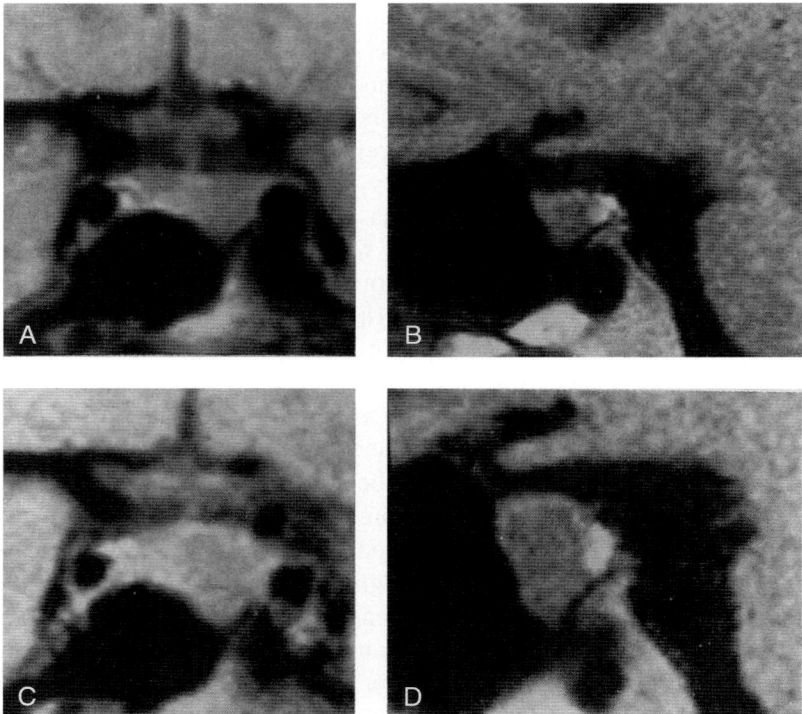

Fig. 1. Coronal and sagittal MR imaging scans of an intrasellar, prolactin-secreting macroadenoma in a woman prior to conception (A and B) and at 7 months gestation (c and D). Note the marked tumor enlargement at the latter point, at which time the patient was complaining of headaches. (Reproduced with permission from Molitch ME. Medical treatment of prolactinomas. Endocrinol Metab Clin N Amer 1999;28:143–169. Copyright Elsevier, 1999).

Table 1
Effect of Pregnancy on Prolactinomas

Tumor Type	Prior Therapy	Number of Patients	Symptomatic Enlargement*
Microadenomas	none	457	12 (2.6%)
Macroadenomas	none	142	45 (31.7%)
Macroadenomas	yes	140	7 (5.0%)

*Headaches and visual disturbances

have compiled data analyzing the risk of symptomatic tumor enlargement in pregnant women with prolactinomas, divided according to their status as microprolactinomas or macroprolactinomas (27–31) (Table 1). For women with microadenomas, only 12 of 457 pregnancies (2.6%) were complicated by symptoms of tumor enlargement (headaches and/or visual disturbances). Surgical intervention was not required in a single case and medical therapy with reinstitution of bromocriptine resolved the symptoms in the five in whom it was tried. In 45 of 142 pregnancies (31.7%) in women who had not undergone prior surgery or radiotherapy for their macroprolactinomas there were symptoms of tumor enlargement (headaches and/or visual disturbances). Of these 45, surgical intervention was undertaken in 12 and medical therapy in 17, leading to resolution of their symptoms. A total of 140 women with macroadenomas who have undergone surgery or radiation prior to pregnancy have been identified. In these individuals, the risk to tumor enlargement was relatively low (5%). If tumor enlargement occurs, reinstitution of bromocriptine and cabergoline is usually successful in reducing the size of the tumor, but transsphenoidal surgery may be necessary (28,32).

2.2. Effects of Hyperprolactinemia and Its Treatment on Pregnancy

Bromocriptine taken for only the first few weeks of gestation has not been associated with any increase in spontaneous abortions, ectopic pregnancies, trophoblastic disease, multiple pregnancies, or congenital malformations (Table 2) (33,34). Long-term follow-up studies of 64 children between the ages of 6 months and 9 years whose mothers took bromocriptine in this fashion have shown no ill effects (35). Experience is limited to only just over 100 women; however, with the use of bromocriptine given throughout gestation; no abnormalities were noted in the infants, except in one with an undescended testicle and in one with a talipes deformity (36). However, because bromocriptine crosses the placenta (37), it should not be used any longer than necessary during pregnancy. Both cabergoline and bromocriptine are considered to be Class B for use during pregnancy.

Table 2
Effect of Bromocriptine on Pregnancies

	Bromocriptine		Normal
	n	%	Population %
Pregnancies	6, 239	100.0	100.0
Spontaneous abortion	620	9.9	10–15
Terminations	75	1.2	
Ectopic	31	0.5	0.5–1.0
Hydatidiform moles	11	0.2	0.05–0.7
Deliveries (known duration)	4, 139	100.0	100.0
At term (>38 weeks)	3, 620	87.5	85
Preterm (<38 weeks)	519	12.5	15
Deliveries (known outcome)	5, 120	100.0	100.0
Single births	5, 031	9.3	8.7
Multiple births	89	1.7	1.3
Babies (known details)	5, 213	100.0	100.0
Normal	5, 030	96.5	95.0
With malformations	93	1.8	3–4
With perinatal disorders	90	1.7	>2

[a]Data from Krupp P, Monka C, Richter K. Program of the Second World Congress of Gynecology and Obstetrics. Rio de Janeiro, 1988, p. 9. *(33)*

Pergolide has been shown to cross the placenta in mice *(38)*. In the discussion of a pregnant patient treated with pergolide for Parkinson's disease, the authors state that "in premarketing studies of pergolide for endocrine disorders, two major and three minor congenital abnormalities were described among 38 pregnancies, but a causal relationship has not been established"

(39). Other information from the manufacturer, Eli Lilly & Co., stated that they had only limited data on pregnancies in which the fetus was exposed to pergolide, finding that 7.2% of pregnancy outcomes resulted in spontaneous abortions, 7.2% in minor malformations, 14.3% in intentional abortions, 28.6% in healthy infants, and 43.4% with no information available *(40)*. This limited information is sufficient to recommend against using pergolide when a women wishes to get pregnant.

Some early publications reported no detrimental effects on pregnancy or fetal development in women who became pregnant during treatment with quinagolide *(41)*. However, a review of 176 pregnancies, in which quinagolide was maintained for a median duration of 37 days, reported 24 spontaneous abortions, 1 ectopic pregnancy, and 1 stillbirth at 31 weeks of gestation *(42)*. Furthermore, nine fetal malformations were reported in this group: spina bifida, trisomy 13, Down's syndrome, talipes, cleft lip, arrhinencephaly, and Zellweger syndrome *(42)*. Therefore, quinagolide should also not be used if pregnancy is desired.

Cabergoline has been shown to cross the placenta in animal studies *(19)*, but such data are lacking in humans. Data on exposure of the fetus or embryo during the first several weeks of pregnancy have been reported in just over 350 cases and such use has not shown an increased percentage of spontaneous abortion, premature delivery, multiple pregnancy, or congenital abnormalities *(31,43–46)*. No alterations in the newborns' weights were observed *(31,43–46)*. Available data from 107 infants followed for 1 to 72 months showed normal physical and mental development *(43)*.

In conclusion, with respect to using a dopamine agonist to facilitate ovulation and fertility, bromocriptine has the largest safety database and has a proven safety record for pregnancy. Although the database for cabergoline use in pregnancy is much smaller, it does not appear to exert any deleterious effects on pregnant women and the incidence of malformation in their offspring is not greater than in the general population. For the woman who is intolerant to bromocriptine and who is doing well with cabergoline, continuation of cabergoline for facilitating pregnancy certainly appears to be reasonable. The safety databases for pergolide and quinagolide are quite limited, but they appear to raise considerable concerns and so these drugs should not be used when fertility is desired. The effects of transsphenoidal surgery during gestation are not known specifically, but would not be expected to be significantly different from the effects of other types of surgery *(47)* (unless hypopituitarism should ensue).

2.3. Management of Prolactinoma in Pregnancy

The risks of surgery versus medical therapy for prolactinoma should be explained in detail to each patient. For patients with microadenomas or intrasellar macroadenomas, bromocriptine or cabergoline therapy is generally preferred to surgery because it is safe for the fetus when discontinued early in gestation and poses only a small risk of tumor enlargement for the mother. Such patients should be seen each trimester and assessed for symptoms such as headaches or visual problems; visual field testing need only be done when clinically indicated. When the tumor is large or extends to the optic chiasm or into the cavernous sinus, the following approaches should be considered: (i) preoperative surgical debulking; (ii) intensive monitoring without dopamine agonist therapy; or (iii) continuous dopamine agonist therapy. The safety of the last approach has not been established, but based on the small number of cases cited earlier, it is probably not harmful. Patients with macroadenomas should be assessed monthly for new symptoms, and visual fields should be tested each trimester. PRL levels, which normally increase in pregnancy, may not rise in women with prolactinomas (48). Furthermore, PRL levels may not always rise with pregnancy-induced tumor enlargement (48); therefore, periodic measurements of PRL levels are of little benefit and may even be misleading.

When there is evidence of tumor enlargement during pregnancy, bromocriptine therapy should be reinstituted immediately and the dosage increased as rapidly as tolerated. Such therapy must be monitored closely and switching to cabergoline, transsphenoidal surgery, or delivery (if the pregnancy is far enough advanced) should be considered if there is no response to bromocriptine (28).

Although suckling stimulates PRL secretion in normal women for the first few weeks to months postpartum, there are no data to suggest that breast-feeding can cause tumor growth. Thus, there seems to be no reason to discourage nursing in women with prolactinomas.

3. ACROMEGALY

Reports of pregnancy in patients with acromegaly are uncommon (49–60), perhaps because 30–40% of such patients have hyperprolactinemia (61). Correction of hyperprolactinemia with bromocriptine may be necessary to permit ovulation and conception in these patients (50,56).

3.1. Diagnosis of Acromegaly During Pregnancy

Conventional immunoassays for GH cannot distinguish between normal pituitary GH and the placental GH variant (8). Special immunoassays using antibodies that recognize specific epitopes on the two hormones (8) must be used. When such specific assays are not available, it may be necessary to wait until after delivery to assess pituitary GH secretion accurately, because the placental variant falls to undetectable levels within 24 h *(8)*. However, there are two differences between the secretion of the placental GH variant and the secretion of pituitary GH during acromegaly that may allow a distinction to be made during pregnancy. First, pituitary GH secretion in acromegaly is highly pulsatile, with 13–19 pulses per 24 h *(62)*, whereas secretion of the pregnancy GH variant is nonpulsatile *(9)*. Second, in acromegaly, about 70% of patients have a GH response to thyrotropin (TSH)-releasing hormone (no longer available in the United States) *(63)*, whereas the placental GH variant does not respond to this hormone *(10)*.

3.2. Effects of Pregnancy on Tumor Size and Acromegaly

Only three patients with tumors secreting GH have been reported to have enlargement of their tumors with a resultant visual field defect in one during pregnancy*(29,60,64)*. However, in one of these three the tumor size had been controlled by somatostatin analogs prior to pregnancy, so how much of the tumor enlargement was due to withdrawal of the somatostatin analog versus the pregnancy cannot be ascertained with certainty *(60)*. In addition, one patient with acromegaly experienced pituitary apoplexy at 33 weeks *(59)*. Therefore, patients with acromegaly should be monitored for symptomatic tumor enlargement in a fashion similar to that for patients with PRL-secreting macroadenomas. There is some evidence that pregnancy may cause an exacerbation of acromegaly in a small number of cases *(50)*, but other series have not reported this *(59,60)*, so this does not appear to be a sufficient enough risk to advise against pregnancy.

3.3. Effects of Acromegaly on the Pregnancy

Certain complications of acromegaly are potentially harmful to both the mother and the fetus. Carbohydrate intolerance is present in as many as 50% of patients with acromegaly, and overt diabetes is seen in 10–20% *(61)*. Insulin resistance secondary to the increased levels of GH may increase the risk of gestational diabetes. There is increased salt retention, and hypertension occurs in 25–35% of patients. In addition, cardiac disease is present in about one-third of patients. There may be a specific cardiomyopathy associated with acromegaly, and coronary artery disease may be increased *(61)*. Thus, the risks for gestational diabetes, hypertension, and heart disease are likely increased in women with acromegaly during pregnancy but there are no specific data to document this.

3.4. Management of Acromegaly and Pregnancy

The considerations regarding the use of bromocriptine and cabergoline in women with prolactinomas also apply to those with acromegaly. For most patients, these drugs should not be continued during pregnancy. Data on the use of octreotide during pregnancy are limited. Only 14 pregnant patients treated with octreotide, octreotide LAR, and lanreotide have been reported; no malformations were found in their children *(57)* Octreotide crosses the placenta *(65)* and therefore can affect developing fetal tissues. On the other hand, it does not bind with high affinity to the placenta and has no effect on the placental GH variant *(66)*. Because octreotide crosses the placenta and there are limited data documenting safety, it is recommended that octreotide and other somatostatin analogs be discontinued if pregnancy is considered and that contraception be used when these drugs are administered. Considering the prolonged nature of the course of most patients with acromegaly, interruption of medical therapy for 9–12 months should not have a particularly adverse effect on the long-term outcome. On the other hand, these drugs can control tumor growth and for enlarging tumors, their reintroduction during pregnancy may be warranted versus operating. Both bromocriptine *(58)* and octreotide *(57)* have been started during pregnancy because of tumor enlargement with successful shrinkage of the tumor.

4. CUSHING'S SYNDROME

Just over 100 cases of Cushing's syndrome in pregnancy have been reported *(67–82)*. The distribution of causes of Cushing's syndrome in pregnancy differs markedly from that in the nonpregnant population. Less than 50% of the pregnant patients described had pituitary adenomas, a similar number had adrenal adenomas, and more than 10% had adrenal carcinomas *(67–82)*. Only three reports have described pregnancies associated with the ectopic ACTH syndrome*(69,73)*.

In many cases, hypercortisolism first became apparent during pregnancy, with improvement after parturition, leading to the speculation that unregulated placental CRH was instrumental in causing this pregnancy-induced exacerbation*(15,68,69,73,79)*. Rarely, recurrent Cushing's syndrome may be associated with pregnancy only to completely remit following delivery; the etiology for this has not been found *(80,81)*.

4.1. Diagnosis of Cushing's Syndrome During Pregnancy

Diagnosing Cushing's syndrome during pregnancy may be difficult. Both conditions may be associated with weight gain in a central distribution, fatigue, edema, emotional upset, glucose intolerance, and hypertension. The striae associated with weight gain and increased abdominal girth are usually white in normal pregnancy and red or purple in Cushing's syndrome. Hirsutism and acne may point to excessive androgen production.

The laboratory evaluation of Cushing's syndrome during pregnancy is not straightforward. Elevated total and free serum cortisol and ACTH levels and urinary free cortisol excretion are compatible with that of normal pregnancy. The overnight dexamethasone test usually demonstrates inadequate suppression during normal pregnancy (70). At least in the latter part of the third trimester, the elevated cortisol levels are not suppressed during the low-dose dexamethasone test but are suppressed during the high-dose test, similar to what is observed in patients with Cushing's disease (68). ACTH levels are normal to elevated in pregnant patients with all forms of Cushing's syndrome (67–72). These "normal" rather than suppressed levels of ACTH in patients with adrenal adenomas may result from the production of ACTH by the placenta or from the nonsuppressible stimulation of pituitary ACTH by placental CRH.

A persistent circadian variation in the elevated levels of total and free serum cortisol during normal pregnancy may be most helpful in distinguishing Cushing's syndrome from the hypercortisolism of pregnancy, because this finding is characteristically absent in all forms of Cushing's syndrome (12). Salivary cortisol measurements may turn out to be useful in this regard but normal limits for midnight levels of salivary cortisol during pregnancy have not yet been standardized (79). In many cases, MRI scanning of the pituitary (without contrast) or ultrasound of the adrenal may be required, although MRIs of the pituitary in patients with Cushing's disease are often nondiagnostic. Little experience has been reported with newer techniques such as CRH stimulation testing or petrosal venous sinus sampling during pregnancy. However, Ross et al. (71) found the typical exaggerated ACTH response to CRH in a woman with Cushing's disease but Mellor et al. (78) found only a doubling of cortisol levels in response to CRH; neither patient had ill effects from such testing. In two patients studied by Lindsay et al. (82), ACTH levels increased more than threefold but cortisol level increases were less than twofold. CRH testing during petrosal sinus sampling was performed without ill effects in one woman by Pinette et al. (74) and in four women by Lindsay et al. (82) but catheterization was performed via the direct jugular vein approach rather than the femoral vein approach to minimize fetal irradiation; in these cases, clearly increased central-to-peripheral ACTH gradients were found.

4.2. Effects of Cushing's Syndrome on the Pregnancy

Cushing's syndrome is associated with a fetal mortality of 25% due to spontaneous abortion, stillbirth, and early neonatal death because of extreme prematurity (67–79,82). Premature labor occurs in more than 50% of cases, regardless of etiology (67–79,82). The passage of cortisol across the placenta occasionally results in suppression of the fetal adrenals (75). This appears to be uncommon, but the neonate should be tested for this potential problem and given exogenous corticosteroids until the results of the evaluation are known.

Maternal complications may also occur. Hypertension develops in most patients. Diabetes and myopathy are frequent. Postoperative wound infection and dehiscence are common after cesarean section. The pregnancy appears to induce an amelioration of Cushing's syndrome in some patients, but an exacerbation in others *(67–73,79)*.

4.3. Management of Cushing's Syndrome During Pregnancy

In data from the literature summarized from two reviews *(67,70)* fetal loss rates of 9% and 24% and premature labor rates of 20% and 47% were found in the 11 and 17 women, respectively, who were treated during pregnancy as compared to fetal loss rates of 30% and 38%, and premature labor rates of 48% and 72% in the 26 and 43 women, respectively, in whom treatment was delayed. Therefore, treatment during pregnancy has been advocated *(67,70,82)*.

Medical therapy for Cushing's disease during pregnancy is not very effective *(69,70,79)*. A few case reports have documented the efficacy of metyrapone *(82)*. Ketoconazole has been given to two patients with complications of intrauterine growth retardation but no malformations or other perinatal disorders *(76,77)*. Use of other drugs such as aminoglutethimide, mitotane, bromocriptine, and cyproheptadine has been very limited *(79)*; because of potential toxicity to the fetus, aminoglutethimide and mitotane should be avoided. Transsphenoidal resection of a pituitary ACTH-secreting adenoma has been carried out successfully in several patients during the second trimester *(68,71,74,75,78,79,82)*. Although any surgery poses risks for the mother and fetus *(47)*, it appears that with Cushing's syndrome, the risks of not operating are considerably higher than those of proceeding with surgery.

5. TSH-SECRETING TUMORS

Only three cases of pregnancy occurring in women with TSH-secreting tumors have been reported *(83–85)*. In one of these cases, octreotide, which had been stopped, had to be reinstituted to control tumor size *(83)* and in a second, octreotide was continued during pregnancy for tumor size control *(84)*. The most pressing issue with such tumors is the need to control hyperthyroidism during pregnancy and that can usually be done with standard antithyroid drugs *(84)*. However, with growing macroadenomas, octreotide may be necessary for tumor size control *(83,84)*.

6. CLINICALLY NONFUNCTIONING ADENOMAS

Pregnancy would not expected to influence tumor size in patients with clinically nonfunctioning adenomas (CNFAs) and only two cases have been reported in which tumor enlargement during pregnancy resulted in a visual field defect *(29,86)*. On the other hand, the lactotroph hyperplasia that occurs during pregnancy can be quite significant *(2,3)*. MRIs obtained during pregnancy and the immediate postpartum period have shown that this hyperplasia may cause the normal pituitary to increase to up to 12 mm in height *(5–7)*. Therefore, it would be expected that if this lactotroph hyperplasia were to occur in a patient with a preexisting CNFA, it could push up the CNFA to cause chiasmal compression or headaches. In the second case reported, the patient responded rapidly to bromocriptine treatment, probably due to shrinkage of the lactotroph hyperplasia with decompression of the chiasm and probably with little or no direct effect on the tumor itself *(86)*. Most CNFAs are actually gonadotroph adenomas *(87)*. Two patients have been reported who had gonadotroph adenomas secreting intact FSH with a resultant ovarian hyperstimulation syndrome *(88,89)*; both became pregnant, one after having the FSH hypersecretion controlled by bromocriptine *(88)* and the second following surgical removal of the tumor *(89)*.

7. HYPOPITUITARISM

Hypopituitarism may occur because of tumor compression of the hypothalamus and/or pituitary stalk or from prior neurosurgery. Hormone deficits can be partial or complete and loss of gonadotropin secretion is common. Induction of ovulation may be difficult and a variety of techniques have been used, including administration of hCG and FSH (in the past as human menopausal gonadotropin *(90–93)*, pulsatile GnRH *(94–96)*, and in vitro fertilization *(97)*.

In adult women the only hormone replacements to be considered during pregnancy are thyroid and adrenal hormones. Because of the increased thyroxine turnover that occurs during pregnancy, T_4 levels fall and TSH levels rise with a fixed thyroxine dose over the course of gestation *(16,98)*. The average increase in thyroxine need in these patients is about 0.05 mg/day. Because patients with hypothalamic/pituitary dysfunction may not elevate their TSH levels normally in the face of increased need for thyroxine, it may be appropriate to increase the thyroxine supplementation by 0.025 mg after the first trimester and by additional 0.025 mg after the second trimester. However, there are no actual data to support this approach.

Because the cortisol production rate is normally increased in pregnancy *(11,12)*, theoretically, the dose of chronic glucocorticoid replacement ought to be increased during pregnancy. However, this does not seem to be necessary in practice and patients usually can be kept on their standard replacement doses of glucocorticoids. Additional glucocorticoids are needed for the stress of labor and delivery, such as 75 mg of hydrocortisone IV every 8 h with rapid tapering postpartum. If there is significant stress during the pregnancy, such as infection, that would require prolonged high doses of glucocorticosteroids, the steroid of choice is prednisolone, which does not cross the placenta *(99)*. However, even high doses of prednisone are generally quite safe *(100)* and suppression of neonatal adrenal function in offspring of women taking prednisone during pregnancy is very uncommon *(101)*. Glucocorticoids may also pass to the neonate in breast milk, but the amounts (0.14% of maternal blood levels) are not sufficient to alter neonatal adrenal function, even with large maternal doses of prednisone *(102)*.

7.1. Lymphocytic Hypophysitis

Lymphocytic hypophysitis usually presents in the peripartum period as a mass lesion indistinguishable from a pituitary adenoma. It is characterized by massive infiltration of the pituitary by lymphocytes and plasma cells with destruction of the normal parenchyma. The disorder is thought to have an autoimmune basis. Most cases occur in association with pregnancy and women present during pregnancy or postpartum either with symptoms of varying degrees of hypopituitarism or with symptoms related to the mass lesion, such as headaches or visual field defects. Mild hyperprolactinemia and DI may also be found. On CT or MRI scan a sellar mass is found, which may extend in an extrasellar fashion and may cause visual field defects. The condition is usually confused with that of a pituitary tumor and, in fact, cannot be distinguished from a tumor except by biopsy. By virtue of the hypopituitarism it produces, lymphocytic hypophysitis can also be confused clinically with Sheehan's syndrome except that there is no history of obstetrical hemorrhage *(103,104)*.

The diagnosis of lymphocytic hypophysitis should be entertained in women with symptoms of hypopituitarism and/or mass lesions of the sella during pregnancy or postpartum, especially in the absence of a history of obstetrical hemorrhage. An evaluation of pituitary function is warranted as well as a CT or an MRI scan. If PRL levels are only modestly elevated (<150 ng/ml) in the presence of a large mass, the diagnosis is unlikely to be an enlarging prolactinoma and more likely to be hypophysitis or a nonsecreting tumor. Hormone replacement therapy should be instituted promptly when hypopituitarism is determined to be present. For unclear reasons, there appears to be a particular predilection for impaired ACTH secretion and this axis must be evaluated carefully and treated to avoid adrenal insufficiency *(105)*. Unless there are visual field defects, uncontrollable headaches, or radiologic evidence of progressive enlargement of the sellar mass, rapid surgical intervention is not warranted, as some women may undergo a spontaneous regression of the mass and return of pituitary function (105–107). Surgery generally does not result in improvement in endocrine function, however (108,109). Although high doses of glucocorticoids have been advocated to reduce the inflammation (109), there have been no controlled studies documenting the benefit of this approach and I do not recommend this.

7.2. Sheehan's Syndrome

Sheehan's syndrome consists of pituitary necrosis secondary to ischemia occurring within hours of delivery (110,111). It is usually secondary to hypotension and shock from an obstetric hemorrhage. Pituitary enlargement during pregnancy apparently predisposes to the risk for ischemia with occlusive spasm of the arteries to the anterior pituitary and stalk (110,111). The degree of ischemia and necrosis dictates the subsequent patient course. Fortunately, modern obstetric techniques have resulted in Sheehan's syndrome being found very rarely in current practice (112).

Acute necrosis is suspected in the setting of an obstetric hemorrhage where hypotension and tachycardia persist following adequate replacement of blood products. In addition, the woman fails to lactate and may have hypoglycemia (110,111,113). Investigation should include levels of ACTH, cortisol, PRL, and free T4. The ACTH stimulation test would be normal, as the adrenal cortex would not be atrophied. T4 levels may prove normal initially, as the hormone has a half-life of 7 days. PRL levels are usually low, although they are generally fivefold to tenfold elevated in the puerperium. Treatment with saline and stress doses of corticosteroids should be instituted immediately after drawing the blood tests. Additional pituitary testing with subsequent therapy should be delayed until recovery. DI may also occur secondary to vascular occlusion with atrophy and scarring of the neurohypophysis (114).

When milder forms of infarction occur, the diagnosis of Sheehan's syndrome may be delayed for months or years (113,114). These women generally have a history of amenorrhea, decreased libido, failure to lactate, breast atrophy, loss of pubic and axillary hair, fatigue, and symptoms of secondary adrenal insufficiency with nausea, vomiting, diarrhea, and abdominal pain (113,114). Some women experience only partial hypopituitarism, and may have normal menses and fertility (115). Although the women may have episodes of transient polydipsia and polyuria, many demonstrate impaired urinary concentrating ability and deficient vasopressin secretion (116). CT or MRI scans generally reveal partial or completely empty sellas (117).

7.3. Synopsis

Hyperprolactinemia and Cushing's disease may interfere with fertility and usually need to be controlled to allow conception. Cushing's syndrome, acromegaly, and hyperthyroidism secondary to TSH hypersecretion may increase maternal morbidity (gestational diabetes, hypertension) and fetal morbidity and mortality. Bromocriptine is generally the preferred treatment for a patient with a prolactinoma desiring pregnancy. Intervention to remove an ACTH-secreting tumor during pregnancy is warranted to reduce fetal loss and medical control of hyperthyroidism is indicated. Surgery or medical therapy for GH-secreting and clinically nonfunctioning adenomas is not indicated during pregnancy. Pregnancy may also cause an increase in PRL-secreting tumors, especially macroadenomas, so that close surveillance is indicated and reinstitution of bromocriptine for tumor size increase may be necessary. Increase in size of other types of tumors is very rare. In patients with hypopituitarism, consideration should be given to increase thyroid hormone doses by 25–50% empirically, as TSH levels cannot be used. However, no increase in glucocorticoid dose is usually needed except to cover the stress of labor and delivery. Lymphocytic hypophysitis may present with mass effects and/or hypopituitarism and often can be managed with hormone replacement and expectant management. When Sheehan's syndrome is suspected, appropriate evaluation and hormone replacement are indicated in both the acute and chronic forms.

REFERENCES

1. Central Brain Tumor Registry of the United States (CTBRUS). Statistical Report. Primary brain tumors in the US 1997–2001. http://www.cbtrus.org/. Accessed April 8, 2005.
2. Goluboff LG, Ezrin C. Effect of pregnancy on the somatotroph and the prolactin cell of the human adenohypophysis. J Clin Endocrinol Metab 1969;29:1533–8.
3. Scheithauer BW, Sano T, Kovacs KT, Young WF, Jr, Ryan N, Randall RV. The pituitary gland in pregnancy. A clinicopathologic and immunohistochemical study of 69 Cases. Mayo Clin Proc 1990;65:461–74.
4. Rigg LA, Lein A, Yen SSC. Pattern of increase in circulating prolactin levels during human gestation. Am J Obstet Gynecol 1977;129:454–6.
5. Gonzalez JG, Elizondo G, Saldivar D, Nanez H, Todd LE, Villarreal JZ. Pituitary gland growth during normal pregnancy: an in vivo study using magnetic resonance imaging. Am J Med 1988;85:217–20.
6. Elster AD, Sanders TG, Vines FS, Chen MYM. Size and shape of the pituitary gland during pregnancy and post partum: Measurement with MR imaging. Radiology 1991;181:531–5.
7. Dinç H, Esen F, Demirci A, Sari A, Gümele HR. Pituitary dimensions and volume measurements in pregnancy and *post partum*. MR assessment. Acta Radiologica 1998;39:64–9.
8. Frankenne F, Closset J, Gomez F, Scippo ML, Smal J, Hennen G. The physiology of growth hormones (GHs) in pregnant women and partial characterization of the placental GH variant. J Clin Endocrinol Metab 1988;66:1171–80.

9. Eriksson L, Frankenne F, Eden S, Hennen G, Von Schoultz B. Growth hormone 24-h serum profiles during pregnancy lack of pulsatility for the secretion of the placental variant. Br J Obstet Gynaecol 1989;106:949–53.

10. Beckers A, Stevenaert A, Foidart J-M, Hennen G, Frankenne F. Placental and pituitary growth hormone secretion during pregnancy in acromegalic women. J Clin Endocrinol Metab 1990;71:725–31.

11. Carr BR, Parker CR, Jr, Madden JD, MacDonald PC, Porter JC. Maternal plasma adrenocorticotropin and cortisol relationships throughout human pregnancy. Am J Obstet Gynecol 1981;139:416–22.

12. Nolten WE, Lindheimer MD, Rueckert PA, Oparil S, Ehrlich EN. Diurnal patterns and regulation of cortisol secretion in pregnancy. J Clin Endocrinol Metab 1980;51:466–72.

13. Rees LH, Burke CW, Chard T, Evans SW, Letchworth AT. Possible placental origin of ACTH in normal human pregnancy. Nature 1975;254:620–2.

14. Sasaki A, Shinkawa O, Yoshinaga K. Placental corticotropin-releasing hormone may be a stimulator of maternal pituitary adrenocorticotropic hormone secretion in humans. J Clin Invest 1989;84:1997–2001.

15. Lindsay JR, Nieman LK. The hypothalamic-pituitary-adrenal axis in pregnancy: challenges in disease detection and treatment. Endocr Rev 2005;26:775–99.

16. Glinoer D. The regulation of thyroid function in pregnancy: pathways of endocrine adaptation from physiology to pathology. Endocr Rev 1997;18:404–33.

17. Jeppsson S, Rannevik G, Liedholm P, Thorell JI. Basal and LHRH stimulated secretion of FSH during pregnancy. Am J Obstet Gynecol 1977;127:32–6.

18. Kredentser JV, Hoskins CF, Scott JZ. Hyperprolactinemia: a significant factor in female infertility. Am J Obstet Gynecol 1981;139:264–7.

19. Gillam MP, Molitch MP, Lombardi G, Colao A. Advances in the treatment of prolactinomas. Endocr Rev 2006.

20. Casanueva FF, Molitch ME, Schlechte JA, et al. Guidelines of the Pituitary Society for the diagnosis and management of prolactinomas. Clin Endocrinol 2006;65:265–73.

21. Webster J, Piscitelli G, Polli A, Ferrari CI, Ismail I, Scanlon MF. A comparison of cabergoline and bromocriptine in the treatment of hyperprolactinemic amenorrhea. N Engl J Med 1994;331:904–9.

22. Bevan JS, Webster J, Burke CW, Scanlon MF. Dopamine agonist and pituitary tumor shrinkage. Endocrine Rev 1992;13:220–40.

23. Biller BMK, Molitch ME, Vance ML, et al. Treatment of prolactin-secreting macroadenomas with the once-weekly dopamine agonist cabergoline. J Clin Endocrinol Metab 1996;81:2338–43.

24. Colao A, DiSarno A, Landi ML, et al. Macroprolactinoma shrinkage during cabergoline treatment is greater in naïve patients than in patients pretreated with other dopamine agonists: a prospective study of 110 patients. J Clin Endocrinol Metab 2000;85:2247–52.

25. Molitch ME. Dopamine resistance of prolactinomas. Pituitary 2003;6:19–27.

26. Schade R, Andersohn F, Suissa S, et al. Dopamine agonists and the risk of cardiac-valve regurgitation. N Engl J Med 2007;356:29–38.

27. Gemzell C, Wang CF. Outcome of pregnancy in women with pituitary adenoma. Fertil Steril 1979;31:363–72.

28. Molitch ME. Pregnancy and the hyperprolactinemic woman. N Engl J Med 1985;312:1364–70.

29. Kupersmith MJ, Rosenberg C, Kleinberg D. Visual loss in pregnant women with pituitary adenomas. Ann Intern Med 1994;121:473–7.

30. Rossi AM, Vilska S, Heinonen PK. Outcome of pregnancies in women with treated or untreated hyperprolactinemia. Eur J Obstet Gynecol Reprod Biol 1995;63:143–6.
31. Musolino NRC, Bronstein MD. Prolactinomas and pregnancy. In: Bronstein MD, editor. Pituitary Tumors and Pregnancy. Norwell, MA: Kluwer Academic Publishers; 2001. pp. 91–108.
32. Liu C, Tyrrell JB. Successful treatment of a large macroprolactinoma with cabergoline during pregnancy. Pituitary 2001;4:179–85.
33. Krupp P, Monka C, Richter K. The safety aspects of infertility treatments. In: Program of the Second World Congress of Gynecology and Obstetrics. Brazil: Rio de Janeiro; 1988. pp. 9.
34. Krupp P, Monka C. Bromocriptine in pregnancy: safety aspects. Klin Wochenschr 1987;65:823–7.
35. Raymond JP, Goldstein E, Konopka P, Leleu MF, Merceron RE, Loria Y. Follow-up of children born of bromocriptine-treated mothers. Horm Res 1985;22:239–46.
36. Konopka P, Raymond JP, Merceron RE, Seneze J. Continuous administration of bromocriptine in the prevention of neurological complications in pregnant women with prolactinomas. Am J Obstet Gynecol 1983;146:935–8.
37. Bigazzi M, Ronga R, Lancranjan I, et al. A pregnancy in an acromegalic woman during bromocriptine treatment: effects on growth hormone and prolactin in the maternal, fetal, and amniotic compartments. J Clin Endocrinol Metab 1979;48:9–12.
38. Buelke-Sam J, Byrd RA, Johnson JA, Tizzano JP, Owen NV. Developmental toxicity of the dopamine agonist pergolide mesylate in CD-1 mice. I: Gestational exposure. Neurotoxicol Teratol 1991;13:283–95.
39. De Mari M, Zenzola A, Lamberti P. Antiparkinsonian treatment in pregnancy. Mov Disord 2002;17:428–9.
40. Acharya V. Review of pregnancy reports in patients on pergolide treatment, July, 2004. Data on file. Eli Lilly & Co.
41. Morange I, Barlier A, Pellegrini I, Brue T, Enjalbert A, Jaquet P. Prolactinomas resistant to bromocriptine: long-term efficacy of quinagolide and outcome of pregnancy. Eur J Endocrinol 1996;135:413–20.
42. Webster J. A comparative review of the tolerability profiles of dopamine agonists in the treatment of hyperprolactinaemia and inhibition of lactation. Drug Saf 1996;14: 228–38
43. Robert E, Musatti L, Piscitelli G, Ferrari CI. Pregnancy outcome after treatment with the ergot derivative, cabergoline. Reprod Toxicol 1996;10:333–7.
44. Data on file, Pharmacia & Upjohn, 1997.
45. Verhelst J, Abs R, Maiter D, et al. Cabergoline in the treatment of hyperprolactinemia: a study in 455 patients. J Clin Endocrinol Metab 1999;84:2518–22.
46. Ricci E, Parazzini F, Motta T, et al. Pregnancy outcome after cabergoline treatment in early weeks of gestation. Reprod Toxicol 2002;16:791–3.
47. Brodsky JB, Cohen EN, Brown BW, Jr, et al. Surgery during pregnancy and fetal outcome. Am J Obstet Gynecol 1980;138:1165–7.
48. Divers WA, Yen SSC. Prolactin-producing microadenomas in pregnancy. Obstet Gynecol 1983;62:425–9.
49. Colao A, Merola B, Ferone D, Lombardi G. Acromegaly. J Clin Endocrinol Metab 1997;82:2777–81.
50. Herman-Bonert V, Seliverstow M, Melmed S. Pregnancy in acromegaly: successful therapeutic outcome. J Clin Endocrinol Metab 1998;83:727–31.

51. Mozas J, Ocón E, López de la Torre M, Suárez AM, Miranda JA, Herruzo AJ. Successful pregnancy in a woman with acromegaly treated with somatostatin analog (octreotide) prior to surgical resection. Int J Gynecol Obstet 1999;65:71–3.

52. DeMenis E, Billeci D, Marton E. Uneventful pregnancy in an acromegalic patient treated with slow-release lanreotide: a case report. J Clin Endocrinol Metab 1999;84:1489.

53. Hierl T, Ziegler R, Kasperk C. Pregnancy in persistent acromegaly. Clin Endocrinol 2000;53:262–3.

54. Neal JM. Successful pregnancy in a woman with acromegaly treated with octreotide. Endocr Pract 2000;6:148–50.

55. Fassnacht M, Capeller B, Arlt W, et al. Octreotide LAR treatment throughout pregnancy in an acromegalic woman. Clin Endocrinol 2001;55:411–5.

56. Bronstein MD, Salgado LR, Musolino NR. Medical management of pituitary adenomas: the special case of management of the pregnant woman. Pituitary 2002;5:99–107.

57. Serri O, Lanoie G. Successful pregnancy in a woman with acromegaly treated with octreotide long-acting release. Endocrinologist 2003;13:17–9.

58. Hisano M, Sakata M, Watanabe N, Kitagawa M, Murashima A, Yamaguchi K. An acromegalic woman first diagnosed in pregnancy. Arch Gynecol Obstet 2006;274:171–3.

59. Atmaca A, Dagdelen S, Erbas T. Follow-up of pregnancy in acromegalic women: different presentations and outcomes. Exp Clin Endocrinol Diabetes 2006;114:135–9.

60. Cozzi R, Attanasio R, Barausee M. Pregnancy in acromegaly: a one-center experience. Eur J Endocrinol 2006;155:279–84.

61. Molitch ME. Clinical manifestations of acromegaly. Endocrinol Metab Clin North Am 1992;21:597–614.

62. Barkan AL, Stred SE, Reno K, et al. Increased growth hormone pulse frequency in acromegaly. J Clin Endocrinol Metab 1989;69:1225–33.

63. Chang-DeMoranville BM, Jackson IMD. Diagnosis and endocrine testing in acromegaly. Endocrinol Metab Clin N Am 1992;21:649–68.

64. Okada Y, Morimoto I, Ejima K, et al. A case of active acromegalic woman with a marked increase in serum insulin-like growth factor-1 levels after delivery. Endocr J 1997;44:117–20.

65. Caron P, Gerbeau C, Pradayrol L. Maternal-fetal transfer of octreotide. N Engl J Med 1995;333:601–2.

66. Caron P, Buscail L, Beckers A, et al. Expression of somatostatin receptor SST4 in human placenta and absence of octreotide effect on human placental growth hormone concentration during pregnancy. J Clin Endocrinol Metab 1997;82:3771–6.

67. Bevan JS, Gough MH, Gillmer MD, Burke CW. Cushing's syndrome in pregnancy. The timing of definitive treatment. Clin Endocrinol 1987;27:225–33.

68. Casson IF, Davis JC, Jeffreys RV, et al. Successful management of Cushing's disease during pregnancy by transsphenoidal adenectomy. Clin Endocrinol 1987;27:423–8.

69. Aron DC, Schnall AM, Sheeler LR. Cushing's syndrome and pregnancy. Am J Obstet Gynecol 1990;162:244–52.

70. Buescher MA, McClamrock HD, Adashi EY. Cushing's syndrome in pregnancy. Obstet Gynecol 1992;79:130–7.

71. Ross RJ, Chew SL, Perry L, Erskine K, Medbak S, Afshar F. Diagnosis and selective cure of Cushing's disease during pregnancy by transsphenoidal surgery. Eur J Endocrinol 1995;132:722–6.

72. Chico A, Manzanares JM, Halperin I, Martinez de Osaba MJ, Adelantado J, Webb SM. Cushing's disease and pregnancy. Eur J Obstet Gynecol Reprod Biol 1996;64:143–6.

73. Guilhaume B, Sanson ML, Billaud L, Bertagna X, Laudat MH, Luton MP. Cushing's syndrome and pregnancy: aetiologies and prognosis in twenty-two patients. Eur J Med 1992;1:83–9.

74. Pinette MG, Pan YQ, Oppenheim D, Pinette SG, Blackstone J. Bilateral inferior petrosal sinus corticotropin sampling with corticotropin-releasing hormone stimulation in a pregnant patient with Cushing's syndrome. Am J Obstet Gynecol 1994;171:563–4.

75. Kreines K, DeVaux WD. Neonatal adrenal insufficiency associated with maternal Cushing's syndrome. Pediatrics 1971;47:516–9.

76. Amado JA, Pesquera C, Gonzalez EM, Otero M, Freijanes J, Alvarez A. Successful treatment with ketoconazole of Cushing's syndrome in pregnancy. Postgrad Med J 1990;66:221–3.

77. Berwaerts J, Verhelst J, Mahler C, Abs R. Cushing's syndrome in pregnancy treated by ketoconazole: case report and review of the literature. Gynecol Endocrinol 1999;13: 175–82.

78. Mellor A, Harvey RD, Pobereskin LH, Sneyd JR. Cushing's disease treated by trans-sphenoidal selective adenomectomy in mid-pregnancy. Brit J Anaesth 1998;80:850–2.

79. Madhun ZT, Aron DC. Cushing's disease in pregnancy. In: Bronstein MD, editor. Pituitary Tumors and Pregnancy. Norwell: Kluwer Academic Publishers; 2001. p. 149–72.

80. Wallace C, Toth EL, Lewanczuk RZ, Siminoski K. Pregnancy-induced Cushing's syndrome in multiple pregnancies. J Clin Endocrinol Metab 1996;81:15–21.

81. Hána V, Dokoupilová M, Marek J, Plavka R. Recurrent ACTH-independent Cushing's syndrome in multiple pregnancies and its treatment with metyrapone. Clin Endocrinol 2001;54:277–81.

82. Lindsay JR, Jonklaas J, Oldfield EH, Nieman LK. Cushing's syndrome during pregnancy: personal experience and review of the literature. J Clin Endocrinol Metab 2005;90: 3077–83.

83. Caron P, Gerbeau C, Pradayrol L, Simonetta C, Bayard F. Successful pregnancy in an infertile woman with a thyrotropin-secreting macroadenoma treated with the somatostatin analog (octreotide). J Clin Endocrinol Metab 1996;81:1164–8.

84. Blackhurst G, Strachan MW, Collie D, Gregor A, Staatham PF, Seckl JER. The treatment of a thyrotropin-secreting pituitary macroadenoma with octreotide in twin pregnancy. Clin Endocrinol 2002;56:401–4.

85. Chaiamnuay S, Moster M, Katz MR, Kim YN. Successful management of a pregnant woman with a TSH secreting pituitary adenoma with surgical and medical therapy. Pituitary 2003;6:109–13.

86. Masding MG, Lees PD, Gawne-Cain ML, Sandeman DD. Visual field compression by a non-secreting pituitary tumour during pregnancy. J Roy Soc Med 2003;96:27–8.

87. Molitch ME. Clinically non-functioning adenomas. In: Bronstein MD, editor. Pituitary Tumors and Pregnancy. Norwell, MA: Kluwer Academic Publishers; 2001. pp. 123–9.

88. Murata Y, Ando H, Nagasaka T, et al. Successful pregnancy after bromocriptine therapy in an anovulatory woman complicated with ovarian hyperstimulation caused by follicle-stimulating hormone-producing plurihormonal pituitary microadenoma. J Clin Endocrinol Metab 2003;88:1988–93.

89. Sugita T, Seki K, Nagai Y, S et al. Successful pregnancy and delivery after removal of gonadotrope adenoma secreting follicle-stimulating hormone in a 29-year-old amenorrheic woman. Gynecol Obstet Invest 2005;59:138–43.

90. Golan A, Abramov L, Yedwab G, David MP. Pregnancy in panhypopituitarism. Gynecol Obstet Invest 1990;29:232–4.

91. Verdu LI, Martin-Caballero C, Garcia-Lopez G, Cueto MJ. Ovulation induction and normal pregnancy after panhypopituitarism due to lymphocytic hypophysitis. Obstet Gynecol 1998;91:850–2.

92. Volz J, Heinrich U, Volz-Köster S. Conception and spontaneous delivery after total hypophysectomy. Fertil Steril 2002;77:624–5.

93. Kitajima Y, Endo T, Yamazaki K, Hayashi T, Kudo R. Successful twin pregnancy in panhypopituitarism caused by suprasellar germinoma. Obstet Gynecol 2003;102:1205–7.

94. Gompel A, Mauvais-Jarvis P. Induction of ovulation with pulsatile GnRH in hypothalamic amenorrhea. Hum Reprod 1988;3:473–7.

95. Martin KA, Hall JE, Adams JM, Crowley WF, Jr. Comparison of exogenous gonadotropins and pulsatile gonadotropin-releasing hormone for induction of ovulation in hypogonadotropic amenorrhea. J Clin Endocrinol Metab 1993;77:125–9.

96. Hall JE, Martin KA, Whitney HA, Landy H, Crowley WF, Jr. Potential for fertility with replacement of hypothalamic gonadotropin-releasing hormone in long term female survivors of cranial tumors. J Clin Endocrinol Metab 1994;79:1166–72.

97. Suganuma N, Furuhashi M, Ando T, Assada Y, Mori O, Kurauchi O. Successful pregnancy and delivery after in vitro fertilization and embryo transfer in a patient with primary hypopituitarism. Fertil Steril 2000;73:1057–8.

98. Mandel SJ, Larsen PR, Seely EW, Brent GA. Increased need for thyroxine during pregnancy in women with primary hypothyroidism. N Engl J Med 1990;323:91–6.

99. Beitins IZ, Bayard F, Ances IG, Kowarski A, Migeon CJ. The transplacental passage of prednisone and prednisolone in pregnancy near term. J Pediatr 1972;81:936–45.

100. Turner ES, Greenberger PA, Patterson R. Management of the pregnant asthmatic patient. Ann Intern Med 1980;93:905–18.

101. Kenny FM, Preeyasombat C, Spaulding JS, Migeon CJ. Cortisol production rate: IV. Infants born of steroid-treated mothers and of diabetic mothers. Infants with trisomy syndrome and with anencephaly. Pediatrics 1966;37:960–6.

102. McKenzie SA, Selley JA, Agnew JE. Secretion of prednisolone into breast milk. Arch Dis Child 1975;50:894–6.

103. Thodou E, Asa SL, Kontogeorgos G, Kovacs K, Horvath E, Ezzat S. Lymphocytic hypophysitis: clinicopathological findings. J Clin Endocrinol Metab 1995;80:2302–11.

104. Pressman EK, Zeidman SM, Reddy UM, Epstein JI, Brem H. Differentiating lymphocytic adenohypophysitis from pituitary adenoma in the peripartum patient. J Reprod Med 1995;40:251–9.

105. Gillam M, Molitch ME. Lymphocytic Hypophysitis. In: Bronstein MD, editor. Pituitary Tumors in Pregnancy. Norwell, MA: Kluwer Academic Publishers; 2001. pp. 131–48.

106. Leiba S, Schindel B, Weinstein R, Lidor I, Friedman S, Matz S. Spontaneous postpartum regression of pituitary mass with return of function. JAMA 1986;255:230–2.

107. McGrail KM, Beyerl BD, Black PM, Klibanski A, Zervas NT Lymphocytic adenohypophysitis of pregnancy with complete recovery. Neurosurgery 1987;20:791–3.

108. Leung GK, Lopes MB, Thorner MO, Vance ML, Laws ER, Jr. Primary hypophysitis: a single-center experience in 16 cases. J Neurosurg 2004;101:262–71.

109. Caturegli P, Newschaffer C, Olivi A, Pomper MG, Burger PC, Rose NR. Autoimmune hypophysitis. Endocr Rev 2005;doi:10.1210/er.2004–0011.

110. Sheehan HL, Davis JC. Pituitary necrosis. Br Med Bull 1968;24:59–70.

111. Kelestimur F. Sheehan's syndrome. Pituitary 2003;6:181–8.

112. Feinberg E, Molitch M, Endres L, Peaceman A. The incidence of Sheehan's syndrome after obstetric hemorrhage. Fertil Steril 2005;84:975–9.

113. Ozbey N, Inanc S, Aral F, et al. Clinical and laboratory evaluation of 40 patients with Sheehan's syndrome. Isr J Med Sci 1994;30:826–9.

114. Sheehan HL. The neurohypophysis in post-partum hypopituitarism. J Pathol Bacteriol 1963;85:145–69.

115. Grimes HG, Brooks MH. Pregnancy in Sheehan's syndrome. Report of a case and review. Obstet Gynecol Surv 1980;35:481–8.

116. Iwasaki Y, Oiso Y, Yamauchi K, et al. Neurohypophyseal function in post-partum hypopituitarism: impaired plasma vasopressin response to osmotic stimuli. J Clin Endocrinol Metab 1989;68:560–5.

117. Bakiri F, Bendib S-E, Maoui R, Bendib A, Benmiloud M. The sella turcica in Sheehan's syndrome: computerized tomographic study in 54 patients. J Endocrinol Invest 1991;14:193–6.

21 Management of Pituitary Incidentalomas

Lawrence A. Frohman, MD

CONTENTS

1. INTRODUCTION
2. PREVALENCE AND INCIDENCE
3. SPECIFIC PATHOLOGIC DISEASES
4. NATURAL HISTORY
5. SCREENING FOR ENDOCRINE DYSFUNCTION
6. APPROACH TO EVALUATION AND MANAGEMENT OF INCIDENTALOMAS

Summary

Pituitary incidentalomas are circumscribed regions of decreased opacity observed in pituitary CT or MRI exams performed in the absence of suspected pituitary disease. Most incidentalomas are pituitary adenomas, although they can be virtually any type of sellar mass. Most are <1 cm in diameter and can be considered microincidentalomas. The incidence of incidentalomas in MRI studies is approximately 10%, similar to the overall incidence of microadenomas in autopsy series. Only a very small percentage (<1%) of incidentalomas are hormonally active, with the most common being prolactinomas. The progression of incidentalomas to clinically significant lesions is infrequent but appears to be greater for nonfunctioning tumors than for pituitary cysts. Screening for hormonal hyperfunction should be based on the clinical suspicion of pituitary disease, and prolactin measurement alone appears to be the most cost-effective strategy for microincidentalomas. Macroincidentalomas have greater growth potential and are more frequently associated with hypopituitarism. Management of incidentalomas unassociated with hormonal disturbances and no increase in size can be conservative. In those with hormonal deficiencies, a more-proactive role can be justified because hypopituitarism is often reversible with removal of the tumor.

Key Words: Pituitary, Incidentaloma.

From: *Contemporary Endocrinology: Diagnosis and Management of Pituitary Disorders*
Edited by: B. Swearingen and B. M. K. Biller © Humana Press, Totowa, NJ

1. INTRODUCTION

Pituitary incidentalomas can be considered a disease of medical progress. The entity has come into existence as a consequence of the dramatic improvement in sensitivity of neuroradiographic imaging techniques, initially with computerized tomography (CT) and subsequent with magnetic resonance imaging (MRI). Whereas the term "incidentalomas" was first popularized in the early 1980s in relation to adrenal lesions discovered on CTs performed for other reasons, pituitary incidentalomas began to enter the medical literature about one decade later *(1)*. The term has not been stringently defined, but in general, refers to a lesion, usually defined as a circumscribed region within the pituitary of reduced opacity on CT or MRI performed in the absence of suspicion of pituitary dysfunction or a mass in the sellar region. During the past decade numerous series of incidentalomas have been reported *(1–5)*, though the different characteristics of patients and lesions in each of the series make overall conclusions of their natural history somewhat variable.

This chapter will address several issues concerning pituitary incidentalomas:

1. What are their prevalence and incidence?
2. What types of specific pathological processes are involved?
3. What is the natural history of incidentalomas?
4. What investigations are warranted and what is the relative cost-effectiveness of different possible strategies?
5. How important is early diagnosis?
6. When and what type is intervention indicated and what is its efficacy?

2. PREVALENCE AND INCIDENCE

The vast majority of incidentalomas are pituitary adenomas, though all of the entities on a differential diagnosis list of sellar masses may be represented, including neural tumors, craniopharyngiomas, and inflammatory, infiltrative, and vascular lesions. Most of the lesions are <1 cm in diameter and, thus, classified as microincidentalomas. The proportion of macroincidentalomas varies among series, depending on the population studied, i.e., surveys of normal populations or patients with other non-pituitary-related disorders that prompt neuroimaging.

In routine autopsy series, the prevalence of pituitary adenomas has ranged from 1.5% to 26.7% *(1)*, with a minimum frequency of 6.5% in all but one study. A meta-analysis of 12,300 autopsies determined the frequency to be 11.3% *(6)*. Less than 1% of the tumors were macroadenomas, and they appeared to be distributed in all age groups and without gender predilection. One study reported that half of all observed lesions consisted of pituitary cysts, foci of metastatic tumors, and pituitary infarcts *(7)*. In a composite of series of autopsy studies previously unsuspected macroadenomas were discovered in less than 0.1% *(1)*. Given the frequency of microadenomas (10–20%) in the population, one can extrapolate that very few will progress to macroadenomas during the lifetime of an individual.

Radiographic (MRI) studies in the normal population have indicated that approximately 10% have findings consistent with a pituitary microadenoma *(8,9)*. Other series have reported a much lower incidence *(10)*, which may be attributable to differences in imaging techniques (MRI versus CT, and "brain" rather than "pituitary" imaging, where a decreased number of pituitary images were generated).

The frequency of pituitary tumors in recent brain tumor registries is approximately 6–8% of all brain tumors, with a prevalence of 1.0 per 100,000 population *(11)*. These figures most likely reflect macroadenomas, although no breakdown by size was reported. This estimate does not include some macroadenomas not treated surgically or by radiotherapy and, for the same reason, does not include the majority of microadenomas.

From the above considerations, the incidentally discovered pituitary microadenoma on neuroimaging studies likely reflects the true prevalence of this disease in the population and further suggests that therapeutic considerations must reflect that only a very small percentage of such lesions are likely to progress to macroadenomas. For these reasons, calculations of the incidence rates are very difficult to make, since precise information on the progression from subclinical to clinical disease is lacking.

3. SPECIFIC PATHOLOGIC DISEASES

In addition to pituitary tumors, incidentally discovered sellar mass lesions may represent other pathological processes. A listing of disorder that should be considered is provided in Table 1. However, with the exception of Rathke's pouch cysts (discussed below), nearly all incidentalomas in which a histopathological diagnosis has been made represent pituitary adenomas.

The best available data on the distribution of tumor cell types among microadenomas are derived from autopsy studies, where up to 46% were shown to exhibit immunostaining for prolactin *(12,13)*. However, no clinical antemortem evidence for prolactin secretion was obtained in nearly all patients. Staining for growth hormone (GH) and ACTH was much less common, again without evidence for clinically active tumors during life. These distributions are similar to those reported in numerous clinical studies, though the latter are much less reliable because of the effects of patient selection and the frequent inability to diagnose "silent" or clinically inactive hormone-secreting tumors. If one assumes that the majority of clinically active tumors are diagnosed during life and the autopsy series reflect primarily those clinically inactive tumors,

Table 1
Pathologic Processes Associated with
Pituitary Mass Lesions

Neoplastic

Pituitary adenomas
  Prolactin-secreting
  GH-secreting
  ACTH-secreting
  TSH-secreting
  LH/FSH-secreting
  Nonfunctioning
      α-Glycoprotein-secreting
      Silent corticotrope adenomas
      Other
  Craniopharyngiomas
  Meningiomas
  Metastatic carcinomas
  Lymphomas
  Hamartomas
  Gliomas
  Germ cell tumors
Developmental—cell rests
  Rathke's pouch cysts
  Dermoid cysts
  Arachnoid cysts
Inflammatory—infectious
  Sarcoidosis
  Lymphocytic hypophysitis
  Granulomatous hypophysitis
  Histiocytosis X
  Tuberculosis
  Other bacterial abscesses
Vascular
  Aneurysms
Other
  Pituitary hyperplasia

the composite results suggest that the distribution of hormone-containing but clinically inactive tumors discovered during life as incidentalomas is similar to those first identified at autopsy. The similarity of the prevalence of incidentalomas discovered during neuroimaging studies with that in autopsy series further suggests that only a very small percentage of incidentalomas identified antemortem should be clinically active (hormone-secreting).

The precise determination of the hormonally active percentage is difficult for several reasons. First, by definition, an incidentalomas can only be defined as such if the neuroimaging examination is performed prior to the physician being aware of any signs or symptoms relating to endocrine dysfunction or of a sellar mass. However, if the history is incomplete, a patient may be considered to have an incidentalomas whereas if a history of amenorrhea or acral enlargement has been elicited, the same imaging results are classified differently. As a result, the best estimates of hormonal activity are derived from epidemiologic studies of the frequency of such tumors in the population. The most common hormonally active pituitary tumor is the prolactinoma, which has been estimated to have a prevalence of ~60 per 100,000 (14,15). Excluding the subgroup of macroprolactinomas (perhaps as high as 20–25%, but probably lower) leaves a prevalence estimate of ~45–50 per 100,000 microprolactinomas in the population. If all have demonstrable defects on MRI and all undergo imaging studies prior to suspicion of the diagnosis, one can calculate that the prevalence rate would be ~4–5 per 1,000 patients in whom an incidentaloma is discovered. Similar estimates have been presented in a study of the cost-effectiveness of evaluation of patients with incidentalomas (16). It is currently not possible from history and laboratory studies to identify which patients with incidentalomas represent those destined to develop clinical significant prolactinomas.

The prevalence of GH-secreting adenomas in the population is considerably lower than that of prolactinomas, with estimates of 6–8 per 100,000 and incidence estimates of 0.16–0.48 per 100,000 per year (17,18). The prevalence of somatotropinomas is thus only about one-sixth to one-eighth that of prolactinomas and there would be an expected prevalence of ~0.5–0.8 per 1,000 patients in whom an incidentalomas is discovered. As with prolactinomas, the identification of those patients with incidentalomas destined to develop acromegaly is an enormous challenge.

Estimates of the prevalence of Cushing's disease in the population are less precise, ranging from 0.6 to 3.2 per 100,000 population (19,20), with the highest value representing half that of somatotropinomas. Similar calculations would predict a prevalence of 0.3–0.6 ACTH-secreting tumors per 1,000 incidentalomas. Their identification in the absence of clinical disease manifestations is equally difficult.

The underlying pathology in those microincidentalomas that do not exhibit hormone hypersecretion is for the most part conjectural because most patients are not subjected to surgery and, thus, no tissue diagnosis is available. However, in one study, patients with nonfunctioning microincidentalomas were subjected to stimulation with TRH *(21)*. Eleven of the 16 patients (72%) exhibited an increase in LH and/or FSH levels, a response similar to that observed in nonfunctioning tumors, suggesting that the majority of microincidentalomas are pituitary adenomas of gonadotrope lineage.

4. NATURAL HISTORY

A separate issue relates to the likelihood of an increase in size of the tumor with time. For the purpose of discussion, microadenomas and macroadenomas require separate consideration.

The best available data on microadenomas are derived from reports of microprolactinomas followed without specific therapy *(22–26)*. Overall, the probability of tumor growth of microprolactinomas is 5% or less.

No comparable data exist for somatotropinomas. However, since 80–90% of such tumors are already macroadenomas by the time of diagnosis, the progression from microadenomas must occur more frequently than that for prolactinomas. Similarly, there is an absence of data for the progression rate of ACTH-secreting tumors from microadenomas to macroadenomas. However, most patients with Cushing's disease are found to have microadenomas, suggesting that the progression rate is fairly low, or that the diagnosis is made at an early stage. In contrast to prolactinomas, the morbidity of acromegaly and Cushing's disease is substantial, thus making it unlikely that data on the progression rate of GH-secreting and ACTH-secreting tumors will be forthcoming. Similarly, patients with TSH-secreting and gonadotropin-secreting tumors, both of which present primarily as macroadenomas, are treated once the diagnosis is established, precluding the generation of information on the natural history of the tumors.

More information is available on the natural history of nonfunctional tumors, which represent the large majority of pituitary incidentalomas. However, the data are derived from retrospective studies of patients referred to neurosurgeons or endocrinologists and therefore may not be representative of the population as a whole. The largest series, consisting of 550 patients with incidentalomas referred to a neurosurgical service, excluded an unreported number of patients with hormone hypersecretion (except for prolactin levels of <100 ng/ml) *(27)*. Nearly half of the group (47%) underwent surgery, primarily because of suprasellar extension, tumor size, or patient preference. The mean maximum tumor diameter was 25 mm, suggesting that nearly all were macroadenomas. The vast majority of the lesions (81%) on histologic examination were nonfunctioning adenomas and most of the remainder (16%) were Rathke's pouch cysts. Also included were a few arachnoid cysts and craniopharyngiomas.

More than half (53%) of the patients were followed by observation only and had presumed diagnoses of nonfunctioning tumors (44%) and Rathke's pouch or other cysts (45%). Among this group of patients, with a mean maximal diameter of 13 mm, an increase in size was observed over a 2-year period in 22% among the presumed adenomas and in only 4% among the presumed Rathke's pouch cysts. Decreases in size were also observed in both presumed adenomas and Rathke's pouch cysts. A small number *(11)* of patients in this group subsequently underwent surgery, primarily for enlargement of the mass lesion. Seven had nonfunctioning adenomas and the others had Rathke's pouch cysts.

In series seen primarily by endocrinologists, the distribution of diagnoses was somewhat different. In two early series reported in the 1980s during the period when the CT radiographic anatomy of the pituitary gland in normals was still being defined, incidentalomas were detected as hypodense or hyperdense lesions in otherwise normal subjects and limited follow-up information was provided *(28,29)*. However, in a more recent series of 46 patients referred to a neuroendocrine service, initial MRIs revealed a macroadenoma in 63% *(4)*. Partial hypopituitarism was found in 41%; 15% had prolactinomas and 22% had hyperprolactinemia from other causes, presumably by loss of dopaminergic inhibition. One-third of the patients underwent surgery because of tumor size and visual impairment. All had pituitary adenomas except for one who had a craniopharyngioma. Of those patients who were followed by observation along, only 1 of 11 microincidentalomas and 1 of 7 macroincidentalomas showed an increase in size. Other reports have also emphasized the relatively slow rate of growth of macroincidentalomas *(30,31)*.

Thus, assessment of the natural history of the non-hormone-secreting incidentaloma must take into consideration the size of the lesion when first encountered (i.e., microincidentaloma versus macroincidentaloma) and the specific pathologic process (e.g., pituitary adenoma versus Rathke's pouch cyst). Furthermore, there is discordance in the underlying pathologic process between those incidentalomas discovered during screening procedures in an otherwise healthy normal population and those discovered during evaluation for central nervous system or behavioral disorders with signs or symptoms not generally associated with pituitary hormonal dysfunction or mass lesions.

5. SCREENING FOR ENDOCRINE DYSFUNCTION

5.1. Hypofunction

Pituitary hormone hypofunction is almost always a consequence of anterior pituitary destruction or compression secondary to a mass effect of the lesion and, therefore, associated with macroincidentalomas. One exception, however, is that of diminished gonadotropin secretion secondary to hyperprolactinemia, which is independent of the size of the lesion. Screening for hypofunction is similar to that for all patients in whom the diagnosis of hypopituitarism is suspected. The pituitary–thyroid axis is evaluated by measuring TSH and free thyroxine, the pituitary–adrenal axis by ACTH and early morning or stimulated cortisol, the pituitary–gonadal axis by LH/FSH and estradiol (females) or testosterone (males), and the GH–IGF-1 axis by IGF-1 and, if appropriate, a GH stimulation test such as insulin hypoglycemia or arginine + GHRH. It is important to diagnose unsuspected hypopituitarism in patients with macroincidentalomas because of its implications for decisions regarding therapy, as discussed below.

5.2. Hyperfunction

Screening should generally be based on a suspicion of hormone hypersecretion from the patient's history and physical examination since hypersecretion rarely occurs in the absence of signs or symptoms. However, it must be recognized that mild hypersecretion, such as may occur in "silent" corticotrope adenomas or occasional prolactinomas, may be unaccompanied by clinical manifestations. The occurrence of pituitary hormone hyperfunction is independent of the size of the lesion and is seen with tumors secreting prolactin, GH, ACTH, and/or TSH.

Prolactin hypersecretion is best assessed by measurement of serum prolactin in a nonstressed state. Prolactin levels >200 ng/ml are virtually diagnostic of a prolactinoma while levels between this value and the upper limit of the normal range are nondiagnostic. Some patients with large tumors may have only minimally elevated prolactin levels, usually attributed to stalk compression with consequent loss of the normal hypothalamic inhibitory dopaminergic tone. In such patients, the measurement should be repeated with diluted serum to exclude the "hook effect," an artificial effect of one-step solid-phase immunoassays (32).

GH hypersecretion is excluded by a normal (for age and gender) serum IGF-1 and by GH suppression to <1 ng/ml after oral glucose. However, some notable exceptions have been reported for the latter criteria, particularly in patients with microadenomas (33).

ACTH hypersecretion is best assessed by measurement of 24-hour urine free cortisol or late-night salivary cortisol. Although opinion varies as to which test is preferred, they appear to have comparable sensitivity and specificity (34).

6. APPROACH TO EVALUATION AND MANAGEMENT OF INCIDENTALOMAS

On the basis of the above information, it is clear that a different approach is indicated for microincidentalomas and macroincidentalomas. Recent surveys have indicated that there are also differences in the approach to investigating both small and large lesions between American and British endocrinologists and that both tend to be more proactive than might have been expected *(35)*.

6.1. Microincidentalomas

The small likelihood that a microincidentaloma in an otherwise asymptomatic individual will develop into clinically significant disease warrants a conservative approach *(36)*. The likelihood of false-positive results from screening procedures must also be considered. Since 2.5% of normal individuals can be expected to have an elevated level of whatever hormone is measured, the risk of unnecessarily extending the workup is considerable. If screening for prolactin and the thyroid, adrenal, GH, and gonadal axes are normal, the patient should be observed and a repeat MRI obtained after 1 year. An analysis of the management of microincidentalomas has concluded that measurement of prolactin alone may be the most cost-effective strategy *(16)*. However, most endocrinologists do not follow this recommendation *(35)*. If there is no significant increase in size of the lesion, a much longer interval can occur before repeat studies are indicated.

6.2. Macroincidentalomas

In addition to the studies recommended for microincidentalomas, it is important to exclude hypopituitarism in patients with macro-sized lesions. In the past it had been considered adequate to treat any hormonal deficiencies and manage the patient conservatively. However, studies have suggested that hypopituitarism associated with a macroadenoma may be due to either stalk compression or increased intrasellar pressure and is often reversible upon removal of the tumor *(37,38)*. Consequently, a more proactive role in management can be justified if hormonal deficiencies are discovered. In addition, the likelihood of growth of the lesion is considerably greater than for microincidentalomas and formal visual field testing and more frequent MRI evaluations are indicated. Nevertheless, conservative management may still be indicated for the macroincidentaloma with no associated hypopituitarism, no encroachment on the visual pathways, and no invasion of surrounding structures, since many of these lesions may remain quiescent for long periods of time.

REFERENCES

1. Molitch ME, Russell EJ. The pituitary "incidentaloma." Ann Intern Med 1990;112:925–31.
2. Chidiac RM, Aron DC. Incidentalomas. A disease of modern technology. Endocrinol Metab Clin North Am 1997;26:233–53.
3. Sanno N, Oyama K, Tahara S, Teramoto A, Kato Y. A survey of pituitary incidentaloma in Japan. Eur J Endocrinol 2003;149:123–7.
4. Fainstein Day P, Guitelman M, Artese R, et al. Retrospective multicentric study of pituitary incidentalomas. Pituitary 2005;7:1–4.
5. Feldkamp J, Santen R, Harms E, Aulich A, Modder U, Scherbaum WA. Incidentally discovered pituitary lesions: high frequency of macroadenomas and hormone-secreting adenomas – results of a prospective study. Clin Endocrinol (Oxf) 1999;51:109–13.
6. Terramoto A, Hirakawa K, Sanno N, Osamura Y. Incidental pituitary lesions in 10000 unselected autopsy specimens. Radiology 1994;193:161–4.
7. Chambers EF, Turski PA, LaMasters D, Newton TH. Regions of low density in the contrast-enhanced pituitary gland: normal and pathologic processes. Radiology 1982;144:109–13.
8. Chong BW, Kucharczyk W, Singer W, George S. Pituitary gland MR: a comparative study of healthy volunteers and patients with microadenomas. AJNR Am J Neuroradiol 1994;15:675–79.
9. Hall WA, Luciano MG, Doppman JL, Patronas NJ, Oldfield EH. Pituitary magnetic resonance imaging in normal human volunteers: occult adenomas in the general population. Ann Intern Med 1994;120:817–20.
10. Katzman GL, Dagher AP, Patronas NJ. Incidental findings on brain magnetic resonance imaging from 1000 asymptomatic volunteers. JAMA 1999;282:36–9.
11. CBTRUS (2005). Statistical Report: Primary Brain Tumors in the United States, 1998–2002. Hinsdale, IL, Central Brain Tumor Registry of the United States; 2006.
12. Burrow GN, Wortzman G, Rewcastle NB, Holgate RC, Kovacs K. Microadenomas of the pituitary and abnormal sellar tomograms in an unselected autopsy series. N Engl J Med 1981;304:156–8.
13. Kovacs K, Corenblum B, Sirek AM, Penz G, Ezrin C. Localization of prolactin in chromophobe pituitary adenomas: study of human necropsy material by immunoperoxidase technique. J Clin Pathol 1976;29:250–8.
14. Miyai K, Ichihara K, Kondo K, Mori S. Asymptomatic hyperprolactinaemia and prolactinoma in the general population – mass screening by paired assays of serum prolactin. Clin Endocrinol (Oxf) 1986;25:549–4.
15. Miyake A, Ikegami M, Chen CF, et al. Mass screening for hyperprolactinemia and prolactinoma in men. J Endocrinol Invest 1988;11:383–4.
16. King JT, Jr, Justice AC, Aron DC. Management of incidental pituitary microadenomas: a cost-effectiveness analysis. J Clin Endocrinol Metab 1997;82:3625–32.
17. Alexander L, Appleton D, Hall R, Ross WM, Wilkinson R. Epidemiology of acromegaly in the Newcastle region. Clin Endocrinol (Oxf) 1980;12:71–9.
18. Bengtsson B-A, Eden S, Ernest I, Oden A, Sjoegren B. Epidemiology and long-term survival in acromegaly. A study of 166 cases diagnosed between 1955 and 1984. Acta Med Scand 1988;223:327–35.
19. Annegers JF, Coulam CB, Abboud CF, Laws ER, Jr, Kurland LT. Pituitary adenoma in Olmsted County, Minnesota, 1935–1977. A report of an increasing incidence of diagnosis in women of childbearing age. Mayo Clin Proc 1978;53:641–3.
20. Etxabe J, Vazquez JA. Morbidity and mortality in Cushing's disease: an epidemiological approach. Clin Endocrinol (Oxf) 1994;40:479–84.

21. Greenman Y, Trostanetsky Y, Somjen D, Tordjman K, Kohen F, Stern N. Effect of TRH on beta-gonadotropin subunits in patients with pituitary microincidentalomas. Eur J Endocrinol 1999;141:17–21.

22. March CM, Kletzky OA, Davajan V, et al. Longitudinal evaluation of patients with untreated prolactin-secreting pituitary adenomas. Am J Obstet Gynecol 1981;139:835–44.

23. Weiss MH, Teal J, Gott P, et al. Natural history of microprolactinomas: six-year follow-up. Neurosurgery 1983;12:180–3.

24. Koppelman MC, Jaffe MJ, Rieth KG, Caruso RC, Loriaux DL. Hyperprolactinemia, amenorrhea, and galactorrhea. A retrospective assessment of twenty-five cases. Ann Intern Med 1984;100:115–21.

25. Sisam D, Redmond G, Sheeler L. The natural history of untreated hyperprolactinemias. Fertil Steril 1987;48:67–72.

26. Schlechte J, Dolan K, Sherman B, Chapler F, Luciano A. The natural history of untreated hyperprolactinemia: a prospective analysis. J Clin Endocrinol Metab 1989;68:412–8.

27. Oyama K, Sanno N, Tahara S, Teramoto A. Management of pituitary incidentalomas: according to a survey of pituitary incidentalomas in Japan. Semin Ultrasound CT MR 2005;26:47–50.

28. Wolpert SM, Molitch ME, Goldman JA, Wood JB. Size, shape, and appearance of the normal female pituitary gland. AJR Am J Roentgenol 1984;143:377–81.

29. Peyster RG, Adler LP, Viscarello RR, Hoover ED, Skarzynski J. CT of the normal pituitary gland. Neuroradiology 1986;28:161–5.

30. Reincke M, Allolio B, Saeger W, Menzel J, Winkelmann W. The 'incidentaloma' of the pituitary gland: Is neurosurgery required. JAMA 1990;263:2772–6.

31. Donovan LE, Corenblum B. The natural history of the pituitary incidentaloma. Arch Intern Med 1995;155:181–3.

32. St-Jean E, Blain F, Comtois R. High prolactin levels may be missed by immunoradiometric assay in patients with macroprolactinomas. Clin Endocrinol (Oxf) 1996;44:305–9.

33. Dimaraki EV, Jaffe CA, DeMott-Friberg R, Chandler WF, Barkan AL. Acromegaly with apparently normal GH secretion: implications for diagnosis and follow-up. J Clin Endocrinol Metab 2002;87:3537–42.

34. Findling JW, Raff H. Screening and diagnosis of Cushing's syndrome. Endocrinol Metab Clin North Am 2005;34:385–402.

35. Howlett TA, Como J, Aron DC. Management of pituitary incidentalomas. A survey of British and American endocrinologists. Endocrinol Metab Clin North Am 2000;29:223–30.

36. Aron DC, Howlett TA. Pituitary incidentalomas. Endocrinol Metab Clin North Am 2000;29:205–21.

37. Arafah BM. Reversible hypopituitarism in patients with large nonfunctioning pituitary adenomas. J Clin Endocrinol Metab 1986;62:1173–79.

38. Arafah BM, Prunty D, Ybarra J, Hlavin ML, Selman WR. The dominant role of increased intrasellar pressure in the pathogenesis of hypopituitarism, hyperprolactinemia, and headaches in patients with pituitary adenomas. J Clin Endocrinol Metab 2000;85: 1789–93.

22 Sellar and Pituitary Tumors in Children

Takara Stanley, MD,
Rajani Prabhakaran, MD,
and Madhusmita Misra, MD, MPH

CONTENTS

1. INTRODUCTION
2. CRANIOPHARYNGIOMAS
3. PITUITARY ADENOMAS
4. SELLAR CYSTS
5. PARASELLAR TUMORS
6. INFILTRATIVE PROCESSES
7. CONCLUSION

Summary

Sellar and parasellar tumors are rare in children and adolescents, but can be associated with significant morbidity. In addition to clinical features resulting from mass effect, and hormonal insufficiencies and excess depending on the nature of the tumor, children with these tumors often present with a slowing of growth velocity and pubertal delay, features unique to children and adolescents. Craniopharyngiomas are the most common sellar/pituitary tumors in children, accounting for 80–90% of these tumors, followed by pituitary adenomas. As in adults, prolactinomas are the most common pituitary adenomas seen in children and adolescents, followed by ACTH secreting adenomas. Suprasellar germinomas in children present classically with diabetes insipidus with or without other pituitary hormone deficiencies and visual field deficits. Treatment for pituitary tumors is typically surgery, with the exception of prolactinomas, treated effectively in most instances with dopamine agonist therapy. Germinomas are very sensitive to chemotherapy and radiotherapy, but use of radiotherapy in children is otherwise limited to tumor recurrence after surgery or tumor occurrence in surgically inaccessible areas.

Key Words: Pediatric pituitary adenomas, Craniopharyngiomas.

From: *Contemporary Endocrinology: Diagnosis and Management of Pituitary Disorders*
Edited by: B. Swearingen and B. M. K. Biller © Humana Press, Totowa, NJ

1. INTRODUCTION

Sellar and parasellar tumors comprise only a small fraction of brain tumors in children. However, when they do occur, they can be associated with significant morbidity including (i) features of raised intracranial pressure or mass effect and (ii) pituitary insufficiency or conditions of hormone excess. In children, craniopharyngiomas and pituitary adenomas make up the vast majority of sellar and parasellar tumors. Overall, these tumors are more likely to occur in adults than in children; however, as many as 26% of craniopharyngiomas and 5% of pituitary tumors present between 0 and 19 years of age *(1)*. Two factors impact significantly on the presentation of these tumors in children as compared with adults: (i) children are actively growing until epiphyseal fusion occurs in late puberty and (ii) pubertal onset and progression are an integral component of childhood after 8–9 years of age. Masses that affect somatotrope or gonadotrope function can thus manifest with a decrease in growth velocity and with pubertal delay or arrest, clinical features that are unique to children. Alterations in growth rate and in the onset and rate of pubertal progression should therefore strongly raise suspicion of pituitary dysfunction and pituitary tumors.

Other masses that may interfere with pituitary function include gliomas, meningiomas (rare in children), sellar and parasellar cysts, germ cell tumors that arise from the infundibulum or posterior pituitary, and infiltrative conditions including Langerhans histiocytosis, tuberculosis, and sarcoidosis. In this chapter, we will review the epidemiology, presentation, diagnosis, and management of common sellar and parasellar masses in children.

2. CRANIOPHARYNGIOMAS

In the pediatric age group, craniopharyngiomas make up 6–10% of all intracranial tumors and 80–90% of tumors in the sellar region *(2,3)*. These are the most common tumors causing hypopituitarism in children, and are 10–20 times more common than pituitary adenomas.

Craniopharyngiomas are slow-growing epithelial neoplasms that arise from embryological remnants of Rathke's pouch. Although histologically benign, they can be invasive and can cause significant morbidity because of their location near the pituitary, optic chiasm, and hypothalamus. These tumors are lined by stratified squamous epithelium and are of two histological types: adamantinomatous and papillary. The former occurs almost exclusively in children, whereas the latter typically occurs in adults. Papillary tumors are entirely solid and usually well circumscribed, and therefore may be difficult to differentiate from pituitary adenomas on imaging. In contrast, adamantinomatous tumors have a characteristic appearance with both cystic and solid components. The cystic components may be multiple and can enlarge, compressing adjacent structures. About 95% of adamantinomatous tumors are calcified (4,5), a feature that contributes to diagnosis on plain film or CT. In one series of 189 pediatric craniopharyngiomas, 99% of the tumors had cystic components and 93% were calcified (5). Karavitaki et al. (6) similarly reported that in 42 children up to 90% of craniopharyngiomas were predominantly cystic or mixed. Craniopharyngiomas can arise anywhere along the path of Rathke's pouch, from the pharynx to the sella and further to the third ventricle. Only 5% of craniopharyngiomas are purely intrasellar, whereas 75% are intrasellar and extrasellar, and 20% are suprasellar (4).

2.1. Epidemiology

Craniopharyngiomas have an incidence of 1.3/1,000,000 person-years, meaning that 338 cases are expected to occur annually in the United States, with 96 occurring in children from 0 to 14 years of age (7). There is a bimodal age distribution for diagnosis, with the first peak occurring between 5 and 14 years and the second peak in the sixth decade of life (7). From one-half to one-third of all craniopharyngiomas occur in children (7). In the pediatric age group, they can occur at any time from infancy to adolescence, but the lowest rates of occurrence are from late adolescence to early adulthood (7).

Craniopharyngiomas are sporadic with no clear familial inheritance. They occur equally in males and females, and no clear racial or ethnic differences in incidence have been observed.

2.2. Presentation

Although craniopharyngiomas often cause endocrine abnormalities, the more common presenting complaint is of the mass effect of the tumor. In several series, headache, vomiting, and visual changes are the most common symptoms, representing between 60% and 86% of initial patient complaints (6,8–11). Symptoms of raised intracranial pressure, in particular, are more common in children than in adults (6). Primary endocrine complaints occur in about 20–30% of patients (6,10–13). Among the more common endocrine complaints are diabetes insipidus (DI, present in 10–25%) (8,9,11,14) and short stature (in about 9%) (8). Other endocrine signs and symptoms include decreased energy, delayed puberty or amenorrhea, precocious puberty, poor weight gain, or rapid weight gain.

Although endocrine abnormalities are not usually the presenting complaint, they are present in ~80% of craniopharyngioma patients at diagnosis (15).

Growth hormone (GH) deficiency is the most common abnormality, occurring in 65–75% of patients at diagnosis *(15–17)*. Growth retardation, which is a symptomatic complaint in <10% of patients, is present in between 25% and 50% of patients *(8,9,14,17)*. In a series from DeVile et al., mean height of 75 patients was one standard deviation below the mean at presentation *(17)*. Müller et al. *(18)* have followed growth from infancy and found that decreases in length standard deviation scores (SDSs) can be observed as early as 10–12 months in patients without hypothalamic involvement and between 3 and 4 years of age in patients with hypothalamic involvement. Although BMI SDS is higher in children with hypothalamic involvement than in those without, some growth retardation appears to occur universally *(18)*.

Abnormality in gonadotropin secretion is the second most common endocrine abnormality, present in about 40% of patients at diagnosis *(15,17)*. Patients may present with either premature or delayed puberty, and some patients present with amenorrhea. Secondary adrenal insufficiency and hypothyroidism are present in 15–30% of patients *(8,15,17,19)*. Hyperprolactinemia due to compression of the pituitary stalk occurs in only 20–30% of cases (despite the often large size of the lesion at diagnosis), and DI in 10–30% *(17,19)*. Management of these abnormalities preoperatively and perioperatively is critical to prevent morbidity and mortality.

2.3. Diagnosis

Imaging with CT or MR confirms the diagnosis of craniopharyngioma in the vast majority of pediatric patients. Since almost all craniopharyngiomas in children are of the adamantinomatous type with calcifications, a calcified, cystic sellar or parasellar mass on CT or MR is suggestive of the diagnosis. MRI can pick up tumors as small as 4 mm, and gadolinium contrast helps distinguish tumor tissue from surrounding edema. Although rarely done and not generally indicated, calcification on plain skull films will sometimes suggest the diagnosis. In one series, only 8.7% of plain films were normal, with 52% showing calcifications, 48% showing erosion and enlargement of the sella, and 28% showing widened sutures *(8)*. In one series of 34 children with craniopharyngioma, invasion of the third ventricular wall or floor and hydrocephalus was reported in 29% and 44% of the children, respectively *(6)*. In this study, hydrocephalus was more commonly observed in children than in adults. Papillary tumors, which are rare in pediatric patients, are more difficult to diagnose on imaging and may be confused with pituitary adenomas. In this case, biopsy is required for definitive diagnosis. Figures 1 and 2 show imaging studies of craniopharyngiomas in two children.

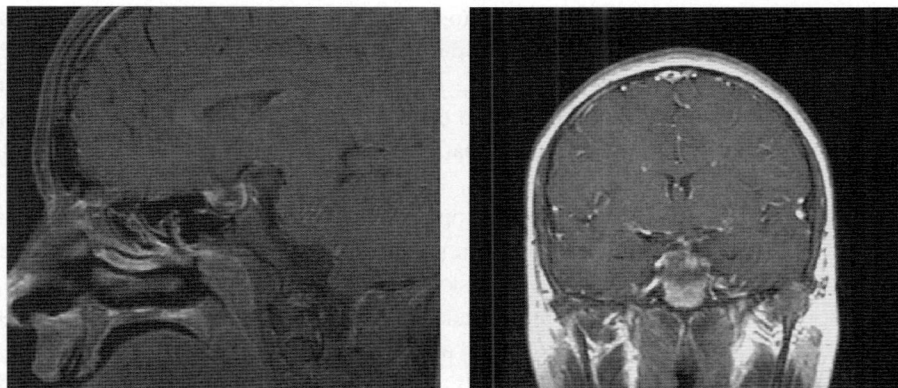

Fig. 1. Craniopharyngioma in a 16-year-old boy. A 1-cm enhancing, cystic lesion was present superior to the planum sphenoidale and tuberculum sella in these T1-weighted post-gadolinium contrast films (sagittal and coronal views). CT was indicative of a craniopharyngioma.

2.4. Treatment and Outcome

All but the smallest craniopharyngiomas require surgical resection, and the approach (transsphenoidal versus transcranial) depends on the site and size of the tumor, as well as proximity to the optic chiasm and hypothalamus. Total resection is possible in small intrasellar and well-circumscribed tumors. Although gross total resection is ideal in all cases, it cannot always be achieved because of tumor invasion or adherence to surrounding structures, particularly the optic chiasm, hypothalamus, and vital neurovascular

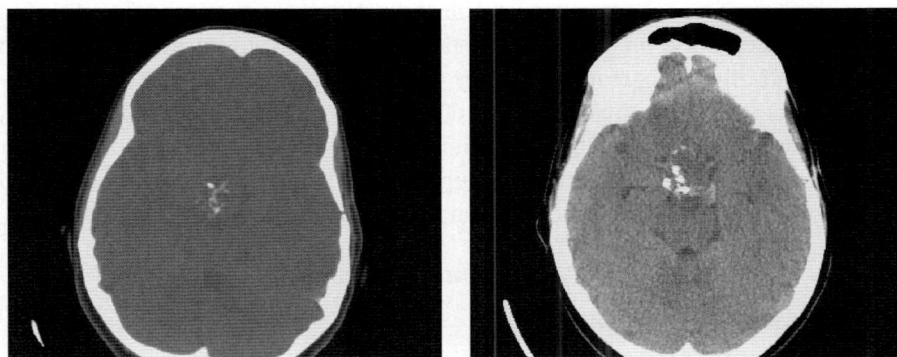

Fig. 2. CT scan of a craniopharyngioma. Chunky peripheral calcifications in a 14-year-old girl are shown.

structures. In these instances, because no clear plane of cleavage exists, subtotal resection is performed, and adjuvant radiation therapy (RT) is usually effective in achieving local control *(11,20,21)*. The recommended dose is 50 Gy in 30–33 daily fractions. Radiation is also effective in cases of tumor recurrence, with no overall survival difference in patients receiving early versus rescue RT *(11,20)*.

As RT has become increasingly sophisticated, controversy has emerged regarding the extent to which surgical resection should be pursued for invasive tumors. Gross total resection avoids risks of radiation to the developing brain, visual apparatus, pituitary, and hypothalamus and the potential risk of second tumors induced by radiation, and may also achieve lower rates of recurrence *(22–24)*. However, it is associated with an increased risk of DI *(11,25,26)* and neurological, cognitive, and ophthalmologic complications *(26)*. The debate continues regarding the benefits and risks associated with complete resection versus less aggressive surgery combined with RT as an effective means to prevent recurrences. The availability of proton beam radiation in some centers is an exciting advance in the field of RT in children, given its ability to target tumor tissue without affecting surrounding healthy tissue. Other treatment modalities that may be used alone or as adjuvant therapy include other forms of radiosurgery, fractionated stereotactic RT, intracavitary radiation, 3D conformal radiation treatment, and, for recurrent, predominantly cystic tumors, the use of intracystic chemotherapy with bleomycin *(27–29)* and interferon-α *(30)* (reviewed in *(31)*), or RT with P^{32} *(32–34)*. With current therapies, overall survival rates are approximately 85–90% at 10 years *(11,20,22,25)*.

Treatment-associated morbidity depends on various factors including size and invasiveness of the tumor, experience of the surgeon, route of surgical approach, and age of the patient. The risk is greatest with large invasive tumors and aggressive attempts at transcranial removal in the hands of a less experienced surgeon. Conversely, the chances of long-term survival with minimal morbidity are greatest in cases of near total excision of the tumor by an experienced surgeon sparing the hypothalamus, carotids, and optic chiasm, followed by fractionated RT. In children over 4 years of age, the best tumor control and least long-term morbidity appear to be achieved with individualized multistaged therapy including conservative surgery followed by local RT.

2.5. Posttreatment Outcome

2.5.1. ENDOCRINE OUTCOME

The majority of patients have endocrine abnormalities after treatment of craniopharyngiomas. Case series show that 75–90% of patients have panhypopituitarism after surgical resection, with the remainder of patients presenting with partial deficits *(10,11,17,35)*. GH deficiency is pervasive; in one series, it was present in all patients following treatment *(8)*. Gonadotropin deficiency is present in 80–100% of patients, and hypothyroidism in 74–94% *(8,9)*. ACTH deficiency occurs in 50–90% *(6,13,17)*, and DI is present in 50–93% of patients postoperatively *(6,9,11,13,17)*. Careful postoperative management of fluid and electrolyte balance is essential, and DI has been described as a cause of postoperative mortality in multiple cases.

Close follow-up is therefore mandated with attention to growth and endocrine function. Replacement therapy needs to be implemented as necessary. Because endocrine deficiencies may evolve over time, ongoing endocrine evaluation is essential for hormones not deficient at initial evaluation after therapy. GH replacement may be initiated after a year from initial treatment in children who develop GH deficiency and slowing of growth, and has not been associated with an increased risk of recurrence *(36)*.

2.5.2. HYPOTHALAMIC MORBIDITY

Despite ubiquitous GH deficiency, children often resume or catch-up growth following resection of craniopharyngioma. This phenomenon of "growth without growth hormone" may have multiple etiologies. In many cases, it is associated with hypothalamic obesity, suggesting that excess insulin acting at IGF-1 receptors may be responsible *(37)*. In one series, only 25% of obese children required GH for growth, whereas 90% of nonobese patients required GH *(9)*. A few cases of "growth without growth hormone" may also be due to hyperprolactinemia, which maintains normal IGF-1 levels despite GH deficiency *(15)*. GH therapy is effective in improving final height in patients with craniopharyngioma *(36,38)*, and it is not an independent risk factor for tumor recurrence *(6)*.

Other features associated with hypothalamic morbidity include hyperphagia, impaired thirst, and changes in behavior and sleep patterns. Müller et al. *(39)* reported a 35% prevalence of increased daytime sleepiness postoperatively in children with craniopharyngioma. Harz et al. *(40)* have suggested that reduced activity levels further contribute to obesity in patients with craniopharyngioma. Hypothalamic obesity is another major morbidity found in ~50% of patients *(9–11)*.

DeVile et al. *(17)* characterized the degree of hypothalamic morbidity in their patients as follows:

  (i) None (45% of patients in the postoperative period and 44% long-term)
 (ii) Mild: postoperative obesity only (19% postoperative and 26% long-term)
(iii) Moderate: hyperphagia, weight gain with/without changes in behavior, memory, and affect (21% postoperative and 13% long-term)

(iv) Severe: extreme weight gain, hyperphagia, rage, impaired thirst, thermoregulation, memory, and sleep-wake patterns (15% postoperative and 16% long-term)

Predictors of increased hypothalamic morbidity included radical resection from the hypothalamus, tumors expanding into the hypothalamus and tumors measuring ≥3.5 cm in the midline.

2.5.3. Cognitive Dysfunction and Learning Disabilities

Significant cognitive deficits have been reported in up to 12% of children after treatment of craniopharyngiomas. DeVile et al. *(17)* reported mild, moderate, or severe learning difficulties (with or without behavioral problems) in 33%, 12%, and 15% of children postoperatively, and 23%, 13%, and 26% of the children long-term. Karavitaki et al. *(6)* similarly reported school performance less than expected for age in 16% of children at 5 years and in 28% 10 years after surgery. Behavioral difficulties include internalizing, attention, somatic, and social difficulties *(41)*. Large tumors, hypothalamic and optic chiasm involvement, retrochiasmatic tumor location, heroic efforts at resection, recurrence, repeat surgery, and young age were important predictors of these difficulties.

2.5.4. Visual and Other Sequelae

Some visual deficit occurs in 35–70% of children postoperatively and long-term, and severe visual compromise may occur in up to 15% of these children *(17,42)*. Other sequelae include neurological symptoms such as hemiparesis or monoparesis, seizure disorders, and depression and other mood disorders, which occur in 10–15% of children postoperatively *(6)*. Complete dependency for daily activities is less common but may occur in 7–10%.

2.5.5. Recurrence

Predictors of recurrence are large size of the tumor, preoperative involvement of the optic chiasm and subtotal resection without subsequent RT, and young age (with sparing use of RT). Even after apparent complete resection, recurrence rates at 10 years are as high as 10–25%. One study reported an overall recurrence-free survival rate of only 55% after radical excision of craniopharyngiomas in 36 children without RT *(43)*. Recurrence is higher with incomplete resection, and in the range of 65–100% *(35)*. Overall, with conservative surgery and RT, recurrence risk is 10–30%. One study reported a higher rate of recurrence with adamantinomatous than with squamous papillary tumors *(35)*.

2.5.6. MORTALITY

In the series by DeVile et al. *(17)*, 9 of 75 children died of tumor-related issues: 6 had hypothalamic symptoms including impaired thirst and DI, 2 may have had an adrenal crisis, 1 had evidence of extrapontine myelinolysis at autopsy. Early and late mortality rates range from 4% to 5% and 6% to 11%, respectively *(42,44)*. One study reported 95% survival at 5, 10, and 15 years, and 80% at 30 years after treatment *(6)*.

3. PITUITARY ADENOMAS

Pituitary adenomas are rare in the pediatric age group, with patients <20 years old accounting for only 2–6% of total cases of adenomas *(45–47)*. Between ages 0 and 19, pituitary adenomas have an incidence rate of 0.12/100,000 person-years, peaking in the pediatric age group between 15 and 19 years of age at 0.39/100,000 person-years *(48)*. These tumors make up only 0.8% of all brain tumors in children aged 0–14, but they constitute 10.1% of brain tumors in the 15–19 year age group *(48)*. As in the adult population, prolactinomas are the most common type of pituitary adenoma. The next most common pituitary adenomas in children are ACTH-secreting pituitary adenomas and somatotropinomas. Prolactinomas typically present in the teenage years, whereas ACTH-secreting pituitary adenomas predominate in children <12 years of age, although the latter can occur at all ages *(46,49)*. Endocrine inactive adenomas, which account for one-fourth to one-third of

Table 1

Occurrence of pediatric pituitary adenomas by age group

Clinical phenotype	No. (%) patients			
	Age 0–11	*Age 12–17*	*Age 18–19*	*Total*
Prolactinoma	5 (16.1)	61 (59.8)	12 (70.6)	78 (52.0)
ACTH-releasing (Cushing's disease)	17 (54.8)	30 (29.4)	3 (17.6)	50 (33.3)
GH-releasing	2 (6.4)	8 (7.8)	2 (11.8)	12 (8.0)
ACTH-releasing (Nelson's syndrome)	5 (16.1)	1 (1.0)	0	6 (4.0)
Endocrine inactive	2 (6.4)	2 (2.0)	0	4 (2.7)
Total[a]	31 (20.7)	102 (68.0)	17 (11.3)	150 (100)

[a] Numbers represent of total of each age group. Percentages are of all 150 patients. Reproduced with permission from Kunwar and Wilson. J Clin Endocrinol Metab 1999;84: 4385–9. Copyright Endocrine Society 1999*(49)*.

adenomas in adults, constitute only 0–5.6% of pediatric adenomas in children in large case series (46,47,49,50). The distribution of pediatric adenomas by age group is represented in Table 1 from Kunwar and Wilson (49). There has been some debate regarding whether pediatric pituitary adenomas are more aggressive than adenomas in adults, but large case series have not supported that assertion (47,50).

Pituitary adenomas have a characteristic presentation in the pediatric population. Adenomas cause not only symptoms from hormone hypersecretion, but also symptoms of hyposecretion caused by compression of the neighboring pituitary cells. Hypersecretory adenomas can present with galactorrhea, menstrual abnormalities, delayed or precocious puberty, Cushingoid features, or gigantism, depending on the hormone secreted. Of the cells in the anterior pituitary, somatotrophs are most sensitive to compression, followed by gonadotrophs then thyrotrophs. Consequently, as with craniopharyngioma, GH is usually the first hormone to be deficient in patients with a macroadenoma. Growth failure, which may be caused either by GH deficiency or by an ACTH-producing adenoma, is a common presentation of a pediatric pituitary adenoma. Irregular menses and amenorrhea are also common presentations, occurring either because of gonadotropin suppression from high prolactin levels or because of compression of gonadotrophs causing decreased levels of FSH, LH, or TSH. Visual symptoms resulting from mass effect may occur, but are less likely in children than in adults because inactive macroadenomas are less prevalent in this younger population. However, particularly in boys, headaches are a common manifestation and visual field defects may occur (51). This appears to be a consequence of greater tumor size at diagnosis.

Two case series describe the frequency of presenting symptoms in pediatric patients with pituitary adenoma (50,51). Headaches are present in 30–52% of children with microadenomas and 52–67% of children with macroadenomas (50,51). Visual field defects are somewhat less common, occurring in only 4% of patients with microadenomas and in 27–44% of patients with macroadenomas (50,51). Short stature is present in 16–27% of patients, and Kane et al. report tall stature in 14% of patients (50,51). Cannavo et al. found menstrual irregularities in 58% and 69% of girls with microadenomas and macroadenomas, while Kane et al. report menstrual dysfunction in 91% of girls and galactorrhea in 41% (50,51). Short stature and pubertal delay were present in 27% and 9% of all children with microadenomas and macroadenomas, respectively (51).

The presence of a pituitary adenoma should bring to mind certain syndromes associated with these tumors. These include the McCune–Albright syndrome, MEN-1, and Carney complex. McCune–Albright syndrome is caused by activating mutations in GNAS1, leading to constitutive activation of Gsα and receptors that are G-protein coupled. Because the GHRH, ACTH, TSH, and

LH/FSH receptors are G-protein coupled, children may present with GH excess (associated with a somatotropinoma), hypercortisolism, hyperthyroidism, and precocious puberty. Precocious puberty with café-au-lait spots and polyostotic fibrous dysplasia is the class triad associated with this syndrome. Mutations in *MENIN* cause MEN-1 associated with parathyroid, pituitary, and pancreatic tumors, and a pituitary tumor may rarely be the first manifestation of this syndrome in a child. The Carney complex is a familial multiple neoplasia syndrome with lentigenes caused by mutations in *PRKAR1A* that is inherited in an autosomal dominant fashion, and associated with primary pigmented nodular adrenocortical disease, GH-secreting adenomas, and atrial and skin myxomas.

MRI of the pituitary before and after gadolinium contrast is the most useful tool in diagnosing the presence of a pituitary adenoma, and T1-weighted sequences of the sagittal and coronal sections (at intervals of 3 mm) are particularly helpful. Adenomas characteristically appear hypointense after gadolinium injection compared with normal gland because of a slower uptake of the contrast agent in adenomatous tissue compared with the normal pituitary. Other features suggestive of an adenoma are deviation of the pituitary stalk away from the side of the lesion and an asymmetric increase in the vertical size of the gland *(19)*. Because a convex upper surface of the pituitary is often seen in the pubertal pituitary gland, it is important to carefully differentiate between apparent pituitary enlargement that may occur at puberty and a true adenoma. A normal pituitary takes up contrast uniformly following gadolinium injection unlike adenomas, although earlier enhancement in the midline of the gland may sometimes be noted in a normal pituitary.

Treatment of pediatric pituitary adenomas is similar to treatment in adults. When surgical resection is indicated, the transsphenoidal approach is safe and effective in the pediatric age group *(45,47,49,52)*. In younger patients, the sphenoid sinus may be incompletely pneumatized, but drilling through the sinus to reach the sella is possible without significant complications *(45,47)*. For large tumors, a transcranial approach may be necessary. Adjuvant therapies such as radiation and pharmacotherapy are also used, but, as in adults, radiation carries a significant risk of hypopituitarism and is reserved for recalcitrant tumors. Treatment specific to each type of adenoma is detailed below.

3.1. Prolactinomas

3.1.1. EPIDEMIOLOGY

Prolactinomas account for 50–75% of the pituitary adenomas seen in pediatric patients, with the great majority of cases presenting in the adolescent years *(46,47,49,50,52,53)*. In one series, 73 of 119 children 12–19 years old with pituitary adenomas had prolactinomas *(49)*. Although prepubertal cases have been reported, only 6.4% of 78 pediatric patients with prolactinomas in

this series were <11 years old *(49)*. Because lactotrophs share lineage with the
somatotrophs and thyrotrophs, prolactin-secreting adenomas may also secrete
GH and to a much lesser extent TSH. In Partington's series, 36% of prolactin-
secreting tumors were plurihormonal *(47)*. As in the adult population, prolactinomas are two to four times more common in females than in males *(47,49)*.
Also consistent with findings in adults, boys tend to have larger tumors and
higher prolactin levels at presentation than do girls *(46,54)*. Colao et al. *(55)*
reported macroadenomas in 8 of 9 boys 7–15 years old with prolactinomas,
whereas only 6 of 17 teenage girls with prolactinomas had macroadenomas.
Cannavo et al. *(51)* similarly reported macroadenomas in all 7 boys presenting
with a prolactinoma in their series, whereas macroadenomas accounted for
only 11 of 23 prolactinomas in girls. Traditionally, this difference has been
attributed to the ease of diagnosing postmenarchal girls relatively early based
on menstrual irregularities, whereas males have less specific symptoms causing
a delay in diagnosis. A study by Delgrange et al. *(54)*, however, showed that
tumors were larger in males independent of age or duration of symptoms, and
that adenomas in males were more likely to be bromocriptine resistant and
invasive, suggesting a more aggressive nature of these tumors in boys.

3.1.2. PRESENTATION

Hypogonadism, caused by the inhibitory effect of high prolactin levels
on GnRH and gonadotropin secretion, is the most common presentation
of prolactinomas in pubertal children *(45,46,52,55,56–58)*. About 90–100%
of female patients present with amenorrhea or oligomenorrhea, and males
typically present with delayed puberty or pubertal arrest *(55–58)*. Arrested
growth is a frequent finding, caused by compression of somatotrophs by the
prolactinoma. About 70–100% of patients are reported to be GH deficient
(57,58). Deficits in ACTH and TSH are less common but occur in a minority of
patients *(57)*. Galactorrhea may be present in either sex, and males may present
with gynecomastia *(49)*. Headache and visual deficits are described in up to
half of patients at presentation and particularly in patients with macroadenomas
(45,55–58). These symptoms are much more common in boys, who tend to
present with larger tumors. Prepubertal patients with prolactinomas are also
more likely to present with macroadenomas, with features of raised intracranial
pressure including headaches and visual deficits, and with decreased growth
velocity. Pubertal children with prolactinomas who are hypogonadal are likely
to have lower bone densities than other children their age, and bone density
improves with treatment and achievement of eugonadism *(59)*.

3.1.3. DIAGNOSIS

The diagnostic approach to prolactinomas does not differ significantly
between adult and pediatric populations. Menstrual irregularities, galactorrhea,

pubertal arrest, or growth delay may prompt measurement of serum prolactin levels. The differential diagnosis of elevated prolactin is discussed in Chapter 6. If a mass is suspected, pituitary MRI is the imaging modality of choice.

Prolactin levels can increase significantly with stress, and some have observed mildly elevated prolactin in children from the stress of venipuncture alone. In such instances, insertion of an indwelling catheter and prolactin measurements at 0 and 60 min can be helpful. High prolactin levels at baseline that normalize 60 min later indicate stress-induced hyperprolactinemia. In addition, nipple stimulation, food intake, and altered sleep patterns can affect prolactin secretion.

Many medications in common use cause elevations in prolactin levels through their dopamine antagonistic effects. These medications include neuroleptics, tricyclic antidepressants, selective serotonin reuptake inhibitors (SSRIs), metoclopramide, opiates, verapamil, and oral contraceptive pills (estrogen component). Neuroleptics, SSRIs, and antidepressants particularly are now being used with increasing frequency in certain pediatric populations. Conventional (typical) neuroleptics cause a threefold to fourfold increase in prolactin levels from a dose-dependent occupancy of D2 receptors (reviewed in (60)). The atypical neuroleptics, conversely, are less likely to cause sustained elevations in prolactin levels, except for risperidone, sulpiride, and amisulpiride (reviewed in (60)). Risperidone is a particularly common offender, and prolactin levels >100 mcg/l have been reported with this medication. Minor elevations in prolactin levels may occur with tricyclic antidepressants. Although long-term elevations of prolactin levels are not common with the SSRIs, short-term elevations can occur (60). In children taking such medications who develop hyperproactinemia, levels should be repeated in 3 months. Temporary elevations of prolactin levels would be expected to resolve in this period. Koves et al. (61) suggest that patients with persistent prolactin elevations in excess of 50 mcg/l in boys and 70 mcg/l in girls should be considered for MRI studies of the pituitary gland regardless of use of medications known to increase prolactin levels.

Compression of the pituitary stalk by a mass prevents the tonic suppression of prolactin by dopamine, and therefore, an elevated prolactin level may be present not only in prolactinomas, but also in craniopharyngiomas and other sellar or suprasellar masses. Prolactinoma size is generally correlated with serum prolactin elevation, so a large mass yielding only a mild elevation in prolactin is probably a tumor causing stalk compression or a plurihormonal adenoma. However, it is important to rule out the "hook" effect in such a situation and to run prolactin levels in dilution to determine whether the lower-than-expected values of prolactin are real or an artifact of the assay. A prolactin value up to 150 mcg/l may be due to stalk compression, whereas a

T1 pre-contrast

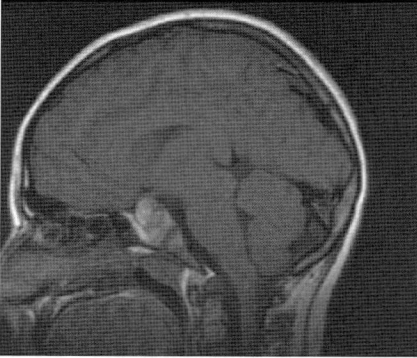

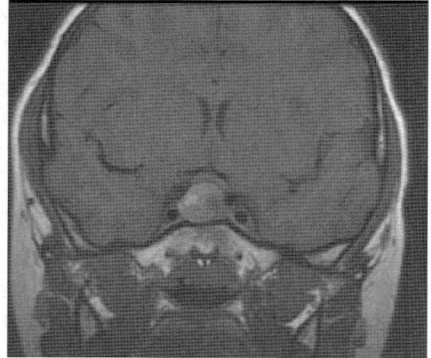

T1 post-contrast

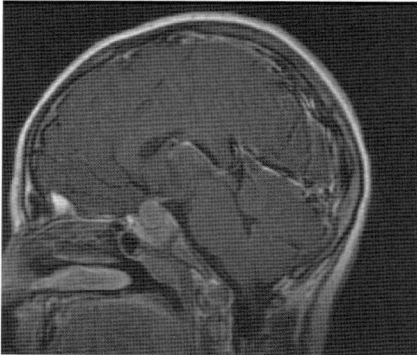

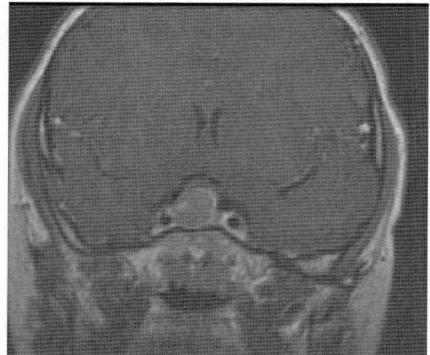

Fig. 3. Cystic macroprolactinoma in a 7-year-old boy. A sellar mass measuring 1.5 × 1.6 × 1.2 cm, with mass effect on the optic chiasm and the proximal optic nerves was present. The pituitary stalk was not well visualized. The mass demonstrated heterogeneous but predominantly hyperintense T1 signal (shown), and a predominantly hypointense T2 signal (not shown). There was apparent enhancement of the left aspect of the mass.

higher value usually indicates a prolactinoma *(62)*. However, a great deal of overlap exists and lower prolactin levels may sometimes be observed in patients with microprolactinomas, and higher values in patients with stalk compression *(63,64)*. Figure 3 shows a cystic macroprolactinoma with a prolactin level of only 280 mcg/l.

3.1.4. TREATMENT AND OUTCOME

As in adults, dopamine agonists are first-line therapy for prolactinomas, both microadenomas and macroadenomas. Studies of bromocriptine therapy in adolescents have shown success in decreasing prolactin levels and reducing tumor size *(57,58)*. Cabergoline is not FDA-approved for use in the pediatric population, but its successful use has been described in adolescent patients, especially those who have tumors resistant to bromocriptine *(55)*. The medical treatment of prolactinomas is discussed in Chapter 6. Of note, there is a case report of pituitary apoplexy in an adolescent patient taking cabergoline *(65)*. Adolescents treated with dopamine agonists usually resume normal pubertal progression *(57)*. Patients do not reliably recover their GH axis, however, and may require GH replacement *(58)*. Concurrent use of GH and bromocriptine without adverse effects on tumor growth has been described *(66)*. A recent study has described cardiac valvular disease as a complication of cabergoline use in patients with Parkinson's disease; the extent to which this risk applies to pediatric patients with prolactinomas is unclear *(67)*.

If patients do not respond to pharmacotherapy or cannot tolerate the side effects, transsphenoidal resection is indicated. Other indications of surgery include pituitary apoplexy, cerebrospinal fluid leak, immediate threat to vision and hydrocephalus. Surgery alone has a good chance of success in curing microadenomas, but macroadenomas often require adjuvant therapy or repeat surgery. Microadenomas have a 70% operative cure rate, whereas the cure rate following surgery for macroadenomas is only 33% *(50)*. Correlating with tumor size, preoperative prolactin level is also a good indictor of potential surgical success. In Kane's pediatric series, patients with a preoperative prolactin level <400 mcg/l had a 69% chance of immediate surgical cure, whereas none of the patients with preoperative values >400 mcg/l had immediate cure. Likewise, patients with preoperative prolactin levels of ≤200 mcg/l achieve up to 90% recurrence-free survival at 5 years, whereas patients with levels >200 mcg/l have approximately 50% 5-year recurrence-free survival *(50)*. Abe et al. *(56)* reported a surgical cure rate of 75% when the preoperative prolactin level was <200 mcg/l. In the hands of an experienced neurosurgeon, transsphenoidal surgery (TSS) in children has extremely low morbidity and mortality *(49,56)*. Postoperative complications include transient DI and CSF rhinorrhea. An unmeasurable prolactin level 1–2 days postoperatively predicts surgical cure with >90% probability *(49)*. In patients with residual or recurrent tumors following surgery, use of a small dose of a dopamine agonist may be sufficient to keep prolactin levels in the normal range and prevent further tumor growth *(49)*. Although patients with microadenomas commonly remain endocrinologically intact, ~50% of patients with macroadenomas require long-term pituitary hormone replacement *(50)*. Second surgeries are sometimes required, and many patients require lifetime treatment with dopamine agonists even after tumor debulking. Microadenomas have a 65% long-term cure rate and a 25% recurrence rate; macroadenomas have a 55% long-term cure rate and a 33% recurrence rate *(50)*. Radiation is sometimes required for control of medication-resistant prolactinomas that enlarge outside surgically accessible areas.

3.2. ACTH-Secreting Pituitary Adenomas

3.2.1. EPIDEMIOLOGY

ACTH-secreting pituitary adenomas are the second most common type of pituitary adenoma in the pediatric age group, and they are the most common type of pituitary adenomas in prepubertal patients. In one series, 15 of 31 pituitary adenomas in children 0–11 years old were ACTH-secreting pituitary adenomas, whereas these tumors accounted for only 33 of 119 pituitary adenomas in children 12–19 years old *(49)*. These tumors are responsible for up to 80% of noniatrogenic Cushing's syndrome in children and adolescents *(68)*. However, in children less than 3 years old, primary adrenal tumors are more likely to cause Cushing's syndrome. Over 90% of ACTH-secreting pituitary adenomas are microadenomas *(68,69)*. The female predominance described in adults is not present in children *(70,71)*, although one study did report a 2.3:1 female to male ratio in children presenting with these adenomas *(49)*. Conversely, Storr et al. *(71)* observed that males comprised 91% of cases in prepubertal patients, whereas there was an equal sex ratio in pubertal patients. In postpubertal patients, as in adults, ACTH-secreting pituitary adenomas are more prevalent in females *(49,71)*.

3.2.2. PRESENTATION

Weight gain and growth retardation are among the most common initial presentations in children with Cushing's disease. Excessive weight gain is present in 90–100% of children with Cushing's disease, and the pattern of weight gain is generalized as opposed to the typical centripetal pattern observed in adults. Decreased linear growth velocity is observed in 83–96% of patients, and often manifests as a dramatic plateauing of the growth curve *(70,72,73)*. The hallmarks of Cushing's disease in adults such as skin thinning and easy bruising typically occur in children only with long-standing disease and are not common early in the course of the disorder *(19,70)*. Osteopenia is an important finding, reported in 74% of patients *(70)*, and fatigue occurs in about 65% *(70,72)*. Skin manifestations are common: striae are present in 36–64%, acne in 44–80%, and hirsutism in 46–60% *(70,72,74)*. Hypertension has been described in 32–63% of children with Cushing's disease *(70,72,73)*. Headache is a less prevalent symptom, described in about one-fifth of patients *(70,72)*. The effect of Cushing's disease on puberty is variable. In the series of Devoe et al. *(70)*, 60% of patients presented with pubertal arrest or delay. Magiakou et al. *(73)* also described pubertal delay in a small percentage of their patients with Cushing's disease, but reported that 40% of their patients who developed the disease in the first decade of life presented with precocious pubarche. Behavioral problems, which are described in 19–44% of patients, differ from the neuropsychiatric effects described in adults *(70,72,73)*. Although poor work performance, depression, poor memory, and sleep disturbances have been reported in adults, children with behavioral changes caused by Cushing's disease tend to be obsessive-compulsive, and often demonstrate improved school performance *(19,49,70,73)*. Depression, moodiness, and irritability are less commonly described *(70)*.

3.2.3. Diagnosis

The diagnostic approach to Cushing's disease is similar to that in adults. The differential diagnosis includes primary adrenal tumors, ectopic ACTH-secreting or (very rarely) CRH-secreting adenomas, and pseudo-Cushing's states. The latter are less common in children than in adults. Twenty-four-hour urine collection for urine free cortisol is the first step in demonstrating elevated cortisol levels. As in the adult population, cortisol secretion may be episodic, and repeat 24-h collections may be necessary to prove cortisol elevation. In children, adjusting cortisol levels for body surface area is necessary *(19,75)*. Adult normal urine free cortisol ranges assume a body surface area of 1.73 m^2. Once hypercortisolism is established, the loss of diurnal variation in cortisol, determined by elevated nighttime serum or saliva measurements, is useful to distinguish Cushing's syndrome from pseudo-Cushing's states. Midnight plasma cortisol levels >208 nmol/l (7.5 mcg/dl) indicate true Cushing's syndrome *(76a)*, although false positives may occur in people with abnormal sleep patterns. A recent paper suggests that a midnight cortisol value greater than 4.4 mcg/dl correctly identifies Cushing's syndrome in almost all children *(76b)*.

Salivary cortisol measurement in children is widely used in the psychiatric literature, and reports suggest that this may be useful in diagnosing Cushing's syndrome as well. An 11 p.m. or midnight salivary cortisol estimation has been validated in adults but not in children. Pediatric norms for salivary cortisol are not well established, and reports differ concerning whether cutoff values for diagnosing Cushing's should vary according to age or pubertal stage. Trilck et al. *(77)* measured 10 p.m. salivary cortisol and achieved high sensitivity and specificity using age-specific cutoffs: <2.8 nmol/l for ages 6–10 years (sensitivity 87.5%, specificity 100%); 4.7 nmol/l for ages 11–15 years (sensitivity 100%, specificity 100%); and 5.2 nmol/l for ages 16–20 years (sensitivity 90.5%, specificity 94.7%). In contrast, two other reports have used a single cutoff for the entire pediatric age group *(78,79)*. Martinelli et al. *(78)* compared patients with Cushing's syndrome with obese controls and found that they could diagnose Cushing's syndrome with 100% sensitivity and specificity by combining an 11 p.m. salivary cortisol measurement with salivary cortisol measured at 9 a.m. following an overnight dexamethasone suppression test (20 mcg/kg to a maximum of 1 mg administered at 11 p.m.), using cutoffs of 7.7 and 2.4 nmol/l, respectively. Likewise, Gafni et al. *(79)* diagnosed Cushing's syndrome with 93% sensitivity using midnight salivary cortisol levels with a cutoff of 7.5 nmol/l.

Finally, the inability of 8 a.m. plasma cortisol levels to suppress to <50 nmol/l (1.8 mcg/dl) following a midnight 15 mcg/kg (0.6 mg/m^2 to a maximum of 1 mg) dose of dexamethasone indicates Cushing's syndrome (19). The dexamethasone-suppressed CRH stimulation test has been reported to have 100% sensitivity, specificity, and accuracy in differentiating Cushing's syndrome from pseudo-Cushing's states in adults (80). Following 2 days of low-dose dexamethasone (0.3 mg/m^2 to a maximum of 0.5 mg) administered six hourly, and 2 h after the last morning dose of dexamethasone, 1 mcg/kg of ovine CRH (oCRH) is injected. Cortisol levels >38 nmol/l (1.4 mcg/dl) 15 min after oCRH administration suggest a diagnosis of Cushing's syndrome. Martin et al. (81), however, have questioned the usefulness of this test, and recently demonstrated that the test had equal sensitivity but lower specificity than the low-dose dexamethasone suppression test in differentiating Cushing's syndrome from pseudo-Cushing's states.

After the diagnosis of Cushing's syndrome is made, morning ACTH levels help differentiate ACTH-independent (ACTH levels unmeasurable) from ACTH-dependent Cushing's (inappropriately normal or elevated ACTH levels). The CRH stimulation test and the high-dose dexamethasone suppression test may be used to differentiate ACTH-secreting pituitary adenomas from ectopic sources of ACTH. Increased ACTH and cortisol secretion following administration of 1 mcg/kg i.v. of oCRH (measurements at −15, −5, −1, 15, 30, 45, 60, 90, and 120 min) (35% increase in basal ACTH values 15 or 30 min after oCRH, and a 20% increase in basal cortisol values 30 and 45 min after oCRH (82) or a 50% increase in peak plasma ACTH and cortisol (83)) is suggestive of an ACTH-secreting pituitary adenoma. Similarly, suppression of 8 a.m. plasma cortisol values by >20% (76b) or >50% (19) following a midnight dose of 120 mcg/kg (5 mg/m^2 to a maximum of 8 mg) of dexamethasone or 24-h urinary cortisol levels by >50% after 2 days of 1.2 mg/m^2 to a maximum of 2 mg of dexamethasone given six hourly suggests an ACTH-secreting pituitary adenoma (83). Increased ACTH following oCRH stimulation identifies 80–90% of patients with Cushing's disease, and suppression of urine or serum cortisol following high-dose dexamethasone identifies between 68% and 92% of patients (70,73,82). Pituitary MRI with gadolinium should be performed on all patients in whom Cushing's disease is suspected, but MRI only detects 29–72% of adenomas (45,68–70,73,84).

For patients whose lesions are not found on MRI, bilateral inferior petrosal sinus sampling (BIPSS) is useful. BIPSS serves two purposes. First, an elevated central to peripheral ACTH gradient confirms the diagnosis of pituitary

ACTH-secreting pituitary adenoma. Bilateral central and peripheral blood samples for ACTH are obtained at baseline before administration of 1 mcg/kg of oCRH and 3, 5, 10, and 15 min after oCRH administration. A central to peripheral ACTH ratio of ≥ 2 pre-oCRH and ≥ 3 post-oCRH are considered indicative of a pituitary ACTH-secreting adenoma (68). Magiakou et al. (73) report that 95% of patients with Cushing's disease have a baseline central to peripheral ACTH ratio ≥ 2, and that 98% of patients have a ratio ≥ 3 following stimulation with oCRH (1 mcg/kg). BIPSS may also be used to localize ACTH-secreting pituitary adenomas, but the reported accuracy of BIPSS in determining laterality varies from 58% to 91% (68,69,72,73). A lateralizing ACTH gradient of ≥ 1.4 may suggest the location of the tumor within the pituitary, particularly when no anomalous venous drainage is present. Magiakou et al. (73) report that this ratio correctly predicts lateralization of microadenomas in 67% of patients before CRH stimulation and in 76% after CRH stimulation. Batista et al. (68) similarly reported correct localization of the tumor based on an elevated lateralization gradient of ≥ 1.4 in 60% of children with Cushing's disease pre-oCRH and 58% post-oCRH. Furthermore, in this series of 94 patients, Batista et al. (68) reported that combined use of MRI and BIPSS did not predict location any better than MRI alone. For cases in which imaging is negative and BIPSS is equivocal, surgical exploration is indicated. One study suggested that bilateral cavernous sinus sampling may be superior to BIPSS in diagnosing ACTH-secreting pituitary adenomas (85). It is important to remember that BIPSS can be technically difficult in very young children, and the procedure and associated anesthesia carry some risk of morbidity. However, the procedure is safe and well tolerated in experienced hands and the gold standard for exclusion of the rare ectopic ACTH-secreting tumor in children with Cushing's syndrome (68).

3.2.4. TREATMENT AND OUTCOME

TSS is the first-line treatment for ACTH-secreting pituitary adenomas in children. Because these adenomas can be small, a comprehensive exploration of the pituitary is necessary. Exploration is begun on the side of radiographic abnormality or ACTH lateralization on BIPSS. If the tumor is not located on this side of the pituitary, the other side is explored. If no tumor is located on either side and a clear lateralization gradient is evident on BIPSS, hemihypophysectomy on the side of lateralization with preservation of the pituitary stalk is an option (49). Storr et al. (86) described 27 pediatric patients with Cushing's disease treated with TSS. Concordance between results of BIPSS and surgical localization of the tumor was observed in 81% of patients, and 75% (12 of 16) of children who showed lateralization of ACTH secretion, as well as 75% (3 of 4) that did not, were cured by surgery.

Patients typically have secondary adrenal insufficiency requiring cortisol replacement for 6–12 months following surgery, after which the hypothalamic–pituitary–adrenal axis may normalize *(87)*. A total daily dose of hydrocortisone equivalent of 8–10 mcg/m^2 is necessary until normal adrenal function has been demonstrated with an ACTH stimulation test. We use a peak cortisol response of greater than 18 mcg/dl 30 or 60 min after administration of 1 mcg/m^2 of ACTH to indicate adrenal sufficiency. In addition to replacement dosing, stress dosing with steroids needs to be reviewed with the patient and parents when a child is determined to be hypoadrenal. Postoperative GH deficiency occurs in 20–36% of patients *(70,72)*, and secondary hypothyroidism has also been reported *(70)*. Lebrethon et al. *(88a)* have successfully used rhGH with or without GnRH analogs to improve adult height potential following treatment of children with Cushing's disease. Other less common postoperative complications are transient DI, transient CSF rhinorrhea, and panhypopituitarism *(72,86)*. Initial remission rates following TSS are reported between 83 and 98%, but long-term remission occurs in 60–75% *(45,69–73)*. Low early morning cortisol or urinary free cortisol 1 week following surgery is a good indicator of initial surgical success, but these values are not predictive of long-term remission *(70)*. Recurrence rates are up to 10% *(19)*.

Patients who are not initially cured by TSS may undergo repeat surgery or RT. Adrenalectomy is not routinely recommended because of the risk of Nelson's syndrome. In a series of pediatric patients with Cushing's disease from Storr et al. *(71)*, 7 of 18 patients were not cured by TSS but were successfully treated with 45 Gy external beam RT. Six of seven developed GH deficiency, but other pituitary function was preserved over a mean follow-up period of 6.9 years. Mean interval from RT to cure was 0.94 years, with time to cure depending on tumor size and RT dose. Recovery of pituitary–adrenal function occurred at an average of 1.2 years *(71)*. However, the range of long-term follow-up varied from 1.4 to 12 years, and a longer period of follow-up with a larger number of patients is necessary to confirm these findings. In patients treated for Cushing's disease, either with surgery alone or surgery and RT, adult height is likely to be compromised, especially in patients treated for adenomas during puberty *(70)*. Medical therapy with ketoconazole (10–15 mg/kg/day) is rarely indicated, but may be necessary in occasional large or recurrent tumors not successfully treated with surgery or radiation.

3.3. Other Pituitary Adenomas

3.3.1. GH-Secreting Adenomas

GH-secreting adenomas are responsible for about 5–15% of the pituitary adenomas in patients <20 years of age *(19,49,51)*. Constitutively activating mutations of *GNAS* (McCune–Albright syndrome) and the *MENIN* gene

(MEN-1) can cause somatotrope hyperplasia, as can the Carney complex, and hypothalamic or ectopic hypersecretion of GHRH *(19)*. They present with symptoms of gigantism or acromegaly depending on whether the condition precedes or follows epiphyseal fusion, with girls also demonstrating menstrual irregularities. Most GH-secreting adenomas are plurihormonal. In the series from Kane et al. *(50)*, none of the GH-secreting adenomas stained only for GH; instead, 8 of 14 stained for GH and prolactin, with the other 6 staining for GH and a glycoprotein hormone. Diagnosis is based on elevated IGF-1 and GH levels, and it is important to consider age-specific and pubertal stage-specific IGF-1 ranges given the marked physiological increase that occurs in IGF-1 levels at puberty. Inability of GH levels to suppress following an oral glucose load of 100 g is the gold standard for diagnosis of acromegaly in adults. Standards for GH suppression following oral glucose are now available for children based on age and pubertal stage *(88b)*. Imaging studies are useful in determining the site of the tumor. Treatment of GH excess in children is similar to that in adults with this condition, and includes surgery (first line of treatment and curative in 83% *(46)*), use of long-acting somatostatin analogs and/or bromocriptine (when surgery alone is not curative) and less commonly RT. There is no experience regarding the use of GH receptor antagonists such as pegvisomant in children, whereas this has been successfully used to treat acromegaly in adults.

3.3.2. THYROTROPE AND GONADOTROPE ADENOMAS

Adenomas that secrete TSH or LH/FSH are extremely rare in children, described only in case reports. Given the paucity of experience in diagnosing and treating such tumors in children, adult norms are used for the management of these rare tumors.

3.3.3. ENDOCRINE INACTIVE TUMORS

Endocrine inactive tumors, which are relatively common in adults, make up only 2–6% of pediatric pituitary adenomas *(19,49)*, although one study reported a prevalence of 20% for nonfunctioning adenomas *(51)*. These tumors are thought to arise from gonadotropes and stain for primarily the α-subunit of glycoprotein hormones, with one or more of the β-subunits and chromogranin A. Diagnosis is usually delayed and the tumors are macroadenomas when diagnosed. Of the various pituitary adenomas, these are often the largest at diagnosis *(49)*. Clinical features include headaches, nausea, visual field deficits, growth failure, and pubertal delay or arrest. Surgery is the mainstay of treatment for large tumors and performed with the aim to release pressure on the optic nerves and chiasm, while preserving pituitary function. Invasion into the cavernous sinus or middle cranial fossa limits surgical resectability.

Lateral displacement of the dural wall of the cavernous sinus without its perforation by a large tumor mimics invasion into the cavernous sinus, but because the dural wall is intact, such tumors are completely resectable *(49)*. A clean surgical plane usually exists between the tumor and the remainder of the compressed pituitary and other structures, and dissection along this plane facilitates complete removal. Anterior pituitary function, if impaired before surgery, usually recovers postoperatively. Smaller tumors may be observed over time. Differentiating these tumors preoperatively from craniopharyngiomas can be a diagnostic challenge.

3.3.4. INCIDENTALOMAS

Incidentally discovered adenomas mandate removal in the following situations: (i) evidence of impaired anterior pituitary function (usually GH deficiency and growth failure), (ii) extension beyond the sella, (iii) greatest diameter >1 cm, (iv) persistent headaches that may be attributable to the tumor, (v) a rapidly growing mass, and (vi) visual field deficits documented on a formal eye examination *(49)*. The evaluation of patients with incidentalomas is discussed in Chapter 21.

4. SELLAR CYSTS

Nonneoplastic cysts of the pituitary include Rathke's cleft cyst, epidermoid cyst, dermoid cyst, and arachnoid cyst. The evaluation of patients with sellar cysts is discussed in detail in Chapter 23. By far, the most common of these are Rathke's cleft cysts, which are congenital cysts located in the pars intermedia. Like craniopharyngiomas, they arise from remnants of Rathke's pouch.

4.1. Rathke's Cleft Cysts

4.1.1. EPIDEMIOLOGY

These cysts are typically asymptomatic and account for a large majority of the incidental pituitary lesions found on neuroimaging. In an autopsy series, 11% of the adult population had incidental Rathke's cleft cysts, with a much lower prevalence of 1.7% in patients 10–29 years of age *(89)*. In this series, no child <9 years old had a Rathke's cleft cyst >2 mm in size. Similarly, in a retrospective review of MRIs, only 1.2% of patients <15 years of age were found to have an asymptomatic Rathke's cleft cyst *(90)*.

4.1.2. PRESENTATION

Although the majority of Rathke's cleft cysts are asymptomatic, some grow large enough to cause symptoms and require treatment. Symptoms typically do not occur until adulthood, but there are case reports of children with symptomatic lesions. Clinical features may include evidence of a mass lesion with headaches and visual deficits, hormonal deficits, or both. Hormonal perturbations include DI, SIADH, precocious puberty, and GH deficiency *(91–93)*.

4.1.3. DIAGNOSIS

Diagnosis is suggested by neuroimaging. Appearance on MRI is characterized by a round or oval well-marginated lesion, usually intrasellar in position between the anterior and posterior pituitary lobes. The cystic lesion is nonenhancing with smooth contour and homogeneous content. The lesion is hypointense to isointense on T1-weighted images, and may be variably hyperintense on T2-weighted images, similar to CSF *(90)*. Another study, however, reported that of 16 cases with Rathke's cleft cyst, on T1-weighted images, 6 were hypointense, 6 were hyperintense, 3 were isointense, and 1 was heterogeneous *(94)*. Conversely, on T2-weighted images, 11 of 13 appeared hyperintense, and 2 were hypointense. Because there may be overlap between the MRI appearance of Rathke's cleft cysts and of cystic craniopharyngiomas, CT is also helpful to assess for calcifications, which are not present in Rathke's cleft cysts but are found in >90% of pediatric craniopharyngiomas. Craniopharyngiomas also have enhancing solid components, which are not observed in Rathke's cleft cysts. Cystic pituitary adenomas may sometimes mimic Rathke's cleft cysts, but the cyst wall of pituitary adenomas is composed of tumor and should enhance with contrast administration. A thin rim of peripheral enhancement may also occur in Rathke's cleft cysts, however, representing the normal pituitary. Cyst contents can be gelatinous or thick and may be dark colored. Sometimes, the contents are CSF like *(94)*. Although most Rathke's cleft cysts are present between the anterior and posterior lobes of the pituitary, on occasion, the location is not constant. Figure 4 shows a suprasellar Rathke's cleft cyst in an 18-year-old girl.

4.1.4. MANAGEMENT AND OUTCOME

Small cysts that are asymptomatic and not compressing the optic nerves and chiasm may be observed with serial MRIs. Treatment for symptomatic cysts is transsphenoidal aspiration of the cyst with a biopsy of the cyst wall to confirm diagnosis. Cysts may recur, and patients should be followed with serial MRIs. Recurrence of a cyst, particularly when the optic nerves and chiasm are compressed, may mandate surgical resection of the cyst.

4.2. Arachnoid Cysts

Arachnoid cysts in children are most commonly suprasellar and present with mass effects. Less commonly, an arachnoid diverticulum may invaginate through an incomplete diaphragma sella, causing an intrasellar cyst. Unlike the

T1 pre-contrast   T1 post-contrast

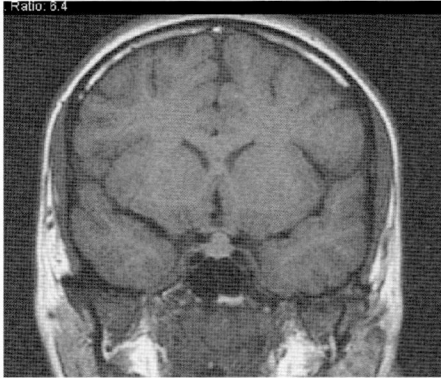

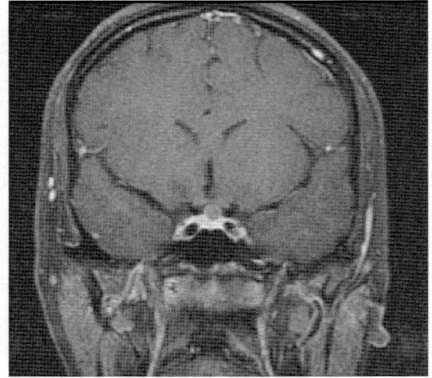

Fig. 4. Rathke's cleft cyst in an 18-year-old girl. Within the suprasellar cistern, just anterior to the pituitary gland and between the pituitary infundibulum and midline optic chiasm, a round, well-circumscribed nonenhancing lesion measuring 7 × 6 × 6 mm was present, which showed signal intensity isointense to gray matter on both T1-weighted (shown) and T2-weighted (not shown) images, relative bright signal on the FLAIR images, and no restricted diffusion. The appearance, signal characteristics and location were most consistent with a Rathke's cleft cyst. The patient was followed with repeat serial MRIs.

Rathke's cleft cyst, intrasellar arachnoid cysts are usually located anterior and superior to the anterior and posterior pituitary lobes, and may cause the partial empty sella syndrome with variable degrees of pituitary insufficiency (95). The cysts appear similar to CSF on T1-weighted and T2-weighted images. Small asymptomatic cysts can be observed, whereas symptomatic cysts require transsphenoidal resection.

5. PARASELLAR TUMORS

These tumors include germ cell tumors as well as other tumors such as meningiomas, gliomas, astrocytomas, lipomas, hamartomas, teratomas, osteoblastomas, and hemangiomas. Only germ cell tumors and hypothalamic hamartomas will be described in detail in this section. Optic nerve gliomas are a component of neurofibromatosis-1, and may involve the optic chiasm. These are very slow-growing tumors and only mandate observation over time with serial MRIs.

5.1. Germ Cell Tumors

5.1.1. EPIDEMIOLOGY

Intracranial germ cell tumors are rare, and in the United States, germ cell tumors account for 3.9% of intracranial tumors from age 0 to 14 years and 6.8%

of intracranial tumors between 15 and 19 years of age *(48)*. This represents an incidence of only 0.2/100,000 person-years between 0 and 19 years of age *(48)*. The pineal gland is the most common site for the origin of these tumors, and pineal germ cell tumors are twice as common as those developing in the suprasellar region *(96,97)*. About 5–10% of these tumors are found at both pineal and suprasellar sites at diagnosis *(98)*, and it is not certain whether this represents simultaneous tumor occurrence at both sites, or spread from one site to the other. Approximately 65% of germ cell tumors are germinomas, with the remainder classified as nongerminomatous germ cell tumors, consisting of teratomas, embryonal carcinomas, endodermal sinus tumors, choriocarcinomas, and mixed germ cell tumors *(98)*. Germinomas comprise the majority of germ cell tumors in the suprasellar region, whereas almost 70% of nongerminomatous germ cell tumors arise in the pineal gland *(98)*. Overall, these tumors exhibit a 2:1 male predominance, but lesions in the sellar region are at least as common (if not more common) in females as in males. Nongerminomatous germ cell tumors more commonly arise in the prepubertal years, whereas germ cell tumors appear between about 10 and 21 years of age, suggesting a hormonal influence on their development *(97,98)*.

5.1.2. PRESENTATION

Suprasellar germinomas, also termed neurohypophyseal germinomas, involve the hypothalamus, pituitary infundibulum, and posterior pituitary, and thus also extend into the sella. They classically present with a triad of DI, pituitary insufficiency, and visual changes, including decreased visual acuity and visual field deficits. DI occurs in 69–92% of patients *(96,99,100)*, and patients initially diagnosed with idiopathic DI may manifest a germinoma on serial neuroimaging *(101)*. Short stature occurs in ~30% of patients <15 years as a result of GH deficiency *(100)*. Likewise, gonadotropin deficiency may delay pubertal development. In the series from Matsutani et al. *(100)*, 93% of the females >12 years of age presented with primary or secondary amenorrhea. Rarely, precocious puberty may be associated, and some but not all children with evidence of early puberty have elevations in β-hCG or LH. Choriocarcinomas are more likely to be associated with precocious puberty than other forms of intracranial germ cell tumors. A small proportion of children with germ cell tumors also have TSH deficiency. In one small series, deficiencies of ADH, GH, ACTH, and TSH were documented in 75%, 42%, 17%, and 8% of patients with suprasellar germinomas, and prolactin levels were elevated in 50% *(102)*. One-third of children with suprasellar tumors will have no symptoms of this disease for up to 6 months, resulting in a delay in diagnosis. Of note, between 6% and 40% of germinomas are reportedly bifocal, with lesions in both the neurohypophysis and the pineal gland *(99,103)*. These tumors also present with symptoms typical of pineal lesions, including hydrocephalus and headaches, Parinaud's syndrome (vertical gaze palsy, impaired light reflex, lid retraction, and convergence or retraction nystagmus), obtundation, pyramidal signs, and ataxia *(98,104)*. Nongerminomatous tumors tend to be larger than germinomas and are associated with greater prevalence and severity of hydrocephalus and visual dysfunction.

5.1.3. DIAGNOSIS

Although biopsy is generally required for definitive diagnosis of suprasellar germinoma, neuroimaging and measurement of tumor markers facilitate initial evaluation. MRI commonly shows (i) infundibular thickening, (ii) absence of a bright T1 signal from the posterior pituitary *(96)*, (iii) strong and homogeneous enhancement with gadolinium contrast. The majority of germinomas are isointense on T1-weighted images, and demonstrate variable intensity on T2-weighted images *(96)*. MRI of the spine helps assess for evidence of metastatic disease. Figure 5 shows a suprasellar germinoma extending into the sella in a 10-year-old girl.

In children with pituitary stalk thickening and central DI, the differential diagnosis should include germ cell tumors, Langerhans histiocytosis, and other infiltrative, autoimmune, or infectious conditions, although some may have idiopathic DI *(105)*. In the series by Leger et al. *(105)*, of 26 patients with a thickened pituitary stalk and DI followed over a mean period of 5.5 years, 4 were diagnosed with a germinoma, 5 had Langerhans histiocytosis, and the remainder had no evidence of pathology, resulting in a diagnosis of idiopathic DI. Stalk thickening may be mistaken for lymphocytic hypophysitis, and biopsies performed early in the course of the disorder have, in fact, been reported as lymphocytic hypophysitis. A germinoma should be strongly considered in children with this diagnosis.

Tumor markers are particularly useful, and β-hCG in CSF is elevated markedly in choriocarcinomas and mixed germ cell tumors, to a lesser extent in syncytiotrophoblastic germinomas, and may be normal or just mildly elevated in pure germinomas and embryonal carcinomas. Germinomas exhibit negative serum and CSF α-fetoprotein, with positive results suggesting an alternative diagnosis of endodermal sinus tumor or mixed germ cell tumor, or rarely embryonal cell carcinoma *(97)*. It is necessary to determine whether or not tumor markers are present in serum and CSF when a germ cell tumor is suspected. In addition, CSF cytology should be performed to determine whether there is evidence of tumor dissemination in the neuroaxis. Schulte et al. *(106)* reported positive CSF cytology in eight of nine children with germinomas, whereas Shibamoto et al. *(107)* reported abnormal CSF cytology in 50% of children and adults.

T1 pre-contrast

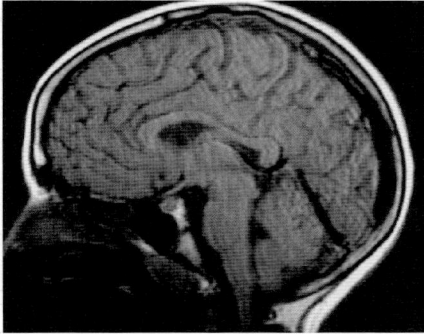

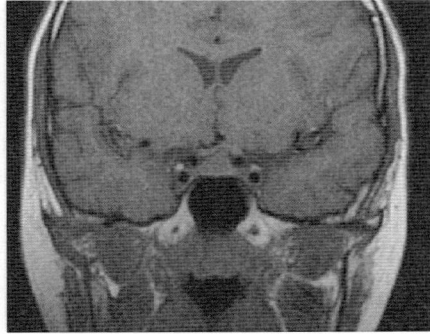

T1 post-contrast

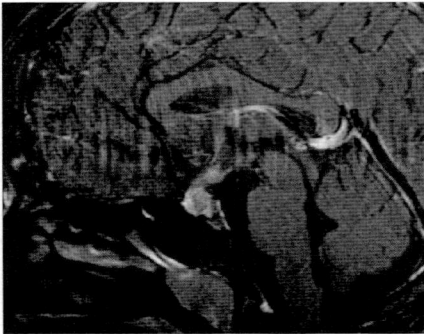

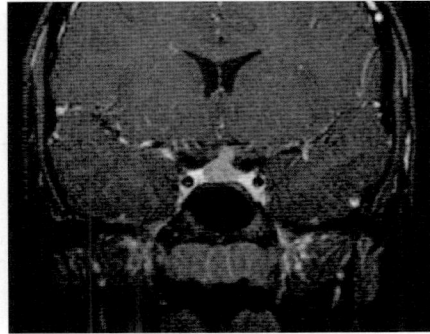

Fig. 5. Germinoma in an 10-year-old girl. The pituitary stalk was thickened and appeared continuous with a sellar mass that measured up to 1.3 × 0.8 × 0.8 cm. The mass abutted the optic chiasm and right cavernous sinus without definite evidence for invasion, and exhibited mild homogeneous enhancement. MRI of the spine did not indicate metastatic spread. CSF was mildly positive for β-hCG. The patient presented with diabetes insipidus and responded to chemotherapy and radiotherapy.

5.1.4. TREATMENT AND OUTCOME

The prognosis is much better for germinomas (pure and syncytiotrophoblastic) compared with nongerminomatous tumors. Among germinomas, pineal tumors may carry a better prognosis than suprasellar tumors, although data are controversial. Germinomas are highly sensitive to both radiation and chemotherapy, and surgery is reserved primarily for diagnostic purposes. Primary site radiation between 4,000 and 5,500 cGy and variable amounts of cranial and spinal radiation for disseminated tumors are described. Although radiation alone is effective treatment, the combination of chemotherapy and radiation is increasingly used because it allows lower radiation exposure, and thus lower potential for neurocognitive and endocrinological sequelae. Lower levels of spinal irradiation also help optimize growth potential. Chemotherapy includes various combinations of cyclophosphamide, vinblastine, bleomycin, cisplatin, carboplatin, etoposide, and ifosfamide. In both strategies, 10-year survival rates are ≥90% *(100,108,109)*. Hormone deficiencies need to be replaced. In contrast, for nongerminomatous tumors, survival rates range only between 40% and 70% *(98,100,104)*. Craniospinal radiation is administered in all patients with nongerminomatous tumors, and chemotherapy is necessary to improve the duration and rate of survival. The presence of high levels of CSF tumor markers and a slowly responding tumor are poor prognostic features.

5.2. Hypothalamic Hamartomas

Hypothalamic hamartomas arise in the tuber cinereum and are a rare but important cause of precocious puberty. These lesions are present at birth and manifest with central precocious puberty usually before 4 years of age. The hamartoma appears to function as an ectopic GnRH pulse generator, thus causing precocious puberty. Large hamartomas may be associated with deficiency of pituitary hormones such as GH, TSH, and ACTH. The diagnosis is usually made with an MRI, and hamartomas are either slow growing or do not grow at all over time. The majority of the masses require no surgical intervention and are followed over time with serial MRIs. Precocious puberty can be treated with depot leuprolide analogs, and hormone replacement carried out as necessary. The Pallister–Hall syndrome is associated with hypothalamic hamartomas and should be ruled out if associated features such as polydactyly, imperforate anus, bifid epiglottis, and pituitary insufficiency exist. This syndrome is caused by mutations in the GLI-Kruppel family member 3 gene, and inherited in an autosomal dominant fashion *(110)*. Features include various combinations of facial defects including multiple buccal frenulae, cleft lip or palate, ear and eye defects, cardiac defects such as VSD, PDA, and aortic coarctation, imperforate anus, renal anomalies, microphallus, limb defects, polydactyly and syndactyly, hypothalamic hamartoma, and varying degrees of holoprosencephaly and hypopituitarism. The phenotype can be very variable. Hypothalamic hamartomas may also be associated with developmental delay and gelastic seizures, which can progress over time to catastrophic seizures *(111,112)*.

6. INFILTRATIVE PROCESSES

Infiltrative processes such as tuberculosis, Langerhans histiocytosis, autoimmune hypophysitis, and sarcoidosis can cause infundibular thickening and are included in the differential diagnosis of this finding. Langerhans histiocytosis, in particular, should be considered in any child with DI, and accounts for 15–20% of cases of stalk thickening and DI *(105)*. Overall, 50%

of children with Langerhans histiocytosis will present with DI. Tuberculosis and sarcoidosis are rare causes of stalk thickening in children.

7. CONCLUSION

Masses affecting pituitary function in children thus have unique features when compared with adults, particularly with regard to epidemiology and presentation. Challenges in management include preservation of neurocognitive function at a time of active neurological growth, particularly in very young children, thus the sparing use of RT except when necessary. The risks of RT as regards neurocognitive function, pituitary dysfunction, growth potential, and second malignancies need to be balanced against morbidity associated with surgery particularly in the case of large craniopharyngiomas. Newer chemotherapeutic modalities are allowing for lower radiation doses in children with germinomas, a tumor that is very radiosensitive and chemosensitive, and far more effectively treated with these modalities than with surgery.

REFERENCES

1. Hoffman S, Propp JM, McCarthy BJ Temporal trends in incidence of primary brain tumors in the United States, 1985–1999. Neuro-oncol 2006;8:27–37.
2. Schoenberg BS, Schoenberg DG, Christine BW, Gomez MR The epidemiology of primary intracranial neoplasms of childhood. A population study. Mayo Clin Proc 1976;51:51–6.
3. Matson DD, Crigler JF, Jr. Management of craniopharyngioma in childhood. J Neurosurg 1969;30:377–90.
4. Harwood-Nash DC. Neuroimaging of childhood craniopharyngioma. Pediatr Neurosurg 1994;21(Suppl 1):2–10.
5. Zhang YQ, Wang CC, Ma ZY. Pediatric craniopharyngiomas: clinicomorphological study of 189 cases. Pediatr Neurosurg 2002;36:80–4.
6. Karavitaki N, Warner JT, Marland A, et al. . GH replacement does not increase the risk of recurrence in patients with craniopharyngioma. Clin Endocrinol (Oxf) 2006;64:556–60.
7. Bunin G, Surawicz T, Witman P, Preston-Martin S, Davis F, Bruner J. The descriptive epidemiology of craniopharyngioma. J Neurosurg 1998;89:547–551.
8. Gonc EN, Yordam N, Ozon A, Alikasifoglu A, Kandemir N. Endocrinological outcome of different treatment options in children with craniopharyngioma: a retrospective analysis of 66 cases. Pediatr Neurosurg 2004;40:112–9.
9. Curtis J, Daneman D, Hoffman HJ, Ehrlich RM. The endocrine outcome after surgical removal of craniopharyngiomas. Pediatr Neurosurg 1994;21(Suppl 1):24–7.
10. Lena G, Paz Paredes A, Scavarda D, Giusiano B. Craniopharyngioma in children: Marseille experience. Childs Nerv Syst 2005;21:778–84.
11. Stripp DC, Maity A, Janss AJ, et al. Surgery with or without radiation therapy in the management of craniopharyngiomas in children and young adults. Int J Radiat Oncol Biol Phys 2004;58:714–20.
12. Bulow B, Attewell R, Hagmar L, Malmstrom P, Nordstrom C, Erfurth E. Post-operative prognosis in craniopharyngioma with respect to cardiovascular mortality, survival and tumor recurrence. J Clin Endocrinol Metab 1998;83:3897–904.
13. Honegger J, Buchfelder M, Fahlbusch R. Surgical treatment of craniopharyngiomas: endocrinological results. J Neurosurg 1999;90:251–7.

14. Scott RM, Hetelekidis S, Barnes PD, Goumnerova L, Tarbell NJ. Surgery, radiation, and combination therapy in the treatment of childhood craniopharyngioma—a 20-year experience. Pediatr Neurosurg 1994;21(Suppl 1):75–81.

15. Sklar C. Craniopharyngioma: endocrine abnormalities at presentation. Pediatr Neurosurg 1994;21(Suppl 1):18–20.

16. Halac I, Zimmerman D. Endocrine manifestations of craniopharyngioma. Childs Nerv Syst 2005;21:640–8.

17. DeVile C, Grant D, Hayward R, Stanhope R. Growth and endocrine sequelae of craniopharyngioma. Arch Dis Child 1996;75:108–14.

18. Müller HL, Emser A, Faldum A, . Longitudinal study on growth and body mass index before and after diagnosis of childhood craniopharyngioma. J Clin Endocrinol Metab 2004;89:3298–3305.

19. Lafferty A, Chrousos G. Pituitary tumors in children and adolescents. J Clin Endocrinol Metab 1999;84:4317–4323.

20. Moon SH, Kim IH, Park SW, . Early adjuvant radiotherapy toward long-term survival and better quality of life for craniopharyngiomas—a study in single institute. Childs Nerv Syst 2005;21:799–807.

21. Fitzek MM, Linggood RM, Adams J, Munzenrider JE. Combined proton and photon irradiation for craniopharyngioma: long-term results of the early cohort of patients treated at Harvard Cyclotron Laboratory and Massachusetts General Hospital. Int J Radiat Oncol Biol Phys 2006;64:1348–54.

22. Fahlbusch R, Honegger J, Paulus W, Huk W, Buchfelder M. Surgical treatment of craniopharyngiomas: experience with 168 patients. J Neurosurg 1999;90:237–50.

23. Scott RM Craniopharyngioma: a personal (Boston) experience. Childs Nerv Syst 2005;21:773–7.

24. Zuccaro G Radical resection of craniopharyngioma. Childs Nerv Syst 2005;21:679–90.

25. Hetelekidis S, Barnes PD, Tao ML, et al.. 20-year experience in childhood craniopharyngioma. Int J Radiat Oncol Biol Phys 1993;27:189–95.

26. Merchant TE, Kiehna EN, Sanford RA, et al. Craniopharyngioma: the St. Jude Children's Research Hospital experience 1984–2001. Int J Radiat Oncol Biol Phys 2002;53:533–42.

27. Takahashi H, Yamaguchi F, Teramoto A. Long-term outcome and reconsideration of intracystic chemotherapy with bleomycin for craniopharyngioma in children. Childs Nerv Syst 2005;21:701–4.

28. Park DH, Park JY, Kim JH, et al. Outcome of postoperative intratumoral bleomycin injection for cystic craniopharyngioma. J Korean Med Sci 2002;17:254–9.

29. Jiang R, Liu Z, Zhu C. Preliminary exploration of the clinical effect of bleomycin on craniopharyngiomas. Stereotact Funct Neurosurg 2002;78:84–94.

30. Cavalheiro S, Dastoli PA, Silva NS, Toledo S, Lederman H, da Silva MC. Use of interferon alpha in intratumoral chemotherapy for cystic craniopharyngioma. Childs Nerv Syst 2005;21:719–24.

31. Kalapurakal JA. Radiation therapy in the management of pediatric craniopharyngiomas – a review. Childs Nerv Syst 2005;21:808–16.

32. Albright AL, Hadjipanayis CG, Lunsford LD, Kondziolka D, Pollack IF, Adelson PD. Individualized treatment of pediatric craniopharyngiomas. Childs Nerv Syst 2005;21:649–54.

33. Hasegawa T, Kondziolka D, Hadjipanayis CG, Lunsford LD. Management of cystic craniopharyngiomas with phosphorus-32 intracavitary irradiation. Neurosurgery 2004;54:813–20; discussion 820–2.

34. Schefter JK, Allen G, Cmelak AJ, et al. The utility of external beam radiation and intracystic 32P radiation in the treatment of craniopharyngiomas. J Neurooncol 2002;56:69–78.
35. Tomita T, Bowman RM. Craniopharyngiomas in children: surgical experience at Children's Memorial Hospital. Childs Nerv Syst 2005;21 729–46.
36. Price DA, Wilton P, Jonsson P, et al. Efficacy and safety of growth hormone treatment in children with prior craniopharyngioma: an analysis of the Pharmacia and Upjohn International Growth Database (KIGS) from 1988 to 1996. Horm Res 1998;49:91–7.
37. Pinto G, Bussieres L, Recasens C, Souberbielle JC, Zerah M, Brauner R. Hormonal factors influencing weight and growth pattern in craniopharyngioma. Horm Res 2000; 53:163–9.
38. Burns EC, Tanner JM, Preece MA, Cameron N. Growth hormone treatment in children with craniopharyngioma: final growth status. Clin Endocrinol (Oxf) 1981;14:587–95.
39. Müller H, Handwerker G, Wollny B, Faldum A, Sorensen N. Melatonin secretion and increased daytime sleepiness in childhood craniopharyngioma patients. J Clin Endocrinol Metab 2002;87:3993–6.
40. Harz KJ, Muller HL, Waldeck E, Pudel V, Roth C. Obesity in patients with craniopharyngioma: assessment of food intake and movement counts indicating physical activity. J Clin Endocrinol Metab 2003;88:5227–31.
41. Sands S, Milner J, Goldberg J, et al. Quality of life and behavioral follow-up study of pediatric survivors of craniopharyngioma. J Neurosurg 2005;103:302–11.
42. Mottolese C, Szathmari A, Berlier P, Hermier M. Craniopharyngiomas: our experience in Lyon. Childs Nerv Syst 2005;21:790–8.
43. Kim SK, Wang KC, Shin SH, Choe G, Chi JG, Cho BK. Radical excision of pediatric craniopharyngioma: recurrence pattern and prognostic factors. Childs Nerv Syst 2001;17:531–6; discussion 537.
44. Caldarelli M, Massimi L, Tamburrini G, Cappa M, Di Rocco C. Long-term results of the surgical treatment of craniopharyngioma: the experience at the Policlinico Gemelli, Catholic University, Rome. Childs Nerv Syst 2005;21:747–57.
45. Dyer EH, Civit T, Visot A, Delalande O, Derome P. Transsphenoidal surgery for pituitary adenomas in children. Neurosurgery 1994;34:207–12; discussion 212.
46. Mindermann T, Wilson CB. Pediatric pituitary adenomas. Neurosurgery 1995;36:259–68; discussion 269.
47. Partington MD, Davis DH, Laws ER, Jr, Scheithauer BW. Pituitary adenomas in childhood and adolescence. Results of transsphenoidal surgery. J Neurosurg 1994;80:209–16.
48. CBTRUS. Statistical Report: Primary Brain Tumors in the United States, 1998–2002. Central Brain Tumor Registry of the United States; 2005.
49. Kunwar S, Wilson CB. Pediatric pituitary adenomas. J Clin Endocrinol Metab 1999;84:4385–9.
50. Kane LA, Leinung MC, Scheithauer BW, et al. Pituitary adenomas in childhood and adolescence. J Clin Endocrinol Metab 1994;79:1135–40.
51. Cannavo S, Venturino M, Curto L, et al. Clinical presentation and outcome of pituitary adenomas in teenagers. Clin Endocrinol (Oxf) 2003;58:519–27.
52. Haddad SF, VanGilder JC, Menezes AH. Pediatric pituitary tumors. Neurosurgery 1991;29:509–14.
53. De Menis E, Visentin A, Billeci D, et al. Pituitary adenomas in childhood and adolescence. Clinical analysis of 10 cases. J Endocrinol Invest 2001;24:92–7.
54. Delgrange E, Trouillas J, Maiter D, Donckier J, Tourniaire J. Sex-related difference in the growth of prolactinomas: a clinical and proliferation marker study. J Clin Endocrinol Metab 1997;82:2102–7.

55. Colao A, Loche S, Cappa M, et al. Prolactinomas in children and adolescents. Clinical presentation and long-term follow-up. J Clin Endocrinol Metab 1998;83:2777–80.
56. Abe T, Ludecke DK. Transnasal surgery for prolactin-secreting pituitary adenomas in childhood and adolescence. Surg Neurol 2002;57:369–78; discussion 378–9.
57. Howlett TA, Wass JA, Grossman A, et al. Prolactinomas presenting as primary amenorrhoea and delayed or arrested puberty: response to medical therapy. Clin Endocrinol (Oxf) 1989;30:131–40.
58. Tyson D, Reggiardo D, Sklar C, David R. Prolactin-secreting macroadenomas in adolescents. Response to bromocriptine therapy. Am J Dis Child 1993;147:1057–61.
59. Galli-Tsinopoulou A, Nousia-Arvanitakis S, Mitsiakos G, Karamouzis M, Dimitriadis A. Osteopenia in children and adolescents with hyperprolactinemia. J Pediatr Endocrinol Metab 2000;13:439–41.
60. Misra M, Papakostas G, Klibanski A. Effects of psychiatric disorders and psychotropic medications on prolactin and bone metabolism. J Clin Psychiatry 2004;65:1607–18.
61. Koves I, Jarman F, Cameron F. Antipsychotic medication and marked hyperprolactinaemia: iatros or true prolactinoma? Acta Paediatr. 2004;93:1543–7.
62. Scott R, Hedley-Whyte E. Case record of the Massachusetts General Hospital. Weekly clinicopathological exercises. Case 35–2002. A nine-year-old girl with cold intolerance, visual-field defects, and a suprasellar tumor. N Engl J Med 2002;347:1604–11.
63. Smith M, Laws EJ. Magnetic resonance imaging measurements of pituitary stalk compression and deviation in patients with nonprolactin-secreting intrasellar and parasellar tumors: lack of correlation with serum prolactin levels. Neurosurgery 1994;34:834–9.
64. Albuquerque F, Hinton D, Weiss M. Excessively high prolactin level in a patient with a nonprolactin-secreting adenoma: case report. J Neurosurg 1998;89:1043–6.
65. Knoepfelmacher M, Gomes MC, Melo ME, Mendonca BB. Pituitary apoplexy during therapy with cabergoline in an adolescent male with prolactin-secreting macroadenoma. Pituitary 2004;7:83–7.
66. Oberfield SE, Nino M, Riddick L, et al. Combined bromocriptine and growth hormone (GH) treatment in GH-deficient children with macroprolactinoma in situ. J Clin Endocrinol Metab 1992;75:87–90.
67. Zanettini R, Antonini A, Gatto G, Gentile R, Tesei S, Pezzoli G. Valvular heart disease and the use of dopamine agonists for Parkinson's disease. N Engl J Med 2007;356:39–46.
68. Batista D, Gennari M, Riar J, et al. An assessment of petrosal sinus sampling for localization of pituitary microadenomas in children with Cushing disease. J Clin Endocrinol Metab 2006;91:221–4.
69. Lienhardt A, Grossman AB, Dacie JE, et al. Relative contributions of inferior petrosal sinus sampling and pituitary imaging in the investigation of children and adolescents with ACTH-dependent Cushing's syndrome. J Clin Endocrinol Metab 2001;86:5711–4.
70. Devoe DJ, Miller WL, Conte FA, et al. Long-term outcome in children and adolescents after transsphenoidal surgery for Cushing's disease. J Clin Endocrinol Metab 1997;82:3196–202.
71. Storr HL, Isidori AM, Monson JP, Besser GM, Grossman AB, Savage MO. Prepubertal Cushing's disease is more common in males, but there is no increase in severity at diagnosis. J Clin Endocrinol Metab 2004;89:3818–20.
72. Joshi SM, Hewitt RJ, Storr HL, et al. Cushing's disease in children and adolescents: 20 years of experience in a single neurosurgical center. Neurosurgery 2005;57:281–5.
73. Magiakou MA, Mastorakos G, Oldfield EH, et al. Cushing's syndrome in children and adolescents. Presentation, diagnosis, and therapy. N Engl J Med 1994;331:629–36.
74. Bickler SW, McMahon TJ, Campbell JR, Mandel S, Piatt JH, Harrison MW. Preoperative diagnostic evaluation of children with Cushing's syndrome. J Pediatr Surg 1994;29:671–6.

75. Legro R, Lin H, Demers L, Lloyd T. Urinary free cortisol increases in adolescent caucasian females during perimenarche. J Clin Endocrinol Metab 2003;88:215–9.
76a. Papanicolaou DA, Yanovski JA, Cutler GB, Jr, Chrousos GP, Nieman LK. A single midnight serum cortisol measurement distinguishes Cushing's syndrome from pseudo-Cushing states. J Clin Endocrinol Metab 1998;83:1163–7.
76b. Batista DL, Riar J, Keil M, Stratakis CA. Diagnostic tests for children who are referred for the investigation of Cushing syndrome. Pediatrics. 2007;120:e575–86.
77. Trilck M, Flitsch J, Ludecke DK, Jung R, Petersenn S. Salivary cortisol measurement—a reliable method for the diagnosis of Cushing's syndrome. Exp Clin Endocrinol Diabetes 2005;113:225–30.
78. Martinelli CE, Jr, Sader SL, Oliveira EB, Daneluzzi JC, Moreira AC. Salivary cortisol for screening of Cushing's syndrome in children. Clin Endocrinol (Oxf) 1999;51:67–71.
79. Gafni RI, Papanicolaou DA, Nieman LK. Nighttime salivary cortisol measurement as a simple, noninvasive, outpatient screening test for Cushing's syndrome in children and adolescents. J Pediatr 2000;137:30–5.
80. Yanovski J, Cutler GJ, Chrousos G, Nieman L. Corticotropin-releasing hormone stimulation following low-dose dexamethasone administration. A new test to distinguish Cushing's syndrome from pseudo-Cushing's states. JAMA 1993;269:2232–8.
81. Martin NM, Dhillo WS, Banerjee A, et al. Comparison of the dexamethasone-suppressed corticotropin-releasing hormone test and low-dose dexamethasone suppression test in the diagnosis of Cushing's syndrome. J Clin Endocrinol Metab 2006;91:2582–6.
82. Nieman L, Oldfield E, Wesley R, Chrousos G, Loriaux D, Cutler GJ. A simplified morning ovine corticotropin-releasing hormone stimulation test for the differential diagnosis of adrenocorticotropin-dependent Cushing's syndrome. J Clin Endocrinol Metab 1993;77:1308–12.
83. Invitti C, Giraldi FP, de Martin M, Cavagnini F. Diagnosis and management of Cushing's syndrome: results of an Italian multicentre study. Study Group of the Italian Society of Endocrinology on the Pathophysiology of the Hypothalamic-Pituitary-Adrenal Axis. J Clin Endocrinol Metab 1999;84:440–8.
84. Batista D, Courkoutsakis N, Oldfield E, et al. Detection of adrenocorticotropin-secreting pituitary adenomas by magnetic resonance imaging in children and adolescents with Cushing disease. J Clin Endocrinol Metab 2005;90:5134–40.
85. Graham K, Samuels M, Nesbit G, et al. Cavernous sinus sampling is highly accurate in distinguishing Cushing's disease from the ectopic adrenocorticotropin syndrome and in predicting intrapituitary tumor location. J Clin Endocrinol Metab 1999;84:1602–10.
86. Storr H, Afshar F, Matson M, et al. Factors influencing cure by transsphenoidal selective adenomectomy in paediatric Cushing's disease. Eur J Endocrinol 2005;152:825–33.
87. Jagannathan J, Dumont AS, Jane JA, Jr, Laws ER, Jr. Pediatric sellar tumors: diagnostic procedures and management. Neurosurg Focus 2005;18:E6.
88a. Lebrethon M-C, Grossman AB, Afshar F, Plowman PN, Besser GM, Savage MO. Linear growth and final height after treatment for Cushing's disease in childhood. J Clin Endocrinol Metab 2000;85:3262–5.
88b. Misra M, Cord J, Prabhakaran R, Miller KK, Klibanski A. Growth hormone suppression after an oral glucose load in children. J Clin Endocrinol Metab. 2007;92:4623–9
89. Teramoto A, Hirakawa K, Sanno N, Osamura Y. Incidental pituitary lesions in 1,000 unselected autopsy specimens. Radiology 1994;193:161–4.
90. Takanashi J, Tada H, Barkovich A, Saeki N, Kohno Y. Pituitary cysts in childhood evaluated by MR imaging. AJNR Am J Neuroradiol 2005;26:2144–7.

91. Setian N, Aguiar C, Galvao J, Crivellaro C, Dichtchekenian V, Damiani D. Rathke's cleft cyst as a cause of growth hormone deficiency and micropenis. Childs Nerv Syst 1999;15:271–3.

92. Cohan P, Foulad A, Esposito F, Martin N, Kelly D. Symptomatic Rathke's cleft cysts: a report of 24 cases. J Endocrinol Invest. 2004;27:943–8.

93. Christophe C, Flamant-Durand J, Hanquinet S, et al. MRI in seven cases of Rathke's cleft cyst in infants and children. Pediatr Radiol 1993;23:79–82.

94. Brassier G, Morandi X, Tayiar E, et al. Rathke's cleft cysts: surgical-MRI correlation in 16 symptomatic cases. J Neuroradiol 1999;26:162–71.

95. Nomura M, Tachibana O, Hasegawa M, et al. Contrast-enhanced MRI of intrasellar arachnoid cysts: relationship between the pituitary gland and cyst. Neuroradiology 1996;38:566–8.

96. Kanagaki M, Miki Y, Takahashi J, et al. MRI and CT findings of neurohypophyseal germinoma. Eur J Radiol 2004;49:204–11.

97. Packer R, Cohen B, Cooney K. Intracranial germ cell tumors. Oncologist 2000;5:312–20.

98. Jennings M, Gelman R, Hochberg F. Intracranial germ-cell tumors: natural history and pathogenesis. J Neurosurg 1985;63:155–67.

99. Hoffman H, Otsubo H, Hendrick E, et al. Intracranial germ-cell tumors in children. J Neurosurg 1991;74:545–51.

100. Matsutani M, Sano K, Takakura K, et al. Primary intracranial germ cell tumors: a clinical analysis of 153 histologically verified cases. J Neurosurg 1997;86:446–55.

101. Mootha S, Barkovich A, Grumbach M, et al. Idiopathic hypothalamic diabetes insipidus, pituitary stalk thickening, and the occult intracranial germinoma in children and adolescents. J Clin Endocrinol Metab 1997;82:1362–7.

102. Oka H, Kawano N, Tanaka T, et al. Long-term functional outcome of suprasellar germinomas: usefulness and limitations of radiotherapy. J Neurooncol 1998;40:185–90.

103. Lafay-Cousin L, Millar B, Mabbott D, et al. Limited-field radiation for bifocal germinoma. Int J Radiat Oncol Biol Phys 2006;65:486–92.

104. Packer R, Sutton L, Rosenstock J, et al. Pineal region tumors of childhood. Pediatrics 1984;74:97–102.

105. Leger J, Velasquez A, Garel C, Hassan M, Czernichow P. Thickened Pituitary Stalk on Magnetic Resonance Imaging in Children with Central Diabetes Insipidus. J Clin Endocrinol Metab 1999;84:1954–60.

106. Schulte F, Herrmann H, Muller D, et al. Pineal region tumours of childhood. Eur J Pediatr 1987;146:233–45.

107. Shibamoto Y, Oda Y, Yamashita J, Takahashi M, Kikuchi H, Abe M. The role of cerebrospinal fluid cytology in radiotherapy planning for intracranial germinoma. Int J Radiat Oncol Biol Phys 1994;29:1089–94.

108. Ogawa K, Shikama N, Toita T, et al. Long-term results of radiotherapy for intracranial germinoma: a multi-institutional retrospective review of 126 patients. Int J Radiat Oncol Biol Phys 2004;58:705–13.

109. Shirato H, Nishio M, Sawamura Y, et al. Analysis of long-term treatment of intracranial germinoma. Int J Radiat Oncol Biol Phys 1997;37:511–5.

110. Boudreau EA, Liow K, Frattali CM, et al. Hypothalamic hamartomas and seizures: distinct natural history of isolated and Pallister-Hall syndrome cases. Epilepsia 2005;46:42–7.

111. Striano S, Striano P, Sarappa C, Boccella P. The clinical spectrum and natural history of gelastic epilepsy-hypothalamic hamartoma syndrome. Seizure 2005;14:232–9.

112. Arita K, Kurisu K, Kiura Y, Iida K, Otsubo H. Hypothalamic hamartoma. Neurol Med Chir (Tokyo) 2005;45:221–31.

23 Cystic Lesions of the Sella

Brian J. Snyder, MD,
Thomas P. Naidich, MD,
and Kalmon D. Post, MD

CONTENTS

Summary

Many lesions that are found within the sella may be cystic in nature. The differential diagnosis for such lesions includes craniopharyngioma, Rathke's cleft cyst, cystic pituitary adenoma, and arachnoid cyst. This chapter describes the evaluation and management of patients who present with these sometimes troublesome lesions.

Key Words: Pituitary cyst, Rathke's cleft cyst, Craniopharyngioma, Arachnoid cyst, Cystic adenoma.

1. INTRODUCTION

Many lesions that are found within the sella may be cystic in nature. The differential diagnosis for such lesions includes craniopharyngioma, Rathke's cleft cyst (RCC), cystic pituitary adenoma, and arachnoid cyst. Many other

From: *Contemporary Endocrinology: Diagnosis and Management of Pituitary Disorders*
Edited by: B. Swearingen and B. M. K. Biller © Humana Press, Totowa, NJ

rarer entities also occur in this region and may be found in a cystic form. Although the specific radiographic findings and presentation are heterogeneous, they share certain common features. Due to anatomic location, the visual and endocrine systems become involved as the lesion grows in size. Although the presentation is varied and is influenced by the pathology, headache, visual complaints, and endocrinopathies are frequently seen at the time of diagnosis and may be the presenting complaint. Neurosurgeons are almost always involved in the management of these lesions, and many patients, if not most, will have surgery. The job of the neurosurgeon in these cases is more complex than merely the technical aspects of surgical resection, which at times is itself a dangerous task due to the unique location of the sella in the center of the skull base. It is incumbent upon the surgeon to weigh the merits of aggressive resection which may involve stripping tumor and/or capsule from the walls of the third ventricle, the optic apparatus, and the arteries along the base of the brain versus a more conservative therapy, potentially leaving tumor but sparing possible greater postoperative morbidity. The reasonable degree of aggressiveness is largely dictated by what the entity is, its known natural history, and an assessment on the likelihood of recurrence. The availability of adjuvant therapies to treat the lesion and the surgeon's familiarity with them are necessary to make the best operative decisions. We present a detailed discussion of the more common entities found in this region and touch on some of the rarer ones.

In a previous review of lesions of the sella, we found that RCC was the most common nonadenomatous lesion, followed by craniopharyngioma. Other cystic lesions also present included arachnoid and epidermoid cysts (1).

RCCs, craniopharyngiomas, epidermoids, dermoids, and neuroepithelial cysts have a common ectodermal lineage. Many of these cystic lesions can be differentiated by modern imaging techniques and present with different rates of recurrence and require different treatment paradigms. These lesions are best seen along some degree of a continuous spectrum with intermediate and indeterminate forms possible (2).

2. CRANIOPHARYNGIOMA

Craniopharyngiomas are benign tumors that arise from the epithelial remnants of Rathke's pouch. They constitute 6–9% of intracranial tumors in children and represent the third most common intracranial tumor in childhood. The peak age at presentation is 8–10 years (3). In adults, the most common age at presentation is in the sixth decade or later. They are slow-growing histologically benign tumors but nonetheless are locally aggressive and may invade the local structures including the optic nerves, blood vessels, pituitary gland, and hypothalamus. There are two main pathologic varieties of craniopharyngiomas:

the adamantinomatous and the papillary. The adamantinomatous is so named because of its hardness, which results from its frequent calcification and which can be visualized on radiographic imaging. This is the more common type in children. The papillary craniopharyngioma, the more common type in adults, rarely calcifies *(4)*.

Common symptoms at presentation include signs of increased intracranial pressure, headache, nausea, and vomiting, as well as visual disturbances. Endocrine abnormalities are present in 80–90% of patients but rarely are the chief complaint *(5)*.

Growth hormone (GH) deficiency is the most common endocrinopathy observed in the pediatric craniopharyngioma population and is found in 75% of such patients *(6)*. GH treatment is recommended in appropriate patients who have been treated and found to be free of residual tumor. Although the long-term implications of GH therapy in patients harboring residual cranio-pharyngioma are unknown, studies have not shown an increased risk of tumor growth *(7)*.

The most common presenting sign in the adult patient is gonadotrophin deficiency and in the adolescent it is delayed puberty, both due to disruptions in secretion of leutinizing hormone LH and FSH *(8)*. Estrogen, testosterone, hCG, FSH, and LH are available in commercially prepared formula for supplementation. Much less common is precocious puberty which has also been reported to occur in patients with craniopharyngiomas *(9)*. Hypothyroidism occurs in a fraction of patients with craniopharyngioma but is much more common in children following surgery and/or radiation therapy *(10)*. Furthermore, many anticonvulsants are known to interfere with thyroid function tests *(11)*. Children (25–71%) with craniopharyngiomas have ACTH dysfunction at presentation and even more on posttreatment assessments *(5,10)*. Replacement of cortisol is necessary as soon as it is recognized, and appropriate stress dosing of the drug should be used as needed. Diabetes insipidus is present in 9–38% of patients at the time of presentation *(5,8)*. The frequency of this disorder is much higher postoperatively, and it has been implicated in some of the early postoperative deaths in the pediatric population due to severe electrolyte abnormalities *(6)*. It is imperative to recognize and aggressively manage DI with DDAVP.

In children, the characteristic radiographic appearance is an enhancing suprasellar mass, with cystic components greater in volume than the solid components, that may be calcified on CT *(12)*. The craniopharyngioma often shows greater superior extension than a pituitary adenoma which may more markedly enlarge the sella. Ninety percent of the tumors calcify on CT in the pediatric age group with approximately 70% doing so in an older population *(12)*. The tumor is classically bright on T1 MR imaging, which is reflective of the high protein content of the tumor cyst (Figs. 1 and 2). On T2 and

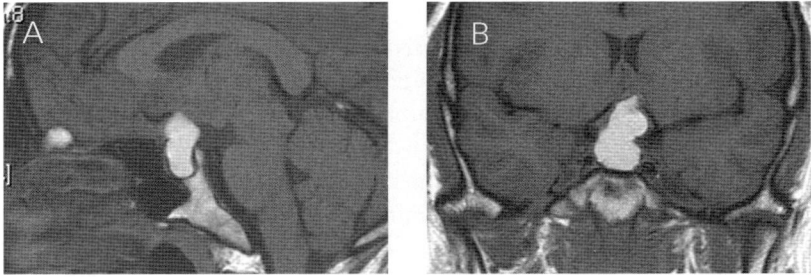

Fig. 1. (A–B)Craniopharyngioma. 25-year-old man.

FLAIR magnetic resonance imaging (MRI), the solid portions of the mass are heterogeneous while the cystic portion is hyperintense. Calcifications appear hypointense on T2-weighted images (WIs) and stand out as susceptibility artifact on gradient echo (GRE) *(13)*. The addition of a diffusion-weighted imaging (DWI) sequence may be useful in differentiating a craniopharyngioma from an epidermoid. MR spectroscopy may reveal a significant lipid

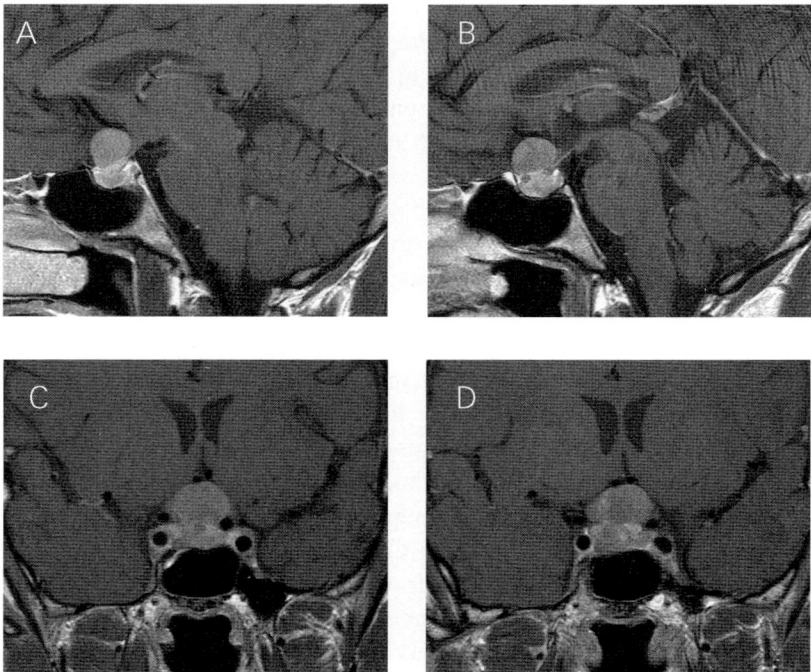

Fig. 2. (A–D)Craniopharyngioma 38-year-old woman.

peak in the cystic cavity. In both CT and MRI, the solid portions and the cyst rim almost invariably enhance. In one study, three of nine patients with craniopharyngiomas were not detected on noncontrast CT scan highlighting the need for contrast if CT is the initial screening tool *(13)*. Angiogram of craniopharyngiomas reveals an avascular mass with displacement of the circle of Willis secondary to the tumor. Craniopharyngiomas may sometimes even be suspected on plain films when the calcification is significant enough.

2.1. Surgical Treatment

The operative resection of a craniopharyngioma usually is tedious as the tumor cyst cavity is typically adherent to the hypothalamus, thalamus, vascular and optic systems. Although a craniopharyngioma may occasionally be entirely intrasellar, and may even be unsuspected at the time of transsphenoidal approach for a sellar mass, it typically has a greater suprasellar component and it is frequently best approached by using craniotomy. The transsphenoidal approach is best suited for smaller tumors, those with the majority of the lesion within the sella and/or when the preference is for cyst drainage, biopsy, or a more conservative operation. The selected approach to the lesion is somewhat dependant on its anatomic extension and surgeon preference. In smaller lesions with minimal superior extension both the pterional and the sub-frontal approaches are reasonable for resection. The fronto-basal interhemispheric approach has been described, which is a modification of a bilateral subfrontal approach. Some authors have found this to yield the best results *(14)*. When the pterional approach is used, some prefer to take the frontal bone opening more medial than is normally done to provide for visualization of the lesion both from a frontal and a temporal direction *(15)*. Tumors that extend further into the interpeduncular cistern are likely to be better approached through the pterional approach with wider splitting of the sylvian fissure. Tumors that have greater superior extension into the third ventricle may be approached from above, through an interhemispheric transcallosal approach. Although gross-total resection is the goal, the consequences of overly aggressive surgery in this very sensitive region of the brain cannot be overstressed. We much prefer to leave tumor adherent to the optic nerves and walls of the hypothalamus than to put undue traction on these regions in efforts to aggressively strip the capsule which may leave the patient with a significantly worse outcome.

Results of surgical resection demonstrate the difficulty operating in this region. In a series of 66 children undergoing surgical resection, a gross total resection was achieved in 50%, subtotal in 36%, and partial in 14%. Thirty-six percent of the patients felt to have achieved gross total resection presented with recurrence over an average follow-up of 7 years and 54% of those with residual tumor progressed. Ninety percent needed postoperative hormonal replacement and 15% had impaired neuropsychological testing *(16)*. Mark et al. *(17)* reported a mortality of 12%, hypothalamic dysfunction in 40%, and visual deterioration in 19%. In Yasargil's series of pediatric tumors, he reported a "good" clinical outcome in only 60% of patients with a 20% morbidity rate *(18)* whereas Laws reported successful results in 81% of patients in his series *(19)*.

2.2. Radiation Therapy

The management strategy for craniopharyngiomas remains complex and is somewhat disputed. As noted above, there is controversy surrounding the degree of aggressiveness the surgeon should adopt in pursuit of a gross total resection. There are many tumors that are not completely resected because of the risk of significant morbidity. These patients are referred for adjuvant therapy, often after a change in the residual tumor.

Traditional external beam-fractionated irradiation has been used to treat craniopharyngiomas with relatively good tumor control. Due to its high morbidity including neuropsychological problems, vasculitis, and visual deterioration, it is relegated as a treatment to those failing most other first- or second-line treatments. Radiation therapy as an adjuvant treatment has been shown to provide better progression-free survival than surgery alone *(20)*. The use of radiation as a salvage therapy in children presenting with recurrent craniopharyngioma is associated with high tumor control rates. Modern three-dimensional conformal radiation treatment utilizes CT and MRI for target localization. With pretreatment planning, higher doses of radiation can be safely given to tumors with lower degrees of morbidity and higher degrees of safety. This is highlighted when comparing the modern 10-year survival in children treated with radiation therapy which is 85–96% with those treated before the availability of such software 56–78% *(21)*.

Stereotactic radiosurgery (SRS) and fractioned stereotactic radiotherapy (SRT) is of increasing importance in the treatment of craniopharyngiomas. Radiosurgery provides the advantage of being able to deliver a high dose of radiation to a more specified region of the brain. The modality is somewhat limited in craniopharyngiomas because of their size and proximity to the optic chiasm, as ideally they need to be <2.5 cm in size and >3 mm in distance from the optic chiasm. Although the tolerance of the optic chiasm to SRT is 54 Gy/30 fractions, it is only 8–9 Gy in a single fraction *(22)*. Control rates of 70–100% have been reported in follow-up of 1–5 years *(23,24)*. SRT delivers radiation in a more precise fashion than conventional external beam in a fractionated fashion. The patient does not need to have a rigid frame placed as is needed for radiosurgery, and due to the fractionated but more precise delivery, there may be a biologic advantage of sparing vital neural structures in the radiation field which is coupled to improved tumor control. Preliminary reports of the use of SRT have demonstrated both the feasibility and the efficacy of SRT in children with brain tumors including craniopharyngiomas *(25,26)*.

The complications due to radiation can include damage to the optic chiasm, endocrinopathy due to damage to the pituitary gland, and neurocognitive and neuropsychological disorders such as appetite and sleep disorders due to damage to the hypothalamus *(27,28)*. Fourteen percent of children treated in one institution with conservative surgery and radiation experienced decline in the periradiation time period with new hydrocephalus, visual deterioration, and neurologic deficit due to cystic enlargement necessitating surgical intervention *(29)*.

2.3. Intracystic Therapies

Stereotactic injection of beta-emitting isotopes has been used as an adjuvant treatment for cystic tumors. The injection of both yttrium-90 (^{90}Y) and phosphorous-32 (^{32}P) are used in Europe and the USA, respectively. In the Pittsburgh experience with ^{32}P, they found cyst control rates at 5 and 10 years to be 76 and 70% when used in a heterogeneous population *(30)*. Visual function improved or stabilized in approximately half of the treatment group. Primary and recurrent treated patients, 48 and 11% respectively, who had normal pituitary function before treatment maintained their normal endocrinologic function *(30)*. Intracystic ^{32}P does not, however, treat the solid component of the lesion. Patients who have both a solid and a cystic component treated with ^{32}P still need to be referred for either surgical or radiation treatment to manage this portion. The results from European studies utilizing ^{90}Y demonstrated similar efficacy to that of ^{32} *(31,32)*.

Intratumoral injections of chemotherapeutics have also been used as a management strategy for craniopharyngiomas. Procedures for injection typically involve the insertion of a catheter with a subcutaneous reservoir (Ommaya reservoir) into the tumor cyst under direct visualization or with the aide of stereotaxy. Following this, the cyst is typically injected to ensure that there is no extrusion or direct continuity with the subarachnoid space and CSF, and following this the treatment is begun.

2.3.1. BLEOMYCIN

Bleomycin is an inhibitor of DNA synthesis and has been demonstrated to be effective in the treatment of various epithelial tumors *(33)*. Early studies demonstrated some degree of efficacy of bleomycin in the treatment of craniopharyngiomas with a large cystic component and minimal response to tumors that were predominately solid in nature *(34,35)*. In a heterogeneous group of patients, some with primary disease and some with recurrence, intracystic bleomycin was found to result in the disappearance of 38% of cysts and a decrease in size by 50–70% in all of the others who were treated *(36)*. Takahashi et al. *(33)* treated their patients underwent primary surgical resection; patients with residual or recurrent solid component were considered for reoperation and/or radiation. Recurrence in the form of cyst was treated by intracystic injection of bleomycin. Three of their four patients with predominately cystic tumors were reported to be disease free 21–26 years posttreatment. The other patient presented with cyst recurrence and was treated with a second injection of bleomycin *(33)*. One of the main risks associated with bleomycin is that it is a neurotoxin, and leakage of bleomycin has been associated with epilepsy and TIAs *(34,37)*. This can be avoided by assessing the cyst for water tightness before the initiation of treatment as well a decreasing the dose and/or volume of injection per treatment.

2.3.2. INTERFERON ALPHA

Interferon (IFN)-α has been previously shown to be active against some squamous cell carcinomas; this prompted investigation of its use in cranio-pharyngiomas *(38)*. Its further advantage over other drugs such as bleomycin is that it is not a neurotoxin. Transient chemical arachnoiditis and chronic fatigue syndrome have been reported to be side effects *(39)*. A series of ten pediatric patients newly diagnosed with a predominantly cystic craniopharyn-gioma underwent placement of Ommaya reservoirs. Of the 9 who began an IFN-α protocol, 7 experienced either a complete response or a >90% disap-pearance in tumor volume, and 2 experienced a partial response (>70% decrease in tumor size) over 1–4 years of follow up *(38)*. One of the patients presented with new onset of depression following initiation of treatment, necessitating oral antidepressants. Although there are few other reports at this time, the use of intracystic agents is appealing if durable levels of control can be documented in larger studies.

3. RATHKE'S CLEFT CYST

RCCs are thought to originate from the embryonic remnants of Rathke's pouch and were named after the German anatomist Martin Heinrich Rathke. They are nonneoplastic in nature and are located in the region of the interme-diate lobe of the pituitary gland. RCCs are found in high frequency in routine autopsy series (3.7–22%), with the majority of these remaining asymptomatic throughout life *(40)*. Eighty percent of these are found at the interface between the anterior and the posterior lobes of the pituitary *(40,41)*. Only 5.4% of RCC were found to increase over time in one series *(42)*. Symptomatic RCCs have been thought of as relatively rare lesions. In the modern era of MRI, RCCs are being more frequently recognized. RCCs are reported to represent 7–15%

of intrasellar/suprasellar lesions and 7–8% in transsphenoidal surgery series *(43,44)*, with the most frequent lesion being the pituitary adenoma.

Histologically, RCCs consist of a single or pseudostratified epithelium with an underlying layer of connective tissue. The epithelium may contain cilia, goblet cells, squamous, and/or basal cells *(45)*.

Embryologically, the development of RCC occurs when a rostral outpouching of the primitive oral cavity occurs at the 3rd or 4th week of gestation meets a downward projection from the diencephalon. Together, these structures form the anterior lobe, pars tuberalis, and intermediate lobe of the pituitary gland *(2)*. In the region of the pars intermedia a cleft exists. When this cleft fails to regress, an RCC is postulated to form *(46)*.

Symptomatic RCCs are found within all age groups, but there are presentation peaks in the fourth through sixth decades. The most common presenting sign in patients with RCC is headache, endocrine disturbance, or visual disturbance depending on the source cited *(44,47)*. Although headache is ubiquitous in the population as a whole, many patients will first be diagnosed with RCCs during evaluation for a headache. In those studies which specifically reviewed this symptom, 63–70% of patients appeared to obtain relief of their headaches when their RCCs were resected or drained *(43,48)*. The most common endocrinologic finding at presentation is hyperprolactinemia *(43)*. Hyperprolactinemia in RCCs is likely due to the cyst growing large enough to interfere with the infundibular system and is more frequently observed in women *(47)*. One series found a 20% incidence of DI in patients presenting with RCCs, and within this series, DI was much more frequent in the older subset of the population that present with the disease versus younger patients *(44)*. DI, as a presenting symptom, was not unique to this report, and in fact, all patients who are reported to present with DI (0–14%) are >35 years of age *(44,49,50)*. Although uncommon, multiple series present a patient or two who present with pituitary dwarfism, due to decreased GH secretion from the gland secondary to compression by the RCC *(43)*.

RCCs are generally heterogeneously appearing on MRI. Whether the cyst wall enhances is a matter of some debate. Most feel that typical RCCs do not enhance after the administration of gadolinium, but this may be difficult to interpret secondary to the enhancement of the nearby normal pituitary gland. Some series present cases with obvious enhancement; these cysts may be more likely to display squamous metaplasia within the cyst wall. The MRI features of the cyst contents in RCC have been reported by multiple authors and are very varied; this is likely to be due to the heterogeneous nature of these contents (Figs 3and 4). It has been postulated that the cyst contents are altered by the activity of secretory cells within the cyst wall and the rate of desquamation of cells into the cyst cavity from the wall *(51)*. Four patterns of cyst intensity

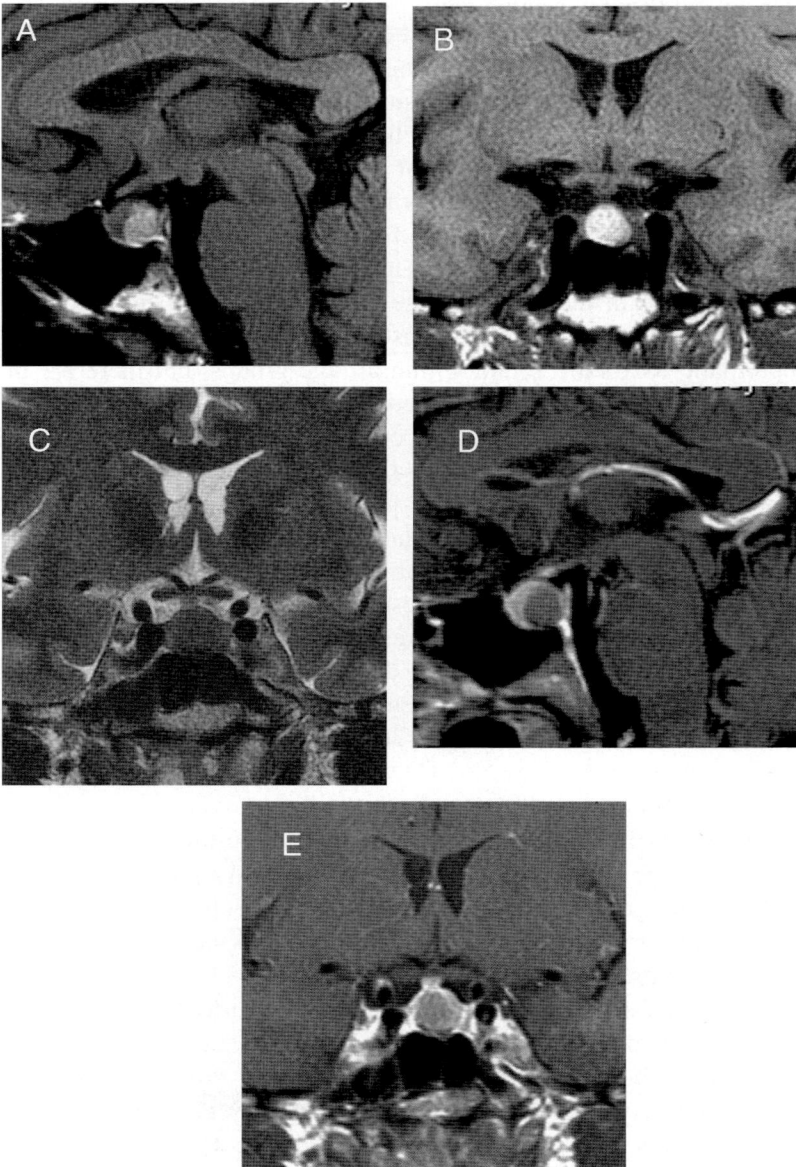

Fig. 3. (A–E) Rathke's cleft cyst. 49-year-old woman.

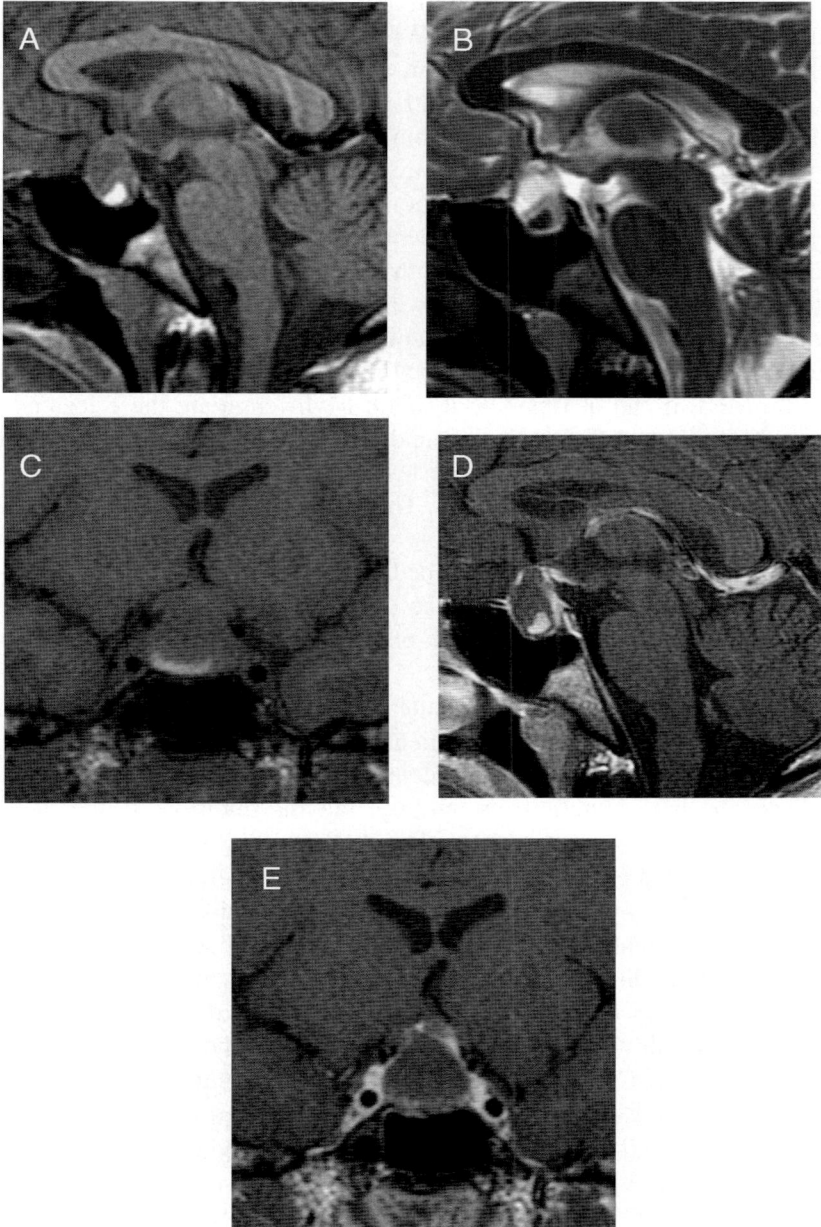

Fig. 4. (A–E) Rathke's cleft cyst. 49-year-old woman.

have been described in RCCs based on the four combinations of high and low T1 and T2 WIs. The T1 WI low/T2 WI high and the T1 iso-to-high/T2 high are the most common patterns with an approximately 30–40% incidence for each *(43,52)*. The high intensity on T1 has been reported to be a product of protein and mucopolysaccharides within the cyst, while the high-intensity T2 is a product of water within the cyst cavity *(53)*. The relationship between the cyst cavity contents and the presentation has not been thoroughly elucidated. One report analyzing a total of 78 patients noted that patients whose RCC had contents similar to CSF presented with larger cysts and visual disturbances (postulated to be due to the slower growing nature of this type of cyst), whereas those cysts appearing more proteinaceous on MRI frequently presented with smaller cysts and other symptoms. *(54)*. Due to the heterogeneous nature of RCCs on MRI, it can at times be difficult to differentiate these lesions from other cystic lesions of the pituitary gland. The lack of strong rim enhancement is the best way of discriminating the lesion from craniopharyngiomas, cystic pituitary adenomas, and other lesions. The presence of an intracystic nodule of low signal intensity on T2 and possible visualization of a high signal intensity nodule on T1 lesion has been described in one study and was found in 40% of cases *(55)*. Other authors have also described nodules within the RCC in some patients *(46,52)*. In up to 8.3% of patients with RCC, the lesion exists as a solely suprasellar mass *(56–58)*.

Patients who present with a visual deficit and/or endocrinopathy need surgical decompression/resection. Patients who present with headache or have asymptomatic cysts discovered incidentally are less straightforward. Those with headache may benefit from surgery, but the duration of and nature of the headache should be fully explored, and the possibility of treatment failure with surgery should be fully explained to the patient before surgical resection. Patients with very small cysts that are incidentally discovered should most likely be followed with interval imaging to assure that there is no progression of their disease. In addition, some patients who present with transient symptoms initially managed in a conservative fashion have had documented regression of the cysts on follow-up imaging with resolution of their symptoms.

Resection of RCC generally will improve the visual function as well as endocrinologic status. Aggressive resection is associated with increased risk of postoperative DI and other endocrine dysfunction. Headache has been found to resolve or improve in 52 and 39% of patients respectively in one series *(47)*. In another, 99% of patients who presented with visual field disturbances had improvement on follow up and in our series 40% had resolution, 30% improvement, and 30% had no significant change *(47,59)*. Resolution of endocrine dysfunction was not as reliable and was varied depending on the preoperative endocrine status. We found 10% of patients developed new anterior pituitary deficiencies postoperatively, while 27% of patient with preoperative dysfunction experienced improvement *(47)*. Others found that 100% of patients with hyperprolactinemia improved following surgery, but only 18, 14, and 18% of patients with GH deficiency, hypocortisolemia, and hypogonadism, respectively, did so *(59)*. Two patients developed new hypogonadism. In the same series, the authors report that in the early cases performed they had a very high rate of postoperative DI (42%) which prompted them to modify their techniques to lower this rate. The subsequent patients who were resected in a less radical fashion only had a 9% rate of DI *(59)*. In our series, we had a 6% rate of permanent DI following surgery but noted a much higher rate (50%) in the patients who underwent a more radical surgery.

The application of absolute alcohol into the cyst cavity, if no violation of the arachnoid is present, has been advocated and adopted by some with the theory that it may effect a cellular death in the cyst wall *(48)*. Caution must be observed, however, as a recent report of a patient who was treated with alcohol developed blindness, anosmia, and a partial third nerve palsy following the fourth resection of a recurrent RCC, when the alcohol mixed with the patient's CSF through a violated arachnoid membrane *(60)*.

Several authors have suggested that RCC and craniopharyngioma exist along a spectrum of aggressiveness. Squamous metaplasia has been found by some to be associated with recurrence *(47,56)*.

Whether to perform an aggressive resection remains controversial. A full evacuation of the cyst contents and liberal opening of the cyst wall was advocated as early as 1966 by Fager and Carter *(61)*. We favor transsphenoidal surgical resection and drainage of RCCs. We adopt an approach in which we prefer to be very conservative in resection of the cyst wall. Although recurrence of RCC has been shown to be linked with incomplete resection or decompression and biopsy of RCC, studies have also shown an increased risk of DI in patients undergoing radical resection of the cyst and wall *(47,56)*. While we found a recurrence in 18% of patients, in our experience re-operation can be performed with minimal morbidity. We generally perform a very conservative operation, leaving the cyst wall along all vital structures and the pituitary gland if a very distinct plane is not evident. We believe that repeated drainage of an RCC is a less morbid procedure than an aggressive resection with possible permanent neurologic or hormonal sequelae.

4. CYSTIC PITUITARY ADENOMA

Pituitary adenomas may be cystic in nature. Their management parallels the management of noncystic pituitary adenomas and is beyond the scope of this chapter and is thoroughly covered in the remainder of this book. Cystic pituitary adenomas are heterogeneous hypodense lesions on CT scan and hypointense on T1-weighted MR imaging with rim enhancement (Fig. 5) *(62)*. They may have large solid components, or more rarely in our experience, are largely cystic with small nodular solid regions. These lesions should be suspected in patients who are noted to have enhancing sellar mass with erosion into the sphenoid. They may have large suprasellar extension as well. The stalk can be noted to be deviated posteriorly with adenomas, which has been proposed as a further method of distinguishing these tumors from RCCs which displace the stalk anteriorly *(57)*.

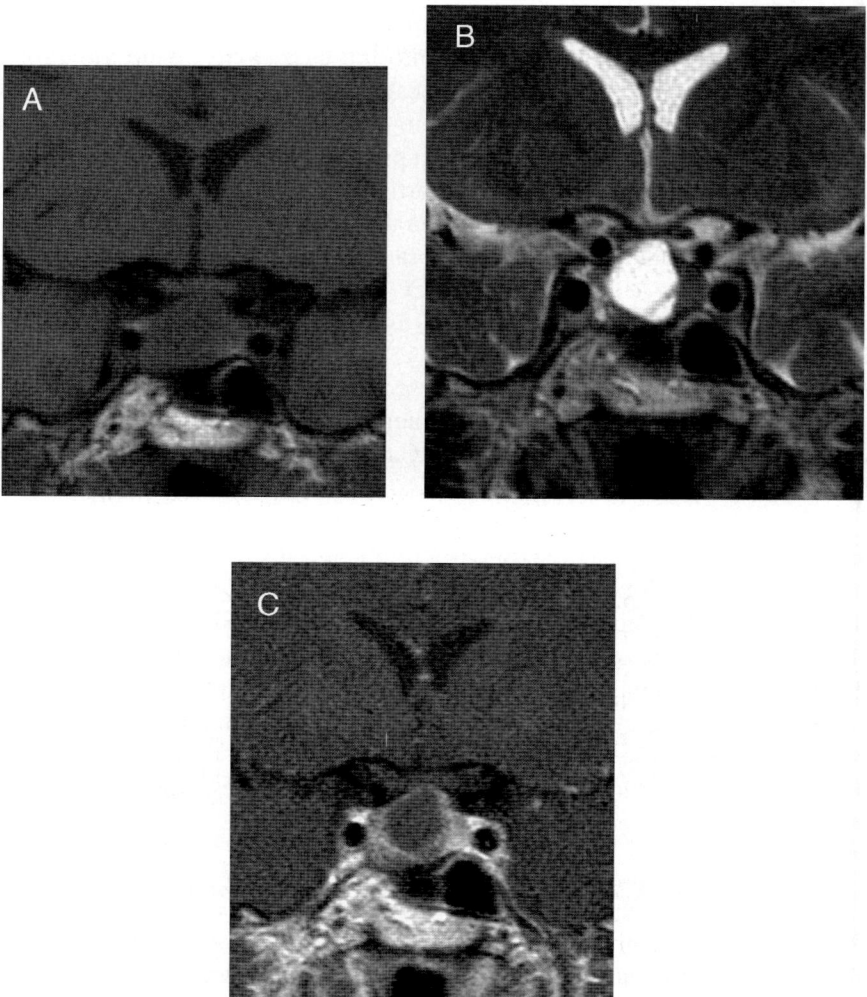

Fig. 5. (A–C) Cystic pituitary adenoma. 73-year-old woman.

5. MENINGIOMA

Meningiomas are known to arise from the tuberculum sella, the planum sphenoidale, the diaphragma sella, and rarely the anterior clinoid process *(63)*. Meningiomas may be cystic in nature with an incidence of 1.6–7%, depending on the series cited *(64–66)*. In these patients, the cyst may represent a region of central necrosis, intratumoral hemorrhage, or loculation of CSF. Differentiating these tumors from other cystic lesion in the region may be complex. Visualization of a dural attachment and the dural "tail" may provide a strong suggestion that the patient has a meningioma *(63)*. Meningiomas are known to calcify in 15–20% of cases which may create difficulty differentiating some from craniopharyngiomas *(67)*. Suprasellar meningiomas are classically approached through a craniotomy, but cases of entirely intrasellar meningiomas may be approached through a transsphenoidal operation, and in some cases, it may be only after pathologic examination that the diagnosis of cystic meningioma of the sella is confirmed.

Incidentally discovered meningiomas in the sella can be observed if they are small and there is no encroachment of the optic apparatus, neurologic deficit, or endocrine dysfunction.

6. ARACHNOID CYSTS

Intrasellar arachnoid cysts are relatively rare. Arachnoid cysts can develop anywhere in the subarachnoid space. Although there is not typically arachnoid tissue below the level of the diaphragma sella, intrasellar arachnoid cysts are thought to arise when arachnoid herniates into the sella through a defect in the diaphragma and then secondarily becomes separated from the subarachnoid space. Others arise from small arachnoid remnants that may exist below the diaphragma sella. Symptomatic arachnoid cysts in adults most typically present with headache followed by decreased visual acuity and less commonly hypopituitarism *(68)*. In children, progressive hydrocephalus and endocrine dysfunction are most common at presentation of *supra*-sellar arachnoid cysts *(69)*.

Arachnoid cysts in other locations are typically recognized on MRI by a cyst-filled cavity with identical imaging characteristics to CSF (Fig. 6) *(70)*. In some cases, the cyst may have a higher protein content or evidence of hemorrhage within it, altering its MRI appearance. Meyer et al. found 2 of 13 cysts had T1-weighted imaging with the fluid characteristics of higher intensity than CSF *(71)*. The superficially similar "empty sella" may be distinguished from an arachnoid cyst by identifying the characteristic extension of the pituitary stalk to the floor of the sella turcica, without deflection, in cases of empty sella (Fig. 7).

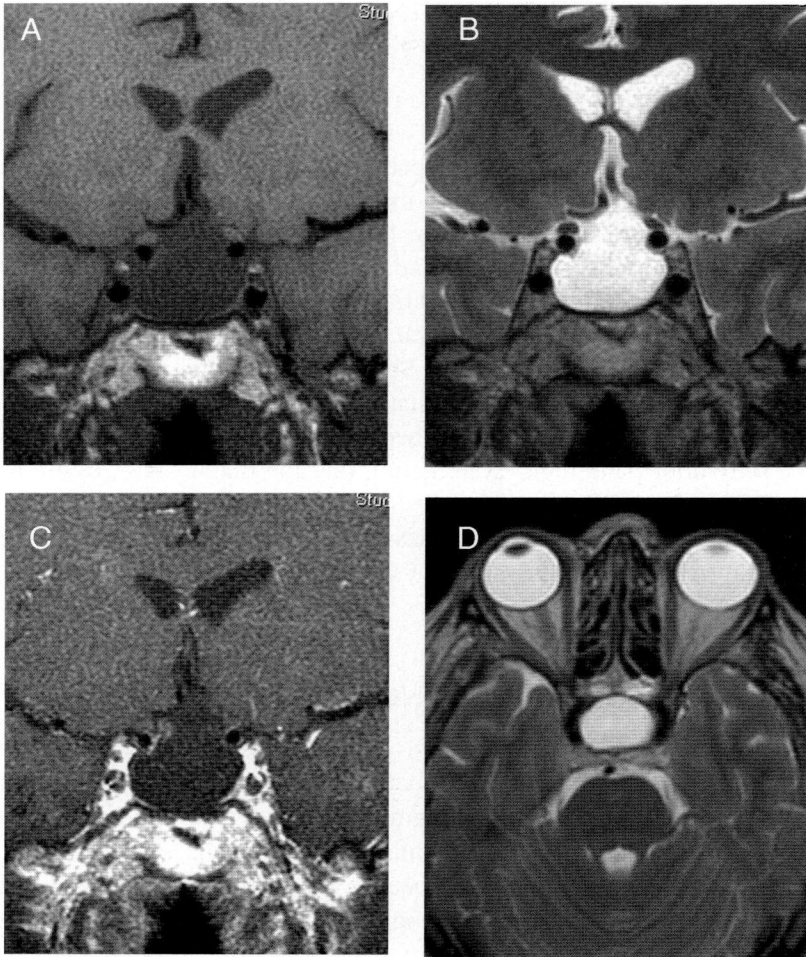

Fig. 6. (A–D) Arachnoid cyst. 63-year-old woman.

The indications for surgical therapy of intrasellar arachnoid cysts are similar to those for other nonsecreting lesions of the region. Patients who present with visual loss or endocrine dysfunction should be offered early surgery. Patients with severe headaches, in similar fashion to the management paradigm for RCCs, may benefit from cyst decompression. The appropriate approach to these lesions is somewhat guided by the exact size and extent of the lesion at diagnosis. We favor a primary approach through a transsphenoidal route with biopsy and drainage of the cyst. If the cyst recurs, it can easily be approached via reoperation through the same route without significant morbidity. We would

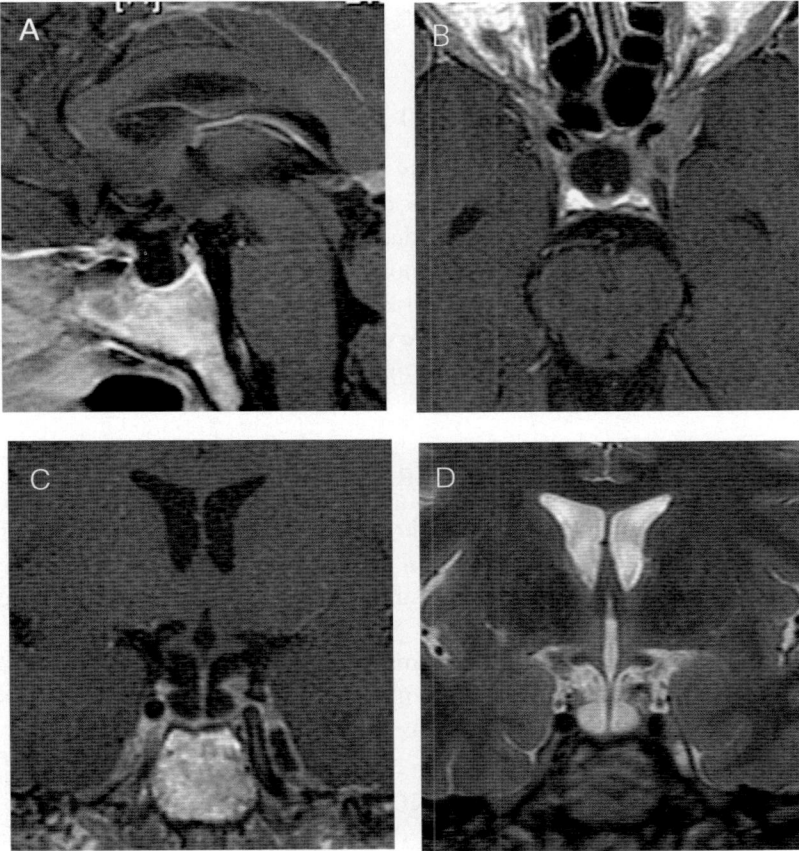

Fig. 7. (A–D). Empty sella. 43-year-old man.

reserve craniotomy for cyst fenestration or placement of shunts into the cyst cavity for patients who fail transsphenoidal decompression and have persistent symptoms, or in the very rare instances where a sellar arachnoid cyst has such extensive superior extension that it may better be approached through a craniotomy.

7. SPHENOID SINUS MUCOCELE

These lesions arise from mucus in the sphenoid sinus when the sphenoid sinus ostium is obstructed. They can extend into the pituitary fossa as well as further into the cranial cavity. Typically, they may present with headache, anosmia, nasal symptoms, and ophthalmoplegia. Plain X-rays and CT scan are helpful in demonstrating bony erosion. A nonenhancing cystic lesion will be visible on CT, with an MRI which has a bright cystic cavity on T2-weighted imaging *(68,72)*.

8. EPIDERMOID AND DERMOID

Both these lesions are very rarely found within the sella. They result from inclusion of epithelial elements during neural tube closure. Dermoids contain desquamated epithelium, sebaceous material dermal appendages and are soft, white, and flaky *(73)*. Epidermoids contain a white cheesy material and most frequently are found in the suprasellar region, cerebello-pontine angle, fourth and lateral ventricles. Both are nonenhancing on CT and are usually hypointense on T1 (unless there is a high lipid content) and hyperintense on T2 WIs.

9. OTHER LESIONS

Cystercercosis is caused by *Taenia solium*. Once the parasite enters the circulation, it can deposit eggs within muscle and brain. These lesions may cause seizure, hydrocephalus, and/or stroke. Lesions in the sella are extremely rare *(74)*.

Pituitary abscesses, giant aneurysms, and aneurysmal bone cysts of the sphenoid are all very rare lesions that must also be considered in a differential diagnosis of cystic lesions of the sella.

10. CONCLUSION

Cystic lesions of the sella and parasellar region are not uncommon. It is imperative to be aware of the differing natural histories of these lesions. It must also be remembered that radiation and other adjuvant therapy are available to augment treatment, especially of craniopharyngiomas and pituitary tumors with significant residual. The decision to approach these lesion transphenoidally or by craniotomy, or from a staged combined approach, is dependent on the anatomy and site and degree of compression. Although techniques for the standard approaches to these lesions are familiar to most neurosurgeons, we believe that large cystic sellar lesions are extremely complex entities to treat, and favor their management by a multidisciplinary team approach which includes endocrinologists and neurosurgeons with experience in the management of lesions of the pituitary. The goal of gross-total resection is no longer acceptable without serious consideration as to the potential sequelae of the proposed approach, alternative treatments, and natural history of the lesion.

We favor surgery to remove as much tumor as is safe, while foregoing further resection if morbidity is likely, even if this necessitates further surgical procedures in the future for recurrence. We believe, and the senior author's personal experience has shown, that reoperation for recurrence is well tolerated and is better for long-term patient outcome, than is leaving a patient with severe permanent visual or hypothalamic dysfunction after an overly aggressive attempt at complete resection.

REFERENCES

1. Freda PU, Wardlaw SL, Post KD. Unusual causes of sellar/parasellar masses in a large transsphenoidal surgical series. J Clin Endocrinol Metab 1996; 81(10):3455–9.
2. Harrison MJ, Morgello S, Post KD. Epithelial cystic lesions of the sellar and parasellar region: a continuum of ectodermal derivatives? J Neurosurg, 1994; 80(6): 1018–25.
3. Russell D, Rubinstein L. Pathology of Tumors of the Nervous System, 5th ed. Baltimore: Williams and Wilkins. 1989, pp. 695–702.
4. Prabhu VC, Brown HG. The pathogenesis of craniopharyngiomas. Childs Nerv Syst 2005;21(8–9):622–7.
5. Sklar CA. Craniopharyngioma: endocrine abnormalities at presentation. Pediatr Neurosurg, 1994;21 Suppl 1:8–20.
6. Halac I, Zimmerman D. Endocrine manifestations of craniopharyngioma. Childs Nerv Syst 2005; 21(8–9):640–8.
7. Moshang T, Jr Rundle AC, Graves DA, et al. Brain tumor recurrence in children treated with growth hormone: the National Cooperative Growth Study experience. J Pediatr 1996;128(5 Pt 2):S4–7.
8. Paja M, Garcia-Uria J, Salame F, et al. Hypothalamic-pituitary dysfunction in patients with craniopharyngioma. Clin Endocrinol (Oxf) 1995;42(5): 467–73.
9. Banna M, Hoare RD, Stanley P, Till K. Craniopharyngioma in children. J Pediatr 1973;83(5):781–5.
10. de Vries L, Lazar L, Phillip M. Craniopharyngioma: presentation and endocrine sequelae in 36 children. J Pediatr Endocrinol Metab 2003;16(5):703–10.
11. Isojarvi JI, Turkka J, Pakarinen AJ, et al. Thyroid function in men taking carbamazepine, oxcarbazepine, or valproate for epilepsy. Epilepsia 2001;42(7):930–4.
12. Curran JG , O'Connor E. Imaging of craniopharyngioma. Childs Nerv Syst 2005;21 (8–9):635–9.
13. Hald JK, Eldevik OP, Skalpe IO. Craniopharyngioma identification by CT and MR imaging at 1.5 T. Acta Radiol 1995;36(2):142–7.
14. Fahlbusch R, et al. Surgical treatment of craniopharyngiomas: experience with 168 patients. J Neurosurg 1999;90(2):237–50.
15. Scott RM. Craniopharyngioma: a personal (Boston) experience. Childs Nerv Syst 2005; 21(8–9):773–7.
16. Sainte-Rose, C, Puget S, Wray A, et al. Craniopharyngioma: the pendulum of surgical management. Childs Nerv Syst, 2005;21(8–9): 691–5.
17. Mark RJ, Lutge WR, Shimizu KT, et al. Craniopharyngioma: treatment in the CT and MR imaging era. Radiology 1995;197(1):195–8.
18. Yasargil MG, Curcic M, Kis M, et al. Total removal of craniopharyngiomas. Approaches and long-term results in 144 patients. J Neurosurg 1990;73(1):3–11.
19. Laws ER, Jr. Transsphenoidal removal of craniopharyngioma. Pediatr Neurosurg 1994;21 Suppl 1:57–63.

20. Kalapurakal JA. Radiation therapy in the management of pediatric craniopharyngiomas – a review. Childs Nerv Syst 2005;21(8–9):808–16.

21. Habrand JL, Ganry O, Couanet D, et al. The role of radiation therapy in the management of craniopharyngioma: a 25-year experience and review of the literature. Int J Radiat Oncol Biol Phys 1999;44(2):255–63.

22. Tishler RB, Loeffler JL, Lunsford LD, et al. Tolerance of cranial nerves of the cavernous sinus to radiosurgery. Int J Radiat Oncol Biol Phys 1993;27(2):215–21.

23. Amendola BE, Wolf A, Coy SR, et al. Role of radiosurgery in craniopharyngiomas: a preliminary report. Med Pediatr Oncol 2003;41(2):123–7.

24. Chung WY, Pan DHC, Shiau CY, et al. Gamma knife radiosurgery for craniopharyngiomas. J Neurosurg 2000;93 Suppl 3:47–56.

25. Kalapurakal JA, Kepka A , Bista T, et al. Fractionated stereotactic radiotherapy for pediatric brain tumors: the Chicago children's experience. Childs Nerv Syst 2000;16(5):296–302, discussion 303.

26. Loeffler JS, Kooy HM, Tarbell NJ. The emergence of conformal radiotherapy: special implications for pediatric neuro-oncology. Int J Radiat Oncol Biol Phys 1999;44(2):237–8.

27. DeVile CJ, Grant DB, Hayward RD, et al. Growth and endocrine sequelae of craniopharyngioma. Arch Dis Child 1996;75(2):108–14.

28. Palm L, Nordin V, Elmqvist D, et al. Sleep and wakefulness after treatment for craniopharyngioma in childhood; influence on the quality and maturation of sleep. Neuropediatrics 1992;23(1):39–45.

29. Rajan B, Ashley S, Gorman C, et al. Craniopharyngioma: improving outcome by early recognition and treatment of acute complications. Int J Radiat Oncol Biol Phys 1997;37(3):517–21.

30. Hasegawa T, Kondziolka D, Hadjipanayis CG, et al. Management of cystic craniopharyngiomas with phosphorus-32 intracavitary irradiation. Neurosurgery 2004;54(4):813–20, discussion 820–2.

31. Van den Berge JH, Blaauw G, Breeman WAP, et al. Intracavitary brachytherapy of cystic craniopharyngiomas. J Neurosurg 1992;77(4):545–50.

32. Voges J, Sturm V, Lehrke R, et al. Cystic craniopharyngioma: long-term results after intracavitary irradiation with stereotactically applied colloidal beta-emitting radioactive sources. Neurosurgery 1997;40(2):263–9, discussion 269–70.

33. Takahashi H, Yamaguchi F, Teramoto A. Long-term outcome and reconsideration of intracystic chemotherapy with bleomycin for craniopharyngioma in children. Childs Nerv Syst 2005;2(8–9):701–4.

34. Broggi G, Giorgi C, Franzini A, et al. Preliminary results of intracavitary treatment of craniopharyngioma with bleomycin. J Neurosurg Sci 1989;33(1):145–8.

35. Takahashi H, Nakazawa S, Shimura T. Evaluation of postoperative intratumoral injection of bleomycin for craniopharyngioma in children. J Neurosurg 1985;62(1):120–7.

36. Mottolese C, Stan H, Hermier M, et al. Intracystic chemotherapy with bleomycin in the treatment of craniopharyngiomas. Childs Nerv Syst 2001;17(12):724–30.

37. Zanon N. Bleomycin Treatment in Cystic Craniopharyngiomas, in Pediatric Neurosurgery, Choux M, et al. editors. Edinburgh: Churchill Livingstone;1999.

38. Cavalheiro S, Dastoli PA, Silva NS, et al. Use of interferon alpha in intratumoral chemotherapy for cystic craniopharyngioma. Childs Nerv Syst 2005;21(8–9):719–24.

39. Chamberlain MC. A phase II trial of intra-cerebrospinal fluid alpha interferon in the treatment of neoplastic meningitis. Cancer 2002;94(10):2675–80.

40. Teramoto A, Hirikawa K, Sanno N, et al. Incidental pituitary lesions in 1,000 unselected autopsy specimens. Radiology 1994;193(1):161–4.

41. Burger P, Scheithauer B, Vogel F. Surgical Pathology of the Nervous System and Its Coverings, 4th ed. Baltimore: Churchill Livingstone;2002.
42. Sanno N, Teramoto A, Osamura RY, et al. Pathology of pituitary tumors. Neurosurg Clin N Am 2003;14(1):25–39, vi.
43. el-Mahdy W, Powell M. Transsphenoidal management of 28 symptomatic Rathke's cleft cysts, with special reference to visual and hormonal recovery. Neurosurgery 1998;42(1): 7–16, discussion 16–7.
44. Isono M, Kamida T, Kobayashi H, et al; Clinical features of symptomatic Rathke's cleft cyst. Clin Neurol Neurosurg 2001;103(2):96–100.
45. Matsushima T, Fukui M, Ohta M, et al. Ciliated and goblet cells in craniopharyngioma. Light and electron microscopic studies at surgery and autopsy. Acta Neuropathol (Berl) 1980;50(3):199–205.
46. Byun WM, Kim OL, Kim D. MR imaging findings of Rathke's cleft cysts: significance of intracystic nodules. AJNR Am J Neuroradiol 2000;21(3): 485–8.
47. Benveniste RJ, King WA, Walsh J, et al. Surgery for Rathke cleft cysts: technical considerations and outcomes. J Neurosurg 2004;101(4):577–84.
48. Ross DA, Norman D, Wilson CB. Radiologic characteristics and results of surgical management of Rathke's cysts in 43 patients. Neurosurgery 1992;30(2):173–8, discussion 178–9.
49. Midha R, Jay V, Smyth HS. Transsphenoidal management of Rathke's cleft cysts. A clinicopathological review of 10 cases. Surg Neurol 1991;35(6): 446–54.
50. Nemoto Y, Inoue Y, Fukuda T, et al. MR appearance of Rathke's cleft cysts. Neuroradiology 1988;30(2):155–9.
51. Saeki N. Sunami K, Sugaya Y, et al. MRI findings and clinical manifestations in Rathke's cleft cyst. Acta Neurochir (Wien) 1999;141(10):1055–61.
52. Sumida M, Uozumi T, Mukada K, et al. Rathke cleft cysts: correlation of enhanced MR and surgical findings. AJNR Am J Neuroradiol 1994;15(3):525–32.
53. Onesti ST, Wisniewski T, Post KD. Pituitary hemorrhage into a Rathke's cleft cyst. Neurosurgery 1990;27(4):644–6.
54. Takeichi Y, Nakasu Y, Handa J. MRI of symptomatic Rathke's cleft cyst: MRI intensity of cyst contents and clinical manifestations. Jpn J Neurosurg 1997;6: 448–55.
55. Binning MJ, Gottfried ON, Osborn AG, et al. Rathke cleft cyst intracystic nodule: a characteristic magnetic resonance imaging finding. J Neurosurg 2005;103(5): 837–40.
56. Kim JE, Kim JH, Kim OL, et al. Surgical treatment of symptomatic Rathke cleft cysts: clinical features and results with special attention to recurrence. J Neurosurg 2004;100(1):33–40.
57. Kleinschmidt-DeMasters BK, Lillehei KO, Stears JC. The pathologic, surgical, and MR spectrum of Rathke cleft cysts. Surg Neurol 1995;44(1):19–26, discussion 26–7.
58. Shin JL, Asa SL, Woodhouse LJ, et al. Cystic lesions of the pituitary: clinicopathological features distinguishing craniopharyngioma, Rathke's cleft cyst, and arachnoid cyst. J Clin Endocrinol Metab 1999;84(11):3972–82.
59. Aho CJ, Liu C, Zelman V, et al. Surgical outcomes in 118 patients with Rathke cleft cysts. J Neurosurg 2005;102(2): 189–93.
60. Hsu HY, Piva A, Sadun AA. Devastating complications from alcohol cauterization of recurrent Rathke cleft cyst. Case report. J Neurosurg 2004;100(6):1087–90.
61. Fager CA Carter H. Intrasellar epithelial cysts. J Neurosurg 1966;24(1):77–81.
62. Sumida M, Migita K, Tominaga A, et al. Concomitant pituitary adenoma and Rathke's cleft cyst. Neuroradiology 2001;43(9):755–9.

63. Goyal A, et al. Suprasellar cystic meningioma: unusual presentation and review of the literature. J Clin Neurosci 2002;9(6):702–4.
64. Fortuna A, et al. Cystic meningiomas. Acta Neurochir (Wien) 1988;90 (1–2):23–30.
65. Kulah A, Ilcayto R, Fiskeci C. Cystic meningiomas. Acta Neurochir (Wien) 1991;111 (3–4):108–13.
66. Odake G. Cystic meningioma: report of three patients. Neurosurgery 1992;30(6):935–40.
67. Osborn AG. Handbook of Neuroradiology. St. Louis, MO: Mosby Year Book. 1991. pp. 302–07.
68. Iqbal J, Kanaan I, Al Homsi M. Non-neoplastic cystic lesions of the sellar region presentation, diagnosis and management of eight cases and review of the literature. Acta Neurochir (Wien) 1999;141(4):389–97, discussion 397–8.
69. Pierre-Kahn A, Capelle L, Brauner R, et al. Presentation and management of suprasellar arachnoid cysts. Review of 20 cases. J Neurosurg 1990;73(3):355–9.
70. Heier L, et al. Magnetic Resonance Imaging of Arachnoid Cysts. Clin Imaging 1989;4: 281–91.
71. Meyer FB, Carpenter SM, Laws ER Jr. Intrasellar arachnoid cysts. Surg Neurol 1987;28(2):105–10.
72. Gore RM, Weinberg PE, Kim KS, et al. Sphenoid sinus mucoceles presenting as intracranial masses on computed tomography. Surg Neurol 1980;13(5):375–9.
73. Yasargil MG, Abernathey CD, Sarioglu AC. Microneurosurgical treatment of intracranial dermoid and epidermoid tumors. Neurosurgery 1989;24(4):561–7.
74. McCormick GF, Zee CS, Heiden J, Cysticercosis cerebri. Review of 127 cases. Arch Neurol 1982;39(9):534–9.

Subject Index

Retinoblastoma tumor suppression gene
    and p27, 142
Retinoid receptors (RXR), 259
Risperidone drug, 129, 423
    See also Hyperprolactinemia
Rosenthal fibers, 30
Rosiglitazone drug for CD, 231
RXR-selective retinoids (rexinoids), 259

Sarcoidosis, 36, 347
    and CNS, 77–78
Schwannomas, 69
Scotoma of visual field, 111
Secretogranin II autoantibodies, 342
Selective serotonin reuptake inhibitors (SSRIs), 423
Sella and parasellar lesions, sign and
    symptoms, 101
Sellar and parasellar tumors, 412
Sellar cyst, 432–434
    arachnoid cysts, 433–434
    Rathke's cleft cysts
        diagnosis, 433
        epidemiology, 432
        management and outcome, 433
        presentation, 432
Sellar gliomas, 32
Sellar lesions, 26–36
    role of neuro-ophthalmologist in diagnosis and
        management, 122–123
Sellar location cystic lesions, 34–35
Sellar mass and hormonal deficiencies, 43
Sellar tumor, surgical approaches
    reoperation for, 300
    surgery for, 296–299
        acromegaly, 297–298
        nonfunctional tumors and CD, 297
        prolactinoma and pituitary apoplexy, 298
        stalk and hypothlmic Lesions, 298–299
    transcranial approaches
        pterional, 296
        unilateral subfrontal, 295–296
    transsphenoidal approaches
        transnasal, 290–294
Sella turcica, 46
    anatomy of, 47, 94–95
Serotonin antagonist cyproheptadine, 231–232
Serotonin reuptake inhibitors, 129
Serum prolactin level, 131
Serum thyroxine-binding globulin concentrations,
    242–243
Sex hormone binding globulin (SHBG), 246
Sheehan's syndrome, 35, 84, 342, 345, 391
Shunt vessels and optic nerve, 106

Signal molecules, 2
Silent adenomas type 1 and type 2, 23
Silent gonadotropin, 273
Slow-release (SR) preparation for octreotide, 154
Snellen chart and visual loss, 102
Sodium homeostasis, 359
Somatostain receptors scintigraphy
    (SRS), 198
Somatostatin analogs therapy, 154
    and clinical development, 159
    efficacy, GH and IGF-I levels, 155–156
    pituitary tumor size and, 157–158
    side effects of, 158
Somatostatin receptor, 230
Somatostatin receptor (sst) type 1–3 and 5, 10
Somatotroph adenomas, 40, 142
Somatotropinomas, 403
Sphenoid periosteum, 48
Sphenoid sinus mucocele, 461–462
Sphenoparietal sinuses, 48
Spina bifida, fetal malformations, 383
Spindle cell oncocytoma, 33
Staircase method for visual field testing, 111
Stereotactic radiotherapy (SRT), 323–324
Steroidogenesis inhibitors, 224, 227–229
Subarachnoid hemorrhage, 362–363, 364
Sublabial transsphenoidal approach, 278–279
Sulpiride drug, 423
Superior hypophyseal artery, 48
Suprasellar germinomas, 435
Sweat gland hypertrophy, 143
Swinging-flashlight test, 105
Syndrome of inappropriate antidiuretic hormone
    secretion (SIADH), 281

Talipes, fetal malformations, 383
Tangent visual field testing, 109
Temporal lobe necrosis, 333
Temporal wedge, visual field defects, 113
Tentorium cerebelli, 48
Teratomas, 30
    See also Germ cell tumors
Testosterone, administration in
    microadenomas, 135
Thiazolidinedione (TZD), 231
Three-dimensional conformal radiation therapy
    (3D-CRT), 324
Thyroid axis testing
    octreotide suppression, 247
    TRH test, 246
    T3 suppression test, 246–247
Thyroid hormone receptor β isoform (TRβ), 9
Thyroiditis, 35

Printed in The United States of America